Strategies for Team Science Success

Kara L. Hall • Amanda L. Vogel
Robert T. Croyle
Editors

Strategies for Team Science Success

Handbook of Evidence-Based
Principles for Cross-Disciplinary
Science and Practical Lessons
Learned from Health Researchers

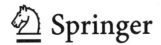 Springer

Editors
Kara L. Hall
Division of Cancer Control
and Population Sciences
National Cancer Institute
National Institutes of Health
Bethesda, MD, USA

Robert T. Croyle
Division of Cancer Control
and Population Sciences
National Cancer Institute
National Institutes of Health
Bethesda, MD, USA

Amanda L. Vogel
Clinical Monitoring Research
Program Directorate
Frederick National Laboratory
for Cancer Research
sponsored by the National
Cancer Institute
Frederick, MD, USA

ISBN 978-3-030-20990-2   ISBN 978-3-030-20992-6   (eBook)
https://doi.org/10.1007/978-3-030-20992-6

Foreword

As a long-term social scientist and recent past director of the Institute for Social Research (ISR) at the University of Michigan, I was asked by the editors of this new book to write a foreword placing team science in the context of social and behavioral sciences research and applications. The ISR is a successful 75-year experiment in the utilization of team science principles to advance high-quality research on basic and applied behavioral and social science problems.

The need for, and implementation of, large research teams has been brought into sharp relief over the last few decades as the complexity and size of scientific problems have grown not only in the social and behavioral sciences but also in the biological and physical sciences. Significant advances in a wide variety of tools, approaches, and technologies combined with rapid growth in computing power, big data, data mining systems, imaging, and geographic information systems, has exponentially increased the need for interdisciplinary teams in order to investigate and address complex scientific questions.

ISR's use of team science did not grow strictly from conceptualization of organizational principles but instead evolved to conduct the work in basic and applied social and behavioral sciences needed to address complex human science problems in business organizations, the military, and other organizational contexts. For 75 years, the nature of problems addressed responded well to the development of interdisciplinary research teams spanning senior investigators to undergraduate students, where the nature of the problem dictated the organizational forms necessary for addressing particular problems. Over this same period, however, the larger context of universities, private and public funders, and public perceptions of science, as well as the size and scope of problems to be addressed, changed substantially. These changes are now dictating the need for more systematic investigations of the nature, context, and structure of the team science enterprise.

There is no reason to believe that science will move backward such that the lone investigator working either in a laboratory or armchair will ever again be the imagined norm for scientific investigation. Thus, the challenges of ensuring cooperation, composition of teams, proximity, scientific credit, reward systems for discoveries, rules of tenure, and promotion are all issues that have to evolve to meet the new reality of team science.

This book is an outstanding product of a massive undertaking examining the multiple facets of team science from a broad array of perspectives. It is a large volume and not meant to be read from cover to cover in one sitting. Instead, the volume is to be used as a scientific and applications sourcebook and to be consulted and employed as a resource manual. The chapters focus on topics ranging from integrative science teams, expanding engagement in science teams, team characteristics, team formation, and team functioning to institutional influences and technological support. Within each of these broad topical areas, the chapters encompass "State of the Science" chapters focused on providing up-to-date evidence and conclusions on what we know scientifically about the nature of effective team science, "Special Topics" chapters that detail and suggest new directions for scientific exploration in team science, and "Practice-Oriented" chapters that are rooted in lived experiences of scientists and administrators – providing insights and examples of successful applications of team science approaches in developing key strategies in organizing, leading, implementing, managing, facilitating, and supporting cross-disciplinary social, behavioral, and health research teams. Each of the chapters within these three broad types discusses implications, lessons learned, and practical strategies for success in order to help guide readers who are interested in applying team science principles and practical action steps in establishing successful team science units.

Knowledge regarding evidence-based principles in the volume is drawn from and applied to team science across the scientific enterprise and research domains. NIH scientists have served as international leaders in studying as well as developing strategies for how to improve the support and conduct of team science. The book has a public health research and application orientation, and nearly half of the chapters draw from, or include, examples of research that integrates behavioral and social science with a broad range of disciplines. So although NIH scientists have utilized and applied their knowledge in the health context, the models, tools, and applications featured in this volume have been developed within and used across the sciences, humanities, and public health arenas.

The National Academies report, *Enhancing the Effectiveness of Team Science*, drew several conclusions addressing the need for more systematic research in the complicated nature, etiology, and context of team science. The growth in the breadth of interdisciplinary areas needed to address evolving scientific problems and questions ranging from the creation of the universe to the nature of cellular activity promoting the growth of cancerous cells portend even further complexity in the future. It is not clear that institutional support systems, policies, organizations, and individual scientists are keeping pace with the evolving needs of these science teams. This volume summarizes current scientific knowledge of effective team science approaches, areas of need for new research on science teams, and, perhaps even more importantly, examples like the ISR organization experiment that have promoted successful (as well as not so successful) team science applications over the years. There are lessons that have been learned, lessons to be learned, and compelling examples of systematic and non-systematic attempts to implement teams of scientists (both inter- and intradisciplinary) working on shared scientific problems.

It is clear that training models for scientists will have to be adapted to meet the new organization of scientific research. In fact, traditional frameworks of individual and group-based contributions will have to be modified. What counts as scientific products may need to be enlarged, and researchers will need to make conscious decisions about their involvement in team science, whether with an interdisciplinary focus or not. Based upon this view, researchers may need to reevaluate what constitute paths to success, especially those in academic settings.

The institutional context of research will need to change as well. The notion of static, enduring research institutions will have to be rethought. Policies around rewards, especially promotion and tenure in universities, will have to be adapted. Business firms will have to rethink traditional private consultation frameworks of collaboration with the universities and government. Studies of alternate organizational structures and management approaches will be needed to inform efforts to integrate team science into scientific operations. Finally, the government, industry, and private funders of research all will need to adjust models for stimulating research to encompass team-based research. They will need to develop new models of awarding funding and monitoring accountability of research expenditures. New collaborative models, e.g., research networks and consortia, will also need to be evolved and tested. This will require the integration of disciplinary perspectives and methods throughout the life of research projects.

The agenda for evolving effective conceptual and practical approaches for implementing cross-disciplinary team science has not been fully written. This volume, however, outlines a roadmap for what the future will require and what the ultimate benefits may be in implementing effective cross-disciplinary team science across public health-related research.

James S. Jackson
Institute for Social Research
University of Michigan,
Ann Arbor, Michigan, USA

Acknowledgements

Many colleagues and friends have made essential contributions to this book, and we are grateful for their vision, expertise, enthusiasm, and commitment.

Heartfelt appreciation and thanks go to our colleagues in the Science of Team Science (SciTS), Science of Teams, and Social and Behavioral Health Research fields, among other diverse areas of scholarship, as well as our colleagues who serve as administrators and leaders at universities, funding agencies, nonprofit organizations, and industry settings around the country, who have contributed to this handbook as chapter authors. They have shared their unique expertise and perspectives, collectively creating what we believe to be a vital resource in translating the evidence base for team science into actionable strategies that can be used to advance collaboration in science. This book would not have been possible without the generosity of more than 100 contributing authors.

Janice Stern, a former senior editor at Springer, was instrumental in championing the initial concept for this book. Her invitation to Kara to propose a Springer Handbook on Team Science inspired the idea for this volume; to pair evidence from the SciTS field and allied fields with the rich experiences of successful leaders in cross-disciplinary team science. With this approach, the book aims to advance the application of evidence-informed strategies for an expansive range of activities in leading, implementing, managing, facilitating, and supporting collaborative scientific initiatives. We also thank Katherine Chabalko, Sara Yanny-Tillar, and Christina Tuballes, of Springer, all of whom contributed in moving this book to publication.

Many peer reviewers also generously donated their time to provide anonymous reviews of chapters for this volume, including incisive feedback that often led to new themes or avenues of thought in the chapters. They, too, contributed to the scientific content of the book, and we sincerely thank them. Listed alphabetically, they include: Nicholas Berente, Mike Conlon, Jay Goodwin, Stan Gully, Susan Jackson, Gaetano Lotrecchiano, Margaret Luciano, Steve Kozlowski, Jonathan Mote, Staša Milojević, Jihad Obeid, Marissa Shuffler, Daniel Stokols, Rick Szostack, Sheila Weber, and Kevin Wooten.

Many thanks go to Elise Rice, a former postdoctoral fellow at the National Cancer Institute (NCI) who, in addition to contributing scientifically as a coauthor, also contributed her organizational skill and diplomatic nature to lead many administrative tasks to facilitate this project. The University of Maryland undergraduate interns Jesse Costa, Jamie Hwang, Katie Dolan,

Jamie Fleishman, and Brandon Estime also made important behind-the-scene contributions to this project.

We also are grateful to the many students, colleagues, and mentors who have had invaluable influence on our work and the Science of Team Science field we value so greatly for its promise to help accelerate science. Foremost, among these is Daniel Stokols. As a pioneer in the SciTS field and a preeminent scholar in both SciTS and social ecology, Dan has been unfaltering in his roles as an intellectual leader, inspirational mentor, and kind-hearted collaborator. Between 2004 and 2011, Dan served as a senior advisor to the NCI Division of Cancer Control and Population Sciences, providing invaluable leadership and guidance for the evaluation and enhancements of large transdisciplinary team science initiatives. Throughout his tenure as a consultant at NCI, and beyond, Dan has been a mentor to two of us (Kara and Amanda) in many ways. His mentorship and collaboration over the years have influenced the development of a number of key ideas that are reflected in this book. In fact, his intellectual influence is reflected throughout our work in the SciTS field.

We are grateful for our colleagues at the National Cancer Institute – Linda Nebeling, Shobha Srinivasan, Bradford Hesse, and Glen Morgan – for their groundbreaking contributions to the development, management, and leadership of the NCI Division of Cancer Control and Population Sciences' flagship transdisciplinary team science initiatives, the Transdisciplinary Research on Energetics and Cancer (TREC) initiative, the Centers for Population Health and Health Disparities (CPHHD) initiative, the Centers of Excellence in Cancer Communication Research (CECCR) initiative, and the Transdisciplinary Tobacco Use Research Centers (TTURC) initiative. Their steadfast support and collaboration in SciTS research provided the opportunity for us to engage with these transdisciplinary team science initiatives to conduct SciTS studies that have contributed to advancing the evidence base for team science. We also thank the following NCI advisors, staff, and fellows who have provided critical leadership and collaboration for novel evaluation studies of team science initiatives: William Trochim, Ginny Hsieh, Scott Marchand, Stephen Marcus, Louise Masse, Rick Moser, Brandie Taylor, and Patrick Weld. We are so grateful to have been a part of this exceptional group of colleagues who, together, generated early SciTS work that helped launch the field by providing new models, measures, and methods to study team science.

Over the next decade, new members joined us and formed the NCI SciTS team. The team continued to conduct research on team science initiatives and advance scholarship in the SciTS field. They brought a diversity of perspectives and subject matter and methodological expertise to the NCI SciTS team that contributed to our work thematically, methodologically, and conceptually. We wish to thank our team members, including: Annie Feng, Grace Huang, Kenny Gibbs, Janet Okamoto, Elise Rice, and Brooke Stipelman for their collaboration over the years. We also thank our long-standing collaborator, Sophia Tsakraklides.

We are also grateful to the SciTS professional community for their commitment to and passion for the development of a collegial and collaborative environment and generative knowledge exchange through their active engagement on the SciTS listserv[1] and at the annual SciTS conference.[2] We thank the founding board of directors of the newly formed International Network for the Science of Team Science (INSciTS), the new professional society for the SciTS field[3]. The founding board members of INSciTS include Maritza Salazar Campo, Holly J. Falk-Krzesinski, Stephen M. Fiore, Andi Hess, Julie Thompson Klein, Gaetano R. Lotrecchiano, Shalini Misra, Zaida Chinchilla Rodriguez, Pips Veazey, and Kevin C. Wooten. With Kara also serving on the founding board and Amanda serving as founding membership chair for the organization, we are honored to have the opportunity to serve alongside these colleagues who provide leadership for maintaining and enhancing the vitality of the growing SciTS community. Their dedication benefits those committed to advancing SciTS research as well as those committed to supporting and conducting cutting-edge cross-disciplinary team science.

So much of the work of building the SciTS field that has been accomplished over the past 10–15 years could not have happened without the vision and support of NCI leaders, including Linda Nebeling, Bill Klein, Bill Riley, and Susan Czajkowski. We thank them for their long-standing support.

Finally, we thank our families for their gift of time that made our work on this book possible. We are deeply grateful for their love and support.

---

[1]https://www.teamsciencetoolkit.cancer.gov/public/RegisterListserv.aspx

[2]https://www.inscits.org/

[3]https://www.inscits.org/inscits-board-of-directors

Contents

The original version of this book was revised. The correction is available at
https://doi.org/10.1007/978-3-030-20992-6_46

Contributors

Gregory D. Abowd, PhD, MS Georgia Institute of Technology, Atlanta, GA, USA

Karen E. Adolph, PhD Department of Psychology, Applied Psychology, and Neural Science, New York University, New York, NY, USA

Anthony J. Alberg, PhD Epidemiology and Biostatistics Department, University of South Carolina, Columbia, SC, USA

Rosa I. Arriaga, PhD Georgia Institute of Technology, Atlanta, GA, USA

Raquel Asencio, PhD Krannert School of Management, Purdue University, West Lafayette, IN, USA

Christine Bachrach, PhD Maryland Population Research Center, University of Maryland, College Park, MD, USA

Bradford S. Bell, PhD Center for Advanced Human Resource Study, Industrial and Labor Relations School, Cornell University, Ithaca, NY, USA

L. Michelle Bennett, PhD Center for Research Strategy, National Cancer Institute, Bethesda, MD, USA

Nicholas Berente, PhD Mendoza College of Business, University of Notre Dame, Notre Dame, IN, USA

Nathan A. Berger, MD Center for Science, Health and Society, Case Western Reserve University School of Medicine, Cleveland, OH, USA

Warren K. Bickel, PhD Virginia Tech and Virginia Tech Carilion School of Medicine, Roanoke, VA, USA

William J. Blot, PhD Vanderbilt University Medical Center, Nashville, TN, USA

Deborah J. Bowen, PhD Bioethics and Humanities, and Health Services, University of Washington, School of Public Health, Seattle, WA, USA

Kathleen T. Brady, MD, PhD South Carolina Clinical and Translational Research Institute, Medical University of South Carolina, Charleston, SC, USA

Sandra A. Brown, PhD Office of Research Affairs and Departments of Psychology and Psychiatry, University of California San Diego, La Jolla, CA, USA

Karen Calhoun, MA Michigan Institute for Clinical & Health Research, University of Michigan, Ann Arbor, MI, USA

Susan Carlson, PhD Office of the President, University of California, Oakland, CA, USA

Dorothy R. Carter, PhD Department of Psychology, University of Georgia, Athens, GA, USA

Susan Carter, JD Santa Fe Institute, Santa Fe, NM, USA

Suzanne P. Christen, JD Simons Center for Systems Biology, School of Natural Sciences, Institute for Advanced Study, Princeton, NJ, USA

Graham Colditz, MD, PhD School of Medicine, Siteman Cancer Center, and Institute for Public Health, Washington University in St. Louis, St. Louis, MO, USA

David E. Conroy, PhD Department of Kinesiology, Penn State University, University Park, PA, USA

Noshir Contractor, PhD Northwestern University, Evanston, IL, USA

Jennifer Couch, PhD Division of Cancer Biology, National Cancer Institute, Bethesda, MD, USA

John Crockett, PhD San Diego State University, San Diego, CA, USA

Michael M. Crow, PhD Office of the President, Arizona State University, Tempe, AZ, USA

Stephen Crowley, PhD Department of Philosophy, Boise State University, Boise, ID, USA

Kevin Crowston, PhD School of Information Studies, Syracuse University, Syracuse, NY, USA

Robert T. Croyle, PhD Division of Cancer Control and Population Sciences, National Cancer Institute, Bethesda, MD, USA

William B. Dabars, PhD School for the Future of Innovation in Society, Arizona State University, Tempe, AZ, USA

Randal Davis, MBA Strategic Research Initiatives, Medical University of South Carolina, Charleston, SC, USA

Leslie A. DeChurch, PhD School of Communication, Northwestern University, Evanston, IL, USA

Kathryn Doiron, MA Claremont Graduate University, Claremont, CA, USA

Milton Eder, PhD Department of Family Medicine and Community Health, Office of Community Engagement to Advance Research and Community Health, Clinical and Translational Science Institute, University of Minnesota, Minneapolis, MN, USA

Mary Falcone, PhD Keck School of Medicine of the University of Southern California, Los Angeles, CA, USA

Holly J. Falk-Krzesinski, PhD Global Strategic Networks, Elsevier Inc., New York, NY, USA

Stephen M. Fiore, PhD Cognitive Sciences, Department of Philosophy, University of Central Florida, Orlando, FL, USA

Cognitive Sciences Laboratory, Institute for Simulation and Training, University of Central Florida, Orlando, FL, USA

Myron F. Floyd, PhD Department of Parks, Recreation and Tourism Management, North Carolina State University, Raleigh, NC, USA

Kenneth R. Fulton, MPA National Academy of Sciences, Washington, DC, USA

Catherine Gabelica, PhD Human Resources Management, IÉSEG School of Management, Paris, France

Howard Gadlin Bethesda, MD, USA

Sarah J. Gehlert, PhD, MSW, MA College of Social Work, University of South Carolina, Columbia, SC, USA

Kenneth D. Gibbs Jr, PhD Division of Training, Workforce Development, and Diversity, National Institute of General Medical Sciences, Bethesda, MD, USA

Elizabeth Gillanders, PhD Division of Cancer Control and Population Sciences, National Cancer Institute, Bethesda, MD, USA

Rick O. Gilmore, PhD Department of Psychology, The Pennsylvania State University, University Park, PA, USA

Kara L. Hall, PhD Division of Cancer Control and Population Sciences, National Cancer Institute, Bethesda, MD, USA

Anna Han, PhD Office of Equity, Diversity and Inclusion, National Institutes of Health, Bethesda, MD, USA

Perry V. Halushka, PhD, MD South Carolina Clinical and Translational Research Institute, Medical University of South Carolina, Charleston, SC, USA

Margaret Hargreaves, PhD Meharry Medical College, Nashville, TN, USA

Christine Ogilvie Hendren, PhD Department of Civil & Environmental Engineering, Duke University, Durham, NC, USA

Robert Hiatt, MD, PhD Department of Epidemiology and Biostatistics and Helen Diller Family Comprehensive Cancer Center, University of California, San Francisco, CA, USA

James Howison, PhD School of Information, University of Texas at Austin, Austin, TX, USA

Patricia D. Hurn, PhD School of Nursing, University of Michigan, Ann Arbor, MI, USA

Praduman Jain Vibrent Health, Fairfax, VA, USA

Peter James, ScD Department of Population Medicine, Harvard Medical School and Harvard Pilgrim Health Care Institute, Boston, MA, USA

Lorraine B. Johnson, JD, MBA LymeDisease.org, San Ramon, CA, USA

Ruth Kanfer, PhD School of Psychology, College of Sciences, Georgia Institute of Technology, Atlanta, GA, USA

Julie Kaplow, PhD, ABPP The Trauma and Grief Center, Texas Children's Hospital, Baylor College of Medicine, Houston, TX, USA

Susan P. Kemp, PhD School of Social Work, University of Washington, Seattle, WA, USA

Faculty of Education and Social Work, University of Auckland, Auckland, New Zealand

Marc T. Kiviniemi, PhD Department of Health, Behavior and Society, University of Kentucky, Lexington, KY, USA

Dave Klein, PhD Vibrent Health, Fairfax, VA, USA

William M. P. Klein, PhD Division of Cancer Control and Population Sciences, National Cancer Institute, Bethesda, MD, USA

Julie Thompson Klein, PhD Department of English, Wayne State University, Detroit, MI, USA

Transdisciplinarity Lab, ETH-Zurich, Switzerland

Steve W. J. Kozlowski, PhD Michigan State University, East Lansing, MI, USA

Sharon Tsai-hsuan Ku, PhD, MA, MS Department of Engineering, University of Virginia, Charlottesville, VA, USA

Theresa K. Lant, PhD Lubin School of Business, Pace University, New York, NY, USA

Bethany Laursen, MS Michigan State University, East Lansing, MI, USA

Margaret S. Leinen, PhD Scripps Institution of Oceanography, and School of Marine Sciences, University of California, San Diego, La Jolla, CA, USA

Caryn Lerman, PhD USC Norris Comprehensive Cancer Center and Keck School of Medicine of USC, Los Angeles, CA, USA

Arnold J. Levine, PhD Simons Center for Systems Biology, School of Natural Sciences, Institute for Advanced Study, Princeton, NJ, USA

Kyle Lewis, PhD Technology Management Program, College of Engineering, University of California Santa Barbara, Santa Barbara, CA, USA

James Loughead, PhD Department of Psychiatry, Neuropsychiatry Section, University of Pennsylvania School of Medicine, Philadelphia, PA, USA

Janetta Lun, PhD Office of Equity, Diversity and Inclusion, National Institutes of Health, Bethesda, MD, USA

Gregory J. Madden, PhD Department of Psychology, Utah State University, Logan, UT, USA

Anne Heberger Marino, MSW The National Academies of Sciences, Engineering, and Medicine, Washington, DC, USA

Maria Elena Martinez, PhD Department of Family and Preventive Medicine, University of California San Diego, La Jolla, CA, USA

Christine Marx, MA Division of Public Health Sciences, Washington University, St. Louis, MO, USA

Samuel McClure, PhD Decision Neuroscience Lab, Department of Psychology, Arizona State University, Tempe, AZ, USA

Rachel Nelan, AIA, LEED AP Flad Architects, Madison, WI, USA

Paula S. Nurius, PhD School of Social Work, University of Washington, Seattle, WA, USA

Jihad S. Obeid, MD South Carolina Clinical and Translational Research Institute, Medical University of South Carolina, Charleston, SC, USA

Michael O'Rourke, PhD MSU Center for Interdisciplinarity, Department of Philosophy and AgBioResearch, and Toolbox Dialogue Initiative, Michigan State University, East Lansing, MI, USA

Angela Fidler Pfammatter, PhD Department of Preventive Medicine, Northwestern University Feinberg School of Medicine, Chicago, IL, USA

Christian Pohl, PhD Transdisciplinarity Lab, Institute for Environmental Decisions, ETH Zürich, Switzerland

Damayanthi Ranwala, PhD South Carolina Clinical and Translational Research Institute, Medical University of South Carolina, Charleston, SC, USA

Susan Redline, MD, MPH Division of Sleep Medicine, Harvard Medical School and Division of Sleep and Circadian Disorders, Brigham and Women's Hospital, Boston, MA, USA

Elise L. Rice, PhD Division of Extramural Research, National Institute of Dental and Craniofacial Research, Bethesda, MD, USA

Stephanie A. Robert, PhD School of Social Work, and Department of Population Health Science, University of Wisconsin-Madison, Madison, WI, USA

Brian Robinson, PhD Department of History, Political Science, and Philosophy, Texas A&M University-Kingsville, Kingsville, TX, USA

Betsy Rolland, PhD, MPH, MLIS Carbone Cancer Center and Institute for Clinical and Translational Research, University of Wisconsin-Madison, Madison, WI, USA

Maritza R. Salazar, PhD, MSW Paul Merage School of Business, University of California, Irvine, CA, USA

James F. Sallis, PhD Family Medicine and Public Health, University of California, San Diego, CA, USA

Jaye Bea Smalley, MPA Global I & I Patient Advocacy and Life Cycle Management, Celgene Corporation, Summit, NJ, USA

Bonnie J. Spring, PhD Department of Preventive Medicine, Northwestern University Feinberg School of Medicine, Chicago, IL, USA

Brad Steeves Operations, Academic Health Sciences Center, University of Saskatchewan, SK, Canada

Brooke A. Stipelman, PhD Abrams and Associates, Rockville, MD, USA

Daniel Stokols, PhD Department of Urban Planning and Public Policy, and Department of Psychological Sciences, School of Social Ecology, University of California Irvine, Irvine, CA, USA

Steffanie A. Strathdee, PhD Division of Infectious Diseases & Global Health Sciences, and Department of Medicine, University of California San Diego School of Medicine, La Jolla, CA, USA

Kimberly A. Suda-Blake The National Academies of Sciences, Engineering, and Medicine, Washington, DC, USA

Katrina Theisz, MS Division of Cancer Biology, National Cancer Institute, Bethesda, MD, USA

Yonette Thomas, PhD Maryland Population Research Center, University of Maryland, College Park, MD, USA

Jim Thornhill, PhD College of Medicine, University of Saskatchewan, SK, Canada

Hayley M. Trainer, MS Department of Psychology, University of Georgia, Athens, GA, USA

Richard J. Traystman, PhD University of Colorado Denver, Anschutz Medical Campus, Aurora, CO, USA

Marlon Twyman II, PhD, MS University of Southern California, Los Angeles, CA, USA

Stephanie E. Vasko, PhD MSU Center for Interdisciplinarity, Michigan State University, East Lansing, MI, USA

Amanda L. Vogel, PhD, MPH Clinical Monitoring Research Program Directorate, Frederick National Laboratory for Cancer Research, Sponsored by the National Cancer Institute, Frederick, MD, USA

Barbara Endemaño Walker, PhD University of California, Santa Barbara, CA, USA

Nina Wallerstein, DrPH, MPH College of Population Health, and Center for Participatory Research, Health Sciences Center, University of New Mexico, Albuquerque, NM, USA

Griffin M. Weber, MD, PhD Beth Israel Deaconess Medical Center and Harvard Medical School, Boston, MA, USA

Karen Widmer, MA Claremont Graduate University, Claremont, CA, USA

Consuelo Hopkins Wilkins, MD, MSCI Department of Medicine, Vanderbilt University Medical Center, Nashville, TN, USA

Travis J. Wiltshire, PhD Department of Cognitive Science and Artificial Intelligence, Tilburg University, Tilburg, Netherlands

Susan Winter, PhD College of Information Studies, University of Maryland, College Park, MD, USA

Gabriela Wuelser, PhD Network for Transdisciplinary Research, Swiss Academies of Arts and Sciences, Bern, Switzerland

Leslie A. Yuan, MPH University of California San Francisco, San Francisco, CA, USA

Stephen J. Zaccaro, PhD College of Humanities and Social Sciences, George Mason University, Fairfax, VA, USA

Wei Zheng, MD, PhD Meharry Medical College, Nashville, TN, USA

Introduction

1

Kara L. Hall, Amanda L. Vogel, and Robert T. Croyle

Contents

1.1 Introduction

Science is the cornerstone of progress, and collaboration is becoming the defining approach in science today. Whether the aim of a given research project is to advance fundamental knowledge or to develop actionable solutions to real-world problems, scientific initiatives are increasingly turning to collaboration to achieve their goals.

Progress in the leading scientific initiatives of our age—including the Human Genome Project, the BRAIN (Brain Research through Advancing Innovative Neurotechnologies) Initiative, the experiments at the Large Hadron Collider, the Mars Exploration Rover Mission, and many others—has been predicated upon collaboration.

K. L. Hall (✉) · R. T. Croyle
Division of Cancer Control and Population Sciences,
National Cancer Institute, Bethesda, MD, USA
e-mail: hallka@mail.nih.gov; croyler@mail.nih.gov

A. L. Vogel
Clinical Monitoring Research Program Directorate,
Frederick National Laboratory for Cancer Research
sponsored by the National Cancer Institute,
Frederick, MD, USA
e-mail: vogelal@mail.nih.gov

Further, when we go beyond the scientific headlines and look at the entirety of the scientific enterprise, we find that it has been driven, increasingly, by collaborative approaches. Since the mid-twentieth century, collaboration has eclipsed solo work as the main approach to generate new scientific knowledge. More scientists are collaborating within and across all disciplines and fields. Scientific articles by co-author teams are more often cited and have greater impact, overall, than individually authored articles, and these advantages have been increasing over time. Further, team authored articles now dominate among exceptionally high impact research (Wuchty et al. 2007).

What has contributed to this trend? Today's ambitious societal and scientific goals, such as eliminating health inequities, understanding nanostructures, arresting climate change, and exploring distant planets have led to increasingly large, complex, and ambitious scientific initiatives. Furthermore, our scientific goals and approaches have been influenced, altered, and enabled by advances in technological and computational capabilities; these include dramatic advances in our ability to capture, store, and analyze data.

As an example, with computing devices embedded in more and more everyday objects in our lives, the Internet of Things (IoT) enables us to collect and connect vast amounts of data. In the domain of health research, we can now monitor and report geocoded health data and use these data, including actively reported behavioral data and passively recorded biological sensor data, to address a wide array of scientific questions. The aggregation of multiple "big data" sources such as, geospatial, environmental exposure, and electronic health record data afford tremendous opportunities to population science but also present methodological challenges inherent to aggregating data from across disciplines and levels of analysis. As another example, unprecedented advances in science and technology enable us to envision and develop healthcare systems and public health strategies of the future that rely upon artificial intelligence systems, provide 3D bioprinted organ transplants, and use genetic engineering to alter disease processes. To capitalize on these opportunities requires cross-disciplinary collaboration.

For science to fully realize its most ambitious goals, scientific perspectives reflecting all influences on the human experience—from genetics to behavior, from individual experiences to interpersonal interactions, from organizational structures to political institutions—must be brought to bear and integrated. As such, novel discoveries and innovative developments increasingly will rely on collaborations that span boundaries and require complex skills and structures. Collaborations will need to include team members with expertise that spans multiple disciplines and fields, crosses organizational and geographic boundaries, and integrates multiple levels of analysis and methodologies. The exciting news is that teams with these characteristics generally yield better outcomes, including greater productivity and scientific impact, compared with less diverse, less distributed teams, or solo scientists (Hall et al. 2018).

Disciplinary specialization has the potential to enrich and deepen scientific knowledge, but it also fragments expertise. Collaboration harnesses the power of specialization by integrating seemingly disparate expertise to address shared research goals. New technological capabilities can facilitate such integration as through dataset integration and collaborative data analysis. All of this can help to answer scientific questions in more novel, holistic, and sophisticated ways. Further, technologies enable virtual communication and support the coordination of tasks among collaborators with the most relevant expertise for a particular scientific question regardless of geographic location (Hall et al. 2018).

While collaboration in science introduces enormous opportunities for scientific advancement, it also introduces greater complexity into the scientific process. In order to maximize the scientific successes of collaborations, we must know how best to manage this complexity. This includes how best to organize, conduct, facilitate, and support collaborative science, given a range of contextual factors, beginning with the scientific problem space, and extending to institutional influences, funding opportunities, and scientific culture and policies. This book offers the state of the art on what we know about how to manage these factors to maximize the effectiveness of team science.

1.1.1 What Is Cross-Disciplinary Team Science?

"Team science" refers to both the *approach* of conducting research in teams, and the complex social, organizational, political, and technological *milieus* that heavily influence how that work occurs (Hall et al. 2018). The team science approaches involves two or more individuals working interdependently toward a shared scientific goal. Team size spans from dyads to small teams, and from large groups to teams of teams. Teams also vary in their disciplinary composition and degree of disciplinary integration. (NRC 2015)

In this book, the term "cross-disciplinary" is used to refer to any type of scientific knowledge integration among disciplines, fields, domains, professions, and other stakeholders in the scientific problem space (see Box 1.1). Collaborators may span scientific disciplines and fields, and work in academia, industry, policy, and community organizations. Cross-disciplinary team science brings together concepts, theories, approaches, and/or methods from across these diverse perspectives. The term "integrative science" is understood similarly to reflect integration of knowledge across disciplines and fields, as well as the expertise of other scientific collaborators, such as translational partners (e.g., practitioners, policy makers, industry, and community organizations). Likewise, the term "convergence research"

(NRC 2014) has been taken up by organizations like the National Science Foundation (NSF) to describe integrative scientific work aimed at addressing scientific and societal challenges through "deep" integration across disciplines (NSF 2018; see also Box 1.1).

Teams vary in the degree or "depth" to which they integrate knowledge, depending on what is needed to address the research problem at hand, with this integration occurring along a continuum from unidisciplinary research (no cross-disciplinary integration) to transdisciplinary research (maximal integration among participating disciplines) (Stokols et al. 2013; Hall et al. 2017). As summarized in Box 1.1, scholars typically define four degrees of cross-disciplinary integration along this continuum: unidisciplinary, multidisciplinary, interdisciplinary, and transdisciplinary.

Cross-disciplinary team science has the potential to produce holistic study designs and findings that often cannot be achieved using unidisciplinary team science. These, in turn, help to advance scientific methods and knowledge relevant to solving complex scientific problems (Vogel et al. 2014). This approach to science offers tremendous opportunity to advance science along the translational continuum, as it has the potential to engage collaborators whose approaches span multiple translational stages.

Support for the cross-disciplinary team science approach is shaping the landscape of science. Universities are developing team-based problem-focused units that cut across disciplines and fields (Crow and Dabars 2015) and are revising their hiring, promotion, and tenure policies to recognize cross-disciplinary team science (Klein and Falk-Krzesinski 2017; Vogel, Hall, Falk-Krzesinski, and Klein 2019), and government agencies are increasing their investments in collaborative and often innovative cross-disciplinary and cross-field approaches (Croyle 2008), to highlight just a few examples. When structures, support, and rewards are aligned, the value-add of team science can be maximized, as reflected in scientific productivity, dissemination of findings across disciplines and fields, and translation of findings into real-world applications in the forms of patents, products, interventions, and policies (Hall et al. 2018).

1.1.2 What Leads to Success in Cross-Disciplinary Team Science?

As with all scientific endeavors, collaborative endeavors vary in their success. Cross-disciplinary science teams can maximize their success by working collectively to ask research questions and utilize scientific approaches that leverage the unique expertise of the group. Yet to maximize the likelihood that the scientific and technical merit of a team science initiative is realized, teams must attend to a range of critical influences on the collaborative process. These occur across multiple levels of influence, including intrapersonal, interpersonal, organizational, social, political, and technological (Stokols et al. 2008). For example, team members' attitudes about team science, their history of prior collaboration, and departmental and institutional policies around cross-disciplinary scholarship all influence the success of cross-disciplinary team science.

For decades, leaders across the scientific enterprise have sought to understand how best to facilitate and support effective cross-disciplinary team science. Yet the research needed to inform development of effective strategies was scant until relatively recently (e.g., NASEM 2005; NRC 2014). Then, over the past fifteen years, a number of strategic efforts emerged to generate evidence-based strategies to maximize the success of team science. These have now coalesced into a relatively new field of scholarship, called the Science of Team Science (c.f., Hall et al. 2018; Kaiser 2017; NRC 2015).

The Science of Team Science (SciTS, pronounced, "sights") field aims to generate evidence for what leads to effective team science through the empirical study of science teams. Studies are informed by theories and methods

from research on teams in other settings and by original theories and methods tailored to the study of science teams, in particular. Ultimately, the "opportunity and promise of SciTS [is] to use science to transform the ways researchers do science" (Hall 2017, p. 563).

Key research questions in the SciTS field include the following: What contextual factors are important influences on team science, such as organizational policies, culture, and workspace, as well as funding opportunities and broader scientific trends? And in what ways do they influence science teams? What team leadership and management approaches contribute to success? And how might these vary based on the scientific goals at hand (e.g., innovation vs. replication)? What are the best approaches to team composition (e.g., team size, diversity, history of collaboration) to maximize the likelihood of success? How does training for scientific collaboration shape success, and what approaches to training are most effective (e.g., individual vs. team training)? What team processes and interactions, such as communication and coordination mechanisms and conflict management approaches, are most effective? What approaches for data sharing, collaborative data analysis, and related attribution/credit contribute to success? What strategies are effective to facilitate integration of multiple discipline-based approaches (e.g., communication strategies, approaches to develop shared terminology and shared mental models of the science)? What are the most effective ways to integrate and leverage knowledge from team members from the professional, policy, and community settings? To what degree are these keys to success stable or variable across organizational settings, teams, and scientific contexts (e.g., disciplines, scientific goals), and what adaptations are effective given particular combinations of team factors and key influences? (Hall 2017; Hall et al. 2018)

The SciTS field seeks to build on research and engage researchers from a wide range of disciplines and fields. The early development of the SciTS field has drawn from fields such as economics, management and organizational science, psychology, science policy, computer science, and the humanities. In particular, the SciTS field has drawn heavily from what has been learned about teamwork over the past half century from the study of groups and teams in other contexts (e.g., military, industry, healthcare) (Fiore 2008). In addition, SciTS studies have integrated analytic methods from network science, perspectives from community stakeholders, theories from economics, and research designs from behavioral and social sciences (Hall et al. 2018).

Although a significant amount of effort has been devoted to studying teams, it is critical to develop evidence for science teams, specifically. Based on literature from teams broadly, we now know that some effective practices apply across many types of teams (e.g., practices around team communication and coordination). But team science operates within the unique conditions of the scientific enterprise, including the legacy structures of academia (e.g., disciplines, departments), sources of financial support, intellectual property issues, rewards and incentives, metrics of success, motivations for collaboration, and collaborators who are also competitors. As such, experts emphasize that while there are opportunities to apply what is known from non-science teams to science teams, it is important to devote resources to studying science teams, in particular (Fiore 2008; Hall et al. 2018; Kozlowski and Bell 2019).

While some scholarship on scientific collaboration emerged prior to 2006 (e.g., Pelz 1967; Pelz and Andrews 1966; Payne 1990), the origins of the SciTS field can be traced to a US National Institutes of Health (NIH) conference held in 2006 entitled *The Science of Team Science: Assessing the Value of Transdisciplinary Research*. The conference led to a special issue of the *American Journal of Preventive Medicine* (Stokols et al. 2008), which provided the conceptual and empirical foundations for the SciTS field. More recently, the National Academies convened a consensus study committee on the Science of Team Science,[1] which culminated in the development of the report *Enhancing the Effectiveness of Team Science* (NRC 2015). This report was recently listed in the top 25 most downloaded reports (out of more than 9000

reports available online) published by the National Academies Press since 1994. This demonstrates the demand for evidence-based guidance for effective team science, as well as growing interest in SciTS scholarship.

Since 2010, the Annual International Science of Team Science Conference[2] has brought together a community of SciTS scholars and team science stakeholders, including practitioners, facilitators, administrators, and funders, to advance SciTS research and evidence-informed team science practices. Overall, the SciTS field is generating and disseminating actionable evidence-based resources and strategies for success that can be used by team science stakeholders across the scientific enterprise to enhance the effectiveness of team science (Hall et al. 2018). Many of these can be found on the US National Cancer Institute's Team Science Toolkit[3] (Vogel et al. 2013).

1.1.3 What You Will Find in This Book

Cumulative developments in the SciTS field and allied fields that study teams in other contexts, as well as growing investments in team science by academia, industry, and government, led us to believe that the time is ripe for a book that pairs scholarship on effective practices in cross-disciplinary team science with practical strategies and lessons learned from those actively involved in conducting, leading, and supporting team science.

Building on more than a decade of work in the SciTS field and decades of research in allied fields, this handbook provides readers with an evidence-based understanding of effective practices in cross-disciplinary team science. It includes practical how-tos for engaging in these teams as well as recommendations for managing, facilitating, and supporting cross-disciplinary research collaborations in varied contexts. The book is therefore relevant to a range of audiences, including principal investigators, science team members, academic administrators, and research funders, among others.

[1] http://sites.nationalacademies.org/dbasse/bbcss/current-projects/dbasse_080231
[2] https://www.inscits.org/
[3] https://www.teamsciencetoolkit.cancer.gov/

The handbook is structured around thematic sections that focus on key influences on the success of cross-disciplinary team science, such as team formation, leadership, communication and coordination, training, and institutional policies and structures. Each section includes one or more *State of the Science* chapters that summarize the evidence base for effective practices for team science from the range of disciplines (e.g., management and organizational sciences, psychology) contributing to the scholarship on that topic. Real-world examples of successful application of these practices are provided in *Practice-Oriented* chapters written by individuals who have engaged in, managed, facilitated, or supported successful cross-disciplinary team science initiatives. In addition, each section highlights Special Topics, including cutting-edge and emerging issues in cross-disciplinary team science. (For more detailed descriptions of each of the three types of chapters, see Box 1.2; and for a list of each State of the Science, Practice-Oriented, and Special Topics Chapters, see Box 1.3).

Following this introductory chapter (Part I), Part II further sets the stage for the book by illuminating how research conducted by *integrative science teams* can lead to unanticipated discoveries and innovative new programs of research. Part II also highlights strategies used by leading researchers to overcome some of the challenges of cross-disciplinary collaboration and facilitate scientific success while moving into new scientific frontiers. The section begins with a chapter that summarizes the state of the science on managing cross-disciplinary diversity in science teams, including practical steps for addressing challenges that emerge with disciplinary diversity. The chapter highlights key processes for identifying appropriate experts, preparing cross-disciplinary teams for collaboration, and enabling the integration of discipline-based perspectives (O'Rourke et al. 2019, Chap. 2). Several chapters in this section are written by experts engaged in cross-disciplinary health research. These chapters showcase the kinds of novel discoveries that can occur with cross-disciplinary team science when scientific perspectives and methods from two or more a different fields or disciplines are integrated into a new or

existing program of research (James and Redline 2019, Chap. 3; Falcone et al. 2019; Chap. 4; Arriaga and Abowd 2019, Chap. 5). For example, chapter 5 (Arriaga and Abowd 2019) highlights collaborative strategies used in a collaboration involving computer science and medicine that led to the design of new technologies as well as the development of clinically significant applications to health behavior. Finally,

---

Box 1.2 Three Types of Handbook Chapters

State of the Science chapters are written by Science of Team Science (SciTS) scholars and/or scholars from allied fields and provide in-depth exploration of the evidence base around key influences on the success of cross-disciplinary team science. Readers can turn to these chapters to find examples of strategies for effective team science, and to get an in-depth understanding of the evidence base that informs effective team science practices.

Practice-Oriented chapters are written by scientists who have successfully used team science approaches in their work; administrators including academic vice presidents, provosts, and center directors, who are involved in the work of facilitating and managing cross-disciplinary team science; and funders with insights to share related to successfully supporting the team science approach. These chapters highlight key strategies for success and lessons learned related to organizing, leading, implementing, managing, facilitating, and supporting cross-disciplinary team science, based on the real-world experiences of their authors.

Special Topics chapters are written by health scientists, SciTS scholars, and scholars in related fields and disciplines. These chapters highlight cutting-edge topics, emerging issues, and current trends in cross-disciplinary team science (e.g., open science, citizen science), as well as other trends in science and technology more broadly, that impact the practice of cross-disciplinary team science.

Box 1.3: A complete listing of the *State of the Science, Practice-Oriented,* and *Special Topics* chapters included in this handbook

Type of chapter	Chapter number	Chapter title
Integrative Science Teams		
State of the Science	2	Disciplinary Diversity in Teams: Integrative Approaches from Unidisciplinarity to Transdisciplinarity
Practice-Oriented: Integrating Disciplines, Fields, and Levels of Analysis	3	The Introduction of a New Domain into an Existing Area of Research: Novel Discoveries Through Integration of Sleep into Cancer and Obesity Research
	4	The Integration of Research from Diverse Fields: Transdisciplinary Approaches Bridging Behavioral Research, Cognitive Neuroscience, Pharmacology, and Genetics to Reduce Cancer Risk Behavior
	5	The Intersection of Technology and Health: Using Human Computer Interaction and Ubiquitous Computing to Drive Behavioral Intervention Research
	6	Research Spanning Animal and Human Models: The Role of Serendipity, Competition, and Strategic Actions in Advancing Stroke Research
	7	Collaborating to Move the Laboratory Findings into Public Health Domains: Maxims for Translational Research
Approaches for Expanding Engagement in Team Science		
State of the Science	8	Methods for Co-Production of Knowledge among Diverse Disciplines and Stakeholders
Special Topics: Engagement Approaches	9	Engaging the Community: Community-Based Participatory Research and Team Science
	10	Engaging the Patient: Patient-Centered Research
	11	Engaging the Practitioner: "But Wait, That's Not All!"— Collaborations with Practitioners and Extending the Reasons You Started Doing Research in the First Place
	12	Engaging the Public: Citizen Science
Individual Competencies and Team Characteristics		
State of the Science	13	Individual-Level Competencies for Team Collaboration with Cross-Disciplinary Researchers and Stakeholders
Special Topics: Personality Traits	14	The Role of Team Personality in Team Effectiveness and Performance
Practice Oriented: Demographic Diversity	15	Demographic Diversity in Teams: The Challenges, Benefits, and Management Strategies
	16	The Added Value of Team Member Diversity to Research in Underserved Populations
Team Formation		
State of the Science	17	Team Assembly
Practice-Oriented: Strategies to Facilitate the Development of New Teams	18	Innovative Collaboration Formation: The National Academies Keck Futures Initiative
	19	Facilitating Cross-Disciplinary Interactions to Stimulate Innovation: Stand Up to Cancer's Matchmaking Convergence Ideas Lab
	20	Retreats to Stimulate Cross-Disciplinary Translational Research Collaborations: Medical University of South Carolina CTSA Pilot Project Program Initiative
Team Functioning and Performance		
State of the Science	21	Evidence-Based Principles and Strategies for Optimizing Team Functioning and Performance in Science Teams
Practice-Oriented: Preventing Conflict	22	Conflict Prevention and Management in Science Teams
	23	Precollaboration Framework: Academic/Industry Partnerships: Mobile and Wearable Technologies for Behavioral Science
Leadership and Management of Teams		
State of the Science	24	Leader Integrative Capabilities: A Catalyst for Effective Interdisciplinary Teams

Special Topics: Leadership Strategies	25	Organizational Perspective on Leadership Strategies for the Success of Cross-Disciplinary Science Teams
Practice-Oriented: Leadership and Management Roles	26	How Leadership Can Support Attainment of Cross-Disciplinary Scientific Goals
	27	The Interdisciplinary Executive Scientist: Connecting Scientific Ideas, Resources, and People
	28	The Role of Research Development Professionals in Supporting Team Science

Facilitating Complex Team Science Initiatives

State of the Science	29	Best Practices for Researchers Working in Multiteam Systems
Practice-Oriented: Strategic Guidance and Support for Centers	30	Developing a Shared Mental Model in the Context of a Center Initiative
	31	The Value of Advisory Boards to Enhance Collaboration and Advance Science
	32	Designing and Developing Coordinating Centers as Infrastructure to Support Team Science

Education, Training, and Professional Development for Cross-Disciplinary Team Science

State of the Science	33	Training to Be a (Team) Scientist
Practice-Oriented: Team Science Training Across Career Stages	34	Continuing Professional Development for Team Science
	35	Training for Interdisciplinary Research in Population Health Science
	36	Cross-Disciplinary Team Science with Trainees: From Undergraduate to Postdoc

Institutional Influences

Practice-Oriented: Changes to Academic Structure and Culture to Advance Team Science	37	Restructuring Research Universities to Advance Transdisciplinary Collaboration
	38	Building a Cross-Disciplinary Culture in Academia Through Joint Hires, Degree Programs, and Scholarships
Special Topics: Recognition, Rewards, and Policies that Facilitate Team Science	39	Broadening our Understanding of Scientific Work for the Era of Team Science: Implications for Recognition and Rewards
	40	The Interrelationship of People, Space, Operations, Institutional Leadership, and Training in Fostering a Team Approach in Health Sciences Research at the University of Saskatchewan
	41	The Development of a New Interdisciplinary Field: Active Living Research—A Foundation-Supported Interdisciplinary Research Funding Program

Technological Supports for Team Science

Special Topics: Technology to Form, Facilitate, and Extend Science Collaborations	42	The Power of Research Networking Systems to Find Experts and Facilitate Collaboration
	43	Strategies for Success in Virtual Collaboration: Structures and Norms for Meetings, Workflow, and Technological Platforms
	44	Open Sharing of Behavioral Research Datasets: Breaking Down the Boundaries of the Research Team

Integration of Team Science Evidence to Guide Practice

| Practice-Oriented | 45 | Comprehensive Collaboration Plans: Practical Considerations Spanning Across Individual Collaborators to Institutional Supports |

White = section heading (i.e. "Part"); blue = state of the science chapters; green = practice-oriented chapters; yellow = special topics chapters

leading researchers share lessons learned distilled from years of experience integrating knowledge across disciplines and levels of analysis (animal models, clinical research, public health) (Hurn and Traystman 2019, Chap. 6; Madden et al. 2019, Chap. 7).

Part III showcases numerous *approaches for expanding engagement in team science*. It emphasizes the importance of including a range of stakeholder perspectives throughout the research process and outlines what it takes to successfully engage varied stakeholders. The section begins with a review of methods used to facilitate the co-production of knowledge to incorporate perspectives among diverse disciplines and stakeholders (Pohl and Wuelser 2019, Chap. 8). The subsequent chapters address needs, opportunities, and strategies for involving community stakeholders (Wallerstein et al. 2019, Chap. 9), patients (Johnson and Smalley 2019, Chap. 10), practitioners (Kiviniemi 2019, Chap. 11), and the broader public (Couch et al. 2019, Chap. 12) in cross-disciplinary research.

Part IV addresses *individual competencies and team characteristics* that facilitate or hinder team science success. The section begins with a chapter that summarizes the literature on individual-level factors—including values, attitudes, knowledge, skills, and habits of mind—critical to the success of cross-disciplinary team science (Nurius and Kemp 2019, Chap. 13). The chapter discusses the importance of understanding these factors when making decisions about team composition, training, coaching, facilitation, and management of differences and conflict. The next chapter focuses on the "big five" personality factors (extraversion, conscientiousness, agreeableness, emotional stability, and openness to experience) and discusses their influence on team effectiveness (Stipelman et al. 2019, Chap. 14). The following chapter provides a review of the literature on the role of demographic diversity in teams and its potential importance for addressing scientific and societal challenges (Gibbs et al. 2019, Chap. 15). Part IV concludes with a chapter that offers reflections on the value of team member demographic diversity in a highly successful program of research conducted in medically underserved populations (Blot et al. 2019, Chap. 16).

Part V addresses how to optimize *team formation*. The section begins with a review of the scientific, individual and interpersonal factors influencing team assembly, and ultimately, functioning and productivity (Twyman and Contractor 2019, Chap. 17). The chapter compares different approaches to team assembly (staff-assembly and self-assembly), includes multiple team assembly perspectives (compositional, relational, and eco-system), and highlights the role of technology (platforms, digital trace data, and recommenda-

tion algorithms) for improving team formation. The subsequent chapters highlight strategies used by different types of organizations to stimulate formation of new cross-disciplinary collaborations to generate innovative advances in science, including strategies used by non-governmental organizations (Marino et al. 2019, Chap. 18), foundations (Christen and Levine 2019, Chap. 19), and academic institutions (Ranwala et al. 2019, Chap. 20).

Part VI delves into the factors that influence *team functioning and performance*. The section begins with a review of the research on effective team functioning and performance in nonscience teams (e.g., military, industry), spanning more than 60 years, and offers insights into how this research can inform our understanding of performance in science teams (Kozlowski and Bell 2019, Chap. 21). The chapter provides a comprehensive set of research recommendations for advancing SciTS evidence on team performance. Part VI also offers frameworks and strategies for heading off conflict among collaborators before it starts and managing conflict when it does arise (Bennett and Gadlin 2019, Chap. 22), and concludes with a framework for preparing for success and preventing conflict in academic-industry partnerships (Jain and Klein 2019, Chap. 23).

Part VII offers guidance for successful *leadership and management of science teams*. The section begins with a chapter that reviews the literature on the role of leaders in enhancing the effectiveness of cross-disciplinary teams (Salazar et al. 2019, Chap. 24). This chapter discusses the critical importance of leaders' integrative capabilities and behaviors to advance knowledge integration, and ultimately, innovation and effectiveness. The following chapter (Winter 2019, Chap. 25) provides guidance to team science leaders on how to navigate within their institutional environments to facilitate the success of science teams. It addresses such practical topics and essential strategies as knowledge of internal operations, resource acquisition, stakeholder analysis, communication approaches, and value-chain analysis. In the next chapter (Berger 2019, Chap. 26), a prominent scientist draws on decades of experience leading cutting-edge cross-disciplinary team science to distill strategies for building and motivating a team, stimulating idea exchange across disciplines, nurturing transdisciplinary collaboration, and supporting sustainability and expansion post-funding. Part VII concludes with two chapters that provide compelling cases for introducing new and/or expanded professional roles to maximize the effectiveness of cross-disciplinary team science. Chapter 27 (Hendren and Ku 2019) highlights emerging roles such as the Interdisciplinary Executive Scientist (IES) who operates at the interstices of organizations, addresses both scientific and interpersonal issues in scientific collaboration, and engages in high-level cross-boundary communication (both cross-disciplinary and cross-organizational), among other scientific and administrative tasks unique to team science.. The following chapter (Carter et al. 2019, Chap. 28) focuses on enhanced roles for existing professionals, such as Research Development Professionals (RDPs), to facilitate team science by helping institutional scientists collaborate with one another, including by creating cross-disciplinary research concepts, building cross-institutional bridges, and developing relationships with external stakeholders and funders.

Part VIII addresses issues related to *facilitating complex initiatives*. The section begins with a review of research on multi-team systems that also offers insights on how best to organize and support collaboration for scientific innovation (Carter et al. 2019, Chap. 29). The following two chapters highlight key elements of effective multi-team systems. Chapter 30 (Gehlert 2019) highlights the role of shared mental models to support team identity and extends the concept of shared mental models to scientific conceptual models. Chapter 31 (Gehlert et al. 2019) demonstrates how internal and external advisory boards can play a pivotal role in supporting the development, maintenance, and sustained implementation of shared mental models. It also showcases the value of using both internal and external advisory boards to increase collaboration and advance science, particularly when there are translational and transdisciplinary aims. The section concludes with a case study that examines the added value introduced by a coordination center to support complex research initiatives (Rolland 2019,

Chap. 32). The case study highlights three key design elements: role clarity, funding structure, and specialized contributions of coordination center staff.

Part IX provides foundational knowledge to guide *education, training, and professional development for cross-disciplinary team science* and examples addressing undergraduates through established researchers. This section begins with a distillation of evidence from a number of relevant fields to provide insights regarding teamwork competencies, curricular strategies, learning approaches, and training methods for developing a scientific workforce capable of collaborating across disciplines (Fiore et al. 2019, Chap. 33). Chapter 34 (Spring et al. 2019) highlights strategies to combine a popular online team science training program with in-person workshops that have the added value of being appropriate to investigators across multiple career stages. The chapter includes materials such as the training protocol, timeline, and workshop materials and provides observations relevant to successful implementation of team science training. Chapter 35 (Bachrach et al. 2019) describes a 14-year-long cross-disciplinary research training program for population health researchers and offers lessons learned from leaders of the training program and from a longitudinal evaluation of trainee outcomes. In addition, recommendations are provided for cross-disciplinary population health training at the pre- and postdoctoral levels, generated from a meeting at the US National Academies. This section concludes with a chapter by a senior researcher offering a personal account of lessons learned collaborating with a wide range of trainees, including undergraduate and graduate students and postdoctoral fellows (Klein 2019, Chap. 36). The chapter highlights strategies to address common challenges specific to collaborating with students and early-career investigators and emphasizes the unique contributions that trainees can make, and the benefits for the science.

Part X delves into the range of *institutional influences* on the success of cross-disciplinary team science, with a focus on how these influences can be leveraged to support team science. The section begins with a case study (Crow and

Dabars 2019, Chap. 37) of the innovative major restructuring of an American university to establish an institutional structure and academic culture that maximally support transdisciplinarity and innovation in research. The authors describe how a structure that de-emphasizes traditional discipline-based departments in favor of novel transdisciplinary configurations can recalibrate the course of inquiry and enhance both discovery and applications. Chapter 38 (Brown et al. 2019) reports on how another American research university has used a different approach to culture change toward the same ends. The authors describe a bevy of interconnected interventions, including changes in academic organization (e.g., cross-departmental institutes and centers), hiring, degree programs, teaching and training approaches, and student scholarships to foster problem-focused cross-disciplinary team science. Chapter 40 (Bennett et al. 2019) describes how a Canadian university implemented its own approaches to advance cross-disciplinary team science within its school of health sciences. An academic restructuring around interdisciplinary biomedical health clusters in lieu of preexisting departments was complemented by developing thematic areas of research and redesigning the physical space. Chapter 39 (Vogel et al. 2019) shines a spotlight on the role of promotion and tenure policies in facilitating or hindering cross-disciplinarity and team science. The authors highlight how traditional tenure and promotion policies reflect longstanding but outdated assumptions that research is a generally solitary pursuit within a single discipline. They respond by offering a taxonomy of a wide range of essential scientific activities for effective team science and discuss how this may inform revisions to promotion and tenure review criteria to expand recognition for team science. The final chapter in this section (Sallis and Floyd 2019, Chap. 41) highlights the role of funding agencies in facilitating cross-disciplinary team science. The chapter describes the successes of the Robert Wood Johnson Foundation's Active Living Research program, which funded cross-disciplinary team science on the interactions of the built environment, policy influences, and physical activity, ultimately leading to the creation of a new trans-

disciplinary field of scholarship that continues to flourish. The chapter describes the methods used to achieve these goals and provides a case study of one grantee's research experiences and career trajectory as a result of participation.

Part XI focuses on *technological supports* for team science, including forming teams, facilitating the work of existing teams, and enabling new research questions to be explored through data sharing. This section begins with a chapter (Weber and Yuan 2019, Chap. 42) that highlights the power of research networking (RN) systems to advance interdisciplinary collaboration. It discusses the value of these tools to facilitate collaboration via a brief history, a wide range of use cases, and detailed guidance based on the authors' experiences using RN systems at two preeminent US research universities. The following chapter (Berente and Howison 2019, Chap. 43) focuses on computer-mediated collaboration, which now characterizes both distance and co-located collaborations. The authors draw on findings from organizational science to provide recommendations for effective virtual collaboration, including steps for structuring work and the use of collaboration platforms. The final chapter in this section (Gilmore and Adolph 2019, Chap. 44) discusses new horizons in data sharing and reuse. The authors describe an innovative data sharing platform for video-based behavioral research datasets, and make the case for data reuse to advance science and hasten development of solutions to health challenges.

The book concludes with a comprehensive framework for planning for team science that *integrates the evidence base for effective team science from across the book in a single practical framework* (Part XII, Hall et al. 2019, Chap. 45). The framework, called Collaboration Planning, is designed to guide potential or current collaborators through a planning process that systematically accounts for the range of multi-level influences on the success of a science team. The Collaboration Planning process leads to the development of a document called a Collaboration Plan, which serves as a guide for ongoing or future team science initiatives. This chapter ties together the entirety of the book by including examples of strategies from each chapter to address each of ten key components that comprise the finished Collaboration Plan. These strategies are summarized in a reference table that links each chapter in the book to one or more components in the Collaboration Plan. Emblematic of the overarching goal of this handbook, Collaboration Planning guides investigators in navigating the team science process to help maximize their likelihood of scientific success.

In closing, this Handbook assembles scholarship on effective practices for team science generated by researchers from a wide range of disciplines and fields and first-person accounts of how evidence-based principles have been implemented successfully in real-world team science initiatives. Authors include internationally renowned scholars, prominent university administrators and leaders for team science and cross-disciplinarity from across nonprofit, industry, and funding organizations. The authors provide insights on key influences on the success of cross-disciplinary team science, and related strategies for success and lessons learned, to enable readers to apply this knowledge in their own contexts, and ultimately advance the solutions to scientific and societal problems that team science aims to produce.

Acknowledgments This project has been funded in whole or in part with federal funds from the National Cancer Institute, National Institutes of Health, under Contract No. HHSN261200800001E. The content of this publication does not necessarily reflect the views or policies of the Department of Health and Human Services, nor does mention of trade names, commercial products, or organizations imply endorsement by the US Government.

References

Arriaga RI, Abowd GD. The intersection of technology and medicine: ubiquitous computing and human computer interaction driving behavioral intervention research to address chronic care management. In: Hall KL, Vogel AL, Croyle RT, editors. Strategies for team science success: handbook of evidence-based principles for cross-disciplinary science and practical lessons learned from health researchers. New York, NY: Springer; 2019.

Bachrach C, Robert SA, Thomas Y. Training for interdisciplinary research in population health science. In: Hall KL, Vogel AL, Croyle RT, editors. Strategies for team science success: handbook of evidence-based principles for cross-disciplinary science and practical lessons learned from health researchers. New York, NY: Springer; 2019.

Bennett M, Gadlin H. Conflict prevention and management in science teams. In: Hall KL, Vogel AL, Croyle RT, editors. Strategies for team science success: handbook of evidence-based principles for cross-disciplinary science and practical lessons learned from health researchers. New York, NY: Springer; 2019.

Bennett M, Nelan R, Steeves B, Thornhill J. The interrelationship of people, space, operations, institutional leadership, and training in fostering a team approach in health sciences research at the University of Saskatchewan. In: Hall KL, Vogel AL, Croyle RT, editors. Strategies for team science success: handbook of evidence-based principles for cross-disciplinary science and practical lessons learned from health researchers. New York, NY: Springer; 2019.

Berente N, Howison J. Strategies for success in virtual collaboration: structures and norms for meetings, workflow, and technological platforms. In: Hall KL, Vogel AL, Croyle RT, editors. Strategies for team science success: handbook of evidence-based principles for cross-disciplinary science and practical lessons learned from health researchers. New York, NY: Springer; 2019.

Berger NA. How leadership can support attainment of cross-disciplinary scientific goals. In: Hall KL, Vogel AL, Croyle RT, editors. Strategies for team science success: handbook of evidence-based principles for cross-disciplinary science and practical lessons learned from health researchers. New York, NY: Springer; 2019.

Blot WJ, Hargreaves M, Zheng W. The added value of team member diversity to research in underserved populations. In: Hall KL, Vogel AL, Croyle RT, editors. Strategies for team science success: handbook of evidence-based principles for cross-disciplinary science and practical lessons learned from health researchers. New York, NY: Springer; 2019.

Brown SA, Leinen MS, Strathdee SA. Building a cross-disciplinary culture in academia through joint hires, degree programs, and scholarships. In: Hall KL, Vogel AL, Croyle RT, editors. Strategies for team science success: handbook of evidence-based principles for cross-disciplinary science and practical lessons learned from health researchers. New York, NY: Springer; 2019.

Carter D, Asencio R, Trainer H, DeChurch L, Zaccaro S, Kanfer R. Best practices for researchers working in multi-team systems. In: Hall KL, Vogel AL, Croyle RT, editors. Strategies for team science success: handbook of evidence-based principles for cross-disciplinary science and practical lessons learned from health researchers. New York, NY: Springer; 2019.

Carter S, Carlson S, Crockett J, Falk-Krzesinski HJ, Lewis K, Walker BE. The role of research development professionals in supporting team science. In: Hall KL, Vogel AL, Croyle RT, editors. Strategies for team science success: handbook of evidence-based principles for cross-disciplinary science and practical lessons learned from health researchers. New York, NY: Springer; 2019.

Christen SP, Levine AJ. Facilitating cross-disciplinary interactions to stimulate innovation: Stand Up To Cancer's matchmaking convergence ideas lab. In: Hall KL, Vogel AL, Croyle RT, editors. Strategies for team science success: handbook of evidence-based principles for cross-disciplinary science and practical lessons learned from health researchers. New York, NY: Springer; 2019.

Couch J, Theisz K, Gillanders E. Engaging the public: citizen science. In: Hall KL, Vogel AL, Croyle RT, editors. Strategies for team science success: handbook of evidence-based principles for cross-disciplinary science and practical lessons learned from health researchers. New York, NY: Springer; 2019.

Crow MM, Dabars WB. Designing the new American University. Baltimore: Johns Hopkins University Press; 2015.

Crow MM, Dabars WB. Restructuring research universities to advance interdisciplinary collaboration. In: Hall KL, Vogel AL, Croyle RT, editors. Strategies for team science success: handbook of evidence-based principles for cross-disciplinary science and practical lessons learned from health researchers. New York, NY: Springer; 2019.

Croyle RT. The National Cancer Institute's transdisciplinary centers initiatives and the need for building a science of team science. Am J Prevent Med. 2008;35(2S):S90–3.

Falcone M, Loughead J, Lerman C. The integration of research from diverse fields: transdisciplinary approaches bridging behavioral research, cognitive neuroscience, pharmacology and genetics to reduce cancer risk behavior. In: Hall KL, Vogel AL, Croyle RT, editors. Strategies for team science success: handbook of evidence-based principles for cross-disciplinary science and practical lessons learned from health researchers. New York, NY: Springer; 2019.

Fiore SM. Interdisciplinarity as teamwork: how the science of teams can inform team science. Small Group Res. 2008;39:251–77. https://doi.org/10.1177/1046496408317797.

Fiore SM, Gabelica C, Wiltshire T, Stokols D. Training to be a (team) scientist. In: Hall KL, Vogel AL, Croyle RT, editors. Strategies for team science success: handbook of evidence-based principles for cross-disciplinary science and practical lessons learned from health researchers. New York, NY: Springer; 2019.

Gehlert S. Developing a shared mental model in the context of center initiative. In: Hall KL, Vogel AL, Croyle RT, editors. Strategies for team science success: handbook of evidence-based principles for cross-disciplinary science and practical lessons learned from health researchers. New York, NY: Springer; 2019.

Gehlert SJ, Bowen D, Martinez ME, Hiatt R, Marx C, Colditz G. The value of advisory boards to increase collaboration and advance science. In: Hall KL,

Vogel AL, Croyle RT, editors. Strategies for team science success: handbook of evidence-based principles for cross-disciplinary science and practical lessons learned from health researchers. New York, NY: Springer; 2019.

Gibbs K, Han A, Lun J. Demographic diversity in teams: the challenges, benefits, and management strategies. In: Hall KL, Vogel AL, Croyle RT, editors. Strategies for team science success: handbook of evidence-based principles for cross-disciplinary science and practical lessons learned from health researchers. New York, NY: Springer; 2019.

Gilmore R, Adolph K. Open sharing of behavioral research datasets – breaking down the boundaries of the research team. In: Hall KL, Vogel AL, Croyle RT, editors. Strategies for team science success: handbook of evidence-based principles for cross-disciplinary science and practical lessons learned from health researchers. New York, NY: Springer; 2019.

Hall KL. What makes teams tick. Nature. 2017;551:562–3.

Hall KL, Stipelman BA, Vogel AL, Stokols D. Understanding cross-disciplinary team-based research: Concepts and conceptual models from the Science of Team Science. In: Frodeman R, Klein JT, Mitcham C, editors. Oxford handbook on interdisciplinarity. 2nd ed. Oxford, UK: Oxford University Press; 2017. p. 338–56.

Hall KL, Stokols D, Moser R, Thornquist M, Taylor B, Nebeling L. The collaboration readiness of transdisciplinary research teams and centers: Findings from the National Cancer Institute TREC year-one evaluation study. Am J Prevent Med. 2008;35(2):S161–72.

Hall KL, Vogel AL, Huang GC, Serrano KJ, Rice EL, Tsakraklides SP, Fiore SM. The science of team science: a review of the empirical evidence and research gaps on collaboration in science. Am Psychol. 2018;73(4):532–48.

Hall KL, Vogel AL, Crowston K. Comprehensive collaboration plans: practical considerations spanning from individual collaborators to institutional supports. In: Hall KL, Vogel AL, Croyle RT, editors. Strategies for team science success: handbook of evidence-based principles for cross-disciplinary science and practical lessons learned from health researchers. New York, NY: Springer; 2019.

Hendren CO, Ku S. The Interdisciplinary Executive Scientist: connecting scientific ideas, resources, and people. In: Hall KL, Vogel AL, Croyle RT, editors. Strategies for team science success: handbook of evidence-based principles for cross-disciplinary science and practical lessons learned from health researchers. New York, NY: Springer; 2019.

Hurn PD, Traystman RJ. Research spanning animal and human models: the role of serendipity, competition, and strategic actions in advancing stroke research. In: Hall KL, Vogel AL, Croyle RT, editors. Strategies for team science success: handbook of evidence-based principles for cross-disciplinary science and practical lessons learned from health researchers. New York, NY: Springer; 2019.

Jain P, Klein D. Precollaboration framework: academic/industry partnerships: mobile and wearable technologies for behavioral science. In: Hall KL, Vogel AL, Croyle RT, editors. Strategies for team science success: handbook of evidence-based principles for cross-disciplinary science and practical lessons learned from health researchers. New York, NY: Springer; 2019.

James P, Redline S. The introduction of a new domain into an existing area of research: novel discoveries through integration of sleep into cancer and obesity research. In: Hall KL, Vogel AL, Croyle RT, editors. Strategies for team science success: handbook of evidence-based principles for cross-disciplinary science and practical lessons learned from health researchers. New York, NY: Springer; 2019.

Johnson LB, Smalley JB. Engaging the patient: patient-centered research. In: Hall KL, Vogel AL, Croyle RT, editors. Strategies for team science success: handbook of evidence-based principles for cross-disciplinary science and practical lessons learned from health researchers. New York, NY: Springer; 2019.

Kiviniemi M. Engaging the practitioner: "but wait, that's not all!" – collaborations with practitioners and extending the reasons you started doing research in the first place. In: Hall KL, Vogel AL, Croyle RT, editors. Strategies for team science success: handbook of evidence-based principles for cross-disciplinary science and practical lessons learned from health researchers. New York, NY: Springer; 2019.

Klein W. Cross-disciplinary team science with trainees: from undergraduate to post-doc. In: Hall KL, Vogel AL, Croyle RT, editors. Strategies for team science success: handbook of evidence-based principles for cross-disciplinary science and practical lessons learned from health researchers. New York, NY: Springer; 2019.

Kozlowski SWJ, Bell BS. Evidence-based principles and strategies for optimizing team functioning and performance in science teams. In: Hall KL, Vogel AL, Croyle RT, editors. Strategies for team science success: handbook of evidence-based principles for cross-disciplinary science and practical lessons learned from health researchers. New York, NY: Springer; 2019.

Madden GJ, McClure S, Bickel WK. Collaborating to move laboratory findings into public health domains: maxims for translational research. In: Hall KL, Vogel AL, Croyle RT, editors. Strategies for team science success: handbook of evidence-based principles for cross-disciplinary science and practical lessons learned from health researchers. New York, NY: Springer; 2019.

Marino AH, Suda-Blake K, Fulton KR. Innovative collaboration formation – the National Academies Keck Futures Initiative. In: Hall KL, Vogel AL, Croyle RT, editors. Strategies for team science success: handbook of evidence-based principles for cross-disciplinary

science and practical lessons learned from health researchers. New York, NY: Springer; 2019.

NASEM (National Academy of Sciences, National Academy of Engineering, and Institute of Medicine). Facilitating interdisciplinary research. Washington, DC: The National Academies Press; 2005. https://doi.org/10.17226/11153.

NRC (National Research Council). Convergence: facilitating transdisciplinary integration of life sciences, physical sciences, engineering, and beyond. Washington, DC: The National Academies Press; 2014. https://doi.org/10.17226/18722.

NRC (National Research Council). Enhancing the effectiveness of team science. Washington, DC: The National Academies Press; 2015.

NSF (National Science Foundation). n.d. https://www.nsf.gov/od/oia/convergence/index.jsp. Accessed 2018 Nov

Nurius PS, Kemp SP. Individual level competencies for team collaboration with cross-disciplinary researchers and stakeholders. In: Hall KL, Vogel AL, Croyle RT, editors. Strategies for team science success: handbook of evidence-based principles for cross-disciplinary science and practical lessons learned from health researchers. New York, NY: Springer; 2019.

O'Rourke M, Crowley S, Laursen B, Robinson B, Vasko SE. Disciplinary diversity in teams: integrative approaches from unidisciplinarity to transdisciplinarity. In: Hall KL, Vogel AL, Croyle RT, editors. Strategies for team science success: handbook of evidence-based principles for cross-disciplinary science and practical lessons learned from health researchers. New York, NY: Springer; 2019.

Payne R. The effectiveness of research teams: a review. In: West MA, Farr JL, editors. Innovation and creativity at work: psychological and organizational strategies. Oxford: John Wiley & Sons; 1990. p. 101–22.

Pelz D, Andrews F. Scientists in organizations: productive climates for research and development. Oxford: John Wiley; 1966.

Pelz DC. Creative tensions in the research and development climate. Science. 1967;157(3785):160–5.

Pohl C, Hirsch Hadorn G. Principles for designing transdisciplinary research. Munich, Germany: Oekom Verlag GmbH; 2007.

Pohl C, Wuelser G. Methods for co-production of knowledge among diverse disciplines and stakeholders. In: Hall KL, Vogel AL, Croyle RT, editors. Strategies for team science success: handbook of evidence-based principles for cross-disciplinary science and practical lessons learned from health researchers. New York, NY: Springer; 2019.

Ranwala D, Alberg AJ, Brady KT, Obeid JS, Davis R, Halushka PV. Retreats to stimulate cross-disciplinary translational research collaborations: Medical University of South Carolina CTSA Pilot Project Program Initiative. In: Hall KL, Vogel AL, Croyle RT, editors. Strategies for team science success: handbook of evidence-based principles for cross-disciplinary science and practical lessons learned from health researchers. New York, NY: Springer; 2019.

Rolland B. Designing and developing coordinating centers as infrastructure to support team science. In: Hall KL, Vogel AL, Croyle RT, editors. Strategies for team science success: handbook of evidence-based principles for cross-disciplinary science and practical lessons learned from health researchers. New York, NY: Springer; 2019.

Salazar M, Widmer K, Doiron K, Lant TK. Leader integrative capabilities: a catalyst for effective interdisciplinary teams. In: Hall KL, Vogel AL, Croyle RT, editors. Strategies for team science success: handbook of evidence-based principles for cross-disciplinary science and practical lessons learned from health researchers. New York, NY: Springer; 2019.

Sallis JF, Floyd MF. The development of a new interdisciplinary field: Active Living Research – a foundation-supported interdisciplinary research funding program. In: Hall KL, Vogel AL, Croyle RT, editors. Strategies for team science success: handbook of evidence-based principles for cross-disciplinary science and practical lessons learned from health researchers. New York, NY: Springer; 2019.

Spring B, Pfammatter A, Conroy DE. Continuing professional development for team science. In: Hall KL, Vogel AL, Croyle RT, editors. Strategies for team science success: handbook of evidence-based principles for cross-disciplinary science and practical lessons learned from health researchers. New York, NY: Springer; 2019.

Stipelman B, Rice E, Vogel AL, Hall KL. The role of team personality on team effectiveness and performance. In: Hall KL, Vogel AL, Croyle RT, editors. Strategies for team science success: handbook of evidence-based principles for cross-disciplinary science and practical lessons learned from health researchers. New York, NY: Springer; 2019.

Stokols D. Toward a science of transdisciplinary action research. Am J Community Psychol. 2006;38:63–77.

Stokols D, Hall KL, Vogel AL. Transdisciplinary public health: definitions, core characteristics and strategies for success. In: Haire-Joshu D, McBride TD, editors. Transdisciplinary public health: research, methods, and practice. San Francisco: Jossey-Bass; 2013. p. 3–30.

Stokols D, Misra S, Moser R, Hall KL, Taylor B. The ecology of team science: understanding contextual influences on transdisciplinary collaboration. Am J Prevent Med. 2008;35(2):S96–S115.

Twyman M, Contractor N. Team assembly. In: Hall KL, Vogel AL, Croyle RT, editors. Strategies for team science success: handbook of evidence-based principles for cross-disciplinary science and practical lessons learned from health researchers. New York, NY: Springer; 2019.

Vogel AL, Stipelman BA, Hall KL, Stokols D, Nebeling L, Spruijt-Metz D. Pioneering the transdisciplinary team science approach: lessons learned from National Cancer Institute grantees. J Transl Med Epidemiol. 2014;2(2):1027.

Vogel AL, Hall KL, Fiore SM, Klein JT, Bennett LM, Gadlin H, Stokols D, Nebeling L, Wuchty S, Patrick K, Spotts EL, Pohl C, Riley WT, Falk-Krzesinski HJ. The team science toolkit: enhancing research collaboration through online knowledge sharing. Am J Prevent Med. 2013;45(6):787–9.

Vogel AL, Hall KL, Falk-Krzesinski HJ, Klein JT. Broadening our understanding of scientific work for the era of team science: implications for recognition and rewards. In: Hall KL, Vogel AL, Croyle RT, editors. Strategies for team science success: handbook of evidence-based principles for cross-disciplinary science and practical lessons learned from health researchers. New York, NY: Springer; 2019.

Wallerstein N, Calhoun K, Eder M, Kaplow J, Wilkins CH. Engaging the community: community-based participatory research and team science. In: Hall KL, Vogel AL, Croyle RT, editors. Strategies for team science success: handbook of evidence-based principles for cross-disciplinary science and practical lessons learned from health researchers. New York, NY: Springer; 2019.

Weber G, Yuan L. The power of research networking systems to find experts and facilitate collaboration. In: Hall KL, Vogel AL, Croyle RT, editors. Strategies for team science success: handbook of evidence-based principles for cross-disciplinary science and practical lessons learned from health researchers. New York, NY: Springer; 2019.

Winter S. Organizational perspectives on leadership strategies for the success of cross-disciplinary science teams. In: Hall KL, Vogel AL, Croyle RT, editors. Strategies for team science success: handbook of evidence-based principles for cross-disciplinary science and practical lessons learned from health researchers. New York, NY: Springer; 2019.

Wuchty S, Jones BF, Uzzi B. The increasing dominance of teams in production of knowledge. Science. 2007;316:1036–9. https://doi.org/10.1126/science.1136099.

Part II

Integrative Science Teams

Michael O'Rourke ⓘ, Stephen Crowley ⓘ,
Bethany Laursen ⓘ, Brian Robinson ⓘ,
and Stephanie E. Vasko ⓘ

Contents

M. O'Rourke (✉)
MSU Center for Interdisciplinarity, Michigan State
University, East Lansing, MI, USA

Toolbox Dialogue Initiative, Michigan State University,
East Lansing, MI, USA

Department of Philosophy and AgBioResearch,
Michigan State University, East Lansing, MI, USA
e-mail: orourk51@msu.edu

S. Crowley
Department of Philosophy, Boise State University,
Boise, ID, USA

B. Laursen
Department of Community Sustainability, College of
Agriculture and Natural Resources, Michigan State
University, East Lansing, MI, USA

Department of Philosophy, Michigan State University,
East Lansing, MI, USA

Laursen Evaluation & Design, LLC, Grand Rapids,
MI, USA

2.1 Introduction: The Challenge of Disciplinary Diversity

Diversity within science teams is both a blessing and a curse. The power of team science derives largely from its ability to leverage individual differences in many forms—e.g., experience, gender, expertise—to enhance the breadth and depth of insight and innovation. But these differences can also manifest as barriers to effective teamwork, giving rise to misunderstanding and mistrust. In this chapter, we focus on beneficial and baneful aspects of a particular type of difference within science teams, namely, difference in expertise, understood roughly and somewhat abstractly as *disciplinary* diversity. By themselves, disciplinary frameworks are narrow and partial, but in combination, they can represent interrelated aspects of complex systems and explain intricate interdependencies. Complex, integrative explanations are powerful, giving us resources to address the grand challenges that confront humanity, such as hunger, infectious disease, and climate change (De Grandis and Efstathiou 2016). Efforts to

B. Robinson
Department of History, Political Science, and
Philosophy, Texas A&M University-Kingsville,
Kingsville, TX, USA

S. E. Vasko
MSU Center for Interdisciplinarity, Michigan State
University, East Lansing, MI, USA

© Springer Nature Switzerland AG 2019
K. L. Hall et al. (eds.), *Strategies for Team Science Success*,
https://doi.org/10.1007/978-3-030-20992-6_2

combine disciplinary frameworks are often motivated by a desire to take full advantage of what we have come to know about ourselves and our world, weaving together complex responses to complex problems.

Although science teams will almost certainly involve members with different relevant expertise, science teams need not involve members from different disciplines. People who represent a single discipline can find value in collaborating in a unidisciplinary team (Stokols et al. 2008); however, team science often combines multiple disciplines, especially for grappling with complex social and behavioral problems such as obesity and cancer prevention and treatment. We call team-based research that combines disciplines *cross-disciplinary team science* (CDTS). CDTS is a mode of research, and as such aims to generate new knowledge. Yet, whether it is unidisciplinary or cross-disciplinary, new knowledge does not emerge from the head fully formed; rather, it takes hard work that unfolds over time in a more or less systematic way. The need for hard work is especially pressing when a team of collaborators looks at research decisions from several different disciplinary perspectives. This is the heart of what we take to be the *challenge of disciplinary diversity*.

Addressing this challenge is a practical problem, but a response can benefit from a theoretical model to guide understanding of the task. Those who conduct CDTS operate against a backdrop of theoretical work in disciplines such as epistemology, interdisciplinary theory, organizational behavior, and social psychology. Although it may not seem as directly relevant to project decisions as practical examples from similar projects, this theoretical work can inform choices about whom to involve as participants, how to structure the effort, and what to regard as appropriate success conditions. Thus, CDTS researchers can profit from consideration of the theory behind CDTS, and this chapter is intended to support such consideration.

In this chapter we highlight research that illuminates the challenge of disciplinary diversity as well as research that describes effective responses to this challenge. After a few preliminary remarks, we unfold this challenge in three steps. First, we discuss the process of *identifying* relevant disciplinary resources. Second, we examine what it is for a team to be *ready* to marshal these resources in integrative CDTS. Finally, we discuss the process of combining, or *integrating*, these resources in a research project.

2.2 Conceptual Scaffolding

In this section, we describe a way of thinking about CDTS as a process, highlighting the trajectory of a typical CDTS experience and using that to emphasize the aspects that are our concern in this chapter. Second, we supply brief, literature-based definitions of concepts that are foundational to this chapter and many of the subsequent chapters as well.

2.2.1 Modeling CDTS

As we consider it here, the challenge of disciplinary diversity can be distilled into three questions:

1. How do you identify the disciplinary experts you need on a project?
2. How do you prepare a cross-disciplinary team to do its work?
3. How should a cross-disciplinary team integrate its perspectives?

Given that these questions rise to prominence at certain times in the life cycle of a CDTS project, it helps to have a dynamic model of a typical team science project as a context within which to consider these questions.

Team science is frequently modeled as a *process* that operates on various *inputs* and produces various *outputs*, in line with the "Input-Process-Output" (or *IPO*) heuristic (McGrath 1964). Research inputs are various and include research questions of the team, disciplinary perspectives and value orientations of the individual collaborators, and contextual factors

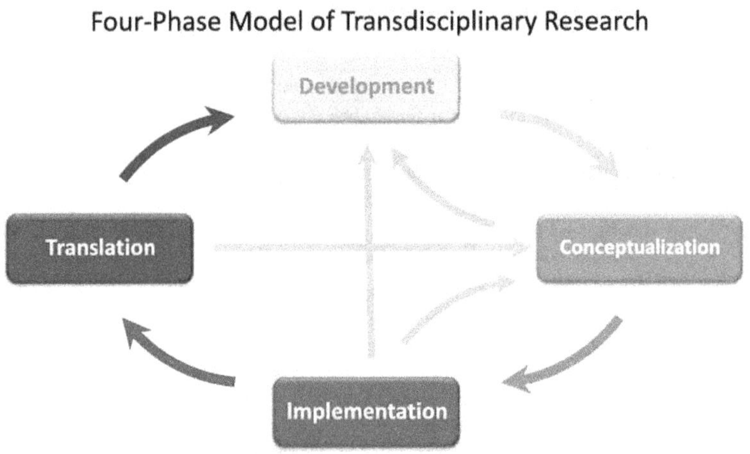

Four-Phase Model of Transdisciplinary Research

Fig. 2.1 A four-phase model of transdisciplinary research, from Hall et al. (2012), p. 417. Teams may move through this along the outside pathways, with the internal arrows representing possible iterative or alternative pathways. Although transdisciplinary research need not be team-based, this model is developed by the authors in the context of team science

such as related work reported in the literature and funding constraints (cf. Cooke and Hilton 2015, p. 62). Outputs include the standard academic deliverables, such as proposals, patents, and publications, intangible impacts such as social learning and trust building, and also nonacademic responses to problems such as new policies and management protocols that reside in the world at large. Following Marks et al. (2001, p. 357), we take the team research process that intervenes between these to be "members' interdependent acts that convert inputs to outcomes through cognitive, verbal, and behavioral activities directed toward organizing taskwork to achieve collective goals." Usefully, the IPO heuristic can be applied to clarify CDTS at different scales, from the life cycle of a project as a whole down to the level of specific decisions that inflect the research at particular moments of time. Further, following Kozlowski (2015, p. 271), it is important that team processes be viewed through the lens of the IPO heuristic as dynamic processes, unfolding in time in ways that are iterative and recursive (Klein 2012).

Among the dynamic, knowledge-focused process models for CDTS teams, there are several that have been developed for transdisciplinary science, with an emphasis on team research. These include the ISOE model (for "Institute for Social-Ecological Research" in Frankfurt, Germany) of Jahn (2008) and the transdisciplinary decision-making model of Hall and O'Rourke (2014). We adopt the model introduced by Hall et al. (2012), who present a dynamic model of transdisciplinary, team-based research that involves four phases: (a) *development*, in which a team representing multiple disciplines forms to address a problem; (b) *conceptualization*, in which the team develops the conceptual infrastructure (e.g., research design) necessary to conduct the research; (c) *implementation*, in which the team conducts the research; and (d) *translation*, in which the team moves the results across levels of analysis and out into the world (see Fig. 2.1). This iterative, recursive model of the life cycle of a transdisciplinary project functions well as a frame for our investigation into the challenge of disciplinary diversity, given its attention to the combination of multiple disciplines in the conduct of team-based research. In subsequent sections, *development* and *conceptualization* will be foregrounded in our discussion of questions (1) and (2) above, while *implementation* and to some extent *translation* will factor into our discussion of question (3).

Table 2.1 Brief definitions of terms that figure centrally into this chapter

Key term	Definition
Axiology	Systematic investigation of value, values, and what makes something valuable
Capacities	Existing abilities to perform certain behaviors or accomplish certain goals (in contrast to *capabilities*, which may only exist potentially)
Collaborate	To interact and coordinate when performing actions, typically toward a common objective (cf. Andrade et al. 2009, p. 302; Crowley et al. 2013)
Cross-disciplinary	A generic cover term for any mode of research that involves the combination of different research perspectives, e.g., multidisciplinarity, interdisciplinarity, and transdisciplinarity (cf. Eigenbrode et al. 2007)
Cross-disciplinary team science (CDTS)	Scientific efforts involving collaborating scientists who work to combine different types of expertise that are often individuated by academic discipline
Discipline (disciplinary)	Quasi-institutional structures, with epistemic dimensions that concern different ways of asking and pursuing research questions, as well as institutional dimensions exhibited by university departments and professional societies (cf. Weingart 2010)
Epistemology	Systematic investigation of knowledge and related concepts (e.g., belief, justification, understanding)
Epistemic culture	"[T]hose sets of practices, arrangements and mechanisms bound together by necessity, affinity and historical coincidence which, in a given area of professional expertise, make up how we know what we know" (Knorr Cetina 2007, p. 363)
Expertise	Skill and knowledge that constitute mastery in a particular domain (Collins and Evans 2002)
Field	Less institutional than disciplines, these typically correspond to the dimensions of disciplines that include "a central problem," "general explanatory factors," and "techniques and methods" (Darden and Maull 1977, p. 44)
Group	A collection of people whose actions are not coordinated and who are not interdependent in their roles and functions (cf. Fisher et al. 1997); cf. *team*
Input-process-output (IPO) heuristic	A way of thinking about change that involves specifying inputs that are processed into outputs (cf. McGrath 1964)
Integrate	To combine elements/inputs into a whole; understood as a kind of process that can figure into an IPO model (cf. O'Rourke et al. 2016)
Methodology	An abstract account that "explains why specific methods work"; often conflated with *method*, understood as a "systematic means to pursue an end" that is (for us) part of a research project (O'Rourke 2017, p. 278–9)
Readiness	Being willing and able to complete a task (cf. Rosas and Camarinha-Matos 2009, p. 4713)
Team	"[T]wo or more individuals with different roles and responsibilities, who interact socially and interdependently within an organizational system to perform tasks and accomplish common goals" (Cooke and Hilton 2015, p. 2); cf. *group*
Worldview	A set of "more or less tacit beliefs held by researchers about what they are studying and how to study it, as well as views about the nature of the output of their inquiry" (O'Rourke and Crowley 2013)

2.2.2 Foundational Concepts for CDTS

The dynamic model of team process in Fig. 2.1 highlights a number of conceptual elements that are foundational to the discussion in this chapter. First, given our focus on the challenge of disciplinary diversity, *discipline* is a central conceptual building block. Further, since the focus of this volume is *team* science, we emphasize disciplinary diversity in the context of team-based research. Teams differ from less cohesive groups

in part because they involve members who *collaborate*. When these teams comprise researchers from different disciplines, the research labor will often aim for *integration* of the different perspectives supplied by the collaborators. Finally, the concept of *readiness* as it has been developed in the team science literature is helpful as a way of highlighting characteristics that can indicate when a team is poised for success. Table 2.1 supplies brief definitions for each of these key terms as well as other terms that figure importantly into subsequent discussions.

2.3   Identifying Appropriate Experts

CDTS involves combining diverse forms of expertise to address complex problems. Given this, an obvious issue is identifying the forms of expertise that should be included in a particular effort. In this section, we concentrate on this identification issue, highlighting a number of considerations that should factor into deliberation about team composition and closing with a table of guiding principles for choosing experts.

2.3.1   Disciplines and Experts

Consider the following scenario, which illustrates a typical way that CDTS teams form (Contractor 2013; Leonelli and Ankeny 2015). A political scientist interested in public attitudes to new technology finds a US National Science Foundation (NSF) request for proposals (RFP) concerning human-robot interaction and decides to submit a proposal. The political scientist recognizes that she needs additional expertise to submit a credible proposal, and so adds a mechanical engineer for robot expertise, a philosopher for ethical expertise, and a sociologist to assist in surveying public attitudes. The team discusses how it would like to respond to the RFP; given their combined expertise, they decide that instead of simply investigating public attitudes to robots, they will identify public and professional attitudes to robots in order to see how attitudes differ between the two communities, thinking that such differences in attitude may have important social consequences. For our purposes the key features of this scenario are (1) that expertise and disciplinary identity are correlated in the team assembly stage, and (2) that the research goals are *revised* to leverage team expertise.

There are several things we can learn from this example. First, while collaborators on CDTS teams are diverse in many ways (e.g., ethnicity, gender, experience with CDTS, career stage; see NAS 2004—e.g., p. 53, Contractor 2013, Cheruvelil et al. 2014, and Cooke and Hilton 2015, Chap. 4), one key dimension of diversity is *disciplinary* diversity, i.e., the disciplines to which they belong

and in terms of which they self-identify. We can think of disciplines as *epistemic cultures* (see Table 2.1). Since disciplinary identity concerns how a person operates as a researcher, knowing the disciplinary identity an individual assigns to him/herself can help make sense of their role in a team (Osbeck and Nersessian 2010).

The second lesson here involves shifting the emphasis from disciplines to expertise. Disciplines per se are not what really matter here; rather, it is the expertise the disciplinary representatives bring with them. Disciplines in this case are proxy for sets of skills that are regarded as essential to the success of the team. The kinds of expertise that might be of interest to a team vary. Collins and Evans (2002) distinguish between *contributory* and *interactional* expertise, with the former held by those who can contribute to research in the field and the latter held by those who cannot contribute to research in the field (i.e., they cannot "do the math") but who can communicate with contributory experts about their work in a way that allows for meaningful, research-relevant interaction. If a CDTS team is engaged in a project that involves community partners or impacts local stakeholders, it is important to recognize *local* expertise alongside academic, disciplinary research expertise, where the former is rooted in knowledge that is "localized, experiential or indigenous" (Raymond et al. 2010, p. 1767). A third helpful distinction for distinguishing different types of expertise of value to CDTS is between *T-shaped* expertise, which involves deep knowledge in one area and breadth in other areas (August et al. 2010), and *shield-shaped* expertise, which combines breadth with depth in multiple areas (Bosque-Pérez et al. 2016).

Third, the expertise required by a team will *co-evolve* with its goals. In some cases, research goals will come first, guiding the selection of experts for the team that will pursue those goals. In other cases, though, the team will already be constituted and will instead be interested in finding research goals to pursue (Gewin 2015; Bosque-Pérez et al. 2016). In the academic context this is the difference between "creating a team for an RFP" and "finding an RFP for our team." In many cases, there will be regular adjustment in both directions over the life cycle of a research effort. The co-evolution of required expertise and team goals is a key element in many models of CDTS, such as the Hall et al. (2012) model discussed above (cf. Lang et al. 2012; Hall and O'Rourke 2014).

2.3.2   Heuristics for Identifying Required Expertise

We now turn to our primary concern, viz., approaching the tandem tasks of assembling both the relevant expertise and team goals necessary for CDTS. In a particular research situation, this concern can take the form of the question, "Do we have the right mix of experts on our team?" There are two different approaches to this question. If the primary goal is to continue work with the team you have, then the answer will of course be *yes* (initially), but the challenge then becomes finding a research problem for which the current composition is the right mix (cf. Bosque-Pérez et al. 2016). Alternatively, if the primary goal is to address a research problem, then it becomes necessary to evaluate research needs in light of the problem you've selected. On either approach (viz., research problem first or team first), it will be necessary to evaluate the problem under consideration to determine how one should understand it. There is no correct way to do this—it will depend on how you describe the problem (Piso 2015), which will be a function of factors such as values and priorities, as well as more practical factors such as what resources are available.

The IPO heuristic introduced in the previous section can help us here. Evaluation of the problem under consideration will typically yield proposals for addressing it, where those proposals describe *outputs* that serve as team goals. Successful pursuit of these goals will require certain *inputs* from the team, e.g., the team in our example must have the capacity to survey the public if it is interested in identifying how the public thinks of robots. These inputs will involve different capacities, e.g., the team will need to know certain things about the problem, will need to be familiar with certain literatures, and will need to have the ability to apply appropriate methods in pursuit of their research objectives.

The task of identifying required expertise, then, can be thought of as the task of matching capacities required by team goals with capacities possessed by team members.

As we noted, if one approaches this matching task with the team in place, then the challenge is to find a problem that the already-constituted team can successfully address. Previous success can help delimit the space of research problems, and of course it is always open to the team to add experts as needed to address its chosen problem. Approaching the matching task from the perspective of the problem can be more difficult (Rittel and Webber 1973). Often interest in the problem will be initiated by an expert who is involved in the matching task from the beginning; their role as team catalyst will privilege their interpretation of the problem (at least initially) as the frame for decisions about what additional experts are required (cf. Andrews et al. 2016). But interest in research problems can also be driven top-down by institutions without having an expert attached in the beginning. In this case, you can find initial assistance in identifying relevant expertise by paying attention to who is talking about the problem in the literature, or who is funding work on the problem—RFPs will often provide guidance on the kinds of expertise required for competitive proposals. Once an expert is attached, though, it is good practice to make sure that additional experts mesh well with them, as the ability to achieve project goals will depend as much on affective considerations such as trust as it will on the presence of the requisite forms of expertise (Fiore et al. 2015; Gewin 2015; Cooke and Hilton 2015, Chap. 4).

Since the matching task takes place in a research context, you can also structure it in terms of the knowledge you will create. For example, one can model the research space with the help of a *knowledge organization system*, i.e., a systematic set of distinctions meant to individuate different knowledge domains and reveal their interrelationships in more or less comprehensive fashion (Szostak et al. 2016). Examples of these include the Library of Congress Classification system used in university libraries, or the Digital Commons Three-Tiered List of Academic Disciplines (bepress 2017). These systems distinguish types of expertise that could be integrated into the research team. Given an understanding of a research problem, one can use systems like these to become aware of the perspectives associated with the disciplines and identify where one might go to find the experts one wants (Repko 2012). One can also go in the other direction. For example, the comprehensive, analytical classification of human phenomena found in Szostak (2004) could be used to aid in the analysis of a research problem, highlighting aspects that require research attention by disciplinary experts. Although he focuses on individuals, Repko (2012, Chap. 5) describes a process combining these directions that can be extended to teams; this process uses "maps" of the phenomena of interest that reveal their disciplinary parts to identify the most relevant types of expertise for a project (cf. Newell 2007).

There are other ways to think about the research process that structure the choice of experts. One can think about the matching task philosophically, in terms of knowledge or methodology-related (i.e., *epistemic*), world-related (i.e., *metaphysical*), and value-related (i.e., *axiological*) aspects of research problems and disciplinary worldviews (Eigenbrode et al. 2007, cf. Patterson and Williams 1998). Phillipson et al. (2009, p. 262), for example, note that "ecologists choose their social science partners based on the various types of expertise and roles that they bring," and in thinking about those partners, they are "guided by their sense of what was methodologically and philosophically compatible with their own research." Focusing on interdisciplinary environmental problem solving, Benda et al. (2002, p. 1127) identify five less abstract categories that constitute the "structure of knowledge" and are intended to help researchers organize their projects and avoid "train wrecks." These categories are:

(1) disciplinary history and attendant forms of available scientific knowledge; (2) spatial and temporal scales at which that knowledge applies; (3) precision (i.e., qualitative versus quantitative nature of understanding across different scales); (4) accuracy of predictions; and (5) availability of data to construct, calibrate, and test predictive models.

Once we move out beyond academic CDTS and involve stakeholders, the rules of the game change somewhat. Bammer (2013) develops a three-area,

five-question approach to identifying areas of focus for a CDTS team that involves nonacademic research partners. The three areas are "(1) synthesising disciplinary and stakeholder knowledge, (2) understanding and managing diverse unknowns, and (3) providing integrated research support for policy and practice change" (p. 15). The five questions concern the synthesis of disciplinary and stakeholder knowledge, focusing on *what* the context, aim, and result of synthesis are, *who* is to benefit, *which* knowledge is synthesized, *how* it is synthesized, and *when* it is synthesized (cf. Bergmann et al. 2012). Identifying relevant experts can be difficult when there are fundamental differences among perspectives, such as when Indigenous knowledge is involved. Murphy (2011, p. 493) focuses on the relation of western and Indigenous knowledge in specifying a six-area framework that could be used to help determine what expertise is required: integrative research, epistemic authority, epistemic power dynamics, Indigenous knowledge positioning, interdisciplinarity, and inter-epistemological acknowledgement. For a summary of principles that can guide identification of appropriate experts for a CDTS project, see Table 2.2.

Table 2.2 Guiding principles for identifying appropriate experts when building (or maintaining) a CDTS project

Guiding principles for choosing experts
1. **Be open to the possibilities**. The process of inviting researchers to a team should be catholic and should be revisited as the project develops—although you need to be careful, *you can always add more experts* (e.g., Hall et al. 2012; Hall and O'Rourke 2014; NAS 2004; Lang et al. 2012).
2. **Use technological resources**. Use resources, both human and technological, for identifying potential collaborators (NAS 2004, Cooke and Hilton 2015, Chap. 4), such as the Elsevier Expert Lookup (Elsevier 2016).
3. **Consider adding generalists**. Teams benefit from the addition of generalists who work to move information around the team and can help with boundary crossing (e.g., Bammer 2013).
4. **Think about team structure**. How the team is structured (e.g., Cheruvelil et al. 2014) and what activities support that structure (e.g., Read et al. 2016) are important aspects of identifying the expertise a team needs to succeed.
5. **Identifying expertise is a wicked problem**. There is no correct answer about who should be on the team, but rather the opportunity to create a collective with a unique set of talents competent to achieve important research objectives (Norris et al. 2016).

2.4 Readiness

Once the team is constituted, attention will naturally turn to the research effort. At this point, early in a team's life cycle, the team should ask, are we *ready* to begin work, and if not, how can we get ready? Our focus in this section will be on the readiness of a team to leverage their disciplinary diversity and produce integrative responses to their research problems. In this section, we use a typology of readiness to address specific epistemic, social, and technological considerations that are well considered before the work of an integrative team commences. We include a table of readiness resources (Table 2.3) and a table of guiding questions (Table 2.4) for assessing a team's readiness.

Table 2.3 A list of tools and associated resources that can be used to enhance the readiness of an integrative team

Readiness tool resources for CDTS
Epistemic tools
1. **Visualization**: *rich pictures* (Fiore et al., 2019); *argument visualization* (Kirschner et al. 2012); *semi-quantitative maps* of the areas of inquiry within each field in their shared epistemic space (Benda et al. 2002); group concept mapping (Kane and Trochim 2007); mental modeling (Gray et al. 2014); constellation mapping (Ohlhorst and Schön 2015)
2. **Dialogue**: general resources—McDonald et al. (2009), Winowiecki et al. (2011); specific resource—the *Toolbox approach* (Eigenbrode et al. 2007; O'Rourke and Crowley 2013)
Social tools
1. **Collaboration plan**: Hall et al. (2019)
2. **TDO Scale**: Misra et al. (2015)
3. **Collaboration Readiness Instrument**: Hall et al. (2008)
4. **The Team Effectiveness Assessment Model**: Webne-Behrman (1998), pp. 135–138
Technological tools
1. **Technological Readiness Plan**: Hall et al. (2014)
2. **Data Management Plan**: DMP Tool 2017

2.4.1 Team Readiness and Integrative Capacity

We take readiness to comprise factors *intrinsic* and *extrinsic* to the team (Fig. 2.2). *Intrinsic* factors are those that belong to a team—specifically, those that bear directly on research-relevant deliberation and decision-making conducted by the team. These include intrapersonal characteristics and interpersonal factors (Hall et al. 2008; Lotrecchiano et al. 2016), as well as material elements that support the collaboration (Olson and Olson 2000). *Extrinsic* factors, by contrast, are factors that are outside of the team, setting the context for their effort and constraining it without being factors that figure directly into decision-making. Hall et al. (2008, p. 162) call these "contextual-environmental" factors, and they include organizational policies, administrative support, cultural norms, institutional infrastructure and resources, and the physical context of the team (cf. Fuqua et al. 2004). Extrinsic factors are reviewed extensively in Sect. 8 of this volume, so we will not review them here (see also Cooke and Hilton 2015, Chaps. 5, 7–9).

In this section, we examine intrinsic individual and collective factors that contribute to a collaborative, integrative culture of knowledge production. Before proceeding we should note that we agree with those (e.g., Hall et al. 2008) who note that these intrinsic factors interact with one another and with extrinsic factors, exhibiting a "dynamic interplay" that influences "the rapidity and ease with which teams develop new outcomes" (Fuqua et al. 2004, p. 1472). As such, the intrinsic/extrinsic distinction is somewhat porous, allowing elements that at one time or for one group count as extrinsic to qualify as intrinsic, or vice versa.

Mapping various readiness constructs to this typology can guide CDTS practitioners to the appropriate construct for self-assessment and improvement. It may also guide CDTS theorists to potential synergies and gaps in the literature. For example, Misra et al. (2015) develop a

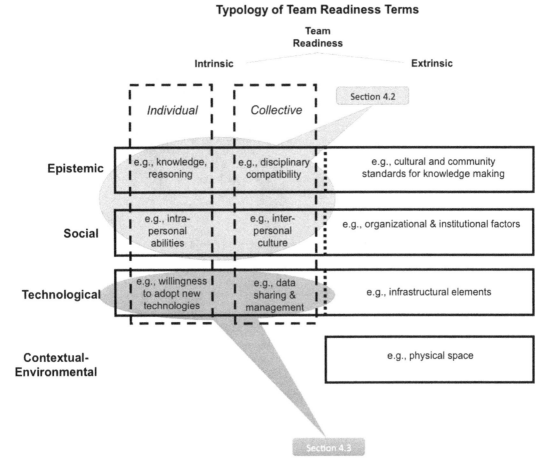

Fig. 2.2 A proposed conceptual typology of team readiness terms. The four horizontal blocks are areas of team structure and environment. The dotted vertical line splits them into intrinsic and extrinsic features. The dashed boxes mark individual and collective aspects of intrinsic team features. In the figure, dots and dashes indicate *porosity*. Thought bubbles indicate coverage in this section

Transdisciplinary Orientation (TDO) Scale that assesses individual epistemic and social factors (cf. Stokols 2013; Lotrecchiano et al. 2016). Epistemic readiness is measured by questions about conceptual skills, such as thinking holistically and knowing about stakeholders. Social readiness is assessed with questions about values, attitudes, beliefs, and behaviors. Members who value inclusivity, diversity, and learning new points of view believe the benefits of transdisciplinary work outweigh the costs, and they are willing to engage in integrative behaviors like reading in other disciplines or professions. Hall et al. (2008) describe *collaborative readiness* in transdisciplinary teams, which covers several domains in the typology with an emphasis on the collective, such as readiness associated with social factors, technology, and the environment (cf. Boix Mansilla et al. 2015). Readiness precedes capacity in their model, so teams that have worked together previously bring some of their former capacity with them to a new project and are potentially more ready than inaugural teams to commence work.

A specific capacity that is especially important for our purposes is *integrative capacity*, which, like collaborative readiness, stretches across both epistemic and social typological domains (Salazar et al. 2012). Since integrative capacity is a *capacity*, it remains relevant at all

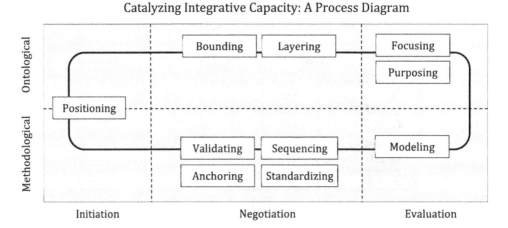

Fig. 2.3 A diagram of processes involved in integrative dialogue, from Piso et al. (2016), p. 87

points in the life cycle of an integrative team (see Fig. 2.1); however, it is important to determine if an integrative team has this in the early stages of its work together—to be successful, they must be ready to engage in research that integrates inputs from multiple disciplinary domains. While Salazar et al. (2012) develop the integrative capacity construct in a way that covers multiple domains in our typology, Piso et al. (2016) develop a version of integrative capacity that foregrounds epistemic readiness (see Fig. 2.3). Focusing on dialogue that catalyzes integrative capacity, they distinguish between the ontological and methodological commitments of collaborators, and how over the course of project discussion they initiate, evaluate, and negotiate these commitments with a view to developing integrated understanding. Whether or not a team has the ability to engage in these processes (e.g., positioning, bounding, modeling) is key to determining whether they are ready to engage in integrative team science.

2.4.2 Intrinsic Team Readiness— Epistemic and Social Factors

A team's readiness to integrate its expertise will be a function primarily of *epistemic* and *social* dimensions of intrinsic readiness. From Fig. 2.2, we note that each of these applies to the team as a collective and to each individual in the team. *Collective epistemic readiness* describes the compatibility of the various disciplinary knowledge structures represented in the team, which manifest as forms of expertise (Benda et al. 2002). *Individual epistemic readiness* includes one's knowledge content and one's ability to reason critically, creatively, and integratively (Misra et al. 2015). *Collective social readiness* describes an *inter*personal culture that supports collaboration, i.e., norms and processes that enable the mutually beneficial exchange of knowledge, emotions, time, finances, and in-kind support (Stokols et al. 2003, 2008). *Individual social readiness* describes the *intra*personal disposition and ability of each team member to support such a team culture (Misra et al. 2015; Lotrecchiano et al. 2016; Sect. 5, this volume). A team that consists of collaborators who are team players capable of supporting one another as people and as experts and who are capable of communicating with one another about their expertise is a team that will exhibit a high degree of readiness along each of these dimensions.

Epistemically, types of expertise can be more or less compatible, i.e., more or less ready to be integrated (Lele and Norgaard 2005). Benda et al. (2002) describe disciplines (including professions and fields) as knowledge structures that can be classified in different ways using the five categories we discussed in the previous section.

Their case study demonstrates how the fields of hydrology, geology, and riverine ecology differ according to the temporal and spatial scales they study, their precision and accuracy, and the data on which they depend. In the social and behavioral sciences, a team might understand constituent knowledge structures in terms of different categories, e.g., population scale, the source of knowledge (stakeholders vs. scientists), and quantitative vs. qualitative findings. When two disciplines are classified in ways that conflict—e.g., when they operate at very different temporal scales—or when there are crucial gaps in theories or data, knowledge "train wrecks" can occur (Benda et al. 2002). These are situations in which attempts to integrate different forms of expertise fail, perhaps spectacularly, because of epistemic incompatibility.

Epistemic incompatibility arises when a team's research argument depends upon a sequence of disciplinary claims but the claims cannot all be justified (perhaps data are lacking) or they are contradictory in their current form (Andersen and Wagenknecht 2013). A newly formed team that manifests epistemic incompatibility exhibits a low level of collective epistemic readiness. Some might reject the possibility of real contradiction due to belief in a "unified universe" (e.g., Benor 1982); however, even if these contradictions are merely apparent, they remain intractable so long as the individuals involved lack the epistemic and social skills to resolve them (Petrie 1976; Klein 2012). These skills include facility with communication and critical thinking (Thompson 2009; Holbrook 2013; Hall and O'Rourke 2014; Laursen 2016), as well as with techniques for creating common ground, such as redefinition, extension, transformation, and organization (Newell 2007; Repko 2012). In fact, much innovation results from resolving apparent disagreements (Monteiro and Keating 2009).

Collective social readiness concerns group norms and processes that guide the interactions among individuals in their roles and support the integrative activity of a team engaged in a cross-disciplinary project. From the beginning, the fundamental currency of a team's culture is trust (Cooke and Hilton 2015, p. 158). This is especially true in a cross-disciplinary collaboration where different disciplinary cultures can make trust difficult to build. Trust can be exchanged for knowledge, emotions, time, finances, and in-kind support (Fiore et al. 2015; Dirks and Ferrin 2001). Yet unlike changing bills at the bank, these mutually beneficial exchanges actually create more currency: the more we use trust the more it grows (cf. Jarvenpaa and Leidner 1999; Bennett and Gadlin 2013; Lotrecchiano et al. 2016). When the team accrues large amounts of trust, members experience psychological safety. Psychological safety is the confidence to take risks—brainstorm a crazy idea, confront conflict, or compromise in an attempt to integrate perspectives—without fear of damaging repercussions. Intuitively and empirically, this is key to productivity and innovation (Cooke and Hilton 2015, p. 67; Duhigg 2016).

Trust can only be exchanged for productive ends in certain team climates. *Team climate* refers to the shared understanding of a team's strategic goals (Cooke and Hilton 2015). Ready teams operate in climates that exhibit (1) robust team efficacy, which is a shared "can-do" attitude that motivates perseverance; (2) team cohesion, which is the net force to remain as a group; and (3) the ability to manage task conflicts without damaging relationships (Cooke and Hilton 2015, pp. 68–70, 158; cf. Kozlowski, 2019). Collective social readiness in an integrative CDTS project includes both a climate conducive to combining expertise and the interpersonal trust necessary to support productive negotiation and compromise. In Table 2.3, we provide a list of resources for enhancing team readiness.

2.4.3 Intrinsic Team Readiness— Technological Factors

Cooke and Hilton (2015) define *technological readiness* as "a disposition to learn new technologies and to access training to make the learning easy" (p. 155). Olson & Olson (2014, p. 32) also point to an idea of "technical readiness," or "the knowledge of how to communicate and coordinate through technology, including the willingness to learn." These definitions emphasize the intrinsic individual aspects of technological readiness; our interest in the remainder of this section is in collective aspects of intrinsic technological readiness that are relevant to integrative CDTS.

Hall et al. (2014, p. 3) distinguish between two types of technological readiness needs. The first type includes *mechanisms to support the scientific process*, such as "technologies for data sharing and analysis (e.g., data sharing agreements, common databases, online collaborative data analysis platforms)." The second type includes *mechanisms to support collaborative processes* "such as communication technologies (e.g., videoconferencing, teleconferencing) and coordination technologies (e.g., calendaring, task management platforms, and work flow or project management tools)." Since integrative CDTS embraces a "richer account of scientific practice" involving data-intensive research (Elliott et al. 2016) and the opportunity to work with collaborators across the globe (Connaughton and Shuffler 2007), both types of readiness are central to success.

Thus, when embarking on a collaboration, two important collective technological hurdles for teams are data management and distance work. First, consider the data collection and data management that are increasingly important parts of scientific research collaboration. Our ability to access large volumes, varieties, and velocities of data (three of the "V's of Big Data") enables new research questions, as well as the creation and use of new tools and techniques including (but not limited to) text analytics, audio analytics, video analytics, social media analytics, and predictive analytics (Gandomi and Haider 2015). Large amounts of data and new ways to process these data require that we have technology in place to manage, access, deploy, and archive the data. Focusing on data integration, Leonelli (2013, p. 504) states that integrative research must "bridge" the many dimensions along which data can vary (e.g., format, mode of production, site, scale) in order to bring together "data obtained in a variety of different settings so that they can be analyzed together and brought to bear on common questions." For Leonelli, data integration "requires extensive scientific labor, including the development of apposite infrastructures, analytic tools, standards, methods and models" (2013, p. 504). This labor can be supported by a data management plan that highlights types of data, formats, locations, storage protocols, metadata, among other things, and is required by many federal agencies on funded projects (e.g., NIH 2003; NSF 2010; DOE 2014).

Second, consider team science that involves distance work. Challenges for teams working at a distance can include geography, infrastructure, willingness to learn, team skills, available technologies, and desired outcomes (Cooke and Hilton 2015; Mirel et al. 2015). Geographically dispersed teams must grapple with "being blind and invisible to one another; time zone differences; differences across institutions, countries, and cultures; and uneven distribution of members across participating locations" (Cooke and Hilton 2015, p. 152). Successfully understanding different perspectives and synthesizing them into coherent, integrative results requires meeting these distance-related challenges and coming together as a group. Technology is a necessary part of a team's response to these challenges, and so becoming technologically ready will help the team avoid early missteps that could compromise the overall effort.

Table 2.4 Five questions for assessing the epistemic, social, and technological readiness of both the team and the participating individuals in a CDTS project

Guiding questions for assessing integrative readiness
1. How compatible are the knowledge structures of our disciplines? (Benda et al. 2002)
2. How strong are the cross-disciplinary reasoning skills of our team members? (Boix Mansilla 2010)
3. How well do our collaborative roles align? (Bennett et al. 2010)
4. Do we trust one another enough to make the compromises necessary for meaningful integration? (Edmondson 1999)
5. Do we have a technological readiness plan in place that reflects constraints and abilities of participants, managers, institutions, and infrastructures? (Hall et al. 2014)

2.5   Integration

In CDTS, readiness must include an openness on the part of collaborators to work with other people and other perspectives. In particular, as we have noted above, a team must be ready to *integrate* both socially and epistemically—a team member must collaborate with other members of the team (Salazar et al. 2012) and must work to develop a coherent, combined point of view on their common project (Piso et al. 2016). One of the most central concepts in CDTS, integration is regarded as critical to interdisciplinary activities (NAS 2004; Klein 2012) and transdisciplinary activities (e.g., Pohl et al. 2008; Bergmann et al. 2012). There is a general agreement that while cross-disciplinary integration is hard (e.g., Lynch 2006; Newell 2007; Sievanen et al. 2011), the importance of the problems that motivate it makes it worthwhile. In this section, we address the notion of *integration*, commenting on its nature, value, and production.

2.5.1   What Is Integration?

Although the prevailing belief among those who investigate the nature of cross-disciplinary research and practice is that integration is of central importance, there is little consensus about exactly what it is. This is reflected in comments from prominent interdisciplinary theorists who bemoan the lack of clarity about what it means or how it works (e.g., Newell 2001), with Repko (2007, p. 7) going so far as to call this lack of clarity the "Achilles' heel of interdisciplinarity." This situation is exacerbated by the multiplicity of metaphors used to describe integration, not all of which are compatible with one another. Moreover, as Boix Mansilla (2010, p. 289) notes, metaphors have not proven especially "productive in their ability to structure strong research agendas or to design empirically grounded programs." Consequently, a cornerstone concept for cross-disciplinary research remains contested and unclear, which has ramifications for our understanding of this mode of research.

For instance, there is debate about whether integration is a process, a product, or both at the same time (e.g., Bruce et al. 2004; Repko 2012). Another point of contention is whether integration within a team is equivalent to the sum of each team member's integrative work, or alternatively is an emergent property attributable only to the team as a whole, where "the interdisciplinary whole is more than the sum of its disciplinary parts" (Boix Mansilla 2006). Furthermore, there is disagreement about whether cross-disciplinary integration should be understood as an instance of a common and generic phenomenon found in a wide range of contexts (O'Rourke et al. 2016) or rather as a phenomenon unique to cross-disciplinary activities.

In recent years, there has been a spate of work on the topic of integration, especially in interdisciplinary theory (e.g., Boix Mansilla 2010; Klein 2012; Bammer 2013) and the philosophy of biology (e.g., Brigandt 2010, 2013; Green and Wolkenhauer 2012). This work has produced a plethora of analyses. Boix Mansilla (2010, p. 299) builds an analysis of integration into a model of interdisciplinary understanding, describing "leveraging integrations" as taking the form of "telling aesthetic interpretations, more comprehensive explanations, predictive integrative models, informative contextualization, and practical problem solving." Klein (2012, p. 293) emphasizes similar themes, noting that the "means of integration" include language, concepts, models, methods, and frameworks, before summarizing her analysis with four "principles of integration": variance, platforming, iteration, and communicative rationality. According to these principles, although there is "no universal formula for integration," it can be achieved by building on a foundation that supports communicative interaction marked by iteration, negotiation, and trade-offs. Repko (2012, pp. 3–4) provides a focused definition of integration as "a process by which ideas, data and information, methods, tools, concepts, and/or theories are synthesized, connected, or blended."

O'Rourke et al. (2016) maintain that cross-disciplinary integration is an instance of the general phenomenon of integration, which they

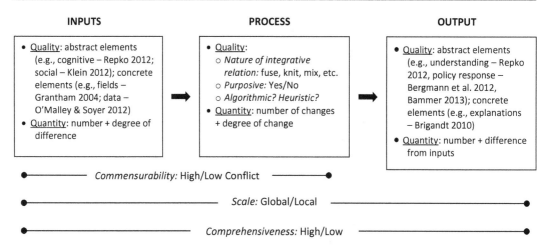

Fig. 2.4 Integration conceived as an input-output process, from O'Rourke et al. (2016), p. 69

conceive according to the IPO heuristic. Conceiving of integration as an input-output process explains why integration exhibits a process/product ambiguity, since when we use the term we can either foreground the *process* of integrating or the integrated *output*. O'Rourke et al. emphasize the *process* interpretation, taking integration to be "a type of putting or bringing together of inputs to produce a whole" (O'Rourke et al. 2016, p. 68). In developing their model, they highlight both qualitative and quantitative aspects of the inputs, process, and outputs, which they take to be variable and instantiated in different ways in different contexts. For example, inputs and outputs could be abstract, such as when the focus is on explanations or methods, or concrete, as when they are objects or certain forms of data, and the process could be rigid and algorithmic, or more heuristic and responsive to context. So understood, integration varies depending on context, and can also vary as a function of constraints that apply across aspects of the process, such as the scale or the comprehensiveness of the integrative activity (see Fig. 2.4).

Whether one thinks of integration as a process or a product, it is important to understand what relation among the inputs is reflected by the output. O'Rourke et al. (2016) call this the *integrative relation*, and it is conceived of in a variety of different forms, e.g., blending (Klein 2008), amalgamation (Pohl et al. 2008), melding (Repko 2012), fusing (Wickson et al. 2006), merging (Plutynski 2013), and even juxtaposition (Rossini and Porter 1979). These relations correspond to different ways in which inputs can be brought together and combined into a single output; for cross-disciplinary integration, this is what Boix Mansilla calls the "productive articulation" of disciplinary insights (2006, p. 19). A prototypical relation is *blending*, reflected in Nissani's (1995) comparison of the process of integration to the preparation of a smoothie. This is consonant with Repko's insistence that when "disciplinary insights are integrated, they generally form something that is truly new" (2012, p. 287). For many commentators, then, integration is a process of *change*, where inputs are more or less unrecoverable in their original form from the output.

2.5.2 What Is Integrated?

We can describe what is integrated—i.e., the *inputs*—with the help of the distinction between *social* and *epistemic* modes of integration (Klein 2008, 2012; Pohl et al. 2008; Armstrong and Jackson-Smith 2013; Szostak et al. 2016; cf. Gerson 2013). For Bergmann et al. (2012, p. 45), social integration "is a matter of differentiating and correlating the participating researchers' different interests and activities, as well as of the sub-projects or organizational units." By contrast, the epistemic mode "is a matter of understanding the methods and terms of other disciplines; clarifying the limits of one's own knowledge; and developing methods and building theories together." In general, *social modes* of integration concern processes that enable individual people to come together as a team and the team to come together with its surrounding institutional and organizational contexts, while *epistemic modes* concern processes that enable team members to combine what they know about the research topic and how they know it. Since CDTS involves people co-constructing knowledge, integration must be both social and epistemic.

On the epistemic side, we can follow Brigandt (2010) in distinguishing between larger and smaller epistemic inputs. Theorists of interdisciplinarity and philosophers of science have concerned themselves with larger inputs, such as disciplines (Klein 1990; van der Steen 1993), fields (Darden and Maull 1977; Grantham 2004), specialties (Gerson 2013), frameworks, and theories (Morse 2013). For integration with these inputs several questions remain open. Should integration of disciplines or domains be contrasted with *unification* and *reduction* (e.g., Plutynski 2013)? Should integration be understood as a "regulative ideal" (e.g., Grantham 2004; Brigandt 2010)?

These questions and the larger inputs on which they focus may be of interest to theoreticians but are not as useful as smaller epistemic inputs to researchers and practitioners who are engaged in integrative research. A more practical approach to integration emphasizes a functional conception of integration that highlights what teams need to think about when they are engaged in cross-disciplinary research (cf., Bennett et al. 2010; Cooke and Hilton 2015; Piso et al. 2016). This is a conception of integration that typically focuses on smaller epistemic inputs, such as "individual methods, concepts, models, explanations" (Brigandt 2010, p. 308). Of course, teams do contemplate the larger inputs of interest to theorists, such as disciplines, but typically that is done in the service of answering more local, practical questions, such as, "Do we have the correct mix of disciplines represented on the team?"

This question of disciplinary mixing underscores an important epistemic input into the integrative process, viz., the disciplinary *worldviews* that structure the contributions of each team member (O'Rourke and Crowley 2013). Experts acquire research worldviews when they acquire a disciplinary identity, and these worldviews frame research deliberation and decision-making by determining what count as appropriate questions and answers and by influencing what one notices and concentrates on. Disciplinary worldviews have many components that can be integrated, including methods (Tress et al. 2004), language (Donovan et al. 2015), concepts (Szostak 2013), mechanisms and systems (Bechtel and Richardson 2010), norms and values (Eigenbrode et al. 2007), explanations (Brigandt 2013), data (Leonelli 2013), models or theories (Mitchell 2002), knowledge (Zierhofer and Burger 2007), and goals (Jantsch 1972). Although we emphasize these as categories of inputs into the integrative process, they also serve to classify integrative outputs. It is important, though, to recognize that categorically heterogeneous inputs may be required to produce a particular output, such as when data, norms, goals, knowledge, and models are required as inputs into an integrative process that aims at an explanation.

Several of these inputs deserve special emphasis. Goals should be jointly defined in CDTS, as this is a crucial part of what helps teammates "assess what they need and expect from each other" (Klein 2012, p. 290). Norms and values similarly influence expectations and constrain decisions—since they are what collaborators take to be *right* or *good*, they are reflected in preferences and in what can and cannot be negotiated (Fisher et al. 2015). Methods that derive from different disciplines must be coordinated so that collaborators can work together and not at cross-purposes (Tress et al. 2004). Of all the inputs to the integrative process, language is perhaps the most critical, as integration of the others is mediated by the use of language in a CDTS context (Thompson 2009; Klein 2013). But it is also a challenge because, as Wear observes, "scientists speak in dialects that are specialised to their disciplines" and "[u]nfortunately, these dialects can at times sound like common language" (Wear 1999, p. 299; cf. Donovan et al. 2015). Given the challenge of linguistic difference, Bracken and Oughton (2006) argue that "what is key to effective research is the development of awareness of language differences and of the time needed to ensure that experts from different disciplines develop a common understanding" (p. 380).

On the social side language also stands out as an input, given that it underwrites communication among collaborators as they pursue their research goals. As the National Academy of Sciences asserts, "[a]t the heart of interdisciplinarity is communication—the conversations, connections, and combinations that bring new insights to virtually every kind of scientist and engineer" (2004, p. 19; cf. Strober 2011). While communication can be understood epistemically, as involving information transactions, it also operates socially, involving relational interactions among communicators (Keyton 1999). Relational communication highlights those aspects of interaction that enable the co-creation of meaning (Hall and O'Rourke 2014), such as *trust*, *respect*, and *openness* (Bennett and Gadlin 2012). The dual nature of inputs like language highlights the interaction between social and epistemic modes of integration (Klein 2008; Pohl et al. 2008). This dual nature is explained in part by the fact that both modes of integration are rooted in the people who construct knowledge collaboratively.

We conclude the discussion of inputs with a caution. As we suggested in Sect. 3, teams are made up of individual experts, not disciplines, and individual experts cannot be reduced to their disciplines or their disciplinary worldviews. Two researchers from the same discipline are different in a myriad of ways, including research worldviews, that reflect what they have studied and where they studied, as well as social capacities, such as the ability to lead (Cooke and Hilton 2015). It is true that individuals are often chosen because of their disciplinary expertise, but stereotyping individuals according to their discipline is a bias that can compromise the effectiveness of a cross-disciplinary project, such as when physical scientists fail to respect social scientists (e.g., Campbell 2005; Gardner 2013).

2.5.3 Degrees of Integration

It is generally held that integration can vary by degrees. From a social perspective, a collaboration could be more or less integrative in terms of the range of participants it involves or the extent to which it requires interaction and interdependence. From an epistemic perspective, the output requires that inputs such as data, concepts, methods, explanations, goals, etc. be more or less blended (Fauconnier 1994; Turner 2001; Morrison 2003). The relation of outputs to inputs in the case of epistemic integration may be such that the inputs are not recoverable from the output, having been changed irrevocably in the process (Boix Mansilla 2006; Armstrong and Jackson-Smith 2013). In the case of social integration, it isn't the recoverability of the inputs (e.g., the activities and interpersonal capacities of the collaborators) from the outputs that marks the degree of integration, but rather how inclusive and interdependent the collaboration is. With both modes, though, the degree of integration will largely be reflected in the integrative relation that underwrites the process in a particular case.

The degree of integration within cross-disciplinary projects is typically marked by modifying the term "disciplinarity" with one of several prefixes, e.g., *uni-, multi-, inter-*, and *trans-*. The resulting terms represent different types of disciplinary combination in theoretical analyses of the degrees of integration (e.g., Miller 1982; Stember 1991; Tress et al. 2004; Huutoniemi et al. 2010; Szostak et al. 2016), and they are also used to locate projects on the map of difference that results from such an analysis (e.g., Stokols et al. 2003, 2008; Eigenbrode et al. 2007; Morse et al. 2007; Hall et al. 2008). Focusing on the former, there are a variety of different terms, and even more maddeningly, various deployments of the same terms. Klein (2010) notes that this has produced "a sometimes confusing array of jargon" (p. 15), an array that has given rise to some skepticism about the value of fine-grained terminological analysis. For example, Rylance finds "unhelpful" the "faintly theological hairsplitting" reflected in "[a]rcane debates about whether research is inter-, multi-, trans-, cross- or post-disciplinary" (Rylance 2015, p. 314).

So articulated, these skeptical concerns suggest that discriminating attention to the nuances of integration is, at best, a theoretical issue that has no implications for practice. However, to the extent that a practitioner is interested in taking advantage of the voluminous work on disciplinary integration that has been conducted over the past 50 years, it would be very helpful to have a map of the different categories into which this work has been classified. Rylance suggests that these debates "complicate data collection" (Rylance 2015, p. 314), but in fact, failure to appreciate them can result in continued fragmentation of effort and, in the worst case, reinvention of the square wheel (Bammer 2013; O'Rourke 2017). Thus, there is a need to organize the labels—without a guide, the swarm of labels can confuse rather than clarify. To this end, Huutoniemi et al. (2010) is especially helpful, and we also provide a table of labels meant to

serve as an "at a glance" guide for the terminology (see Table 2.5).

The labels in most common use are *disciplinarity* (or *unidisciplinarity*), *multidisciplinarity*, *interdisciplinarity*, and *transdisciplinarity*. These are often discussed in combination (e.g., Klein 1990, 2010; Stokols et al. 2003; Hall et al. 2008; Huutoniemi et al. 2010; Leavy 2011), arrayed as presented in a way that represents increasing integration. Disciplinarity is the default condition, involving contributions from a single discipline. The rest involve multiple disciplines in combination, but the nature of the integration can be quite low and perhaps ad hoc, as in the case of multidisciplinarity (Stember 1991), to more significant and perhaps even transformative, as in the case of transdisciplinarity (Tress et al. 2004).

It should be noted, though, that adopting a uniform understanding of the spectrum of integration results in unhelpful conflation. This is

Table 2.5 A sample of labels used to refer to modes of disciplinary combination, arranged alphabetically

Label	Characterization(s)	Select source(s)
Antedisciplinarity	1. "The science that precedes the organization of new disciplines, the Wild West frontier stage that comes before the law arrives" (p. 0004)	1. Eddy (2005)
Cross-disciplinarity	1. A mode of disciplinary combination in which one discipline's perspective is privileged and serves to ground contributions from the others 2. A generic cover term for all forms of disciplinary combination (hereafter, "cover term")	1. Jantsch (1972), Stember (1991) 2. Eigenbrode et al. (2007), Hall et al. (2008)
Disciplinarity (*also* unidisciplinarity)	1. Research conducted by those in "stable systemic communities" where experience is concentrated "into a particular worldview" (*p. 458*) 2. "A process in which researchers from a single discipline work together to address a common research problem" (p. S79)	1. *Bruce et al.* (2004), Berger (1972), Miller (1982) 2. Stokols et al. (2008)
Interdisciplinarity	1. "An interactive process in which researchers work jointly, each drawing from his or her own discipline-specific perspective, to address a common research problem" (p. S79) 2. "Integrates knowledge and modes of thinking from two or more disciplines" (p. 3)	1. *Stokols et al.* (2008), Klein and Newell (1996), NAS (2004) 2. *Boix Mansilla and Gardner* (2003), Brewer 1999, Karlqvist (1999), Ramadier (2004)
Intradisciplinarity	1. "Mutually exclusive levels of theoretical integration … within one single discipline" (p. 85) 2. "Within disciplinary work" (p. 4)	1. Heckhausen (1972) 2. Stember (1991)
Multidisciplinarity	1. "Research that involves more than a single discipline in which each discipline makes a separate contribution" (*p. 27*), typically from their discipline-specific perspective in a way that does not result in a change to the disciplines 2. "Examines the appropriate relationships of the disciplines to each other and to the larger intellectual terrain" (2) 3. Occasionally a cover term, although less so recently	1. *NAS* (2004), Piaget (1972), Jantsch (1972), Rosenfield (1992), Ramadier (2004) 2. Kline (1995) 3. Blackwell (1955)

(continued)

Table 2.5 (Continued)

Label	Characterization(s)	Select source(s)
Pluridisciplinarity	1. "Juxtaposition of disciplines assumed to be more or less related" (*p. 25*)	1. *Berger (1972)*, Jantsch (1972)
Polydisciplinarity	1. A generic cover term	1. Shalinsky (1989)
Post-disciplinarity	1. An "approach that reflects the crisis in the received categories of analysis and the disciplines that correspond to them" (*p. 132*)	1. Jessop and Sum (2001)
Supradisciplinarity	1. "A collective term for all forms of scientific collaboration where the field of a single discipline is transgressed" (pp. 99–100)	1. Kötter and Balsiger (1999)
Transdisciplinarity	1. Efforts that combine disciplines in creating "novel conceptualizations and methodologic approaches that transcend or move beyond the individual disciplines represented among team members" (*p.S164*) 2. Efforts that "bridge the academic world and the needs of different social bodies to address real-world issues and problems" (*p. 26*)	1. *Hall et al. (2008)*, Stember (1991), Stokols et al. (2003, 2008), Hall et al. (2012) 2. *Leavy (2011)*, Pohl and Hirsch Hadorn (2007), Pohl (2008), Bergmann et al. (2012)

Boldface indicates the most prominent categories in the literature. *Italics* indicates the source of a quote if there are multiple sources listed

illustrated by the competing conceptions of *transdisciplinarity* as transformative interdisciplinarity (e.g., Stokols et al. 2008) and as stakeholder-involving problem-focused research (e.g., Bergmann et al. 2012). To be sure, there are different meanings or "trendlines" (Klein 2010) for each of these terms, some of which are on display in Table 2.5.[1] In keeping with the distinction we have emphasized in this chapter, we recommend teasing apart two different integrative dimensions along which these modes of cross-disciplinarity can be located, the *epistemic* dimension and the *social* dimension. Along the epistemic dimension we emphasize *identity*, specifically, the assumptions and commitments that constitute contributing worldviews. As we move from unidisciplinarity to transdisciplinarity, we move from worldviews that remain in place (e.g., unidisciplinarity and multidisciplinarity) to worldviews that hybridize with others (e.g., interdisciplinarity) to those that fundamentally transform in combination with other worldviews (e.g., transdisciplinarity). The social

dimension corresponds to *diversity*, with integration increasing according to the number of different types of worldviews contributing to the project. Here, the lowest levels of integration are marked by projects in which there is but a single disciplinary worldview (viz., unidisciplinarity) to those in which there are several of more or less the same kind (e.g., multidisciplinarity or interdisciplinarity involving academic disciplines) to those that involve nonacademic perspectives alongside academic ones (viz., transdisciplinarity). Here *transdisciplinary* would involve transgressing academic boundaries.

2.5.4 How to Integrate

Once one understands integration as a priority for a cross-disciplinary team, there is still the problem of figuring out how to integrate. Klein (2012) argues that "[t]here is no universal formula for integration," in part because it is "influenced by the goals of a particular program, the participants who are involved, their disciplinary and professional backgrounds, and institutional settings" (pp. 293–294). The contextual nature of integration implies that there is no easy way to integrate

---

[1]For additional discussion of term meanings, see Boden (1999) and Huutoniemi et al. (2010) for *interdisciplinarity* and Carew and Wickson (2010) and Klein (2014) for *transdisciplinarity*.

the diverse worldviews of an interdisciplinary research team. How to integrate will at least somewhat be determined by the specific characteristics of each team and each project. The best way to integrate for two different teams working on the same project could well be different, and likewise for the same team working on two different projects.

Although it is highly contextual at the level of detail, integration is clearly a phenomenon that can be discussed in general, as this section indicates. Further, careful consideration of the nature of integration can guide project planning and enable the development of project infrastructure that supports the kind of combination required to achieve project goals. Nevertheless, there is disagreement about whether there can be any general guidelines or methods for integration. For example, O'Rourke et al. (2016) note disagreement about whether integration can be accomplished *algorithmically* or is better approached *heuristically*. According to those who favor an algorithmic approach (e.g., Repko 2007, 2012; Newell 2001, 2007; Klein 1990; Cosens et al. 2011), there is a clear set of steps for integration that can be employed in a wide range of contexts. On the other hand, those who favor a heuristic approach (e.g., Bammer 2013; Klein 2012; Huutoniemi 2014) contend that integration is a creative process for which there are no generalizable steps; to integrate, we must respect the multidimensional complexities of each distinct interdisciplinary context.

However, this debate is resolved, there are a number of methods that have been developed or adapted to foster integration, and these can be helpful if employed in ways that respect the exigencies of a situation (O'Rourke 2017). We close this section with a set of suggestions meant to aid the process of cross-disciplinary integration in CDTS projects (Table 2.6).

2.6   Conclusion

This chapter provides CDTS with a conceptual vocabulary for identifying and leveraging the varieties of expertise required to address complex problems, i.e., the *challenge of disciplinary diversity*. Our vocabulary highlights three concepts: identification of disciplinary expertise, readiness, and integration. Identification of disciplinary expertise requires treating disciplinary identity as a proxy variable for the kinds of expertise we require, and the task of identifying relevant expertise is a dynamic one that changes interactively with project goals. Readiness is key to capacity building, focusing on how prepared a team is to engage in integrative CDTS. We have concentrated on readiness factors that bear directly on a team's research decisions, including epistemic, social, and technological factors. Finally, the notion of *integration* is a success term for the task of combining resources. Integration can be modeled as an input-output process, with its nature and value revealed by systematic attention to the integrative inputs, a process that varies by degree, and the outputs that exhibit different integrative relationships among the inputs.

Social and behavioral research efforts are increasingly collaborative and cross-disciplinary (Wuchty et al. 2007; van Noorden 2015). As a result, more and more social and behavioral scientists will need to address the epistemic, social, and technological challenges of integrating research contributions from representatives of different disciplines. The conceptual vocabulary we propose in this chapter systematically associates a number of relevant literatures that address aspects of these challenges. As such, the vocabulary informs and orients theorists and practitioners who must identify and manage the epistemic and social resources required for successful CDTS.

Table 2.6 Five suggestions for conducting integrative CDTS

Guiding suggestions for integrating disciplinary perspectives
1. Attend to process.
• Complex CDTS projects involve people with different beliefs and priorities working together typically over an extended period of time. With so many moving parts, there are many ways a project can fail. By attending to the *process* of the research, leaders can stay attuned to what the project needs to achieve its objectives (Cooke and Hilton 2015)
• Build opportunities into the life of the team to engage in structured reflection on what they have done and where they are going, and also encourage participants to think about their collaborator's perspectives on their common problem (Salazar et al., 2019)
2. Watch your language.
• Complex research is communication intensive (NAS 2004), with technical terminology playing a central role. This entails use of different terms that strike some collaborators as mysterious, but also similar terms that everyone mistakenly thinks they understand, e.g., "hypothesis" or "dynamic" (Donovan et al. 2015; Bracken and Oughton 2006)
• Don't be complacent—it is easy to operate under the mistaken assumption that certain important technical terms are understood in the same way by all collaborators. Consider having a structured dialogue about central technical concepts (Eigenbrode et al. 2007) or producing a dynamic glossary of central terms and concepts
3. Emphasize dialogue.
• Structured, facilitated dialogue among collaborators can foster mutual understanding (Winowiecki et al. 2011; O'Rourke and Crowley 2013; Palmer et al. 2016) and assist in the integration of many different inputs, such as expertise, ethical implications, power differentials, and "change stories" (McDonald et al. 2009)
• Teammates can use dialogue to discover worldview differences, such as differences in language use, norms, methods, and explanations, and collectively develop a way of communicating with less ambiguity or confusion
4. Use metaphor.
• Metaphor can enable the framing and bridging of difference (e.g., Lakoff and Johnson 1980), including disciplinary difference (e.g., Cooke and Hilton 2015; Szostak et al. 2016). Metaphors can function as "evocative approximations to interdisciplinary cognition" (Boix Mansilla 2010, p. 289) and can helpfully substitute for technical jargon (Vogel et al. 2012)
• Metaphors can serve as *boundary objects* (Star and Griesemer 1989), providing different disciplines with the means to work together even though they understand, interpret, and operationalize that metaphors differently (Bechtel 2013)
5. Map the project.
• There are a range of *concept mapping* methods for graphically representing concepts and their relationships (e.g., Trochim and Kane 2005; Morse 2013; Okada et al. 2014). Concept mapping can help reveal points of contact between expert worldviews, and also highlight possible trade-offs that can move the project forward (Hirsch and Brosius 2013)
• These techniques for "knowledge elicitation and evaluation" (Falk-Krzesinski et al. 2011, p. 146) can be more informal (e.g., Heemskerk et al. (2003) describe a technique involving pen and paper for mapping conceptual relationships in a project) or more formal (e.g., quantitative, computer-based modeling as a replicable method—Olabisi et al. 2013)

References

Andersen H, Wagenknecht S. Epistemic dependence in interdisciplinary groups. Synthese. 2013;190(11):1881–98.

Andrade HB, de los Reyes López H, Martín TB. Dimensions of scientific collaboration and its contribution to the academic research groups' scientific quality. Res Eval. 2009;18(4):301–11.

Andrews AC, Clawson RA, Gramig BM, Raymond L. Finding the right value: framing effects on domain experts. Political Psychol. 2016;38:261. https://doi.org/10.1111/pops.12339.

Armstrong A, Jackson-Smith D. Forms and levels of integration: evaluation of an interdisciplinary team-building project. J Res Pract. 2013;9(1):M1. http://jrp.icaap.org/index.php/jrp/article/view/335/297

August PV, Swift JM, Kellogg DQ, Page G, Nelson P, Opaluch J, Cobb JS, Foster C, Gold AJ. The T assessment tool: a simple metric for assessing multidisciplinary graduate education. J Nat Res Life Sci Educ. 2010;39:15–21.

Bammer G. Disciplining interdisciplinarity: Integration and implementation sciences for researching complex real-world problems. Canberra: ANU E-Press; 2013.

Bechtel W. From molecules to behavior and the clinic: integration in chronobiology. Stud Hist Phil Biol Biomed Sci. 2013;44:493–502.

Bechtel W, Richardson R. Discovering complexity: decomposition and localization as strategies in scientific research. Cambridge, MA: MIT Press; 2010.

Benda LE, Poff LN, Tague C, Palmer MA, Pizzuto J, Cooper S, et al. How to avoid train wrecks when using science in environmental problem solving. Bioscience. 2002;52(12):1127–36.

Bennett LM, Gadlin H. Collaboration and team science: from theory to practice. J Investig Med. 2012;60(5):768–75.

Bennett LM, Gadlin H. Supporting interdisciplinary collaboration: the role of the institution. In: O'Rourke M, Crowley S, Eigenbrode SD, Wulfhorst JD, editors. Enhancing communication and collaboration in interdisciplinary research. Thousand Oaks, CA: Sage Publications; 2013. p. 356–84.

Bennett LM, Gadlin H, Levine-Finley S. Collaboration and team science: a field guide. Washington, DC: National Institutes of Health; 2010.

Benor DE. Interdisciplinary integration in medical education: theory and method. Med Educ. 1982;16:355–61.

bepress. Digital commons three-tiered list of academic disciplines. 2017. https://www.bepress.com/wp-content/uploads/2016/12/Digital-Commons-Disciplines-taxonomy-2017-01.pdf

Berger G. Opinions and facts. In: Apostel L, Berger G, Briggs A, Michaud G, editors. Interdisciplinarity: problems of teaching and research in universities. Paris: Organization for Economic Cooperation and Development; 1972. p. 21–74.

Bergmann M, Jahn T, Knobloch T, Krohn W, Pohl C, Schramm E. Methods for transdisciplinary research. Frankfurt/New York: Campus Verlag; 2012.

Blackwell GW. Multidisciplinary team research. Soc Forces. 1955;33:367–74.

Boden M. What is interdisciplinarity? In: Cunningham R, editor. Interdisciplinarity and the organization of knowledge in Europe. Luxembourg: European Communities; 1999. p. 13–24.

Boix Mansilla V. Assessing expert interdisciplinary work at the frontier: an empirical exploration. Res Eval. 2006;15(1):17–29.

Boix Mansilla V. Learning to synthesize: the development of interdisciplinary understanding. In: Frodeman R, Klein JT, Mitcham C, editors. The Oxford handbook of interdisciplinarity. Oxford: Oxford University Press; 2010. p. 288–306.

Boix Mansilla V, Gardner H. Assessing interdisciplinary work at the frontier: an empirical exploration of "symptoms of quality". In: GoodWork project report series, vol. 26. Cambridge, MA: Harvard University; 2003.

Boix Mansilla V, Lamont M, Sato K. Shared cognitive-emotional-interactional platforms: markers and conditions for successful interdisciplinary collaborations. Sci Technol Hum Values. 2015;41:1–42. https://doi.org/10.1177/0162243915614103.

Bosque-Pérez NA, Klos PZ, Force JE, Waits LP, Cleary K, Rhoades P, Galbraith SM, Bentley Brymer AL, O'Rourke M, Eigenbrode SD, Finegan B, Wulfhorst JD, Sibelet N, Holbrook JD. A pedagogical model for team-based, problem-focused interdisciplinary doctoral education. BioScience. . http://bioscience.oxford-journals.org/content/early/2016/04/08/biosci.biw042. 2016;66:477. https://doi.org/10.1093/biosci/biw042.

Bracken LJ, Oughton EA. 'What do you mean?' The importance of language in developing interdisciplinary research. Trans Inst Br Geogr. 2006;31(3):371–82.

Brewer GD. The challenges of interdisciplinarity. Policy Sci. 1999;32:327–37.

Brigandt I. Beyond reduction and pluralism: toward an epistemology of explanatory integration in biology. Erkenntnis. 2010;73:295–311.

Brigandt I. Integration in biology: philosophical perspectives on the dynamics of interdisciplinarity. Stud Hist Phil Biol Biomed Sci. 2013;44:461–5.

Bruce A, Lyall C, Tait J, Williams R. Interdisciplinary integration in Europe: the case of the fifth framework programme. Futures. 2004;36:457–70.

Campbell LM. Overcoming obstacles to interdisciplinary research. Conserv Biol. 2005;19:574–7.

Carew AL, Wickson F. The TD wheel: a heuristic to shape, support and evaluate transdisciplinary research. Futures. 2010;42:1146–55.

Cheruvelil KS, Soranno PA, Weathers KC, Hanson PC, Goring SJ, Filstrup CT, Read EK. Creating and maintaining high-performing collaborative research teams: the importance of diversity and interpersonal skills. Front Ecol Environ. 2014;12(1):31–8.

Collins HM, Evans R. The third wave of science studies: studies of expertise and experience. Soc Stud Sci. 2002;32(2):235–96.

Connaughton SL, Shuffler M. Multinational and multicultural distributed teams: a review and future agenda. Small Group Res. 2007;38(3):387–412.

Contractor N. Some assembly required: leveraging web science to understand and enable team assembly. Phil Trans R Soc A. 2013;371:20120385. https://doi.org/10.1098/rsta.2012.0385.

Cooke NJ, Hilton ML. Enhancing the effectiveness of team science. Washington, DC: The National Academies Press; 2015.

Cosens B, Fiedler F, Boll J, Higgins L, Johnson G, Kennedy B, Strand E, Wilson P. Interdisciplinary methods in water resources. Issues Integr Studies. 2011;29:118–43.

Crowley S, Eigenbrode SD, O'Rourke M, Wulfhorst JD. Introduction. In: O'Rourke M, Crowley S, Eigenbrode SD, Wulfhorst JD, editors. Enhancing communication and collaboration in interdisciplinary research. Thousand Oaks, CA: Sage Publications; 2013.

DMP Tool. California Digital Library. University of California. 2017. https://www.cdlib.org/services/uc3/dmpt.html.

Darden L, Maull N. Interfield theories. Philos Sci. 1977;44:43–64.

De Grandis G, Efstathiou S. Introduction—grand challenges and small steps. Stud Hist Phil Biol Biomed Sci. 2016;56:39–47.

Dirks KT, Ferrin DL. The role of trust in organizational settings. Organ Sci. 2001;12(4):450–67.

Donovan SM, O'Rourke M, Looney C. Your hypothesis or mine? Terminological and conceptual variation across disciplines. SAGE Open. 2015;5(2):1–13.

Duhigg C. What Google learned from its quest to build the perfect team. The New York Times Magazine, (the work issue). 2016. http://nyti.ms/20WG1yY

Eddy SR. "Antedisciplinary" science. PLoS Comput Biol. 2005;1(1):e6. https://doi.org/10.1371/journal.pcbi.0010006.

Edmondson AC. Psychological safety and learning behavior in work teams. Adm Sci Q. 1999;44(2):350–83.

Eigenbrode S, O'Rourke M, Wulfhorst JD, Althoff DM, Goldberg CS, Merrill K, Morse W, Nielsen-Pincus M, Stephens J, Winowiecki L, Bosque-Pérez NA. Employing philosophical dialogue in collaborative science. Bioscience. 2007;57:55–64.

Elliott KC, Cheruvelil KS, Montgomery GM, Soranno PA. Conceptions of good science in our data-rich world. Bioscience. 2016;66(10):880–9.

Elsevier BV. Expert lookup. 2016. https://www.elsevier.com/solutions/expert-lookup.

Falk-Krzesinski HJ, Contractor N, Fiore SM, Hall KL, Kane C, Keyton J, et al. Mapping a research agenda for the science of team science. Res Eval. 2011;20(2):145–58.

Fauconnier G. Mental spaces: aspects of meaning construction in natural language. Cambridge: Cambridge University Press; 1994.

Fiore SM, Carter DR, Asencio R. Conflict, trust, and cohesion: examining affective and attitudinal factors in science teams. In: Salas E, Vessey WB, Estrada AX, editors. Team cohesion: advances in psychological theory, methods and practice. Bingley: Emerald Group Publishing; 2015. p. 271–301.

Fiore SM, Gabelica C, Wiltshire T, Stokols D. Training to be a (Team) scientist. In: Hall KL, Vogel AL, Croyle RT, editors. Strategies for team science success: handbook of evidence-based principles for cross-disciplinary science and practical lessons learned from health researchers. New York, NY: Springer; 2019. p. 421–444.

Fisher SG, Hunter TA, Macrosson WDK. Team or group? Managers' perceptions of the differences. J Manag Psychol. 1997;12(4):232–42.

Fisher E, O'Rourke M, Evans R, Kennedy EB, Gorman ME, Seager TP. Mapping the integrative field: taking stock of socio-technical collaborations. J Responsible Innovation. 2015;2(1):39–61.

Fuqua J, Stokols D, Gress J, Phillips K, Harvey R. Transdisciplinary collaboration as a basis for enhancing the science and prevention of substance use and "abuse". Subst Use Misuse. 2004;39(10–12):1457–514.

Gandomi A, Haider M. Beyond the hype: big data concepts, methods, and analytics. Int J Inf Manag. 2015;35(2):137–44.

Gardner S. Paradigmatic differences, power, and status: a qualitative investigation of faculty in one interdis-

ciplinary research collaboration on sustainability science. Sustain Sci. 2013;8(2):241–52.

Gerson EM. Integration of specialties: an institutional and organizational view. Stud Hist Phil Biol Biomed Sci. 2013;44:515–24.

Gewin V. Recipe for a team: a scientific collaboration is vulnerable to derailment unless members learn to trust each other at the outset. Nature. 2015;523:245–7.

Grantham TA. Conceptualizing the (dis)unity of science. Philos Sci. 2004;71:133–55.

Gray SA, Zanre E, Gray SRJ. Fuzzy cognitive maps as representations of mental models and group beliefs. In: Fuzzy cognitive maps for applied sciences and engineering, vol. 54. Berlin, Heidelberg: Springer Berlin Heidelberg; 2014. p. 29–48.

Green S, Wolkenhauer O. Integration in action. EMBO Rep. 2012;13:769–71.

Hall KL, Crowston K, Vogel AL. How to write a collaboration plan. Draft. 2014. https://www.team-sciencetoolkit.cancer.gov/public/TSResourceBiblio.aspx?tid=3&rid=3119

Hall KL, Stokols D, Moser RP, Taylor BK, Thornquist MD, Nebeling LC, Ehret CC, Barnett MJ, McTiernan A, Berger NA, Goran MI, Jeffery RW. The collaboration readiness of transdisciplinary research teams and centers: findings from the National Cancer Institute's TREC year-one evaluation study. Am J Prev Med. 2008;35(2S):S161–72.

Hall KL, Vogel AL, Stipelman BA, Stokols D, Morgan G, Gehlert S. A four-phase model of transdisciplinary team-based research: goals, team processes, and strategies. Transl Behav Med. 2012;2:415–30.

Hall KL, Vogel AL, Crowston K. Comprehensive collaboration plans: practical considerations spanning from individual collaborators to institutional supports. In: Hall KL, Vogel AL, Croyle RT, editors. Strategies for team science success: handbook of evidence-based principles for cross-disciplinary science and practical lessons learned from health researchers. New York, NY: Springer; 2019. p. 587–611.

Hall KL, O'Rourke M. Responding to communication challenges in transdisciplinary sustainability science. In: Huutoniemi K, Tapio P, editors. Transdisciplinary sustainability studies: a heuristic approach. New York, NY: Routledge; 2014. p. 119–39.

Heckhausen H. Discipline and interdisciplinarity. In: Apostel L, Berger G, Briggs A, Michaud G, editors. Interdisciplinarity: problems of teaching and research in universities. Paris: Organization for Economic Cooperation and Development; 1972. p. 83–90.

Heemskerk M, Wilson K, Pavao-Zuckerman M. Conceptual models as tools for communication across disciplines. Conserv Ecol. 2003;7(3):8. http://www.consecol.org/vol7/iss3/art8/

Hirsch PD, Brosius JP. Navigating complex trade-offs in conservation and development: an integrative framework. Issues Integr Studies. 2013;31:99–122.

Holbrook JB. What is interdisciplinary communication? Reflections on the very idea of disciplinary integration. Synthese. 2013;190:1865–79.

Huutoniemi K. Introduction: sustainability, transdisciplinarity and the complexity of knowing. In: Huutoniemi K, Tapio P, editors. Transdisciplinary sustainability science: a heuristic approach. Oxon/New York: Routledge; 2014. p. 1–20.

Huutoniemi K, Klein JT, Bruun H, Hukkinen J. Analyzing interdisciplinarity: typology and indicators. Res Policy. 2010;39:79–88.

Jahn T. Transdisziplinarität in der Forschungspraxis. In: Bergmann M, Schramm E, editors. Transdisziplinäre Forschung. Integrative Forschungsprozesse verstehen und bewerten. Frankfurt Campus: Verlag; 2008. p. 21–37.

Jantsch E. Towards interdisciplinarity and transdisciplinarity in education and innovation. In: Apostel L, Berger G, Briggs A, Michaud G, editors. Interdisciplinarity: problems of teaching and research in universities. Paris: Organization for Economic Cooperation and Development; 1972. p. 97–121.

Jarvenpaa SL, Leidner DE. Communication and trust in global virtual teams. Organ Sci. 1999;10(6):791–815.

Jessop B, Sum N. Pre-disciplinary and post-disciplinary perspectives. New Political Economy. 2001;6(1):89–101.

Kane M, Trochim WMK. Concept mapping for planning and evaluation. Thousand Oaks, CA: SAGE Publications Limited; 2007.

Karlqvist A. Going beyond disciplines: the meanings of interdisciplinarity. Policy Sci. 1999;32:379–83.

Keyton J. Relational communication in groups. In: Frey LR, Gouran DS, Poole MS, editors. The handbook of group communication theory and research. Thousand Oaks, CA: Sage; 1999. p. 192–222.

Kirschner PA, Buckingham Shum SJ, Carr CS. Visualizing argumentation. Berlin: Springer Science & Business Media; 2012.

Klein JT. Interdisciplinarity: History, theory, and practice. Detroit, MI: Wayne State University Press; 1990.

Klein JT. Evaluation of interdisciplinary and transdisciplinary research: a literature review. Am J Prev Med. 2008;35(2S):S116–23.

Klein JT. A taxonomy of interdisciplinarity. In: Frodeman R, Klein JT, Mitcham C, editors. The Oxford handbook of interdisciplinarity. Oxford: Oxford University Press; 2010. p. 15–30.

Klein JT. Research integration: a comparative knowledge base. In: Repko AF, Newell WH, Szostak R, editors. Case studies in interdisciplinary research. Thousand Oaks, CA: Sage Publications; 2012. p. 283–98.

Klein JT. Communication and collaboration in interdisciplinary research. In: O'Rourke M, Crowley S, Eigenbrode SD, Wulfhorst JD, editors. Enhancing communication and collaboration in interdisciplinary research. Thousand Oaks, CA: Sage Publications; 2013. p. 11–30.

Klein JT. Discourses of transdisciplinarity: looking back to the future. Futures. 2014;63:68–74.

Klein JT, Newell W. Advancing interdisciplinary studies. In: Gaff J, Ratcliff J, editors. Handbook of the undergraduate curriculum: comprehensive guide to purposes, structures, practices, and change. San Francisco: Jossey-Bass; 1996. p. 393–415.

Kline SJ. Conceptual foundations for multidisciplinary thinking. Stanford: Stanford University Press; 1995.

Knorr Cetina K. Culture in global knowledge societies: knowledge cultures and epistemic cultures. Interdiscip Sci Rev. 2007;32(4):361–75.

Kötter R, Balsiger PW. Interdisciplinarity and transdisciplinarity: a constant challenge to the sciences. Issues Integr Studies. 1999;17:87–120.

Kozlowski SWJ. Advancing research on team process dynamics: theoretical, methodological, and measurement considerations. Organ Psychol Rev. 2015;5(4):270–99.

Kozlowski SWJ, Bell BS. Evidence-based principles and strategies for optimizing team functioning and performance in science teams. In: Hall KL, Vogel AL, Croyle RT, editors. Strategies for team science success: handbook of evidence-based principles for cross-disciplinary science and practical lessons learned from health researchers. New York, NY: Springer; 2019. p. 269–293.

Lakoff G, Johnson M. Metaphors we live by. Chicago: University of Chicago Press; 1980.

Lang DJ, Wiek A, Bergmann M, Stauffacher M, Martens P, Moll P, Swilling M, Thomas CJ. Transdisciplinary research in sustainability science: practice, principles, and challenges. Sustain Sci. 2012;7(Suppl 1):25–43.

Laursen B. Explicating and negotiating bias in interdisciplinary argumentation using abductive tools. Presented at the Argumentation, Objectivity, and Bias Eleventh Annual International Conference of the Ontario Society for the Study of Argumentation, Windsor, Ontario, Canada; 2016. pp. 1–8. http://scholar.uwindsor.ca/ossaarchive/OSSA11/

Leavy P. Essentials of transdisciplinary research. Walnut Creek, CA: Left Coast Press; 2011.

Lele S, Norgaard RB. Practicing interdisciplinarity. Bioscience. 2005;55(11):967–75.

Leonelli S. Integrating data to acquire new knowledge: three modes of integration in plant science. Stud Hist Phil Biol Biomed Sci. 2013;44:503–14.

Leonelli S, Ankeny RA. Repertoires: how to transform a project into a research community. Bioscience. 2015;65(7):701–8.

Lotrecchiano GR, Mallinson TR, Leblanc-Beaudoin T, Schwartz LS, Lazar D, Falk-Krzesinski HJ. Individual motivation and threat indicators of collaboration readiness in scientific knowledge producing teams: a scoping review and domain analysis. Heliyon. 2016;2(5):e00105.

Lynch J. It's not easy being interdisciplinary. Int J Epidemiol. 2006;35:1119–22.

Marks MA, Mathieu JE, Zaccaro SJ. A temporally based framework and taxonomy of team processes. Acad Manag Rev. 2001;26(3):356–76.

McDonald D, Bammer G, Deane P. Research integration using dialogue methods. Canberra: Australian National University Press; 2009.

McGrath JE. Social psychology: a brief introduction. New York: Holt, Rinehart, and Winston; 1964.

Miller RC. Varieties of interdisciplinary approaches in the social sciences: a 1981 overview. Issues Integr Studies. 1982;1:1–37.

Mirel B, Luo A, Harris M. Research infrastructure for collaborative team science: challenges in technology-supported workflows in and across laboratories, institutions, and geographies. Semin Nephrol. 2015;35(3):291–302.

Misra S, Stokols D, Cheng L. The transdisciplinary orientation scale: factor structure and relation to the integrative quality and scope of scientific publications. J Transl Med Epidemiol. 2015;3(2):1042–51.

Mitchell SD. Integrative pluralism. Biol Philos. 2002;17:55–70.

Monteiro M, Keating E. Managing misunderstandings: the role of language in interdisciplinary scientific collaboration. Sci Commun. 2009;31(1):6–28.

Morrison JL. Conceptual integration in online interdisciplinary study: current perspectives, theories, and implications for future research. Int Rev Res Open Distributed Learn. 2003;4:2. http://www.irrodl.org/index.php/irrodl/issue/view/16

Morse WC. Integration of frameworks and theories across disciplines for effective cross-disciplinary communication. In: O'Rourke M, Crowley S, Eigenbrode SD, Wulfhorst JD, editors. Enhancing communication and collaboration in interdisciplinary research. Thousand Oaks, CA: Sage Publications; 2013. p. 244–70.

Morse WC, Nielsen-Pincus M, Force JE, Wulfhorst JD. Bridges and barriers to developing and conducting interdisciplinary graduate-student team research. Ecol Soc. 2007;12(2):8. http://www.ecologyandsociety.org/vol12/iss2/art8/

Murphy BL. From interdisciplinary to inter-epistemological approaches: confronting the challenges of integrated climate change research. Can Geogr. 2011;55(44):490–509.

National Academy of Sciences, Committee on Facilitating Interdisciplinary Research and Committee on Science Engineering and Public Policy (NAS). Facilitating interdisciplinary research. Washington, DC: National Academies Press; 2004.

National Institutes of Health (NIH). NIH data sharing policy and implementation guidance. 2003. http://grants.nih.gov/grants/policy/data_sharing/data_sharing_guidance.htm

National Science Foundation (NSF). Data management & sharing frequently asked questions (FAQs). 2010. https://www.nsf.gov/bfa/dias/policy/dmpfaqs.jsp

Newell WH. A theory of interdisciplinary studies. Issues Integr Studies. 2001;19:1–25.

Newell WH. Decision-making in interdisciplinary studies. In: Morçöl G, editor. Handbook of decision making. Boca Raton, FL: CRC/Taylor & Francis; 2007. p. 245–64.

Nissani M. Fruits, salads, and smoothies: a working definition of interdisciplinarity. J Educ Thought. 1995;2:121–8.

Norris PE, O'Rourke M, Mayer AS, Halvorsen KE. Managing the wicked problem of transdisciplinary team formation in socio-ecological systems. Landsc Urban Plan. 2016;154:115–22.

O'Rourke M. Comparing methods for cross-disciplinary research. In: Frodeman R, Klein JT, Dos Santos Pacheco R, editors. The Oxford handbook of interdisciplinarity. Oxford: Oxford University Press; 2017. p. 276–90.

O'Rourke M, Crowley S. Philosophical intervention and cross-disciplinary science: the story of the toolbox project. Synthese. 2013;190:1937–54.

O'Rourke M, Crowley S, Gonnerman C. On the nature of cross-disciplinary integration: a philosophical framework. Stud Hist Phil Biol Biomed Sci. 2016;56:62–70.

Ohlhorst D, Schön S. Constellation analysis as a means of interdisciplinary innovation research–theory formation from the bottom up. Hist Soc Res. 2015;40(3):258–78.

Okada A, Buckingham Shum SJ, Sherborne T. Knowledge cartography: software tools and mapping techniques. 2nd ed. London: Springer; 2014.

Olabisi LS, Blythe S, Ligmann-Zielinska A, Marquart-Pyatt S. Modeling as a tool for cross-disciplinary communication in solving environmental problems. In: O'Rourke M, Crowley S, Eigenbrode SD, Wulfhorst JD, editors. Enhancing communication and collaboration in interdisciplinary research. Thousand Oaks, CA: Sage Publications; 2013. p. 271–90.

Olson GM, Olson JS. Distance matters. Hum Comput Interact. 2000;15(2/3):139–78.

Olson J, Olson G. How to make distance work. Interactions. 2014;XXI(2):28–35.

Osbeck LM, Nersessian NJ. Forms of positioning in interdisciplinary science practice and their epistemic effects. J Theory Soc Behav. 2010;40(2):136–61.

Palmer MA, Kramer JG, Boyd J, Hawthorne D. Practices for facilitating interdisciplinary synthetic research: the National Socio-Environmental Synthesis Center (SESYNC). Curr Opin Environ Sustain. 2016;19:111–22.

Patterson ME, Williams DR. Paradigms and problems: the practice of social science in natural resource management. Soc Nat Res Int J. 1998;11(3):279–95.

Petrie HG. Do you see what I see? The epistemology of interdisciplinary inquiry. Educ Res. 1976;5(2):9–15.

Phillipson J, Lowe P, Bullock JM. Navigating the social sciences: interdisciplinarity and ecology. J Appl Ecol. 2009;46:261–4.

Piaget J. The epistemology of interdisciplinary relationships. In: Apostel L, Berger G, Briggs A, Michaud G, editors. Interdisciplinarity: problems of teaching and research in universities. Paris: Organization for Economic Cooperation and Development; 1972. p. 127–39.

Piso Z. Integration, language, and practice: Wittgenstein and interdisciplinary communication. Issues Interdisciplinary Studies. 2015;33:14–38.

Piso Z, O'Rourke M, Weather KC. Out of the fog: catalyzing integrative capacity in interdisciplinary research. Stud Hist Phil Sci. 2016;56:84–94.

Plutynski A. Cancer and the goals of integration. Stud Hist Phil Biol Biomed Sci. 2013;44:466–76.

Pohl C. From science to policy through transdisciplinary research. Environ Sci Pol. 2008;11:46–53.

Pohl C, Hirsch Hadorn G. Principles for designing transdisciplinary research. Munich: Oekom Verlag; 2007.

Pohl C, van Kerkhoff L, Hirsch Hadorn G, Bammer G. Integration. In: Hirsch Hadorn G, Hoffman-Riem H, Biber-Klemm S, Grossenbacher-Mansuy W, Joye D, Pohl C, Wiesmann U, Zemp E, editors. Handbook of transdisciplinary research. Berlin: Springer; 2008. p. 411–24.

Ramadier T. Transdisciplinarity and its challenges: the case of urban studies. Futures. 2004;36:423–39.

Raymond CM, Fazey I, Reed MS, Stringer LC, Robinson GM, Evely AC. Integrating local and scientific knowledge for environmental management. J Environ Manag. 2010;91:1766–77.

Read EK, O'Rourke M, Hong GS, Hanson PC, Winslow LA, Crowley S, Brewer CA, Weathers KC. Building the team for team science. Ecosphere. 2016;7(3):e01291. https://doi.org/10.1002/ecs2.1291.

Repko AF. Integrating interdisciplinarity: how the theories of common ground and cognitive interdisciplinarity are informing the debate on interdisciplinary integration. Issues Integrative Studies. 2007;25:1–31.

Repko AF. Interdisciplinary research: process and theory. 2nd ed. Los Angeles: Sage; 2012.

Rittel HW, Webber MM. Dilemmas in a general theory of planning. Policy Sci. 1973;4(2):155–69.

Rosas J, Camarinha-Matos LM. An approach to assess collaboration readiness. Int J Prod Res. 2009; 47(17):4711–35.

Rosenfield PL. The potential for transdisciplinary research for sustaining and extending linkages between the health and social sciences. Soc Sci Med. 1992;35(11):1343–57.

Rossini FA, Porter AL. Frameworks for integrating interdisciplinary research. Res Policy. 1979;8:70–9.

Rylance R. Global funders to focus on interdisciplinarity. Nature. 2015;525:313–5.

Salazar MR, Lant TK, Fiore SM, Salas E. Facilitating innovation in diverse science teams through integrative capacity. Small Group Res. 2012;43(5):527–58.

Salazar M, Widmer K, Doiron K, Lant T. Leader integrative capabilities: a catalyst for effective interdisciplinary teams. In: Hall KL, Vogel AL, Croyle RT, editors. Strategies for team science success: handbook of evidence-based principles for cross-disciplinary science and practical lessons learned from health researchers. New York, NY: Springer; 2019. p. 313–328.

Shalinsky W. Polydisciplinary groups in the human services. Small Group Behav. 1989;20(2):203–19.

Sievanen L, Campbell LM, Leslie HM. Challenges to interdisciplinary research in ecosystem-based management. Conserv Biol. 2011;26(2):315–23.

Star SL, Griesemer JR. Institutional ecology, 'translations' and boundary objects: amateurs and professionals in Berkeley's Museum of Vertebrate Zoology, 1907–39. Soc Stud Sci. 1989;19(387–420):393.

Stember M. Advancing the social sciences through the interdisciplinary enterprise. Soc Sci J. 1991;28(1):1–14.

Stokols D. Training the next generation of transdisciplinarians. In: O'Rourke M, Crowley S, Eigenbrode SD, Wulfhorst JD, editors. Enhancing communication and collaboration in interdisciplinary research. Thousand Oaks, CA: Sage Publications; 2013. p. 56–81.

Stokols D, Fuqua J, Gress J, Harvey R, Phillips K, Baezcondi-Garbanati L, et al. Evaluating transdisciplinary science. Nicotine Tob Res. 2003;5:S21–39.

Stokols D, Hall KL, Taylor BK, Moser RP. The science of team science: overview of the field and introduction to the supplement. Am J Prev Med. 2008;35(2S):S77–89.

Strober M. Interdisciplinary conversations: challenging habits of thought. Stanford: Stanford University Press; 2011.

Szostak R. Classifying science: phenomena, data, theory, method, practice. Dordrecht: Springer; 2004.

Szostak R. Communicating complex concepts. In: O'Rourke M, Crowley S, Eigenbrode SD, Wulfhorst JD, editors. Enhancing communication and collaboration in interdisciplinary research. Thousand Oaks, CA: Sage Publications; 2013. p. 271–90.

Szostak R, Gnoli C, López-Huertas M. Interdisciplinary knowledge organizations. Cham: Springer International Publishing; 2016.

Thompson JL. Building collective communication competence in interdisciplinary research teams. J Appl Commun Res. 2009;37(3):278–97.

Tress G, Tress B, Fry G. Clarifying integrative research concepts in landscape ecology. Landsc Ecol. 2004;20:479–93.

Trochim W, Kane M. Concept-mapping: an introduction to structured conceptualization in health care. Int J Qual Health Care. 2005;17:187–91.

Turner M. Cognitive dimensions of social science. New York: Oxford University Press; 2001.

United States Department of Energy (DOE). Statement on digital data management. 2014. http://science.energy.gov/funding-opportunities/digital-data-management/

van der Steen WJ. Towards disciplinary disintegration in biology. Biol Philos. 1993;8:259–75.

van Noorden R. Interdisciplinary research by the numbers. Nature. 2015;525:306–7.

Vogel AL, Feng A, Oh A, Hall KL, Stipelman BA, Stokols D, Okamoto J, Perna FM, Moser R, Nebeling L. Influence of a National Cancer Institute transdisciplinary research and training initiative on trainees' transdisciplinary research competencies and scholarly productivity. Transl Behav Med. 2012;2:459–68.

Wear DN. Challenges to interdisciplinary discourse. Ecosystems. 1999;2:299–301.

Webne-Behrman H. The practice of facilitation. Charlotte, NC: Information Age Publishing; 1998.

Weingart P. A short history of knowledge formations. In: Frodeman R, Klein JT, Mitcham C, editors. The Oxford handbook of interdisciplinarity. Oxford: Oxford University Press; 2010. p. 3–14.

Wickson F, Carew AL, Russell AW. Transdisciplinary research: characteristics, quandaries and quality. Futures. 2006;38:1046–59.

Winowiecki L, Smukler S, Shirley K, Remans R, Peltier G, Lothes E, King E, Comita L, Baptista S, Alkema L. Tools for enhancing interdisciplinary communication. Sci Pract Policy. 2011;7:74–80.

Wuchty S, Jones BF, Uzzi B. The increasing dominance of teams in production of knowledge. Science. 2007;316:1036–8.

Zierhofer W, Burger P. Disentangling transdisciplinarity: an analysis of knowledge integration in problem-oriented research. Sci Stud. 2007;20(1):51–74.

The Introduction of a New Domain into an Existing Area of Research: Novel Discoveries Through Integration of Sleep into Cancer and Obesity Research

3

Peter James and Susan Redline

Contents

3.1 Introduction

Cancer is a spectrum of diseases with multifactorial determinants, including the inter-related areas of sleep, energy balance, and obesity. Studies exploring single risk factors explain only a small amount of the variation in cancer risk, and because behaviors are not conducted in isolation, targeting individual behavioral risk factors for cancer has proven challenging. Interventions aimed at only one risk factor and not adapted to the social and physical environment of the targeted population are less potent and durable than interventions that address inter-related behaviors operative in the real-world conditions of given populations. Multi- and transdisciplinary approaches to understanding the role of health behaviors on cancer risk show promise, as they bring together complementary expertise needed to evaluate multiple correlated factors operating in concert. Cross-disciplinary teams also provide the engines to integrate approaches and knowledge from basic, clinical, behavioral, and epidemiological sciences to catalyze new discoveries addressing etiology, intervention, and dissemination.

The following chapter explores how the application of cross-disciplinary approaches to inter-related behavioral factors of sleep, energy balance, and obesity has coalesced to enable new perspectives on these novel contributors to cancer risk. The chapter provides an overview of the emerging science that supports the importance of sleep as integral to energy balance, as well as influential on cancer incidence and progression through alterations in hormonal and inflammatory pathways. The challenges in integrating sleep into energetics and cancer research are discussed, as is the role that the National Cancer Institute

P. James (✉)
Department of Population Medicine, Harvard
Medical School and Harvard Pilgrim Health Care
Institute, Boston, MA, USA
e-mail: pjames@hsph.harvard.edu

S. Redline
Division of Sleep Medicine, Harvard Medical School
and Division of Sleep and Circadian Disorders,
Brigham and Women's Hospital,
Boston, MA, USA

© Springer Nature Switzerland AG 2019
K. L. Hall et al. (eds.), *Strategies for Team Science Success*,
https://doi.org/10.1007/978-3-030-20992-6_3

played in catalyzing transdisciplinary teams that embraced studies of sleep in cancer and energetics-related research. The chapter then reviews a sample of ongoing transdisciplinary studies focusing on sleep, energy balance, and cancer. Finally, the chapter discusses approaches for measuring energy balance and sleep, noting particular opportunities for diverse scientists to collaborate in developing and implementing better measurements of inter-related behaviors of physical activity, diet, sleep, and circadian rhythms using methods that span across disciplines.

3.2 Energy Balance: Interdependent Influences of Physical Activity, Diet, and Sleep on Cancer

Obesity has consistently been shown to increase risk of multiple cancers, including esophageal, pancreatic, colorectal, breast, endometrial, kidney, thyroid, and gallbladder cancer (Wolin et al. 2010; Arnold et al. 2015; Calle and Kaaks 2004; Calle and Thun 2004; McTiernan 2008; Wu et al. 2013; Blask 2009). Obesity is thought to affect cancer risk by influencing immune function and inflammation; changing hormone levels and hormone metabolism, including insulin and estradiol; altering factors that regulate cell proliferation and growth, such as insulin-like growth factor (IGF)-1; and modifying proteins that make hormones more or less available to tissues, such as sex hormone-binding globulin and IGF-binding proteins (Kushi et al. 2012). Substantial evidence has emerged explaining that the interdependent behaviors of inadequate physical activity, diet, and insufficient sleep act in concert to drive obesity (Patel and Hu 2008; Patel et al. 2006). Diet is a major contributor to positive energy balance and is therefore closely linked to obesity. There also is considerable evidence supporting the role of physical activity in preventing obesity and obesity-related diseases through increased energy expenditure (Bouchard and Katzmarzyk 2010). Physical activity has consistently been determined to reduce the risk of breast and colon cancer (Slattery 2004; IARC Handbooks of Cancer

Prevention 2002; Ballard-Barbash et al. 2006; Lee 2003), and suggestive evidence indicates that inadequate physical activity is associated with endometriosis and lung cancer risk (Latino-Martel et al. 2016). Evidence is growing that physical activity may reduce the risk of many other cancer types (Moore et al. 2016). Mechanistically, it is hypothesized that higher levels of physical activity and negative energy balance reduce cancer risk by decreasing plasma levels of estrogens, insulin, and IGF-1, influencing cell proliferation (McTiernan 2008), improving immune function, and decreasing adipokine levels, oxidative stress, and inflammatory markers (Wu et al. 2013; Friedenreich et al. 2010). In addition to influencing cancer risk, energy balance may also affect cancer survivorship (Li et al. 2016). Studies have explained that increasing levels of physical activity after diagnosis of breast cancer can improve quality of life and mental health, lower fatigue, aid with energy balance, and increase survival rates (Holmes et al. 2005; Ibrahim and Al-Homaidh 2011; Holick et al. 2008; Bradshaw et al. 2014; Borch et al. 2015; Schmid and Leitzmann 2014; Zhu et al. 2016). Physical activity and a healthy diet after diagnosis of colorectal cancer also appear to reduce cancer recurrence and improve chances of survival (Schmid and Leitzmann 2014; Meyerhardt et al. 2006; Golshiri et al. 2016; Van Blarigan and Meyerhardt 2015). Studies also suggest that physical activity could have benefits for survival after diagnosis of a number of other cancers (Li et al. 2016; Friedenreich et al. 2016).

3.2.1 Sleep: An Emerging Risk Factor for Cancer

Sleep and circadian rhythms are more recently recognized factors that influence both obesity and cancer through direct effects on diet and weight, as well as through metabolic, hormonal, and inflammatory mechanisms. Emerging research indicates that maintaining sleep of sufficient quantity and quality is a fundamental component of health, and insufficient sleep, including short sleep duration, fragmented sleep, and sleep disorders, is associated with all-cause mortality, chronic heart disease, diabetes, metabolic syndrome, obesity, and cancer (Patel and Hu 2008; Ayas et al. 2003; Patel et al. 2004, 2006; Kripke et al. 2002). More specifically, evidence supports a link between insufficient sleep, circadian disruption, nocturnal melatonin suppression, and sleep disturbances with breast (Hansen 2001; Davis et al. 2001; Schernhammer et al. 2001; Wang et al. 2013; Lie et al. 2013; He et al. 2014; Xiao et al. 2016), colon (Schernhammer et al. 2003; Papantoniou et al. 2014), prostate (Kubo et al. 2006; Gapstur et al. 2014; Sigurdardottir et al. 2012), and endometrial cancer (Viswanathan et al. 2007). Shift work, a known disruptor of healthy sleep and circadian rhythms, has been declared a probable human carcinogen by the International Agency for Research on Cancer (IARC) (Straif et al. 2007). Sleep disturbances are hypothesized to increase cancer risk through immune suppression, impairments in melatonin production, and a shift to the predominance in cancer-stimulatory cytokines (Blask 2009).

3.2.1.1 Sleep Deficiency vs. Sleep Health

Sleep is a fundamental and complex neurobehavioral state influenced by homeostatic and circadian processes, with behavioral and physiological manifestations. Researchers have traditionally focused on studying the negative impact of poor sleep, conceptualized in the 2011 National Institutes of Health Sleep Disorders Research Plan as *sleep deficiency*: "a deficit in the quantity or quality of sleep obtained versus the amount needed for optimal health, performance, and well-being; sleep deficiency may result from prolonged wakefulness leading to sleep deprivation, insufficient sleep duration, sleep fragmentation, or a sleep disorder, such as in obstructive sleep apnea, that disrupts sleep and thereby renders sleep non-restorative" (National Institutes of Health 2011). In contrast, Buysse has put forth an alternative framework for conceptualizing the positive attributes of sleep health, defined as: "....a multidimensional pattern of sleep-wakefulness, adapted to individual, social, and environmental demands, that promotes physical

and mental well-being. Good sleep health is characterized by subjective satisfaction, appropriate timing, adequate duration, high efficiency, and sustained alertness during waking hours" (Buysse 2014). An advantage to this perspective is its applicability to all people—not just those with sleep disorders—and potential to serve as a population-health target and to integrate with other initiatives addressing behaviors and social and environmental factors influencing health and disease.

Buysse noted that sleep health can be measured across multiple dimensions and in various time scales and at various levels of analysis, including self-report, behavioral, and physiological. He proposed that there are five to six salient sleep domains, each of which has been associated with health outcomes:

1. Duration—the total amount of sleep obtained in 24 h.
2. Continuity or efficiency—the extent of time in the sleep period spent asleep (vs. waking).
3. Timing—when in the 24 h period sleep occurs.
4. Alertness/Sleepiness—ability to maintain attentive wakefulness.
5. Satisfaction/Quality—subjective assessment of sleep (poor-good).
6. Depth—measured physiologically, reflecting the patterns of EEG activity.

The extent to which each of these dimensions contribute to health generally (or to specific health problems specifically, such as cancer) and the validity of alternative measurement approaches requires investigation. Figure 3.1, adapted from Buysse (2014), illustrates the relationship between sleep dimensions and cancer outcomes within the context of social, environmental, and behavioral factors.

Disruption of circadian rhythm is thought to be a key driving factor behind sleep disturbances and cancer risk. The endogenous circadian rhythm is regulated by the suprachiasmatic nuclei (SCN), and the circadian system is responsible for synchronizing external environment signals (light, eating) with daily cyclical physiology, from gene expression to behavior (Kang and

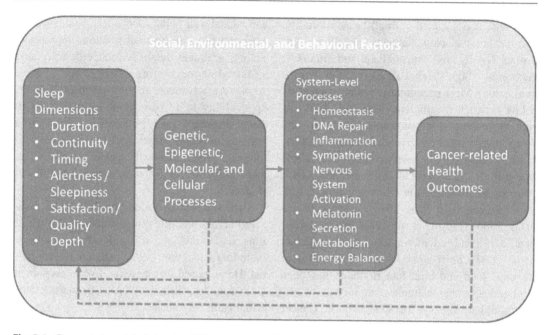

Fig. 3.1 Conceptual model of sleep health in the context of cancer (adapted from Buysse 2014)

Sancar 2009). Laboratory-based research suggests that circadian disruption may amplify adverse effects of prolonged sleep restriction on insulin and glucose secretion (Buxton et al. 2012). Circadian rhythm disruption may influence tumorigenesis through a number of mechanisms, including disturbed homeostasis and metabolism, suppression of melatonin secretion, reduced capacity in DNA repair, and energy imbalance. Experimental studies demonstrate that disruption of circadian rhythms promotes carcinogenesis in animals (Straif et al. 2007), and evidence is building that disrupted circadian rhythms in shift workers associate with increased breast and prostate cancer risk (Schernhammer et al. 2001, 2006; Kubo et al. 2006; Sigurdardottir et al. 2012; Straif et al. 2007), with suggestive evidence for colorectal (Schernhammer et al. 2003) and endometrial cancer (Viswanathan et al. 2007). These studies also provide support that energy imbalance and obesity play a role in mediating the relationship between shift work and cancer. Shift workers tend to gain weight more rapidly than non-shift workers (Morikawa et al. 2007; Suwazono et al. 2008; Zhao et al. 2011; Pan et al. 2011; Itani et al. 2011), and it is thought that shift work influences glucose and

lipid metabolism and reduced thermogenesis related to eating food at night (Antunes et al. 2010). Individuals with delayed sleep timing (later bedtimes) have also been reported to shift work have higher weight (Golley et al. 2013).

Short sleep duration is another mechanism linking sleep and cancer. Short sleep duration has been associated with colorectal (Thompson et al. 2011; Jiao et al. 2013), prostate (Kakizaki et al. 2008), and endometrial cancer (Sturgeon et al. 2012), as well as breast cancer (Kakizaki et al. 2008; Verkasalo et al. 2005; McElroy et al. 2006; Wu et al. 2008), although evidence is not completely consistent (Girschik et al. 2013; Pinheiro et al. 2006). Insufficient sleep is thought to influence obesity risk through sympathetic nervous system activation, alterations of the hypothalamic pituitary adrenal axis influencing secretion of cortisol and the renin-angiotensin system, and augmented systemic levels of inflammation, such as elevations in C reactive protein (Cappuccio and Miller 2011; Cappuccio et al. 2008). Inconsistencies in the literature may reflect differences in measurement and sample variation.

Sleep disorders have also been implicated in driving cancer risk, in particular insomnia and sleep apnea. Insomnia, a disorder defined by difficulties in falling asleep, staying asleep, and/ or early morning awakenings, is a chronic disorder observed in approximately 10% of adults for one or more years, and affects as many as 30% of adults transiently (Saddichha 2010). Chronic insomnia is associated with daytime dysfunction and often with psychiatric diseases (Roth 2007). Insomnia is considered to be a disorder of "hyperarousal," with associated abnormalities in autonomic nervous system function and increased hypothalamic pituitary adrenal activity, including hypersecretion of cortisol (Floam et al. 2015). In addition to its association with physiological disturbances, insomnia is associated with altered dietary behaviors. For example, a large cohort study has revealed that insomnia was associated with higher dietary energy intake as well as higher intake of trans fat and lower intake of vegetables (Cheng et al. 2016). Given these links, it is not surprising that insomnia has been identified as a risk factor for diabetes (Vgontzas et al. 2001) and incident hypertension (Fernandez-Mendoza et al. 2012), myocardial infarction (Laugsand et al. 2011), heart failure (Laugsand et al. 2014), and depression (Buysse et al. 2008), as well as mortality (Li et al. 2014). Recent evidence also suggests that women with insomnia have an increased risk of breast cancer (Fang et al. 2015) and of thyroid cancer (Luo et al. 2013). Insomnia may or may not be accompanied by short sleep duration; however, insomnia associated with short sleep duration appears to more adversely affect metabolism and contributes more to chronic disease than insomnia or short sleep duration each do alone (Vgontzas et al. 2009). It is likely that a "short sleep-insomnia" phenotype is also associated with cancer risk, but this has not been well studied. Insomnia also frequently occurs in patients with cancer (Engstrom et al. 1999; Savard and Morin 2001), contributing to reduced quality of life, and possibly negatively affects other outcomes, including survival.

Sleep apnea, a disorder characterized by recurrent episodic disturbances of breathing during sleep (apneas and hypopneas: full and partial episodes of upper airway closure), affects over 15% of the adult population (Young et al. 2002), with an increased prevalence with advancing age,

with obesity, and in ethnic and racial minorities (Chen et al. 2015). As a result of intermittent airway closure, the individual is exposed to chronic intermittent hypoxemia and sleep fragmentation, both of which contribute to sympathetic-parasympathetic nervous system imbalance, insulin resistance, oxidative stress, and inflammation. Sleep apnea-associated intermittent hypoxemia (IH) may play a particularly important role in cancer incidence and progression. IH is known to activate key pathways that influence tumor growth through effects on apoptosis, cell proliferation, migration, angiogenesis, and tumor metastases. Specifically, IH (1) activates the transcriptional factor hypoxia inducible factor (HIF)-1 that causes release of proangiogenic factors such as vascular endothelial growth factor; (2) stimulates free oxygen radicals release, increasing oxidative stress, damages DNA, and alters gene expression; (3) activates NF-kB inflammatory pathways, increasing release of TNFa, CRP, and other inflammatory mediators; (4) increases insulin resistance; and (5) alters DNA methylation and transcriptional regulation. In addition, IH can exacerbate tumor hypoxia, causing local over-expression of HIF-1A, leading to aggressive tumor activity and resistance to chemotherapy. The evidence supporting this includes cell culture studies, animal studies, and epidemiological investigations. Cell culture studies have shown that IH exposure can cause tumor cells to resist apoptosis, leading to higher metastatic potential (Almendros et al. 2012). Severity of IH has been linked to histological evidence of tumor aggressiveness, including higher mitotic index, tumor ulceration, and stage at excision (Martinez-Garcia et al. 2014). Animal models also indicate that hypoxia may be linked to increased tumor growth (Almendros et al. 2012). Sleep apnea also may influence cancer risk through alterations in energy balance. One of the strongest risk factors for sleep apnea is obesity (Fang et al. 2015), and obesity may amplify the effects of IH on cancer-related pathways. In addition, sleep apnea is associated with sleepiness and fatigue, which may contribute to lower levels of physical activity and positive energy balance. Epidemiologic studies support an association between sleep apnea and risk for total and cancer-related mortality (Nieto et al. 2012; Campos-Rodriguez et al. 2013). In two studies of approximately 5000 predominantly middle-aged patients referred to a sleep center and followed for 4.5 years, cancer incidence and mortality were increased by at least twofold for those with low oxyhemoglobin saturation levels (Nieto et al. 2012; Campos-Rodriguez et al. 2013). Similar associations were reported in a US cohort study which reported 20 years of follow-up data for 1552 middle-aged participants in the Wisconsin Sleep Cohort and found a 3.4-fold increase in cancer mortality in association with severe sleep apnea, with even stronger associations with overnight hypoxemia (Martinez-Garcia et al. 2014). Although results have been less consistent for analyses that use self or medical record reports of sleep apnea, a large medical record study from Taiwan has shown that sleep apnea was associated with increased risks of breast, prostate, and nasal cancers (Fang et al. 2015).

Sleep disturbances, particularly insomnia, are prevalent in patients with cancer (Savard et al. 2011). Diagnosis of cancer is associated with mood changes that can contribute to insomnia and sleep disturbances (Hoyt et al. 2016; Otte et al. 2016). Furthermore, insufficient sleep, poor sleep quality and efficiency, disturbed circadian rhythms, and sleep disorders may negatively influence cancer survival (Phipps et al. 2016; Palesh et al. 2014; Levi et al. 2014). These effects may be mediated through a number of pathways: (a) by contributing to obesity, metabolic, and neurohumoral effects that promote tumor aggressiveness and metastases; and (b) by contributing to fatigue, poor quality of life, anxiety, depression, and stress. A mouse model demonstrated that chronic sleep disturbance accelerated tumor growth and invasiveness (Hakim et al. 2014), and suggested this occurs through a pro-inflammatory TKR4 pathway. Two longitudinal studies reported poorer breast and colorectal cancer survival in patients with low sleep efficiency or quality, respectively (Palesh et al. 2014; Levi et al. 2014). In the Women's Health Initiative, among the sleep exposures, the combination of short sleep (<6 h/night) and snoring (a symptom of sleep

apnea) was associated with a more than twofold increased risk of cancer-specific death in women with breast cancer (Phipps et al. 2016). There is also emerging evidence that behavioral treatment of sleep disturbances, particularly insomnia, may have beneficial health effects in patients with cancer (Savard et al. 2016). Physical activity has also been shown to protect against sleep disruption among breast cancer survivors (Roveda et al. 2016), although evidence is not completely consistent (Zhu et al. 2016).

Many attributes of sleep, such as sleep duration and timing, may vary greatly within individuals, and this variation, possibly by causing circadian disruption, may itself be a risk factor for many health-related outcomes, including obesity (Patel et al. 2014). One approach to measuring across-week variation in sleep timing is to compare the "mid-sleep" point (between bed and wake times) on weekdays compared to weekends. Individuals with differences of greater than 2 h are classified with "social jet lag," indicating misalignment between ones' social and biological clock has been associated with increased weight (Roenneberg et al. 2012).

3.2.2 Intersecting Pathways: Opportunities for Transdisciplinary Research Teams

Pioneering cross-disciplinary work merging sleep medicine, physical activity research, and nutritional epidemiology has elucidated how energy balance and sleep interact to influence obesity risk, and subsequently cancer (Fig. 3.2). Studies have observed consistent links between short sleep duration and higher total energy intake, higher total fat intake, and irregular eating behavior (Dashti et al. 2015). The association between sleep duration and dietary intake is thought to be driven by differences in the appetite-related hormones leptin and ghrelin, hedonic pathways and centrally mediated reward responses, extended hours for intake, and altered time of intake (and misalignment of sleep and eating with circadian rhythms). Epidemiologic

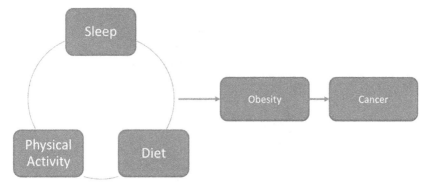

Fig. 3.2 Conceptual diagram of interrelationships between physical activity, diet, and sleep in driving obesity and cancer risk

and experimental evidence underscores the role of sleep disturbances as important risk factors for obesity (Patel and Hu 2008), primarily through metabolic and endocrine alterations, including decreased glucose tolerance, decreased insulin sensitivity, increased evening concentrations of cortisol, increased levels of ghrelin, decreased levels of leptin, and increased hunger and appetite (Patel and Hu 2008; Beccuti and Pannain 2011; Shlisky et al. 2012; Cermakian and Boivin 2009). Evidence also points to benefits of physical activity to improving total sleep time and sleep efficiency, sleep onset latency, and sleep quality (Kredlow et al. 2015). However, exercise too close to bedtime may increase core body temperature and prolong sleep onset. Increased walking, and living in "walkable" neighborhoods also have been associated with reducing sleep apnea severity (Billings et al. 2016), attributed to favorable effects on fluid distribution in the body, reducing nocturnal fluid accumulation in the airway. There is also interest in the bidirectional relationships between physical activity and sleep. Although improved sleep may lead to less fatigue and more activity, some epidemiological data indicate that the reverse may also occur (Pesonen et al. 2011; Soric et al. 2015; Lang et al. 2016). The basis for this is not understood, but suggests that individuals may view sleeping and exercise as "competing" activities and curtail one to spend more time in the other. Such phenomena provide a strong motivation for considering the co-occurrence of multiple behaviors in assessing and intervening on health behaviors.

Sleep, energy balance, and obesity may play an important role in driving cancer risk and could potentially serve as promising targets for intervention. A full understanding of these intersecting behaviors and their impact on obesity, metabolism, and cancer requires transdisciplinary teamwork.

3.3 Transdisciplinary Approaches to Understanding Physical Activity, Diet, Obesity, and Sleep and Their Relationships to Cancer

Studies of the interacting influences of diet and physical activity on risk of obesity and cancer have long been fundamental to energetics research. In contrast, appreciable interest in sleep as an inter-related risk factor for these outcomes did not occur until recently. Although disturbed sleep was long recognized to significantly impact well-being, mood, and cognition, it was only in the last decade that the influence of sleep and circadian rhythms on energy balance and obesity was fully recognized. In the early part of this millennium, landmark human studies reported that appetitive hormone levels respond to experimental sleep restriction or extension, suggesting novel biological mechanisms linking sleep duration to obesity in healthy adults (Spiegel et al. 2004, b). The idea that sleep is a "novel obesity risk factor" attracted significant interest of researchers, although mostly from those already dedicated to sleep research. In parallel, animal models identified marked metabolic effects resulting from circadian disruption (Turek et al. 2005). These studies, accompanied by marked advances in the basic science of circadian rhythms, also catalyzed a wide variety of clinical and translational research addressing the roles of circadian misalignment on metabolic health. Sleep health was increasingly identified as representing the "third pillar" of health, with an expressed need to consider the triad of physical activity, diet, and sleep as fundamental and complementary health behaviors.

Despite growing multidisciplinary research addressing the relationships between sleep and obesity, and between obesity and cancer, much less research addressed the interrelationships among cancer, obesity, and sleep. Figure 3.3 shows the number of articles addressing both "sleep and obesity" and also "sleep, obesity, and cancer" based on a PubMed search (March 9, 2017). Consistent with the emergence of research described earlier, a notable increase in publications indexing "sleep and obesity" occurred after

about the year 2000. In contrast, a delayed and slower increase in publications that also address cancer is seen, with 18 articles on these combined topics published in the year 2004, increasing to 45 in 2016. The multiple reasons for the paucity of research include the challenges in bringing together not two, but three or more distinct disciplines; barriers in establishing collaboration among investigators without a tradition of working together and addressing topics that do not fit clearly (and thus recognized) by a single discipline; and finding support for topics that may not "belong" to a single funding agency. Although tremendous advances were made in characterizing mechanistic pathways potentially linking sleep to cancer (needed to support the scientific premise for further research), it can take time to both disseminate new knowledge across diverse scientific areas and to translate knowledge into "actionable" research. In addition, generation of epidemiological data lagged due to the time required to add sleep measures to studies measuring the incidence of cancer outcomes. In comparison to decades of epidemiological studies that measured diet, physical activity, and health

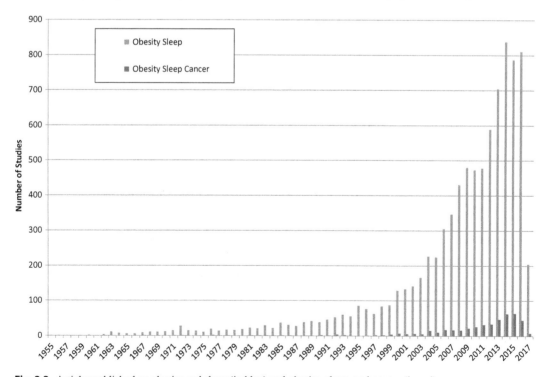

Fig. 3.3 Articles published on obesity and sleep (in blue) and obesity, sleep, and cancer (in red)

outcomes, many fewer studies measured sleep, thus limiting the available epidemiological data needed to characterize interrelationships in the population, and limiting the number of research studies utilizing secondary data analysis. Finally, the number of investigators conducting sleep research is modest and unevenly distributed across academic institutions, and many strong cancer and obesity centers have limited access to local sleep medicine expertise, reducing the ability to expand research foci.

3.3.1 Catalyst: The Transdisciplinary Research on Energy Balance and Cancer (TREC) Program

In 2004, the National Cancer Institute (NCI) funded the Transdisciplinary Research on Energy Balance and Cancer (TREC) program, catalyzing further collaborative research in cancer and energetics through an initiative that explicitly encouraged inclusion of new disciplines, such as sleep medicine, in studies of obesity, energetics, and cancer. In its first funding cycle (2004–2010), TREC included four academic medical centers (Case Western Reserve University, University of Minnesota, University of Southern California, and Fred Hutchison Cancer Center). The program was designed and incentivized to deliberately foster the involvement of both new scientists and new disciplines in a full range of research and training activities aimed at identifying novel and translational discoveries relating to energy balance and cancer. Investigators, trainees, and approaches from "nontraditional" areas, such as geography, system networks, and sleep medicine, were incorporated into the core research programs. In addition, funds were allocated to specifically support pilot projects that prioritized involvement of trainees committed to transdisciplinary science, a group who were felt likely to adopt enduring approaches for conducting transdisciplinary research and likely to serve as role models for a new generation of researchers. TREC aimed to enhance transdisciplinary research in several ways, including establishing incentives to encourage investigators and trainees

across institutions to collaborate in developmental projects; providing support for transdisciplinary working groups to meet regularly by conference calls and at periodic study meetings; and promoting team science through projects such as those addressing new methods development and writing of position articles. A supportive culture, with opportunities to build comradery and for new investigators to interact with a wide range of senior investigators and to visit collaborating institutions, was embraced. Similar priorities and strategies for promoting collaboration, especially supporting activities aimed at supporting trainees, were later adopted and further extended by the TREC program during its second cycle. This second cycle began in 2010, and involved centers at Harvard University, University of California San Diego, University of Pennsylvania, and Washington University in St. Louis.

TREC provided numerous opportunities for investigators to discuss their projects and provide perspectives across diverse scientific areas to members of the collaborative. One major project in each of the first and second TREC cycles (at Case Western Reserve University and Harvard University, respectively) was specifically focused on the role of sleep in influencing adiposity and cancer-related biomarkers. With these projects as foci, sleep science was regularly discussed at local and at cross-institutional meetings, and evolved to also include broader overviews of mechanisms, epidemiology, and measurement. Learning about sleep and circadian science was enthusiastically received by investigators and trainees across all institutions, some of whom had prior interests in these areas, and others in whom this was a novel and appealing area. Investigators across institutions recognized that the complex and correlated relationship between energy balance, sleep, obesity, and cancer provided an impetus for developing integrated approaches spanning multiple fields, encouraging collaboration among researchers trained in sleep medicine, metabolism, epidemiology, public health, and other areas. These interactions also identified measurement challenges that overlapped other areas (e.g., physical activity) and opportunities to measure multiple behaviors concurrently using state-of-the-art devices and software. Synergies were leveraged, such as linking individuals with measurement expertise with those with knowledge of sleep health and physical activity.

The following sections discuss several examples of TREC-funded pilot studies that helped build cross-disciplinary teams to tackle research questions that clarify the influences on and relationship between these behavioral risk factors for cancer.

3.3.1.1 Integrating Measures of Physical Activity, Sedentary Behavior, Sleep, and the Built Environment

The TREC initiative funded many projects across centers, including a study entitled "Integrating measures of physical activity, sedentary behavior, sleep, and the built environment." In this study, 373 women (mean age 55.3+ 10.2) across the four sites were asked to wear an accelerometer on their wrist for 24 h, and an accelerometer and global positioning systems (GPS) device on their hip during waking hours for 7 days. Participants were recruited from existing TREC studies, which included varying recruitment strategies (local community samples and national US samples), methods (observational and intervention studies), and populations (participants were recruited as breast cancer survivors, nurses, or from the general population). Participants completed surveys and wore the suite of devices over at least five consecutive days and nights in combination with self-reported sleep logs reporting the times they were in and out of bed for the corresponding sleep periods. Expertise varied widely across sites, with some centers focused primarily on observational environmental epidemiology in large cohort studies, while other centers focused on objective measurement of location, physical activity, and sleep. Across centers, a transdisciplinary study team engaged epidemiologists, behavioral scientists, biostatisticians, geographers, sociologists, and data scientists to tackle novel data streams, collaborated to develop new approaches, and answer new questions about the interaction between environment, energy balance, and sleep. Catalyzed by TREC, members from each center met multiple times and developed protocols so that all sites were trained extensively on questionnaire development, accelerometry data collection, participant interactions, and data analysis and processing techniques. The resulting data on time-matched location, physical activity, sedentary behavior, and sleep on a nationwide sample is unparalleled and is beginning to provide new insights into the relationships between these behavioral influences on obesity and cancer. Numerous publications are in process examining the relationship between activity and sleep (Mitchell et al. 2016), patterns of sleep and activity (Mitchell et al. 2016), the relationship between location of activity and sleep (Murray et al. 2017), environmental influences on activity (James et al. 2017) and sleep, and new ways of processing accelerometry data to accurately identify physical activity patterns (Kerr et al. 2016).

3.3.1.2 Impact of Nocturnal Zeitgebers on Energy in TREC

Improving knowledge about the interplay between circadian rhythms and energy balance may identify novel interventions to reduce obesity and cancer-related morbidities, which can make evidence-based prevention and treatment strategies more effective. The Impact of Nocturnal Zeitgebers on Energy in TREC (INZEIT) study was another cross-center project funded by NCI's TREC initiative that aims to examine the associations between circadian rhythms, behaviors, and energy balance. The INZEIT team integrated a mobile smartphone app to gather questionnaire data in real time over multiple days on key "zeitgebers," or environmental cues for circadian patterns, including light exposure, meal timing and activity by sharing knowledge and expertise on mobile technology, health behaviors and measurement (Fig. 3.4).

A collaborating biomedical engineer adapted and tested algorithms for deriving both parametric and nonparametric parameters from the accelerometry data, enabling comprehensive assessment of circadian rest-activity patterns and sleep timing in existing TREC samples of children

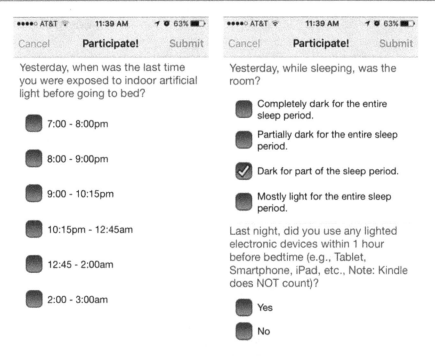

Fig. 3.4 Screenshots of smartphone application for the INZEIT study

and adults. The team integrated these data with the app-based information and physiological measurements evaluating the strength of the associations of these accelerometry-derived circadian parameters with demographics, activity, and sleep with markers of cardio-metabolism. The researchers merged these data with accelerometry data and assessed the impact of these factors on circadian rhythm. Data gathered through INZEIT supported the feasibility of integrating data from state-of-the-art accelerometers and mobile applications, and established preliminary data on the impact of "zeitgebers" measured in field settings on circadian rhythm, as well as the role of variations in parametric and nonparametric rhythm measures on energy balance. Finally, the project afforded interdisciplinary training in circadian rhythm and large data integration to TREC researchers, which they are already using to publish on this novel study (Mitchell et al. 2017).

3.3.1.3 Implementing Mobile Health Technology in the Nurses' Health Study 3

Environmental measures, including neighborhood walkability and access to green space, are sug-

gested to affect physical activity, sleep patterns, and obesity. Novel mobile health technologies (mHealth), such as GPS-enabled smartphones and consumer wearable accelerometry devices, can provide efficient, rigorous, and objective measures of environment, physical activity, and sleep with high spatio-temporal resolution. However, managing, processing, and analyzing streaming high-dimensional data presents significant logistical and analytical challenges, especially when linking these data to existing data from large prospective cohorts. A new mHealth-based pilot within the Nurses' Health Study 3 (NHS3) prospective cohort is confronting these challenges through transdisciplinary approaches and assessing the effect of dynamic measures of geographic context on objective measures of physical activity and sleep, as well as subsequent obesity and cancer risk. NHS3 is a web-based, nationwide, prospective open cohort with a current enrollment of ~44,000 male and female nurses aged 19–46 years old. Building on lessons learned from the TREC initiative, this ongoing substudy is piloting measures of the interdependent relationships between geographic context, physical activity, sleep, and obesity by testing the feasibility of deploying smartphone applications and wearable devices within 500 NHS3 participants. The mobile technologies collect streaming, high spatio-temporal resolution measures of geographic environment (e.g., walkability and green space), physical activity, and sleep over a 7-day monitoring period, four times over 1 year. Investigators are applying state-of-the-science statistical methods to examine the interrelationships between these high-dimensional, big data measures of environment and behavior. Ultimately, investigators will use these data to develop error-corrected measures of environment, physical activity, and sleep that can be applied to the full NHS3 cohort. A team of data scientists, sleep medicine experts, biostatisticians, epidemiologists, obesity experts, environmental health researchers, software programmers, and experts in sensor-based technologies have been assembled to rigorously quantify contextual exposures, physical activity, and sleep, and effectively evaluate the influence of environmental factors on interdependent behavioral risk factors for cancer and obesity.

3.4   Measurement Approaches: Opportunities for the Transdisciplinary Team

As the above examples illustrate, research addressing measurement of energy balance and sleep presented, and continues to present, challenges to the evolving teams of TREC early investigators. The following sections further discuss ongoing challenges in reliably measuring energy balance and sleep over long time periods that provide exemplars for further transdisciplinary collaboration. Improving on these measures will provide cross-disciplinary researchers with increasing insights into how energy balance and sleep interact to influence cancer risk. In turn, insights derived from improved measurement may provide translational data to inform actionable interventions on energy balance and sleep that may favorably impact cancer incidence and outcomes, as well as prove beneficial for other health outcomes related to these important health behaviors.

3.4.1   Measuring Energy Balance

Energy balance consists of energy expenditure, a combination of resting metabolic rate, the thermogenic effect of food, adaptive thermogenesis, and physical activity (Willett 2013); and energy intake, through diet. Many prospective studies use self-reported measures to measure energy balance, which have potential for subjective errors; record behavioral factors at fixed time periods, often only a few times over follow-up, and therefore cannot effectively evaluate time-varying behaviors; and often estimate associations between individual behavioral factors and cancer, without accounting for other potentially correlated lifestyle factors. These measurement shortcomings lead to errors in assessing energy balance, which may bias findings on energy balance and cancer risk. Improving measures of energy balance will decrease biases and deliver a more accurate picture of the relationship between energy balance and cancer.

Accelerometers or actigraphs, movement sensors worn on the body capable of objectively measuring physical activity at a fine temporal resolution (e.g., 50 measures per second), have been commonly employed in the past few decades to estimate physical activity (Rothney et al. 2010; Troiano et al. 2008, 2014). Self-report measures of physical activities are also widely used, such as a log of activities throughout the day or questionnaires where participants report their routine participation in common physical activity categories (e.g., average hours spent walking, running, or biking in the past week) (Wolf et al. 1994). Self-report methods are applied most commonly in prospective studies investigating the incidence of cancer, where the expense and intrusiveness of accelerometry and doubly labeled water over long periods of time are prohibitive. While the foundational focus of measuring physical activity is estimating energy expenditure, there are multiple domains and dimensions of physical activity that might be relevant for cancer. Domains of physical activity may include leisure, occupational, and travel-related physical activity, while different dimensions of physical activity might include duration, frequency, timing, intensity, and type of activity (Kelly et al. 2016). Each of these domains and dimensions may have important specific influences on behaviors, such as sleep, as well as health outcomes, such as cancer. In addition, specific environmental factors, such as the built environment, access to green space, and safety from crime, may influence levels of physical activity (Sallis et al. 2012; James et al. 2015; Casagrande et al. 2009). It should also be noted that sedentary behavior, independent of physical activity, may have independent effects on sleep and health outcomes (Lynch et al. 2010; Owen et al. 2010, b), including cancer (Shen et al. 2014). Finally, there is evidence that increased physical activity may reduce cancer risk independent of preventing weight gain (Moore et al. 2016).

3.4.2 Measuring Sleep

Many of the concepts discussed for measuring physical activity apply to sleep measurement, including its multidimensionality, variation over time, and the broad range of assessment tools that include subjective self-reports and precise physiological monitoring. Similar to challenges in measuring energy balance, errors in measuring sleep contribute to uncertainty over how sleep might influence cancer risk. Improved sleep measures will enhance our understanding of how the various dimensions of sleep health interact with energy balance to drive cancer.

The gold standard for measuring sleep is in-laboratory overnight polysomnography (PSG), which records multiple physiological signals simultaneously, such as the electroencephalogram (EEG), electrocardiogram, chin and leg electromyograms (EMG), electro-oculogram (EOG), pulse oximetry, respiratory excursions, airflow, leg movements, body position, and snoring. Concurrent measurement of EEG, EOG, and EMG is required for accurately classifying sleep stages. Autonomic output, blood pressure, and hormone release vary by sleep stage and selective restriction of given stages can result in memory and mood impairments (N2, REM) (Smith and MacNeill 1994; Stickgold and Walker 2007), increased insulin resistance (N3) (Tasali et al. 2008), and increased incidence of hypertension (N3) (Fung et al. 2011). Measurement of breath-

ing and oxygen saturation provides the ability to detect and quantify sleep apnea and other sleep-related breathing abnormalities. Leg movement monitoring allows detection of periodic limb movement disorder.

Although comprehensive, PSG can be burdensome and it can be difficult and expensive to collect multiple nights of data, which might be crucial to characterize chronic sleep behaviors that are relevant to cancer and other chronic diseases. In addition, laboratory-based PSG may be limited by "first-night" effects, referring to poor sleep experienced by the individual who is not habituated to a laboratory sleeping environment. Advances in technology now allow full PSG to be performed in home settings, where night to night variability has been shown to be low, with minimal first-night effect (Quan et al. 2002), and provides results comparable to lab-based PSG (Iber et al. 2004). More limited monitoring devices, such as home sleep apnea tests which measure a few channels of respiratory informative data, provide reliable means to assess sleep apnea at relatively minimal burden (Rosen et al. 2012). Single channel monitors, such as finger oximeters, also can provide useful information on markers of sleep apnea severity (hypoxemia), which may be the prime sleep drivers for certain outcomes such as diabetes and cancer.

Questionnaires and other methods for obtaining self-report data are most relevant for assessing sleep quality and insomnia, which is defined based on subjective experience. However, they also can be used to obtain information on sleep duration, timing, habits, and behaviors; assess associated daytime functioning (alertness, sleepiness); characterize chronotype; and provide screening for sleep disorders (sleep apnea, insomnia, periodic limb movement disorder, hypersomnolence). These types of questionnaires might also be relevant for assessing long-term sleep health, which again might be most relevant to chronic disease, such as cancer. Commonly used sleep questionnaires are illustrated in Table 3.1. Questionnaires include daily sleep diaries (in paper or electronic format), survey instruments, and screening instruments. A major challenge in sleep questionnaires is that often the behaviors of interest occur during sleep or during

Table 3.1 Sleep questionnaires

Commonly used sleep questionnaires
Pittsburgh Sleep Quality Index
Women's Health Study Insomnia Severity Index
Sleep Health Heart Study Sleep Habits Questionnaire
Epworth Sleepiness Scale
Specialized sleep questionnaires
Eveningness Morningness
Sleep Timing Questionnaire
Sleep Habits Survey (used primarily for teenage populations)
Adolescent Sleep Habits/Adolescent Sleep Wake Scale/Adolescent Sleepiness Scale
Cleveland Adolescent Sleep Questionnaire
Functional Outcomes of Sleep Apnea Questionnaire
Sleep Apnea Quality of Life Questionnaire
Insomnia Severity Index
International RLS Questionnaire

the sleep-wake transition, which are difficult to self-report. Some attributes, such as sleep duration, are poorly standardized across instruments.

Wrist accelerometry is increasingly used in research studies to characterize sleep-wake behaviors. Similar to the accelerometers used to measure physical activity, devices contain piezoelectric sensors that measure digitized acceleration signals over time periods such as 30 to 60 s, and apply algorithms that translate these movement features to classify given epochs as sleep or wake. Actigraphs have advantages over questionnaires in eliminating recall and reporting biases and providing the temporal resolution and repeated measurements needed to characterize sleep timing, sleep efficiency, sleep latency, wake after sleep onset time, napping periods, and variability in sleep duration. Circadian rest-activity rhythms also can be estimated from multiple days of accelerometry data (Van Someren 2011; Paudel et al. 2010), providing information on the stability, timing, and robustness of rhythms across days. However, as reviewed before (Quante et al. 2015), devices differ in hardware and software and interpretation of data requires careful consideration of accelerometer model, placement, cut-points, epoch length, filters, and wear-time definitions, as well as an appreciation for the differences introduced by the manual editing procedures that are applied to the data.

Furthermore, accelerometry has well-known measurement errors, with generally good ability to detect sleep and poorer ability to identify wake periods. These errors do not appear to be random; rather, sleep is generally underestimated in short sleepers and overestimated in those will low sleep efficiency (Blackwell et al. 2008).

Concurrent use of the same accelerometer to measure both physical activity and sleep provides an attractive approach for collecting and integrating data on both of these activities, as well as sedentary behavior, while minimizing subject burden and cost. One challenge is that physical activity algorithms have been developed using data from hip or waist placement while sleep algorithms have been developed from data obtained from wrist-placed devices. Total sleep time is systematically overestimated with hip compared to wrist placement (Zinkhan et al. 2014). Subjects are more compliant with wrist compared to hip placement (van Hees et al. 2011), suggesting value in using the wrist as the single placement site. The recent development of cutoffs for translating wrist movements to levels of physical activity shows promise for estimating light, moderate, and vigorous physical activity from wrist-worn devices (Chandler et al. 2016).

3.4.3 Challenges in Measuring Chronic Sleep and Energy Balance

Measuring the multiple dimensions of sleep and energy balance over long periods of time presents numerous challenges to researchers and ultimately demands cross-disciplinary approaches to estimate substantive linkages to cancer. These behavioral factors are highly variable over time and may require measures of fine temporal resolution. This resolution alone presents logistical, technological, and statistical obstacles that must be overcome. Logistically, research employing devices to measure sleep and energy balance requires designing and executing studies where staff can feasibly manage device initialization and distribution, where participants adhere to study protocols and return devices to researchers, and where staff can process device data. In the context of large-scale studies evaluating cancer outcomes, this can quickly become a massive logistical undertaking (Lee and Shiroma 2014). In addition, studies involving precise and intrusive measurement of health behaviors, such as PSG, may require access to specialized sleep laboratories and sleep technologists. Logistical concerns are compounded by the fact that maximal information may be achieved by measuring sleep and energy balance over multiple days and multiple nights, and to sample repeatedly over multiple years. Researchers must tailor their study designs and measurement approaches to meet the needs of different populations, including children, adults, elderly, and individuals with sleep disorders. Different populations may experience measurement burden differently, and different devices and signal processing and other algorithms may vary by age, sex, and underlying disease characteristics.

The measurement of chronic sleep and energy balance, as well as their role in driving cancer, has required researchers to build cross-disciplinary expertise in technologies that can accurately and reliably record these behaviors. Epidemiologists, physicians, and behavioral scientists have engaged with experts in PSG, accelerometry, and other technologies, as well as individuals with expertise in studying diverse populations, to create multidisciplinary teams. The rapidly changing landscape of technology to measure sleep and energy balance can present opportunities in hand with pitfalls. While devices to measure behaviors that may be relevant to cancer evolve each day (Evenson et al. 2015), the rate of development for these devices often outpaces validation studies. This leaves researchers to choose whether to use devices that have not been formally evaluated, or devices that may be outdated and have lower participant acceptability. Therefore, it is imperative that researchers stay up to date with the latest technology, understand what each device measures, and remain persistent in validating new devices as they hit the market.

Analyzing fine temporal resolution data can also present concerns for researchers. Much like other types of "Big Data," these behavioral measures are high in volume, as the sheer amount of data can be massive. The velocity, or speed of data generation, can be difficult to keep up with, as devices can provide hundreds of measures per second. The variety, or range of data types and sources, can multiply the complexity of these high-volume and high-velocity measures. For instance, each second an accelerometer can gather 50 measures on 3 axes per participant, and when you measure hundreds of participants over a week, these data become extremely complex very quickly. To address these analytical concerns, researchers in this field have developed data analytics, or analysis tools to process data efficiently, to identify new behavioral patterns, and to create predictive algorithms. Also, high resolution data with densely repeated measures on individuals violate assumptions of traditional statistical models. Therefore, sleep and energetics researchers have begun to collaborate with data scientists to develop novel statistical methods that can appropriately account for the correlation structure of these data streams. Only through these collaborations will researchers obtain measures of chronic sleep and energy balance that are operationalizable for integrative analyses that address how these health behaviors influence cancer risk.

3.4.4 Recent Advances in Technology to Measure Physical Activity, Diet, and Sleep

There is an array of methods to measure physical activity, diet, and sleep—all major contributors to energy balance. Each approach has applications to answer different research questions. In the context of estimating contributions to cancer risk, questionnaire-based approaches have traditionally dominated. However, as technology and computational methods advance, studies are beginning to incorporate accelerometers (Lee and Shiroma 2014) and other mobile health technologies to assess physical activity, diet, and sleep (Evenson et al. 2015; Martin et al. 2014). For instance, consumer wearable devices (such as the Fitbit, Apple Watch, Jawbone UP, or MisFit Shine) (Worldwide Wearable Computing Market 2014; Adam Noah et al. 2013; Lee et al. 2014;

Takacs et al. 2013) that utilize wrist-worn accelerometers are available for less than 50% the cost of accelerometers commonly used in research. These devices have been shown to perform as well as or better than "research-grade" accelerometry to measure physical activity in lab settings (Evenson et al. 2015; Lee et al. 2014; Diaz et al. 2015), and have been tested for validity and usability in free-living subjects (Adam Noah et al. 2013; Diaz et al. 2015; Vooijs et al. 2014). While exhibiting the same potential measurement errors as research-grade accelerometry, wearable devices have also shown moderate agreement with PSG to measure certain sleep domains (Evenson et al. 2015; de Zambotti et al. 2016); however, evidence is not completely consistent (Mantua et al. 2016), with overestimation of sleep time a limitation. Wearable devices can stream wireless physical activity and sleep data in near-real time, alleviating the need for the expensive and time-consuming mailing of devices back to researchers. In addition, smartphone applications are increasingly used to track dietary intake (Martin et al. 2014), physical activity, and sleep (Pew Internet Project Health Fact Sheet 2014). While evaluation of these approaches is an ever-evolving process, the popularization of consumer technologies has brought an abundant flow of high resolution data on sleep and energy balance which holds great potential in articulating the role of these behaviors to influence cancer risk.

3.4.5 Future Directions

The rapid adoption of smartphone applications and consumer wearable devices to measure sleep and energy balance (Worldwide Wearable Computing Market 2014; Adam Noah et al. 2013; Lee et al. 2014; Takacs et al. 2013) has the capacity to provide researchers with tremendous new data streams to explore patterns in these behavioral risk factors for cancer across the general population at an unprecedented scale. To take advantage of these novel technologies, researchers are rapidly developing groundbreaking methodologic approaches and are beginning to work in coordination with private industry. Progress in computer science, engaging machine learning

and signal processing techniques, has empowered researchers to process massive datasets that may enable the identification of patterns of behavior that might be relevant for cancer outcomes. As these applications, devices, and approaches evolve, cross-disciplinary collaborations will facilitate new perspectives on the interrelations between sleep and energy balance and their contribution to cancer.

3.5 Conclusions

This chapter describes the contributions of cross-disciplinary research to improve knowledge on how sleep and energy balance influence cancer and cancer survivorship. There are numerous logistical, technical, and analytical challenges that have been confronted in examining these behavioral risk factors for cancer. The integration of approaches across disparate fields, including but not limited to epidemiology, sleep medicine, behavioral science, technological development, and computer science, demonstrates immense potential for better characterizing these complex behaviors. In the coming years, these cross-disciplinary approaches will reveal a better understanding of how these behaviors are related to cancer incidence and cancer survivorship, and the identification of upstream influences on these behaviors with the aims of reducing the cancer-related disease burden.

References

Adam Noah J, Spierer DK, Gu J, Bronner S. Comparison of steps and energy expenditure assessment in adults of Fitbit tracker and ultra to the actical and indirect calorimetry. J Med Eng Technol. 2013;37:456–62.

Almendros I, Montserrat JM, Ramirez J, et al. Intermittent hypoxia enhances cancer progression in a mouse model of sleep apnoea. Eur Respir J. 2012;39:215–7.

Almendros I, Montserrat JM, Torres M, et al. Obesity and intermittent hypoxia increase tumor growth in a mouse model of sleep apnea. Sleep Med. 2012;13:1254–60.

Antunes LC, Levandovski R, Dantas G, Caumo W, Hidalgo MP. Obesity and shift work: chronobiological aspects. Nutr Res Rev. 2010;23:155–68.

Arnold M, Pandeya N, Byrnes G, et al. Global burden of cancer attributable to high body-mass index in 2012: a population-based study. Lancet Oncol. 2015;16(1):36–46.

Ayas NT, White DP, Al-Delaimy WK, et al. A prospective study of self-reported sleep duration and incident diabetes in women. Diabetes Care. 2003;26:380–4.

Ballard-Barbash R, Friedenreich C, Slattery M, Thune L. Obesity and body composition. In: Schottenfeld D, Fraumeni J, editors. Cancer epidemiology and prevention, vol. 3. New York: Oxford University Press; 2006.

Beccuti G, Pannain S. Sleep and obesity. Curr Opin Clin Nutr Metab Care. 2011;14:402–12.

Billings ME, Johnson D, Simonelli G, et al. Neighborhood walking environment and activity level are associated with obstructive sleep apnea: the multi-ethnic study of atherosclerosis. Chest. 2016;150:1042.

Blackwell T, Redline S, Ancoli-Israel S, et al. Comparison of sleep parameters from actigraphy and polysomnography in older women: the SOF study. Sleep. 2008;31:283–91.

Blask DE. Melatonin, sleep disturbance and cancer risk. Sleep Med Rev. 2009;13:257–64.

Borch KB, Braaten T, Lund E, Weiderpass E. Physical activity before and after breast cancer diagnosis and survival – the Norwegian women and cancer cohort study. BMC Cancer. 2015;15:967.

Bouchard C, Katzmarzyk PT, editors. Physical activity and obesity. 2nd ed. Baton Rouge, LA: Human Kinetics; 2010.

Bradshaw PT, Ibrahim JG, Khankari N, et al. Post-diagnosis physical activity and survival after breast cancer diagnosis: the Long Island Breast Cancer Study. Breast Cancer Res Treat. 2014;145:735–42.

Buxton OM, Cain SW, O'Connor SP, et al. Adverse metabolic consequences in humans of prolonged sleep restriction combined with circadian disruption. Sci Transl Med. 2012;4:129ra43.

Buysse DJ. Sleep health: can we define it? Does it matter? Sleep. 2014;37:9–17.

Buysse DJ, Angst J, Gamma A, Ajdacic V, Eich D, Rossler W. Prevalence, course, and comorbidity of insomnia and depression in young adults. Sleep. 2008;31:473–80.

Calle EE, Kaaks R. Overweight, obesity and cancer: epidemiological evidence and proposed mechanisms. Nat Rev Cancer. 2004;4:579–91.

Calle EE, Thun MJ. Obesity and cancer. Oncogene. 2004;23:6365–78.

Campos-Rodriguez F, Martinez-Garcia MA, Martinez M, et al. Association between obstructive sleep apnea and cancer incidence in a large multicenter Spanish cohort. Am J Respir Crit Care Med. 2013;187:99–105.

Cappuccio FP, Miller MA. Is prolonged lack of sleep associated with obesity? BMJ. 2011;342:d3306.

Cappuccio FP, Taggart FM, Kandala NB, et al. Meta-analysis of short sleep duration and obesity in children and adults. Sleep. 2008;31:619–26.

Casagrande SS, Whitt-Glover MC, Lancaster KJ, Odoms-Young AM, Gary TL. Built environment and health behaviors among African Americans: a systematic review. Am J Prev Med. 2009;36:174–81.

Cermakian N, Boivin DB. The regulation of central and peripheral circadian clocks in humans. Obes Rev. 2009;10(Suppl 2):25–36.

Chandler JL, Brazendale K, Beets MW, Mealing BA. Classification of physical activity intensities using a wrist-worn accelerometer in 8-12-year-old children. Pediatr Obes. 2016;11:120–7.

Chen X, Wang R, Zee P, et al. Racial/ethnic differences in sleep disturbances: The Multi-Ethnic Study of Atherosclerosis (MESA). Sleep. 2015;38:877–88.

Cheng FW, Li Y, Winkelman JW, Hu FB, Rimm EB, Gao X. Probable insomnia is associated with future total energy intake and diet quality in men. Am J Clin Nutr. 2016;104:462.

Dashti HS, Scheer FA, Jacques PF, Lamon-Fava S, Ordovas JM. Short sleep duration and dietary intake: epidemiologic evidence, mechanisms, and health implications. Adv Nutr. 2015;6:648–59.

Davis S, Mirick DK, Stevens RG. Night shift work, light at night, and risk of breast cancer. J Natl Cancer Inst. 2001;93:1557–62.

de Zambotti M, Baker FC, Willoughby AR, et al. Measures of sleep and cardiac functioning during sleep using a multi-sensory commercially-available wristband in adolescents. Physiol Behav. 2016;158:143–9.

Diaz KM, Krupka DJ, Chang MJ, et al. Fitbit(R): an accurate and reliable device for wireless physical activity tracking. Int J Cardiol. 2015;185:138–40.

Engstrom CA, Strohl RA, Rose L, Lewandowski L, Stefanek ME. Sleep alterations in cancer patients. Cancer Nurs. 1999;22:143–8.

Evenson KR, Goto MM, Furberg RD. Systematic review of the validity and reliability of consumer-wearable activity trackers. Int J Behav Nutr Phys Act. 2015;12:159.

Fang HF, Miao NF, Chen CD, Sithole T, Chung MH. Risk of cancer in patients with insomnia, parasomnia, and obstructive sleep apnea: a Nationwide Nested Case-Control Study. J Cancer. 2015;6:1140–7.

Fernandez-Mendoza J, Vgontzas AN, Liao D, et al. Insomnia with objective short sleep duration and incident hypertension: the Penn State Cohort. Hypertension. 2012;60:929–35.

Floam S, Simpson N, Nemeth E, Scott-Sutherland J, Gautam S, Haack M. Sleep characteristics as predictor variables of stress systems markers in insomnia disorder. J Sleep Res. 2015;24:296–304.

Friedenreich CM, Neilson HK, Lynch BM. State of the epidemiological evidence on physical activity and cancer prevention. Eur J Cancer. 2010;46:2593–604.

Friedenreich CM, Wang Q, Neilson HK, Kopciuk KA, McGregor SE, Courneya KS. Physical activity and survival after prostate cancer. Eur Urol. 2016;70:576.

Fung MM, Peters K, Redline S, et al. Decreased slow wave sleep increases risk of developing hypertension in elderly men. Hypertension. 2011;58:596–603.

Gapstur SM, Diver WR, Stevens VL, Carter BD, Teras LR, Jacobs EJ. Work schedule, sleep duration, insomnia, and risk of fatal prostate cancer. Am J Prev Med. 2014;46:S26–33.

Girschik J, Heyworth J, Fritschi L. Self-reported sleep duration, sleep quality, and breast cancer risk in a population-based case-control study. Am J Epidemiol. 2013;177:316–27.

Golley RK, Maher CA, Matricciani L, Olds TS. Sleep duration or bedtime? Exploring the association between sleep timing behaviour, diet and BMI in children and adolescents. Int J Obes. 2013;37:546–51.

Golshiri P, Rasooli S, Emami M, Najimi A. Effects of physical activity on risk of colorectal cancer: a case-control study. Int J Prev Med. 2016;7:32.

Hakim F, Wang Y, Zhang SX, et al. Fragmented sleep accelerates tumor growth and progression through recruitment of tumor-associated macrophages and TLR4 signaling. Cancer Res. 2014;74:1329–37.

Hansen J. Increased breast cancer risk among women who work predominantly at night. Epidemiology. 2001;12:74–7.

He C, Anand ST, Ebell MH, Vena JE, Robb SW. Circadian disrupting exposures and breast cancer risk: a meta-analysis. Int Arch Occup Environ Health. 2014;88:533–47.

Holick CN, Newcomb PA, Trentham-Dietz A, et al. Physical activity and survival after diagnosis of invasive breast cancer. Cancer Epidemiol Biomark Prev. 2008;17:379–86.

Holmes MD, Chen WY, Feskanich D, Kroenke CH, Colditz GA. Physical activity and survival after breast cancer diagnosis. JAMA. 2005;293:2479–86.

Hoyt MA, Bower JE, Irwin MR, Weierich MR, Stanton AL. Sleep quality and depressive symptoms after prostate cancer: the mechanistic role of cortisol. Behav Neurosci. 2016;130:351–6.

IARC Handbooks of Cancer Prevention. Weight control and physical activity, vol. 601. Lyon: International Agency for Research on Cancer; 2002.

Iber C, Redline S, Kaplan Gilpin AM, et al. Polysomnography performed in the unattended home versus the attended laboratory setting--Sleep Heart Health Study methodology. Sleep. 2004;27:536–40.

Ibrahim EM, Al-Homaidh A. Physical activity and survival after breast cancer diagnosis: meta-analysis of published studies. Med Oncol. 2011;28:753–65.

Itani O, Kaneita Y, Murata A, Yokoyama E, Ohida T. Association of onset of obesity with sleep duration and shift work among Japanese adults. Sleep Med. 2011;12:341–5.

James P, Banay RF, Hart JE, Laden F. A review of the health benefits of greenness. Curr Epidemiol Rep. 2015;2:131–42.

James P, Hart JE, Hipp JA, et al. GPS-based exposure to greenness and walkability and accelerometry-based physical activity. Cancer Epidemiol Biomark Prev. 2017;26:525–32.

Jiao L, Duan Z, Sangi-Haghpeykar H, Hale L, White DL, El-Serag HB. Sleep duration and incidence of colorectal cancer in postmenopausal women. Br J Cancer. 2013;108:213–21.

Kakizaki M, Inoue K, Kuriyama S, et al. Sleep duration and the risk of prostate cancer: the Ohsaki Cohort Study. Br J Cancer. 2008;99:176–8.

Kakizaki M, Kuriyama S, Sone T, et al. Sleep duration and the risk of breast cancer: the Ohsaki Cohort Study. Br J Cancer. 2008;99:1502–5.

Kang TH, Sancar A. Circadian regulation of DNA excision repair: implications for chrono-chemotherapy. Cell Cycle. 2009;8:1665–7.

Kelly P, Fitzsimons C, Baker G. Should we reframe how we think about physical activity and sedentary behaviour measurement? Validity and reliability reconsidered. Int J Behav Nutr Phys Act. 2016;13:32.

Kerr J, Marinac C, Ellis K, et al. Comparison of accelerometry methods for estimating physical activity. Med Sci Sports Exerc. 2016;49:617–24.

Kredlow MA, Capozzoli MC, Hearon BA, Calkins AW, Otto MW. The effects of physical activity on sleep: a meta-analytic review. J Behav Med. 2015;38:427–49.

Kripke DF, Garfinkel L, Wingard DL, Klauber MR, Marler MR. Mortality associated with sleep duration and insomnia. Arch Gen Psychiatry. 2002;59:131–6.

Kubo T, Ozasa K, Mikami K, et al. Prospective cohort study of the risk of prostate cancer among rotating-shift workers: findings from the Japan collaborative cohort study. Am J Epidemiol. 2006;164:549–55.

Kushi LH, Doyle C, McCullough M, et al. American Cancer Society Guidelines on nutrition and physical activity for cancer prevention: reducing the risk of cancer with healthy food choices and physical activity. CA Cancer J Clin. 2012;62:30–67.

Lang C, Kalak N, Brand S, Holsboer-Trachsler E, Puhse U, Gerber M. The relationship between physical activity and sleep from mid adolescence to early adulthood. A systematic review of methodological approaches and meta-analysis. Sleep Med Rev. 2016;28:32–45.

Latino-Martel P, Cottet V, Druesne-Pecollo N, et al. Alcoholic beverages, obesity, physical activity and other nutritional factors, and cancer risk: a review of the evidence. Crit Rev Oncol Hematol. 2016;99:308–23.

Laugsand LE, Strand LB, Platou C, Vatten LJ, Janszky I. Insomnia and the risk of incident heart failure: a population study. Eur Heart J. 2014;35:1382–93.

Laugsand LE, Vatten LJ, Platou C, Janszky I. Insomnia and the risk of acute myocardial infarction: a population study. Circulation. 2011;124:2073–81.

Lee IM. Physical activity and cancer prevention--data from epidemiologic studies. Med Sci Sports Exerc. 2003;35:1823–7.

Lee JM, Kim Y, Welk GJ. Validity of consumer-based physical activity monitors. Med Sci Sports Exerc. 2014;46:1840–8.

Lee IM, Shiroma EJ. Using accelerometers to measure physical activity in large-scale epidemiological studies: issues and challenges. Br J Sports Med. 2014;48:197–201.

Levi F, Dugue PA, Innominato P, et al. Wrist actimetry circadian rhythm as a robust predictor of colorectal cancer patients survival. Chronobiol Int. 2014;31:891–900.

Li T, Wei S, Shi Y, et al. The dose-response effect of physical activity on cancer mortality: findings from 71 prospective cohort studies. Br J Sports Med. 2016;50:339–45.

Li Y, Zhang X, Winkelman JW, et al. Association between insomnia symptoms and mortality: a prospective study of U.S. men. Circulation. 2014;129:737–46.

Lie JA, Kjuus H, Zienolddiny S, Haugen A, Kjaerheim K. Breast cancer among nurses: is the intensity of night work related to hormone receptor status? Am J Epidemiol. 2013;178:110–7.

Luo J, Sands M, Wactawski-Wende J, Song Y, Margolis KL. Sleep disturbance and incidence of thyroid cancer in postmenopausal women the Women's Health Initiative. Am J Epidemiol. 2013;177:42–9.

Lynch BM, Healy GN, Dunstan DW, Owen N. Sedentary versus inactive: distinctions for disease prevention. Nat Rev Cardiol 2010;7:11 https://doi.org/10.1083/nrcardio2010.68-c1; author reply https://doi.org/10.1083/nrcardio2010.68-c2.

Mantua J, Gravel N, Spencer RM. Reliability of sleep measures from four personal health monitoring devices compared to research-based Actigraphy and polysomnography. Sensors (Basel). 2016;16(5):E646.

Martin CK, Nicklas T, Gunturk B, Correa JB, Allen HR, Champagne C. Measuring food intake with digital photography. J Hum Nutr Diet. 2014;27(Suppl 1):72–81.

Martinez-Garcia MA, Campos-Rodriguez F, Duran-Cantolla J, et al. Obstructive sleep apnea is associated with cancer mortality in younger patients. Sleep Med. 2014;15:742–8.

Martinez-Garcia MA, Martorell-Calatayud A, Nagore E, et al. Association between sleep disordered breathing and aggressiveness markers of malignant cutaneous melanoma. Eur Respir J. 2014;43:1661–8.

McElroy JA, Newcomb PA, Titus-Ernstoff L, Trentham-Dietz A, Hampton JM, Egan KM. Duration of sleep and breast cancer risk in a large population-based case-control study. J Sleep Res. 2006;15:241–9.

McTiernan A. Mechanisms linking physical activity with cancer. Nat Rev Cancer. 2008;8:205–11.

Meyerhardt JA, Giovannucci EL, Holmes MD, et al. Physical activity and survival after colorectal cancer diagnosis. J Clin Oncol. 2006;24:3527–34.

Mitchell JA, Godbole S, Moran K, et al. No evidence of reciprocal associations between daily sleep and physical activity. Med Sci Sports Exerc. 2016;48:1950.

Mitchell JA, Quante M, Godbole S, et al. Variation in actigraphy-estimated rest-activity patterns by demographic factors. Chronobiol Int. 2017;34:1042–56.

Moore SC, Lee IM, Weiderpass E, et al. Association of leisure-time physical activity with risk of 26 types of cancer in 1.44 million adults. JAMA Intern Med. 2016;176:816–25.

Morikawa Y, Nakagawa H, Miura K, et al. Effect of shift work on body mass index and metabolic parameters. Scand J Work Environ Health. 2007;33:45–50.

Murray K, Godbole S, Natarajan L, et al. The relations between sleep, time of physical activity, and time outdoors among adult women. PLoS One. 2017;12:e0182013.

National Institutes of Health. National Institutes of health sleep disorders research plan. Bethesda, MD: National Institutes of Health; 2011.

Nieto FJ, Peppard PE, Young T, Finn L, Hla KM, Farre R. Sleep-disordered breathing and cancer mortality: results from the Wisconsin Sleep Cohort Study. Am J Respir Crit Care Med. 2012;186:190–4.

Otte JL, Davis L, Carpenter JS, et al. Sleep disorders in breast cancer survivors. Support Care Cancer. 2016;24:4197.

Owen N, Healy GN, Matthews CE, Dunstan DW. Too much sitting: the population health science of sedentary behavior. Exerc Sport Sci Rev. 2010;38:105–13.

Owen N, Sparling PB, Healy GN, Dunstan DW, Matthews CE. Sedentary behavior: emerging evidence for a new health risk. Mayo Clin Proc. 2010;85:1138–41.

Palesh O, Aldridge-Gerry A, Zeitzer JM, et al. Actigraphy-measured sleep disruption as a predictor of survival among women with advanced breast cancer. Sleep. 2014;37:837–42.

Pan A, Schernhammer ES, Sun Q, Hu FB. Rotating night shift work and risk of type 2 diabetes: two prospective cohort studies in women. PLoS Med. 2011;8:e1001141.

Papantoniou K, Kogevinas M, Martin Sanchez V, et al. 0058 Colorectal cancer risk and shift work in a population-based case-control study in Spain (MCC-Spain). Occup Environ Med. 2014;71(Suppl 1):A5–6.

Patel SR, Ayas NT, Malhotra MR, et al. A prospective study of sleep duration and mortality risk in women. Sleep. 2004;27:440–4.

Patel SR, Hayes AL, Blackwell T, et al. The association between sleep patterns and obesity in older adults. Int J Obes. 2014;38:1159–64.

Patel SR, Hu FB. Short sleep duration and weight gain: a systematic review. Obesity (Silver Spring). 2008;16:643–53.

Patel SR, Malhotra A, White DP, Gottlieb DJ, Hu FB. Association between reduced sleep and weight gain in women. Am J Epidemiol. 2006;164:947–54.

Paudel ML, Taylor BC, Ancoli-Israel S, et al. Rest/activity rhythms and mortality rates in older men: MrOS Sleep Study. Chronobiol Int. 2010;27:363–77.

Pesonen AK, Sjosten NM, Matthews KA, et al. Temporal associations between daytime physical activity and sleep in children. PLoS One. 2011;6:e22958.

Pew Internet Project Health Fact Sheet. 2014. http://www.pewinternet.org/fact-sheets/health-fact-sheet/. Accessed 1 Aug 2016

Phipps AI, Bhatti P, Neuhouser ML, et al. Pre-diagnostic sleep duration and sleep quality in relation to subsequent cancer survival. J Clin Sleep Med. 2016;12:495–503.

Pinheiro SP, Schernhammer ES, Tworoger SS, Michels KB. A prospective study on habitual duration of sleep and incidence of breast cancer in a large cohort of women. Cancer Res. 2006;66:5521–5.

Quan SF, Griswold ME, Iber C, et al. Short-term variability of respiration and sleep during unattended non-laboratory polysomnography--the Sleep Heart Health Study. [corrected]. Sleep. 2002;25:843–9.

Quante M, Kaplan ER, Rueschman M, Cailler M, Buxton OM, Redline S. Practical considerations in using accelerometers to assess physical activity, sedentary behavior, and sleep. Sleep Health. 2015;1:275–84.

Roenneberg T, Allebrandt KV, Merrow M, Vetter C. Social jetlag and obesity. Curr Biol. 2012;22:939–43.

Rosen CL, Auckley D, Benca R, et al. A multisite randomized trial of portable sleep studies and positive airway pressure autotitration versus laboratory-based polysomnography for the diagnosis and treatment of obstructive sleep apnea: the HomePAP study. Sleep. 2012;35:757–67.

Roth T. Insomnia: definition, prevalence, etiology, and consequences. J Clin Sleep Med. 2007;3:S7–10.

Rothney MP, Brychta RJ, Meade NN, Chen KY, Buchowski MS. Validation of the ActiGraph two-regression model for predicting energy expenditure. Med Sci Sports Exerc. 2010;42:1785–92.

Roveda E, Vitale JA, Bruno E, et al. Protective effect of aerobic physical activity on sleep behavior in breast cancer survivors. Integr Cancer Ther. 2016;

Saddichha S. Diagnosis and treatment of chronic insomnia. Ann Indian Acad Neurol. 2010;13:94–102.

Sallis JF, Floyd MF, Rodriguez DA, Saelens BE. Role of built environments in physical activity, obesity, and cardiovascular disease. Circulation. 2012;125:729–37.

Savard J, Ivers H, Savard MH, Morin CM. Long-term effects of two formats of cognitive behavioral therapy for insomnia comorbid with breast cancer. Sleep. 2016;39:813–23.

Savard J, Ivers H, Villa J, Caplette-Gingras A, Morin CM. Natural course of insomnia comorbid with cancer: an 18-month longitudinal study. J Clin Oncol. 2011;29:3580–6.

Savard J, Morin CM. Insomnia in the context of cancer: a review of a neglected problem. J Clin Oncol. 2001;19:895–908.

Schernhammer ES, Kroenke CH, Laden F, Hankinson SE. Night work and risk of breast cancer. Epidemiology. 2006;17:108–11.

Schernhammer ES, Laden F, Speizer FE, et al. Rotating night shifts and risk of breast cancer in women participating in the nurses' health study. J Natl Cancer Inst. 2001;93:1563–8.

Schernhammer ES, Laden F, Speizer FE, et al. Night-shift work and risk of colorectal cancer in the nurses' health study. J Natl Cancer Inst. 2003;95:825–8.

Schmid D, Leitzmann MF. Association between physical activity and mortality among breast cancer and colorectal cancer survivors: a systematic review and meta-analysis. Ann Oncol. 2014;25:1293–311.

Shen D, Mao W, Liu T, et al. Sedentary behavior and incident cancer: a meta-analysis of prospective studies. PLoS One. 2014;9:e105709.

Shlisky JD, Hartman TJ, Kris-Etherton PM, Rogers CJ, Sharkey NA, Nickols-Richardson SM. Partial sleep deprivation and energy balance in adults: an emerging issue for consideration by dietetics practitioners. J Acad Nutr Diet. 2012;112:1785–97.

Sigurdardottir LG, Valdimarsdottir UA, Fall K, et al. Circadian disruption, sleep loss, and prostate cancer risk: a systematic review of epidemiologic studies. Cancer Epidemiol Biomark Prev. 2012;21:1002–11.

Slattery ML. Physical activity and colorectal cancer. Sports Med. 2004;34:239–52.

Smith C, MacNeill C. Impaired motor memory for a pursuit rotor task following Stage 2 sleep loss in college students. J Sleep Res. 1994;3:206–13.

Soric M, Starc G, Borer KT, et al. Associations of objectively assessed sleep and physical activity in 11-year old children. Ann Hum Biol. 2015;42:31–7.

Spiegel K, Leproult R, L'Hermite-Baleriaux M, Copinschi G, Penev PD, Van Cauter E. Leptin levels are dependent on sleep duration: relationships with sympathovagal balance, carbohydrate regulation, cortisol, and thyrotropin. J Clin Endocrinol Metab. 2004;89:5762–71.

Spiegel K, Tasali E, Penev P, Van Cauter E. Brief communication: sleep curtailment in healthy young men is associated with decreased leptin levels, elevated ghrelin levels, and increased hunger and appetite. Ann Intern Med. 2004;141:846–50.

Stickgold R, Walker MP. Sleep-dependent memory consolidation and reconsolidation. Sleep Med. 2007;8:331–43.

Straif K, Baan R, Grosse Y, et al. Carcinogenicity of shift-work, painting, and fire-fighting. Lancet Oncol. 2007;8:1065–6.

Sturgeon SR, Luisi N, Balasubramanian R, Reeves KW. Sleep duration and endometrial cancer risk. Cancer Causes Control. 2012;23:547–53.

Suwazono Y, Dochi M, Sakata K, et al. A longitudinal study on the effect of shift work on weight gain in male Japanese workers. Obesity (Silver Spring). 2008;16:1887–93.

Takacs J, Pollock CL, Guenther JR, Bahar M, Napier C, Hunt MA. Validation of the fitbit one activity monitor device during treadmill walking. J Sci Med Sport. 2013;17:496–500.

Tasali E, Leproult R, Ehrmann DA, Van Cauter E. Slow-wave sleep and the risk of type 2 diabetes in humans. Proc Natl Acad Sci U S A. 2008;105:1044–9.

Thompson CL, Larkin EK, Patel S, Berger NA, Redline S, Li L. Short duration of sleep increases risk of colorectal adenoma. Cancer. 2011;117:841–7.

Troiano RP, Berrigan D, Dodd KW, Masse LC, Tilert T, McDowell M. Physical activity in the United States measured by accelerometer. Med Sci Sports Exerc. 2008;40:181–8.

Troiano RP, McClain JJ, Brychta RJ, Chen KY. Evolution of accelerometer methods for physical activity research. Br J Sports Med. 2014;48:1019–23.

Turek FW, Joshu C, Kohsaka A, et al. Obesity and metabolic syndrome in circadian clock mutant mice. Science. 2005;308:1043–5.

Van Blarigan EL, Meyerhardt JA. Role of physical activity and diet after colorectal cancer diagnosis. J Clin Oncol. 2015;33:1825–34.

van Hees VT, Renstrom F, Wright A, et al. Estimation of daily energy expenditure in pregnant and non-pregnant women using a wrist-worn tri-axial accelerometer. PLoS One. 2011;6:e22922.

Van Someren EJ. Actigraphic monitoring of sleep and circadian rhythms. Handb Clin Neurol. 2011;98:55–63.

Verkasalo PK, Lillberg K, Stevens RG, et al. Sleep duration and breast cancer: a prospective cohort study. Cancer Res. 2005;65:9595–600.

Vgontzas AN, Bixler EO, Lin HM, et al. Chronic insomnia is associated with nyctohemeral activation of the hypothalamic-pituitary-adrenal axis: clinical implications. J Clin Endocrinol Metab. 2001;86:3787–94.

Vgontzas AN, Liao D, Pejovic S, Calhoun S, Karataraki M, Bixler EO. Insomnia with objective short sleep duration is associated with type 2 diabetes: a population-based study. Diabetes Care. 2009;32:1980–5.

Viswanathan AN, Hankinson SE, Schernhammer ES. Night shift work and the risk of endometrial cancer. Cancer Res. 2007;67:10618–22.

Vooijs M, Alpay LL, Snoeck-Stroband JB, et al. Validity and usability of low-cost accelerometers for internet-based self-monitoring of physical activity in patients with chronic obstructive pulmonary disease. Interact J Med Res. 2014;3:e14.

Wang F, Yeung KL, Chan WC, et al. A meta-analysis on dose-response relationship between night shift work and the risk of breast cancer. Ann Oncol. 2013;24:2724–32.

Willett W. Nutritional Epidemiology. 3rd ed. New York, NY: Oxford University Press; 2013.

Wolf AM, Hunter DJ, Colditz GA, et al. Reproducibility and validity of a self-administered physical activity questionnaire. Int J Epidemiol. 1994;23:991–9.

Wolin KY, Carson K, Colditz GA. Obesity and cancer. Oncologist. 2010;15:556–65.

Worldwide Wearable Computing Market Gains Momentum with Shipments Reaching 19.2 Million in 2014 and Climbing to Nearly 112 Million in 2018, Says IDC. 2014. http://www.idc.com/getdoc.jsp?containerId=prUS24794914. Accessed 31 July 2014.

Wu AH, Wang R, Koh WP, Stanczyk FZ, Lee HP, Yu MC. Sleep duration, melatonin and breast cancer among Chinese women in Singapore. Carcinogenesis. 2008;29:1244–8.

Wu Y, Zhang D, Kang S. Physical activity and risk of breast cancer: a meta-analysis of prospective studies. Breast Cancer Res Treat. 2013;137:869–82.

Xiao Q, Signorello LB, Brinton LA, Cohen SS, Blot WJ, Matthews CE. Sleep duration and breast cancer risk among black and white women. Sleep Med. 2016;20:25–9.

Young T, Peppard PE, Gottlieb DJ. Epidemiology of obstructive sleep apnea: a population health perspective. Am J Respir Crit Care Med. 2002;165:1217–39.

Zhao I, Bogossian F, Song S, Turner C. The association between shift work and unhealthy weight: a cross-sectional analysis from the Nurses and Midwives' e-cohort Study. J Occup Environ Med. 2011;53:153–8.

Zhu G, Zhang X, Wang Y, Xiong H, Zhao Y, Sun F. Effects of exercise intervention in breast cancer survivors: a meta-analysis of 33 randomized controlled trails. Onco Targets Ther. 2016;9:2153–68.

Zinkhan M, Berger K, Hense S, et al. Agreement of different methods for assessing sleep characteristics: a comparison of two actigraphs, wrist and hip placement, and self-report with polysomnography. Sleep Med. 2014;15:1107–14.

The Integration of Research from Diverse Fields: Transdisciplinary Approaches Bridging Behavioral Research, Cognitive Neuroscience, Pharmacology, and Genetics to Reduce Cancer Risk Behavior

4

Mary Falcone, James Loughead,
and Caryn Lerman

Contents

M. Falcone (✉)
Keck School of Medicine of the University
of Southern California, Los Angeles, California, USA
e-mail: Mary.Falcone@med.usc.edu

J. Loughead
Department of Psychiatry, Neuropsychiatry Section,
University of Pennsylvania School of Medicine,
Philadelphia, PA, USA

C. Lerman
USC Norris Comprehensive Cancer Center and
Keck School of Medicine of USC,
Los Angeles, CA, USA

4.1   Introduction

Many health risks can be reduced or avoided by changing behavior. Quitting smoking, maintaining a healthy weight, and engaging in regular physical activity have been shown to reduce the risk of developing cardiovascular disease, cancer, and other chronic diseases by a significant margin (Arem et al. 2015; Centers for Disease Control and Prevention 2015; NIH Consensus Development Conference 1996; US Department of Health and Human Services 1990). Unfortunately, changing the behaviors that may increase health risk is difficult, even with the best available pharmacotherapies and behavioral treatments (Centers for Disease Control and Prevention 2010, 2011b; Yanovski and Yanovski 2014). Although many behavior modification interventions have been tested, the benefits are sometimes modest and often not sustained (An et al. 2008; Calfas et al. 2000; Elder et al. 1993; Greaves et al. 2011; Hutfless et al. 2013a; b; Lin et al. 2010). Pharmacologic interventions are only marginally better, with long-term success rates of <30% for smoking cessation (Cahill et al. 2013) and <20% for obesity (Wing and Phelan 2005). Thus, there is a need for novel behavior change interventions.

© Springer Nature Switzerland AG 2019
K. L. Hall et al. (eds.), *Strategies for Team Science Success*,
https://doi.org/10.1007/978-3-030-20992-6_4

The mechanisms supporting behavior change are complex; cognitive, social, biological, genetic, and environmental factors all contribute to an individual's ability to initiate and maintain healthy behaviors such as smoking cessation or weight loss. Effective interventions are therefore likely to require a comprehensive approach that takes several or all of these factors into account. In light of this, there is substantial opportunity for transdisciplinary research to generate novel hypotheses that could lead to more effective interventions.

Illustrating one such approach, this chapter presents strategies for transdisciplinary science that have been successfully employed to facilitate a program of research on cognitive and neural mechanisms underlying smoking relapse, using the four phase (development, conceptualization, implementation, and translation) model of transdisciplinary research to provide context (Hall et al. 2012). We discuss the challenges encountered during each phase, and present methods our team used to overcome these challenges in order to identify neural biomarkers of smoking relapse and translate these findings to novel neuroscience-based interventions for tobacco dependence.

4.2   Development

Tobacco smoking is the leading preventable cause of death worldwide (World Health Organization 2011). Quitting smoking significantly reduces the risk of smoking-related health problems, and 70% of adult smokers in the United States report a desire to quit smoking completely (Centers for Disease Control and Prevention 2011a). Despite this, only 3% of smokers are able to successfully quit in the long term without assistance (Benowitz 2010). Nicotine is the psychoactive substance in tobacco responsible for its addictive properties. Long-term nicotine exposure results in neurobiological changes, and nicotine withdrawal is associated with impaired cognitive function as well as subjective symptoms of craving (Leventhal et al. 2010). Withdrawal symptoms contribute to high rates of relapse during the first week of a quit attempt (Hughes 2007; Piasecki 2006). Currently,

there are only three FDA-approved pharmacological treatments for smoking cessation: nicotine replacement therapy, bupropion, and varenicline. All of these treatments mitigate withdrawal symptoms to some degree, but even with the best treatment less than a third of smokers are able to remain quit for more than a year (Benowitz 2010). To address this challenge, we embarked on a transdisciplinary research program to (1) improve understanding of the cognitive and neural mechanisms that promote relapse, and (2) apply this new knowledge about therapeutic targets to develop innovative smoking cessation interventions. Because nicotine withdrawal and smoking relapse are complex multifactorial phenomena, we sought to integrate knowledge from diverse fields including behavioral science, pharmacology, genetics, and cognitive neuroscience. One of the first challenges to creating our transdisciplinary research program was selecting the team of scientists who would be involved. Although it may seem straightforward to identify potential investigators with the desired expertise, we found that some researchers lacked the time or the inclination to engage in a long-term transdisciplinary collaboration. It was also necessary to seek out individuals who would be able to accommodate the unique demands of team science and contribute to positive interactions with other team members. We found a number of personal qualities which contribute to success in a transdisciplinary team science effort, including:

A commitment to transparency: Willingness to share ideas, techniques, and research findings with other members of the team.

Cognitive flexibility: Ability to integrate new conceptual perspectives and develop new and broader ways of thinking about problems.

Dependability: Responsivity to communication, and motivation to meet important project deadlines.

Patience: Patience to communicate complex concepts to diverse groups of scientists and perseverance in the face of the inevitable challenges that arise during the project.

In order to attract potential team members who possessed the necessary expertise, qualities that promote teamwork, and an interest in transdisciplinary research, we began hosting a series of seminars and lunch meetings on topics of interest. These gatherings helped to foster creative discussion and provided a sense of who might work well together. However, many of the potential team members were already very busy with their own research. One strategy that was successful to incentivize participation was offering the opportunity to obtain small pilot grants. This initiative focused on collaborative studies (investigators in at least two disciplines) addressing a common problem of relevance to smoking cessation treatment. For those who received pilot grant awards (and some who did not), the process led to increased engagement and the funds were leveraged for NIH grant submissions (and projects within the future Center grant renewal). Pilot awardees were asked to join the monthly research team meetings and to present their work. Most researchers found that they enjoyed the interaction with colleagues from other disciplines, and this provided intrinsic motivation to continue. Over time, these methods led to the coalescence of a convivial group of scientists with a shared interest in tobacco research and excitement for transdisciplinary science. This group became one of the first seven Transdisciplinary Tobacco Use Research Centers sponsored by the National Cancer Institute and National Institute on Drug Abuse.

4.3 Conceptualization

Once the team was assembled, the next step was to create a focused and integrated scientific vision and plan. The goal was to identify a common problem related to tobacco dependence treatment and a unifying conceptual framework that would leverage the strengths of a transdisciplinary approach to generate novel hypotheses and potential interventions. One of the first challenges encountered was the need to develop a common vocabulary to use when talking about the problem. A neuroscientist may approach the concept of "cognitive control" differently than a behavioral scientist, and this can lead to confusion during brainstorming sessions. To address this, we hosted a series of introductory lectures wherein team members had the opportunity to present fundamental concepts from their discipline and familiarize others with the technologies utilized in their research. These cross-education efforts helped to bridge the gap and establish a common language among group members. Strong consensus-based leadership was necessary to maintain focus on group objectives. Finally, it was important to maintain an open, friendly atmosphere during group interactions so that team members felt comfortable asking questions and sharing ideas.

After careful consideration of the existing body of knowledge, the interests of the investigators on the team, and the types of questions that could be approached using the techniques provided by each discipline, our efforts to identify a unifying theme converged on the cognitive and neural effects of early nicotine withdrawal and the influence of these processes on smoking relapse.

In order to frame our approach consistently across projects, we sought to develop a common conceptual model of self-control as it relates to smoking relapse. A major interest of our research team centered around self-control as an interaction between "bottom-up" reward-driven impulses and "top-down" executive cognitive control. Executive control refers to a core set of cognitive processes (including working memory, attentional control, and response inhibition) that support self-control and guide goal-directed behavior (Botvinick et al. 2001). Working memory is required to focus on goal-related information and on one's goals for behavior change (Baddeley 2003, 2007). Response inhibition requires effortful control to inhibit a "pre-potent" response (i.e., a habit or automatic behavior) (Logan 1994; Logan et al. 1977). The ultimate choices people make are thought to be influenced by an interplay between bottom-up reward and affective responses and top-down executive control processes in the brain.

In the context of tobacco dependence, executive control contributes to a smoker's ability to quit smoking. Smoking cessation requires self-control in order to inhibit habitual, automated behaviors (such as lighting a cigarette) and replace them with new goal-oriented behaviors (Sun et al. 2007). Working memory in particular facilitates top-down executive control through active maintenance of task-related goals (Mecklinger et al. 2003). When executive control is strong, choices are biased toward long-term rewards and goal-directed behavior such as quitting smoking, whereas when executive control is weaker, choices are biased toward immediate rewards and impulsive behavior, leading to smoking relapse (Fig. 4.1). Importantly, working memory is a limited cognitive resource which can be depleted by efforts to manage cravings (Kemps et al. 2008; Meule et al. 2012; Muraven and Baumeister 2000; Scharmuller et al. 2012; Tiggemann et al. 2010). Areas of the brain associated with working memory and executive control are active when smokers are attempting to resist craving (Hartwell et al. 2011), and individuals with poorer working memory are less able to resist smoking when cravings are strong (Day et al. 2015). However, smokers frequently report subjective deficits in cognitive function during nicotine withdrawal (Hughes 2007), and objectively measured deficits in executive processes such as working memory are apparent in laboratory studies (Mendrek et al. 2006;

Patterson et al. 2009). It seemed possible that withdrawal-induced deficits in cognitive control could negatively impact a smoker's ability to override reward-driven cravings and urges to smoke that promote relapse. The neural mechanisms underlying withdrawal-induced deficits were not clear, and the role of these deficits in smoking relapse had not been investigated. Our team therefore decided to apply their combined experience to test the hypothesis that executive cognitive control processes are compromised during early nicotine withdrawal, and the extent of these effects would predict smoking relapse.

4.4   Implementation

Having selected a unifying theme, our transdisciplinary approach allowed us to examine mechanisms involved in withdrawal-induced cognitive deficits at behavioral, neural, and genetic levels. We began by examining withdrawal-induced deficits during early abstinence using a behavioral pharmacology approach. Deficits in executive processes such as working memory and attention emerge during the first 24–72 h after stopping

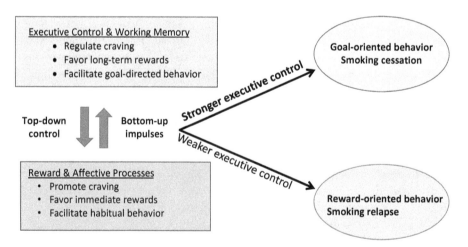

Fig. 4.1 An integrated model of neural processes contributing to smoking cessation. We developed a common conceptual model framing behavioral self-control as the product of an interaction between "bottom-up" reward-driven impulses and "top-down" executive cognitive control processes in the brain. Smoking cessation requires self-control in order to override habitual behaviors and

replace them with goal-oriented behaviors. When executive control is strong, choices are biased toward long-term rewards and goal-directed behavior such as quitting smoking, whereas when executive control is weaker, choices are biased toward immediate rewards and impulsive behavior, leading to smoking relapse smoking (Hughes 2007; Mendrek et al. 2006). This is a critical time period for smoking cessation, since most relapses to smoking behavior occur during this time frame (Piasecki 2006). Efficacious smoking cessation medications such as varenicline had been shown to reduce craving and somatic symptoms of withdrawal, but their effects on cognitive symptoms had not been well characterized. We utilized a within-subject crossover design to assess withdrawal-induced cognitive deficits and smoking behavior during two study periods. Each period consisted of a 10-day medication run-up period (varenicline or placebo) followed by a simulated quit attempt. This model involved 3 days of mandatory abstinence followed by a scheduled "lapse" where participants were instructed to return to smoking for a day. The next 7 days comprised a "practice quit attempt," during which participants were instructed to try to remain abstinent. Cognitive performance was assessed using a working memory task administered at baseline and on the third day of the mandatory abstinence period. In two studies utilizing this approach, we showed that withdrawal-induced deficits in working memory predicted the ability to remain abstinent during the 7-day practice quit attempt (Patterson et al. 2010); furthermore, treatment with varenicline mitigated these deficits (Patterson et al. 2009). These studies provided support for the hypothesis that cognitive deficits were an important facet of withdrawal that could contribute to smoking relapse.

From there, we decided to examine the neural underpinnings of withdrawal-induced cognitive deficits in order to gain a better understanding of the mechanisms. We initiated a new study incorporating functional magnetic resonance imaging (fMRI) into the smoking lapse model. This was similar to the prior studies, but on the third day of mandatory abstinence, participants also completed a working memory task during an fMRI scan. By incorporating neuroimaging, we were able to examine differences in working memory-related neural processes during abstinence. We found that varenicline increased brain activation in regions important to executive function (including the dorsolateral prefrontal cortex [DLPFC] and the medial frontal/cingulate gyrus [MF/CG]) when participants were completing the more difficult portions of the task. Varenicline also improved performance of the task in highly dependent smokers; among this group, better response times on the task were associated with higher levels of brain activity in the executive control regions (Loughead et al. 2010).

We then examined withdrawal-induced cognitive deficits from a genetic perspective. Catechol-o-methyltransferase (COMT) is an enzyme that inactivates the neurotransmitter dopamine, and individuals with a common variant in the gene encoding this enzyme (the Val allele of the *COMT* Val158Met variant) have been shown, in some studies, to have a higher risk of smoking relapse (Berrettini et al. 2007; Colilla et al. 2005; Johnstone et al. 2007; Munafo et al. 2008). This may be attributable to increased dopamine levels in brain, including in the prefrontal cortex where dopamine transporter levels are low (Chen et al. 2004). Because of the importance of dopamine in executive cognitive function (Logue and Gould 2014), we hypothesized that individuals with the Val allele might be more susceptible to withdrawal-induced working memory deficits and corresponding reductions in working-memory related activity in the prefrontal cortex. The results of our neuroimaging study comparing participants who were screened a priori for the *COMT* variant supported this hypothesis (Loughead et al. 2009). Unfortunately, however, these findings were not replicated in an independent study from our lab (Ashare et al. 2013a). Nor did we find evidence for the efficacy of a COMT-inhibitor medication, tolcapone, on withdrawal-related cognitive deficits or brain activity (Ashare et al. 2013b).

Despite the disappointing pharmacogenetic results, our studies continued to provide consistent support for an effect of abstinence on working memory-related brain activity. Based on this, we hypothesized that smokers who experienced greater withdrawal-induced deficits in working memory-related brain activity would be at greater risk of relapse during smoking cessation. To test our hypothesis, we incorporated neuroimaging into a clinical trial for treatment-seeking smokers (Loughead et al. 2015). Prior to taking part in a counseling-based smoking cessation program, participants completed two separate fMRI scanning sessions (one while they had been smoking as usual, and one following 24 h of biochemically confirmed abstinence), during which they performed a working memory task and a cue reactivity task. Consistent with the prior studies, during the working memory task, we observed abstinence-induced decreases in goal-directed neural activity in the bilateral DLPFC and medial frontal/cingulate gyrus (Falcone et al. 2014), as well as reduced suppression of goal-irrelevant brain activity in the default mode network, which is normally active when the brain is at rest and suppressed during performance of a task (Falcone et al. 2014; Fox et al. 2005). We also found reduced coupling between large-scale brain networks, leading to increases in clinical symptoms of nicotine withdrawal and craving (Lerman et al. 2014). Furthermore, reductions in working memory-related DLPFC activity predicted smoking relapse above and beyond standard clinical measures, with up to 81% accuracy (Loughead et al. 2015). Additional data suggest that abstinence-induced brain responses may be modified by individual differences. During the cue reactivity task, smokers who metabolize nicotine faster (and who would presumably be experiencing more rapid withdrawal) showed enhanced responses to smoking-related cues during abstinence, whereas slower metabolizers demonstrated slightly reduced responses (Falcone et al. 2016).

Moving from behavioral pharmacology studies to neuroimaging and genetics and then to a clinical trial was not without difficulty. Some of the challenges we faced will be familiar to anyone who has undertaken a collaborative research project: determining the appropriate staff allocations from each research group, coordinating schedules to ensure that the appropriate resources are available for each session, and ensuring that each team understands exactly which tasks they will be responsible for so that data are collected and processed in a timely fashion. Although we were all very familiar with the techniques within our own disciplines, we had to rely on each other to interpret the data from techniques unique to the others' disciplines, and had to be able explain our own interpretations clearly to the rest of the team. For example, although the behavioral scientists were confident in the interpretation of the behavioral and cognitive testing data, a collaborative approach with the neuroimaging experts was necessary to understand the brain data, and both groups contributed to the design of the clinical trial; the entire team had to work closely together to understand the data as a whole. We found that frequent meetings to discuss project updates and data analysis as well as ongoing cross-education efforts were very important as the projects progressed. These efforts paid off, and by the end of the clinical trial we had evidence from multiple lines of research supporting the hypothesis that withdrawal-induced reductions in brain activity in regions essential to executive cognitive function contribute to an increased risk of smoking relapse. Taken in conjunction with the research showing that an efficacious smoking cessation medication mitigates the effects of withdrawal on brain activity, these findings suggested that enhancing DLPFC activity might offer a novel approach to smoking cessation.

4.5   Translation

With this hypothesis in mind, we consulted the literature for methods of enhancing DLPFC activity. Once thought to be fixed by adulthood, recent evidence shows that executive cognitive function can be enhanced through training of working memory, attention, response inhibition, or problem solving (Ball et al. 2002; Jaeggi et al. 2008, 2011; Nouchi et al. 2013; Willis et al. 2006). Moreover, improvements in performance in one cognitive domain may transfer to others (Buschkuehl et al. 2012; Dahlin et al. 2008; b; Willis et al. 2006). However, debate over whether improvements on specific trained tasks contribute to improvements only in similar tasks (called "near transfer") or to other domains of executive function (called "far transfer") is ongoing (Barnett and Ceci 2002). For example, some studies have shown that computer-based training programs targeting working memory can improve performance on untrained tasks such as verbal learning (Richmond et al. 2011), selective attention and reading comprehension (Chein and Morrison 2010), and fluid intelligence (Jaeggi et al. 2008, 2011). However, other studies show no benefits beyond improvements on the trained task (Gomar et al. 2015; Owen et al. 2010; Thompson et al. 2013). Only a few studies had investigated cognitive training as an adjunctive treatment for addiction. For example, a study of 27 stimulant addicts compared active working memory training with a control training program that provided answers to participants (so that the working memory system was not engaged) (Bickel et al. 2011). Participants in the active training group, but not the control group, showed decreased delay discounting rates (a measure of impulsivity) post-training compared to pre-training rates (Bickel et al. 2011). A study of 48 problem drinkers who completed 25 training sessions over at least 25 days demonstrated that working memory training decreased short-term alcohol intake (Houben et al. 2011).

Based on our findings, we undertook a clinical trial examining whether cognitive training could be used as an adjunctive smoking cessation treatment (Loughead et al. 2016). In this study, 213 treatment-seeking smokers received either 12 weeks of computerized cognitive training targeting multiple executive function domains (including working memory, attention, and response inhibition) or 12 weeks of computerized relaxation exercises (control group). Both groups received nicotine replacement therapy and smoking cessation counseling beginning on week 4 of the training program. Unfortunately, although the active training group showed some improvement in cognitive performance at the end of the training period, there were no differences in smoking cessation rates between groups (Loughead et al. 2016).

A second clinical trial in healthy young adults examined whether cognitive training could improve executive cognitive function, thereby shifting risk sensitivity and decision-making (Kable et al. 2017). This trial compared a commercially available training program (Lumosity®, www.lumosity.com) to an active control group in which participants played video games that required motor coordination but did not specifically target working memory. Both groups completed five 30-min sessions of their assigned training per week for 10 weeks. Participants completed fMRI neuroimaging sessions before and after training. During these sessions they completed a delay discounting task and a risk sensitivity task in the scanner, in addition to a computerized battery of executive function tasks administered out of the scanner. This study also found no evidence for relative improvements in cognitive function, delay discounting or risk sensitivity, and no changes in brain response during these tasks from pre- to post-training. Furthermore, both groups showed similar improvement on the executive function tasks to a degree comparable to a no-contact control group, suggesting that the improvements in the active conditions reflected simple practice effects (Kable et al. 2017). In conjunction with the smoking cessation study, these results suggest that cognitive training may not produce sufficient transfer effects to modulate risky decision-making or addictive behavior.

Although these studies did not support the use of cognitive training alone as an adjunctive smoking cessation treatment, we still wanted to explore other methods of cognitive enhancement, such as noninvasive brain stimulation. Transcranial direct current stimulation (tDCS) is a noninvasive technique in which electrodes are placed on the scalp and a low current (i.e., 1–2 mA) is passed through the underlying tissue to stimulate brain activity (Coffman et al. 2014). Importantly, changes in brain activity persist after stimulation has ended, an effect attributed to long-term potentiation of stimulated synapses (Nitsche et al. 2003). The safety of tDCS is also well documented. Subjective effects tend to be mild and transient (tingling, itching, or warm sensation at the electrode site, fatigue during stimulation but not after) (Iyer et al. 2005; Poreisz et al. 2007).

A growing body of evidence supports the potential efficacy of active tDCS (vs. sham tDCS) for improving executive cognitive function in healthy individuals, as well as those with psychiatric or neurological disorders (Brevet-Aeby et al. 2016; Demirtas-Tatlidede et al. 2013; Spagnolo and Goldman 2017). Even a single session of tDCS targeted to the DLPFC can improve memory, planning ability, functional brain connectivity, and neural efficiency during cognitive processing (Dockery et al. 2009; Keeser et al. 2011; Meinzer et al. 2014). Improvements in cognitive function and clinical symptoms result from multi-session tDCS for depression and schizophrenia (Boggio et al. 2008; Brunelin et al. 2012; Fregni et al. 2006; Goder et al. 2013; Vercammen et al. 2011), Parkinson's disease (Benninger et al. 2010; Boggio et al. 2006; Fregni et al. 2006), and Alzheimer's disease (Boggio et al. 2012; Ferrucci et al. 2008). Cravings for food or cigarettes also appear to decrease immediately following active tDCS (vs. sham) (Fregni et al. 2008; b; Goldman et al. 2011; Val-Laillet et al. 2015).

Although we were interested in pursuing tDCS as a potential treatment for smoking cessation, our existing team lacked experience with neurostimulation. In order to follow up on our lead, we sought new collaborators with expertise in clinical applications of neurostimulation. The challenges of finding and integrating a new neurologist collaborator into an existing transdisciplinary team were similar to those encountered during the initial development phase. We found that our ability to offer incentives such as effort support, co-authorship, and new grant collaborations helped us to entice new collaborators to become involved with our translational research efforts. Once involved, we integrated them into our regular team meetings, offering both the opportunity to learn about our ongoing research efforts and to teach the rest of the team about their field.

With the support of our new collaborators, we examined the effects of tDCS on smoking behavior using a validated laboratory-based smoking lapse paradigm (Falcone et al. 2016). In this paradigm, smokers who were abstinent overnight were given a chance to smoke or to earn money by not smoking ($1 for every 5 min they resisted) (McKee et al. 2012). Smokers who received active tDCS during this paradigm were able to resist smoking longer than those who received sham tDCS (Falcone et al. 2016). These promising results reflected acute effects of a single session of tDCS; however, repeated tDCS administration has been shown to have a cumulative effect on reducing cue-induced cigarette craving (Boggio et al. 2009), and multiple sessions of tDCS can reduce food intake and self-reported appetite (Jauch-Chara et al. 2014). The next step will be to examine effects of repeated sessions of tDCS on smoking behavior; should this prove successful, this evidence will provide support for undertaking a larger clinical trial of tDCS for smoking cessation.

4.6 Conclusions and Future Directions

To summarize, each phase of our transdisciplinary research program presented unique challenges which required thoughtful solutions in order to proceed with the research. Carefully selecting the group of scientists who will make up the core of the transdisciplinary team is critical to the success of the project. These scientists must have a shared interest in transdisciplinary collaboration, and must also be able to accommodate the unique demands of transdisciplinary work and contribute to positive interactions with other team members. Informal seminars on interesting topics can entice busy researchers to engage with the project, spark creative discussions, and provide a sense of who will work well together. Next, it is important to determine a collective vision for the group prior to initiating research activities. Establishing consensus on the overarching goals of the collaboration will help to maintain focus on group objectives, rather than encouraging individual contributors to split off into their own projects. Developing a common conceptual model and engaging in cross-education is key to establishing a common language among group members. Finally, frequent personal interaction is important in building interdisciplinary relationships and encouraging a true "team science" approach. Regular meetings to discuss research progress not only keep group members informed but also encourage feedback and spark creative discussions that inspire innovative approaches to research problems. As with any professional relationship, ongoing effort to encourage a team mentality will help keep members invested in the outcomes of the collaboration.

Our interdisciplinary research efforts allowed us to investigate the neural substrates of the cognitive effects of nicotine withdrawal and to apply this knowledge to develop novel smoking cessation treatments, a topic that would have been difficult to address from a single disciplinary perspective. Once we identified a novel potential target for smoking cessation treatment, our transdisciplinary collaboration allowed us to progress quickly to translational studies, rather than simply publishing the information and hoping that another research group with the necessary expertise would pick up the thread. If successful, this treatment approach could have applications to other health behaviors. For example, working memory-related DLPFC activity plays a central role in obesity. Much like smoking, obesity is also associated with reduced function in the executive control network, possibly due to brain changes in cardiovascular and metabolic function (Gunstad et al. 2007; Spitznagel et al. 2015). Working memory-related brain activity predicts weight loss outcomes (Hege et al. 2013), and successful dieters show greater activation in the DLPFC following food intake compared to unsuccessful dieters, which may suggest engagement of cognitive control circuits to downregulate reward-driven responses (DelParigi et al. 2007). It is therefore possible that treatments designed to increase executive control processes in the brain could benefit individuals who are trying to lose weight.

Although great strides have been made in leveraging our understanding of the brain in order to facilitate behavior change, there is still much research to be done to bring these findings to clinical use. Mechanistic imaging studies could offer insight into whether specific executive domains are more or less effective at supporting self-control. This information would aid in the development of treatments that engage those domains to facilitate behavior change. Further development is also needed to optimize current targets of behavioral interventions. Although initial studies suggest that cognitive training and brain stimulation may be valuable tools for treating addiction, research evaluating the efficacy of these interventions for obesity and other risky health behaviors is still limited. Finally, larger clinical trials are necessary to evaluate the efficacy of behavioral interventions and brain stimulation in promoting healthy decision-making before implementing these treatments in a clinical setting. Integrating interdisciplinary teams into each stage of research will optimize the development of novel treatments by offering broader perspectives on complex health behavior interventions.

Acknowledgment This work was supported by NCI grants R35-CA197461, R01-CA170297, and R01-DA030819.

References

An LC, et al. The RealU online cessation intervention for college smokers: a randomized controlled trial. Prev Med. 2008;47:194–9.

Arem H, et al. Leisure time physical activity and mortality: a detailed pooled analysis of the dose-response relationship. JAMA Intern Med. 2015;175:959–67.

Ashare RL, et al. Association of abstinence-induced alterations in working memory function and COMT genotype in smokers. Psychopharmacology. 2013a;230:653–62.

Ashare RL, et al. Effects of tolcapone on working memory and brain activity in abstinent smokers: a proof-of-concept study. Drug Alcohol Depend. 2013b;133:852–6.

Baddeley A. Working memory: looking back and looking forward. Nat Rev Neurosci. 2003;4:829–39.

Baddeley A. Working memory, thought, and action. Oxford: Oxford University Press; 2007.

Ball K, et al. Effects of cognitive training interventions with older adults: a randomized controlled trial. JAMA. 2002;288:2271–81.

Barnett SM, Ceci SJ. When and where do we apply what we learn? A taxonomy for far transfer. Psychol Bull. 2002;128:612–37.

Benninger DH, Lomarev M, Lopez G, Wassermann EM, Li X, Considine E, Hallett M. Transcranial direct current stimulation for the treatment of Parkinson's disease. J Neurol Neurosurg Psychiatry. 2010;81:1105–11.

Benowitz NL. Nicotine addiction. N Engl J Med. 2010;362:2295–303.

Berrettini WH, et al. Catechol-O-methyltransferase (COMT) gene variants predict response to bupropion therapy for tobacco dependence. Biol Psychiatry. 2007;61:111–8.

Bickel WK, Yi R, Landes RD, Hill PF, Baxter C. Remember the future: working memory training decreases delay discounting among stimulant addicts. Biol Psychiatry. 2011;69:260–5.

Boggio PS, Ferrucci R, Rigonatti SP, Covre P, Nitsche M, Pascual-Leone A, Fregni F. Effects of transcranial direct current stimulation on working memory in patients with Parkinson's disease. J Neurol Sci. 2006;249:31–8.

Boggio PS, Liguori P, Sultani N, Rezende L, Fecteau S, Fregni F. Cumulative priming effects of cortical stimulation on smoking cue-induced craving. Neurosci Lett. 2009;463:82–6.

Boggio PS, Rigonatti SP, Ribeiro RB, Myczkowski ML, Nitsche MA, Pascual-Leone A, Fregni F. A randomized, double-blind clinical trial on the efficacy of cortical direct current stimulation for the treatment of major depression. Int J Neuropsychopharmacol. 2008;11:249–54.

Boggio PS, et al. Prolonged visual memory enhancement after direct current stimulation in Alzheimer's disease. Brain Stimul. 2012;5:223–30.

Botvinick MM, Braver TS, Barch DM, Carter CS, Cohen JD. Conflict monitoring and cognitive control. Psychol Rev. 2001;108:624–52.

Brevet-Aeby C, Brunelin J, Iceta S, Padovan C, Poulet E. Prefrontal cortex and impulsivity: interest of noninvasive brain stimulation. Neurosci Biobehav Rev. 2016;71:112–34.

Brunelin J, et al. Examining transcranial direct-current stimulation (tDCS) as a treatment for hallucinations in schizophrenia. Am J Psychiatry. 2012;169:719–24.

Buschkuehl M, Jaeggi SM, Jonides J. Neuronal effects following working memory training. Dev Cogn Neurosci. 2012;2(Suppl 1):S167–79.

Cahill K, Stevens S, Perera R, Lancaster T. Pharmacological interventions for smoking cessation: an overview and network meta-analysis. Cochrane Database Syst Rev. 2013;5:CD009329.

Calfas KJ, et al. Project GRAD: two-year outcomes of a randomized controlled physical activity intervention among young adults. Graduate ready for activity daily. Am J Prev Med. 2000;18:28–37.

Centers for Disease Control and Prevention. Exercise or physical activity. 2010. http://www.cdc.gov/nchs/fastats/exercise.htm

Centers for Disease Control and Prevention. Quitting smoking among adults--United States, 2001–2010. MMWR Morb Mortal Wkly Rep. 2011a;60:1513–9.

Centers for Disease Control and Prevention. Vital signs: current cigarette smoking among adults aged >/=18 years--United States, 2005–2010. MMWR Morb Mortal Wkly Rep. 2011b;60:1207–12.

Centers for Disease Control and Prevention. Adult obesity causes & consequences. 2015. http://www.cdc.gov/obesity/adult/causes.html

Chein JM, Morrison AB. Expanding the mind's workspace: training and transfer effects with a complex working memory span task. Psychon Bull Rev. 2010;17:193–9.

Chen J, et al. Functional analysis of genetic variation in catechol-O-methyltransferase (COMT): effects on mRNA, protein, and enzyme activity in postmortem human brain. Am J Hum Genet. 2004;75:807–21.

Coffman BA, Clark VP, Parasuraman R. Battery powered thought: enhancement of attention, learning, and memory in healthy adults using transcranial direct current stimulation. NeuroImage. 2014;85(Pt 3):895–908.

Colilla S, et al. Association of catechol-O-methyltransferase with smoking cessation in two independent studies of women. Pharmacogenet Genomics. 2005;15:393–8.

Dahlin E, Neely AS, Larsson A, Backman L, Nyberg L. Transfer of learning after updating training mediated by the striatum. Science. 2008;320:1510–2.

Dahlin E, Nyberg L, Backman L, Neely AS. Plasticity of executive functioning in young and older adults: immediate training gains, transfer, and long-term maintenance. Psychol Aging. 2008;23:720–30.

Day AM, Kahler CW, Metrik J, Spillane NS, Tidey JW, Rohsenow DJ. Working memory moderates the association between smoking urge and smoking lapse behavior after alcohol Administration in a Laboratory Analogue Task. Nicotine Tob Res. 2015;17:1173–7.

DelParigi A, Chen K, Salbe AD, Hill JO, Wing RR, Reiman EM, Tataranni PA. Successful dieters have increased neural activity in cortical areas involved in the control of behavior. Int J Obes. 2007;31:440–8.

Demirtas-Tatlidede A, Vahabzadeh-Hagh AM, Pascual-Leone A. Can noninvasive brain stimulation enhance cognition in neuropsychiatric disorders? Neuropharmacology. 2013;64:566–78.

Dockery CA, Hueckel-Weng R, Birbaumer N, Plewnia C. Enhancement of planning ability by transcranial direct current stimulation. J Neurosci. 2009;29:7271–7.

Elder JP, Sallis JF, Woodruff SI, Wildey MB. Tobacco-refusal skills and tobacco use among high-risk adolescents. J Behav Med. 1993;16:629–42.

Falcone M, Cao W, Bernardo L, Tyndale RF, Loughead J, Lerman C. Brain responses to smoking cues differ based on nicotine metabolism rate. Biol Psychiatry. 2016;80:190–7.

Falcone M, et al. Age-related differences in working memory deficits during nicotine withdrawal. Addict Biol. 2014;19:907–17.

Falcone M, et al. Transcranial direct current brain stimulation increases ability to resist smoking. Brain Stimul. 2016;9:191–6.

Ferrucci R, et al. Transcranial direct current stimulation improves recognition memory in Alzheimer disease. Neurology. 2008;71:493–8.

Fox MD, Snyder AZ, Vincent JL, Corbetta M, Van Essen DC, Raichle ME. The human brain is intrinsically organized into dynamic, anticorrelated functional networks. Proc Natl Acad Sci U S A. 2005;102:9673–8.

Fregni F, Boggio PS, Nitsche MA, Rigonatti SP, Pascual-Leone A. Cognitive effects of repeated sessions of transcranial direct current stimulation in patients with depression. Depress Anxiety. 2006;23:482–4.

Fregni F, Liguori P, Fecteau S, Nitsche MA, Pascual-Leone A, Boggio PS. Cortical stimulation of the prefrontal cortex with transcranial direct current stimulation reduces cue-provoked smoking craving: a randomized, sham-controlled study. J Clin Psychiatry. 2008;69:32–40.

Fregni F, et al. Noninvasive cortical stimulation with transcranial direct current stimulation in Parkinson's disease. Mov Disord. 2006;21:1693–702.

Fregni F, et al. Transcranial direct current stimulation of the prefrontal cortex modulates the desire for specific foods. Appetite. 2008;51:34–41.

Goder R, Baier PC, Beith B, Baecker C, Seeck-Hirschner M, Junghanns K, Marshall L. Effects of transcranial direct current stimulation during sleep on memory performance in patients with schizophrenia. Schizophr Res. 2013;144:153–4.

Goldman RL, et al. Prefrontal cortex transcranial direct current stimulation (tDCS) temporarily reduces food cravings and increases the self-reported ability to resist food in adults with frequent food craving. Appetite. 2011;56:741–6.

Gomar JJ, et al. A multisite, randomized controlled clinical trial of computerized cognitive remediation therapy for schizophrenia. Schizophr Bull. 2015;41:1387–96.

Greaves CJ, et al. Systematic review of reviews of intervention components associated with increased effectiveness in dietary and physical activity interventions. BMC Public Health. 2011;11:119.

Gunstad J, Paul RH, Cohen RA, Tate DF, Spitznagel MB, Gordon E. Elevated body mass index is associated with executive dysfunction in otherwise healthy adults. Compr Psychiatry. 2007;48:57–61.

Hall KL, Vogel AL, Stipelman B, Stokols D, Morgan G, Gehlert S. A four-phase model of transdisciplinary team-based research: goals, team processes, and strategies. Transl Behav Med. 2012;2:415–30.

Hartwell KJ, Johnson KA, Li X, Myrick H, LeMatty T, George MS, Brady KT. Neural correlates of craving and resisting craving for tobacco in nicotine dependent smokers. Addict Biol. 2011;16:654–66.

Hege MA, Stingl KT, Ketterer C, Haring HU, Heni M, Fritsche A, Preissl H. Working memory-related brain activity is associated with outcome of lifestyle intervention. Obesity (Silver Spring). 2013;21:2488–94.

Houben K, Wiers RW, Jansen A. Getting a grip on drinking behavior: training working memory to reduce alcohol abuse. Psychol Sci. 2011;22:968–75.

Hughes JR. Effects of abstinence from tobacco: valid symptoms and time course. Nicotine Tob Res. 2007;9:315–27.

Hutfless S, et al. Strategies to prevent weight gain in adults: a systematic review. Am J Prev Med. 2013a;45:e41–51.

Hutfless S, et al. Strategies to prevent weight gain among Adults. Comparative effectiveness review No. 97. (Prepared by The Johns Hopkins University Evidence-based Practice Center under Contract No. 290-2007-10061-I.). Rockville, MD: Agency for Healthcare Research and Quality; 2013b.

Iyer MB, Mattu U, Grafman J, Lomarev M, Sato S, Wassermann EM. Safety and cognitive effect of frontal DC brain polarization in healthy individuals. Neurology. 2005;64:872–5.

Jaeggi SM, Buschkuehl M, Jonides J, Perrig WJ. Improving fluid intelligence with training on working memory. Proc Natl Acad Sci U S A. 2008;105:6829–33.

Jaeggi SM, Buschkuehl M, Jonides J, Shah P. Short- and long-term benefits of cognitive training. Proc Natl Acad Sci U S A. 2011;108:10081–6.

Jauch-Chara K, Kistenmacher A, Herzog N, Schwarz M, Schweiger U, Oltmanns KM. Repetitive electric brain stimulation reduces food intake in humans. Am J Clin Nutr. 2014;100:1003–9.

Johnstone EC, Elliot KM, David SP, Murphy MF, Walton RT, Munafo MR. Association of COMT Val108/158Met genotype with smoking cessation in a nicotine replacement therapy randomized trial. Cancer Epidemiol Biomark Prev. 2007;16:1065–9.

Kable JW, et al. No effect of commercial cognitive training on brain activity, choice behavior, or cognitive performance. J Neurosci. 2017;37:7390–402.

Keeser D, et al. Prefrontal transcranial direct current stimulation changes connectivity of resting-state networks during fMRI. J Neurosci. 2011;31:15284–93.

Kemps E, Tiggemann M, Grigg M. Food cravings consume limited cognitive resources. J Exp Psychol Appl. 2008;14:247–54.

Lerman C, Gu H, Loughead J, Ruparel K, Yang Y, Stein EA. Large-scale brain network coupling predicts acute nicotine abstinence effects on craving and cognitive function. JAMA Psychiat. 2014;71:523–30.

Leventhal AM, Waters AJ, Moolchan ET, Heishman SJ, Pickworth WB. A quantitative analysis of subjective, cognitive, and physiological manifestations of the acute tobacco abstinence syndrome. Addict Behav. 2010;35:1120–30.

Lin JS, O'Connor E, Whitlock EP, Beil TL. Behavioral counseling to promote physical activity and a healthful diet to prevent cardiovascular disease in adults: a systematic review for the U.S. Preventive Services Task Force. Ann Intern Med. 2010;153:736–50.

Logan GD. On the ability to inhibit thought and action: a user's guide to the stop signal paradigm. In: Dagenbach D, Carr TH, editors. Inhibitory processes in attention, memory, and language. San Diego, CA: Academic Press; 1994. p. 189–238.

Logan GD, Schachar RJ, Tannock R. Impulsivity and inhibitory control. Psychol Sci. 1977;8:60–6.

Logue SF, Gould TJ. The neural and genetic basis of executive function: attention, cognitive flexibility, and response inhibition. Pharmacol Biochem Behav. 2014;123:45–54.

Loughead J, Wileyto EP, Ruparel K, Falcone M, Hopson R, Gur R, Lerman C. Working memory-related neural activity predicts future smoking relapse. Neuropsychopharmacology. 2015;40:1311–20.

Loughead J, et al. Effect of abstinence challenge on brain function and cognition in smokers differs by COMT genotype. Mol Psychiatry. 2009;14:820–6.

Loughead J, et al. Effects of the alpha4beta2 partial agonist varenicline on brain activity and working memory in abstinent smokers. Biol Psychiatry. 2010;67:715–21.

Loughead J, et al. Can brain games help smokers quit?: Results of a randomized clinical trial. Drug Alcohol Depend. 2016;168:112–8.

McKee SA, Weinberger AH, Shi J, Tetrault J, Coppola S. Developing and validating a human laboratory model to screen medications for smoking cessation. Nicotine Tob Res. 2012;14:1362–71.

Mecklinger A, Weber K, Gunter TC, Engle RW. Dissociable brain mechanisms for inhibitory control: effects of interference content and working memory capacity. Brain Res Cogn Brain Res. 2003;18:26–38.

Meinzer M, et al. Transcranial direct current stimulation over multiple days improves learning and maintenance of a novel vocabulary. Cortex. 2014;50:137–47.

Mendrek A, et al. Working memory in cigarette smokers: comparison to non-smokers and effects of abstinence. Addict Behav. 2006;31:833–44.

Meule A, Skirde AK, Freund R, Vogele C, Kubler A. High-calorie food-cues impair working memory performance in high and low food cravers. Appetite. 2012;59:264–9.

Munafo MR, Johnstone EC, Guo B, Murphy MF, Aveyard P. Association of COMT Val108/158Met genotype with smoking cessation. Pharmacogenet Genomics. 2008;18:121–8.

Muraven M, Baumeister RF. Self-regulation and depletion of limited resources: does self-control resemble a muscle? Psychol Bull. 2000;126:247–59.

NIH Consensus Development Conference. Physical activity and cardiovascular health. NIH consensus development panel on physical activity and cardiovascular health. JAMA. 1996;276:241–6.

Nitsche MA, et al. Pharmacological modulation of cortical excitability shifts induced by transcranial direct current stimulation in humans. J Physiol. 2003;553:293–301.

Nouchi R, et al. Brain training game boosts executive functions, working memory and processing speed in the young adults: a randomized controlled trial. PLoS One. 2013;8:e55518.

Owen AM, et al. Putting brain training to the test. Nature. 2010;465:775–8.

Patterson F, et al. Varenicline improves mood and cognition during smoking abstinence. Biol Psychiatry. 2009;65:144–9.

Patterson F, et al. Working memory deficits predict short-term smoking resumption following brief abstinence. Drug Alcohol Depend. 2010;106:61–4.

Piasecki TM. Relapse to smoking. Clin Psychol Rev. 2006;26:196–215.

Poreisz C, Boros K, Antal A, Paulus W. Safety aspects of transcranial direct current stimulation concerning healthy subjects and patients. Brain Res Bull. 2007;72:208–14.

Richmond LL, Morrison AB, Chein JM, Olson IR. Working memory training and transfer in older adults. Psychol Aging. 2011;26:813–22.

Scharmuller W, Ubel S, Ebner F, Schienle A. Appetite regulation during food cue exposure: a comparison of normal-weight and obese women. Neurosci Lett. 2012;518:106–10.

Spagnolo PA, Goldman D. Neuromodulation interventions for addictive disorders: challenges, promise, and roadmap for future research. Brain. 2017;140:1183–203.

Spitznagel MB, Hawkins M, Alosco M, Galioto R, Garcia S, Miller L, Gunstad J. Neurocognitive effects of obesity and bariatric surgery. Eur Eat Disord Rev. 2015;23:488–95.

Sun X, Prochaska JO, Velicer WF, Laforge RG. Transtheoretical principles and processes for quitting smoking: a 24-month comparison of a representative sample of quitters, relapsers, and non-quitters. Addict Behav. 2007;32:2707–26.

Thompson TW, et al. Failure of working memory training to enhance cognition or intelligence. PLoS One. 2013;8:e63614.

Tiggemann M, Kemps E, Parnell J. The selective impact of chocolate craving on visuospatial working memory. Appetite. 2010;55:44–8.

US Department of Health and Human Services. The health benefits of smoking cessation: a report of the surgeon general. US Department of Health and Human Services Office on Smoking and Health DHHS Publication No (CDC) YO-K-116; 1990.

Val-Laillet D, et al. Neuroimaging and neuromodulation approaches to study eating behavior and prevent and treat eating disorders and obesity. Neuroimage Clin. 2015;8:1–31.

Vercammen A, Rushby JA, Loo C, Short B, Weickert CS, Weickert TW. Transcranial direct current stimulation influences probabilistic association learning in schizophrenia. Schizophr Res. 2011;131:198–205.

Willis SL, et al. Long-term effects of cognitive training on everyday functional outcomes in older adults. JAMA. 2006;296:2805–14.

Wing RR, Phelan S. Long-term weight loss maintenance. Am J Clin Nutr. 2005;82:222S–5S.

World Health Organization. WHO report on the global tobacco epidemic. Geneva: World Health Organization; 2011. p. 2011.

Yanovski SZ, Yanovski JA. Long-term drug treatment for obesity: a systematic and clinical review. JAMA. 2014;311:74–86.

The Intersection of Technology and Health: Using Human Computer Interaction and Ubiquitous Computing to Drive Behavioral Intervention Research

Rosa I. Arriaga and Gregory D. Abowd

Contents

5.1 Introduction: Case Study of a Research Collaboration Between a Psychologist and Computer Scientist

In the last decade, our research group has made interesting strides in coupling computer science, psychology, and behavioral science. However, this was not a mechanistic process where we had a roadmap for how a psychologist and a computer scientist could collaborate and simply embarked on the journey. We had to articulate what the research values and methods were in each area and then derive an approach that could help us move forward. We were able to move forward because we respected the skill set that each brought to the questions at hand. It was not the case that either the computer scientist or the psychologist had the upper hand. We had the understanding that together we could address questions in a more productive manner. Also important was our conviction that for our work to have impact we needed to find domain experts outside our respective fields. Thus, we have had successful collaborations with public health researchers, pulmonologists, endocrinologists, cardiologists, and community entities both governmental and nongovernmental. In reaching outside of our disciplinary boundaries we developed a set of heuristics that were at first implicit. These guided our goal setting approach for embarking on these collaborations. We are now at a point where we can articulate these heuristics.

In this chapter, we share what we have learned about how to derive successful teams. Our hope is that other teams will benefit from our lessons learned and that this will make setting up these collaborations more efficient and effective. In our experience efficient collaborations are those that can quickly articulate a research question, a set of reasonable milestones, and a timeline for meeting these goals. We say a collaboration is effective if each disciplinary team has a desired deliverable that they can point to at the end of the collaboration. We have also found that success requires that the expectations of the various team members are managed early on. It is often a miscon-

R. I. Arriaga (✉) · G. D. Abowd
Georgia Institute of Technology, Atlanta, GA, USA
e-mail: arriaga@cc.gatech.edu

© Springer Nature Switzerland AG 2019
K. L. Hall et al. (eds.), *Strategies for Team Science Success*,
https://doi.org/10.1007/978-3-030-20992-6_5

ception that the computer scientists will be able to build a fully functional system for the domain expert. Likewise, we have found that the domain experts (especially physicians) are a deep source of knowledge but have hard constraints on their time. Knowing these two facts can help articulate what the deliverable will be for a given timeline. As academics, our deliverables are often in lock-step with the academic calendar. Will this be something we can finish in a semester in the context of a course we teach? If we have two or three semesters can we get a master's student to do their thesis on the project? Could this be the basis of doctoral work? The deliverables include artifacts such as research publications (in each other's domains), reports about the problem space, proof of concept designs, pilot studies, random control trials, etc.

This chapter is organized as follows. First, we will describe the set of values that we bring to the table as a computer scientist and psychologist. We then show how we have coupled these values to deepen our understanding about chronic care management and wellness. Finally, we will describe a set of lessons learned from our decade of collaboration.

5.2 Integrating Disciplinary Values

In this section, we describe how the interplay of disciplinary strengths can drive impactful research. On one hand, computing can alleviate some of the negative impact of chronic illness by leveraging the proliferation of new technologies to serve individuals with chronic illness and their care providers. Behavioral science, on the other hand, has a plethora of theories readily available to drive health interventions. Collaboration at the intersection of computing and behavioral science requires an understanding of methodologies that drive both fields. Computing and in particular the areas called ubiquitous computing and human computer interaction (HCI) derive technology via a User-Centered Design Approach. Behavioral research is driven by the scientific method, but

few researchers in this field know about User-Centered Design. In this section, we provide an overview of the User-Centered Design Approach. We also highlight two theories that have helped us bridge the computing and behavioral research divide. We discuss successful collaborations at the service of technology development for asthma and for autism spectrum disorder. But first, we will situate our discussion about computing by providing a brief history.

5.2.1 A Brief History of Computing and a Cautionary Tale

We will frame our conversation of the history of computing in terms of the people to device ratio, the canonical technology that defined a given era, and the kinds of applications that were developed at the time. The advent of computing as we know it came in the early 1930s with mainframe computers that would fill up a room. Many scientists would have to queue up with punch cards in hand in order to get these behemoths to run calculations that would previously be impossible to manage. The personal computer (PC) ushered in the second generation of computing in the late 1960. Personal computers were defined as, "… non (time) shared system containing sufficient processing power and storage capabilities to satisfy the needs of an individual user." The third generation of computing started in the 1980s, where some individuals not only had laptop but could have a car phone and even a mobile phone or a "palm pilot." We were able to start to envision a future where humans and sensors interact seamlessly.

In his seminal 1991 paper, Mark Weiser described an emerging area of "ubiquitous computing," what has been defined by others as the third generation of computing (after the mainframe and personal computing generations) Weiser (1991). Central to Weiser's vision was that by the late 1980's it was clear that computing devices were going to take on many different shapes and sizes beyond the mainframe and desktop/laptop form that was then familiar. By the middle of the first decade of the 21st century,

Weiser's vision of these computing devices had come true in the form of inch-scale handheld devices, foot-scale tablets and yard-scale (and larger) interactive displays. In 2016, Abowd wrote of a fourth generation of technologies that began to emerge by 2004 and that were distinctly different from what Weiser had predicted. These technologies included: "cloud" technologies of unlimited storage and computation made accessible via the network; "crowd" technologies that more intimately and programmatically brought human abilities into the computational loop; and "shroud" technologies that combine Internet of Things and wearable devices to create a layer of digital devices over the physical world to connect it to the digital world Abowd (2016). Arriaga noted that recognition technologies (primarily speech and vision) also started to see a dramatic increase in practical effectiveness around this time due to deep learning techniques Arriaga (2017). The combination of these technologies created what Abowd called "collective computing", or the ability for individuals to harness and acquire real-time expertise in domains for which they had no significant training. This now presents an opportunity in important domains, such as finance, education, and most important to this chapter, health.

The notion that sensors can provide data that improves quality of life is particularly appealing for researchers that work in healthcare. We can now imagine how technology can help a child with severe asthma to live a healthy happy life. She can have a wearable sensor on her chest to collect data about her current lung health as well as coughing episodes and sleep disruptions. This information would be fed to an algorithm that would update her medication regiment for the day via a mobile phone application. At the same time, the app would have information about the air quality and pollen counts for the day and provide advice about the kind of activity that would be safe. Whenever the child takes a puff from her inhaler, spatial and temporal data would be recorded. This would allow the caregiver to track medication adherence. As the child rides her bike to school, an environmental sensor on her wrist-watch tracks the air quality around her. Beyond the objective data, there could also be subjective data about symptoms the child is experiencing. Meta-data from all the sensors could recommend a route home from school to minimize exposure to poor quality air. Likewise, the child's parents could get correlational data for dairy intake and the child's asthma exacerbation. All of the information about the child's health, activity, and asthma exacerbation symptoms would be uploaded into a system that would start to come up with a profile and recommendations to improve his asthma management. If the child was part of a network of children in her city, we can also envision that the asthma system could make recommendations based on the collective data.

The example above highlights how simple it is to come up with ideas for systems that "could be built." This brings us to a major pitfall in computing and behavioral science collaborations: the false expectation of what computer scientist will do. Most computer scientists are not in a position to build whole systems. Further, most behavioral scientists are not in a position to know what system should be built. This brings us to the next section where instead of a generic computer scientist, we introduce behavioral scientists to human computer interaction (HCI) researchers. We then detail the value that comes from employing their paradigms to design computing systems. This approach is called User-Centered Design and it will be described in the next section.

5.2.2   An Introduction to Human Computer Interaction (HCI) and User-Centered Design

In the second generation of computing, the status quo became one person to one computer. This led to a new field in computer science called human computer interaction (HCI). HCI investigates the divide between technology and the individual using it. Given that humans are a primary focus, the field borrows methods from anthropology, sociology, and psychology; however, it is not driven by the scientific approach. It is driven by the goal of designing "interfaces" that are useful and usable (Dix et al. 2004). In this section, we provide a brief overview of definitions and methodology that are most commonly adopted by HCI researchers to develop interfaces or technologies (i.e., systems) for individual to meet their goals. Once again, we present these concepts because it allows behavioral scientists to mitigate their expectations of what deliverables the HCI researchers can provide.

A core concept in HCI is that "Users use interfaces to accomplish tasks." HCI researchers move from the premise that if we understand the individual using the system (i.e., user) and the task she wants to accomplish, then the best design can be developed (Dix et al. 2004). Figure 5.1 highlights the interplay of users, tasks, and interfaces. It shows that the "interface" is the mediation of the user's task ("Ut") and the technological system's core function ("S"). It also shows that the user must provide some input and that this leads to some output by the system. Figure 5.1 reminds us that sometimes accomplishing a task (like calling someone on our cell) requires us to engage a whole system (the mobile phone). Our cell phone (system) has a core function (communicate with others, Ut); however the cell phone has various input options for communicating with others (call via keypad, voice activation, or text, or email). Additionally each of these tasks requires input that will lead to the desired output—in the case of making a call the input can be pressing the contact icon for the desired person and the output is the other person's cell phone will ring. Note that in placing a call, I opted to try to reach the person on their cell phone, though I could have decided to call their office line instead.

User-Centered Design is the preferred paradigm in HCI. Figure 5.2 shows the typical 4-step design cycle which includes (1) Requirements Gathering, (2) Designing Alternatives (3) Prototyping, and (4) Evaluation. Each of these steps has a set of established techniques. While it is beyond the scope of this chapter to go into detail of the various techniques used in each of the steps, we will provide examples of how we have incorporated a variety of them in our published work. It should also be noted that there are slight variations of this 4-step process referred to by other names, including *Interaction Design* (Preece et al. 2015), Design Thinking (prominently promoted by the Stanford Design School), and Human-Centered Design (Norman 2013). One important consideration for behavioral scientists is that deliverables in collaboration with an HCI researcher can result from each of these steps.

The first step of the design process requires that the researcher obtain an in-depth understanding of the user, and the way she currently accomplishes the relevant set of tasks to meet her goals. In this step, HCI researchers employ a variety of techniques to understand the users and their current practices. These include naturalistic observation, ethnographies, survey, interviews, etc. The point is to gather as much qualitative and quanti-

S   O utput   U t
         interface
              I nput

Fig. 5.1 The relationship between users, interfaces, and systems

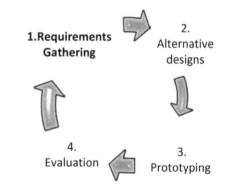

Fig. 5.2 The User-Centered Design cycle. Requirements Gathering is in bold to denote that this step is called by other names (e.g., analyses, needs assessment, research, etc). The same is true for the other steps

tative data as is needed to gain a thorough understanding of how the user is currently accomplishing a given task. In the second step, the researcher will gather the data collected via the requirement gathering phase and through inductive and deductive analyses develop a set of alternative designs to meet the user's goals. In one of our early asthma research projects (Jeong et al. 2011), we employed these first two steps to understand how children and their caregivers (i.e., users) manage asthma (i.e., task). During the requirement gathering phase, we went to the users' home and conducted interviews with both the caregiver and the child. We also observed where and how they kept track of the medicine and paraphernalia associated with their asthma management practices. We found that families commonly created their own asthma-care kits that include inhalers, peak flow meters, asthma action plan, and medication instructions. However, one of the problems they mentioned was that these kits were often incomplete or misplaced. Thus, we *designed* a smart kit whereby all of the items in the kit would have RFID tags and the bag would "keep track" of all of the items. The kit would be able to send text message alerts whenever any of the items were not back in the kit within a given set of time. Additionally, the bag could have a sensor that captured location information so the families could track the misplaced kit. The tracking system could ensure that the kit itself is not left behind. From Jeung et al.'s study we gain insights into the process of HCI/Ubicomp research. Notice that we never actually built the kit. In HCI both requirements gathering and designing alternatives constitute research contributions.

In the previous example we saw how researchers could take requirements gathering phase information and develop design alternatives for the user's current practices. In the Prototyping Step the researchers actually build models of the interfaces they designed. Building Prototypes serves a variety of purposes. First, it allows the researcher to envisage the various contexts where the design can be used. Second, it can be used to elicit feedback from the user to facilitate iterative design. We can see all three steps at work in Hong

et al. (2012). Here we were interested in how individuals with high-functioning autism (i.e., the users) could use technology to improve their quality of life. During the requirement gathering phase, we found that the individuals with autism wanted to increase their independence from their primary caregivers. We also found that their primary caregivers were often overburdened by the need to constantly address their child's needs and concerns. We proposed a system whereby an individual with autism could get support for their daily tasks remotely from friends and family. The system allowed friends and family to access the individual's calendar as well as other information (e.g., photographs) that was posted to this specialized social network. We built two prototypes of the system. Social Mirror was a physical prototype with limited functionality. We were able to share this with the users to collect feedback about how it could be improved. We then took what we learned from steps 1, 2, and 3, and iterate on the design. This led to a second video prototype that showed the system being "used" in various scenarios (see video here: https://www.youtube.com/watch?v=91-JnTq3MhA).

We started this section by stating that the goal of HCI was to build systems that were useful and usable. In the evaluation phase, step 4, researchers quantify if the system is useful and usable. By useful we mean that it actually meets the users' needs. By usable we mean that the user can accomplish the task (via the interface) in an effective, efficient, and satisfying manner. We must measure the degree to which the tasks are met with the new design. Evaluation is generally divided into two categories, formative and summative. Formative Evaluation is conducted early on in the design process with low-fidelity prototypes while Summative Evaluation is conducted with high-fidelity prototypes on a nearly final interface. Data collected in the evaluation phase can be qualitative data in the form of user interviews or quantitative in the form of surveys, or system log data that indicates how the user interacted with the system (e.g., number of mistakes the user made, amount of time the user spent on the system).

We can ascertain if the design is efficient by evaluating various task-related measures—these include time to completion, number of clicks, and number of errors while performing a task. We also need to have indicators of the subjective *user satisfaction* while executing the task—these can be both cognitive or emotional aspects. Cognitive measures can include mental effort required to complete the task, for example were the steps required to complete the task intuitive? For the emotional component, we want to have a sense of the feelings the user experienced as she completed the task.

Earlier we introduced you to SocialMirror (Hong et al. 2012). This study included three of the four phases in the design process: requirement gathering, designing alternatives, and prototyping. We were able to evaluate the main concept from SocialMirror via a field deployment with an off-the-shelf system called GroupMe (Hong et al. 2013). In this field deployment individuals with high functioning autism interacted with friends and families to garner social, emotional, and functional support. The system we used was a pre-existing text message-based social network system (a contemporary of WhatsApp) that allowed the individual to post question to their support network. The users (individuals with autism and their primary caregivers) found that the system effectively allowed an individual with autism to communicate their questions to the group members. The caregivers told us that they were happy that other people could answer their child's queries. In fact, there were times when other group members were able to provide more relevant information. Results also indicated that using the system fostered real-world interactions between the individuals with autism and their GroupMe supporters.

In this section, we reviewed the User-Centered Design process. As we saw from the research examples this process is not binding in the sense that all four steps need to be completed. Nor does it have to be followed in a particular order. We also showed that good HCI research need not apply the scientific method. In fact none of the studies we shared included experiments. The goal of the research was to have a deep understanding of the user and the task and thereby to develop novel technology designs. Moreover, the

examples showed that none of the systems were actually fully functional. It was enough to model the critical aspect of the design. Finally, the studies we presented in this section were not driven by any theoretical perspectives. In the next section, we share two theories that we have used in our research. One has guided our entry into experimental behavioral interventions and the other has allowed us to envision a Ubicomp solution to improve chronic care management.

5.2.3 Theories in Action: Case Studies from Our Work in Chronic Care Management

Thus far we have introduced the reader to two fields in computer science, ubiquitous computing (Ubicomp) and HCI, as well as the predominant paradigm in HCI, User-Centered Design. In this section we focus on how we integrated the psychological perspective into our research and how this led to impactful collaborations with our clinical partners. We discuss how we have conceptualized research at the crossroads of computing and behavioral science that leverages both fields. We also present a theory-based approach for closing important gaps in chronic care management. We show that the same theories that drive our research in pediatric health and developmental disabilities allow us to venture into the area of adult mental health.

As we mentioned earlier, our strength as a collaborative team comes from the fact that we can merge our competencies as a psychologist and as a computer scientist. When we employed User-Centered Design, many of our deliverables were novel/futuristic designs that were for the most part proof-of-concepts. These deliverables were interesting for our partners because it allowed them to have a broader understanding of their users (children with asthma or individuals with autism) and to conceptualize how the technology might change their practices in the future. However, it did not help them with their primary task, which is to improve chronic care management among their patients. However, coupling our computational strengths with a theoretical approach allowed us to build robust systems that could be brought to the clinical practice.

Our theory-based approach allows us to address three major gaps in chronic care management. These are (a) the medical care provider's lack of awareness of the patient's symptoms between scheduled visits, (b) the scarcity of tools to promote communication and support decision-making between patients and medical care providers, and (c) the lack of models that predict when a patient will have an exacerbation. In our research we have addressed the first two by (1) implementing a method for continuous patient monitoring between scheduled visits that includes timely recognition of symptom exacerbation and (2) developing a set of decision-support tools based on the symptoms the patient reports and their knowledge of the disease. We have also conceptualized how to solve the third gap, building predictive models, by integrating a variety of psychosocial, environmental, biological, and clinical data. We maintain that these computational models could predict the occurrence of negative events and can provide more personalized and timely interventions.

Our approach for improving chronic care management has three components: psycho-social theories,[1] a patient-centered continuous assessment system (P-CCAS), and a computational model. Two theories are central to our conceptualization of how to transform chronic care management; these are the Health Belief Model (HBM, Rosenstock 1974) and Bronfenbrenner's Ecological Systems Theory (EST, Bronfenbrenner 1977, 1979).

The Health Belief Model (HBM) is well known and used widely in the field of Behavioral Science. In HCI we are the first group that has used it extensively in technology design. The HBM explains and predicts health-related behavior in terms of the psychological and experiential factors that lead to positive behavior change (see Fig. 5.3). The HBM views the individual as the primary catalyst for change. It proposes that knowledge and perceived severity of the disease are two factors that influence whether an individual engages in beneficial

health behavior. It suggests that enhancing symptom awareness and knowledge through appropriate communication channels can positively impact the individual. We took all of these factors into account in developing the P-CCAS.

Our entrée into technology-based interventions was in the area of pediatric asthma. Our goal was to provide useful asthma education and queries about asthma symptoms (Yun et al. 2012). We opted for text message delivery because it was the preferred mode of communication for children. Text messages also made it possible to include children from a broader demographic base than could be reached via a mobile phone application (when we first conducted these studies).

As opposed to previous examples where our designs were driven by the user-centered approach, P-CCAS (see Fig. 5.4) was designed based on the HBM. Thus, we prioritized the asthmatic child's role in her asthma management and delivered the text messages directly to her, as opposed to her parent/caregiver. We hypothesized that by asking her about her symptoms we would raise her awareness of potential discomfort, or inconvenience (see Fig. 5.4A, first "symptom" text message) caused by asthma. In addition to making the patient aware of her symptoms we also gave her information about asthma (see Fig. 5.4A, second "knowledge" text messages). Data collected via the child's text message responses were fed into a dashboard that could be viewed by the pulmonologist (see Fig. 5.4B). This allowed communication to the physician that allowed continuous patient monitoring between scheduled visits and system alerts (see Fig. 5.4C) when the patient reported that they were not able to control their asthma. The ability for the medical care provider to access the child's responses also served to promote communication during scheduled visit following the intervention. The pulmonologist could discuss knowledge questions the child got wrong or symptoms the child had reported since their last visit.

The fact that our team now included clinical partners and patients meant that we had to alter our practices beyond our HCI objectives. We now

---

[1] These are not traditional HCI theories; see Rogers (2012) for a discussion of HCI theories.

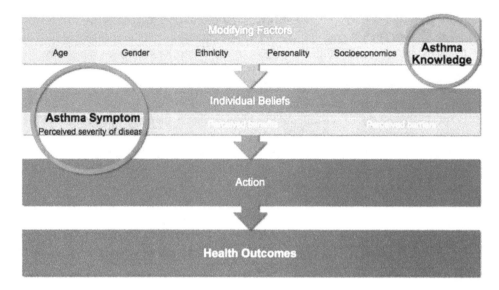

Fig. 5.3 The HBM modified for the asthma context

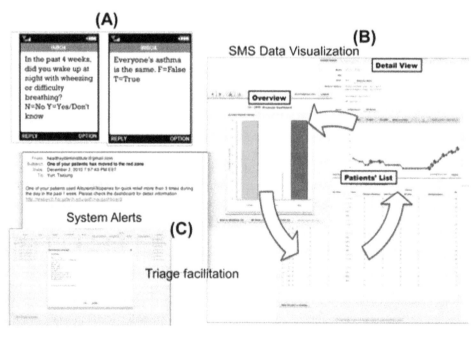

Fig. 5.4 The Asthma P-CCAS includes: text messages for patients (**A**), a physician dashboard (**B**) and communication interface (**C**)

had to include physiological and psychological outcomes. It was no longer enough that we had traditional HCI measures of system usability. It was also necessary that we move beyond proof of concept. We built robust computational systems that could function in the real world for extended periods of time. The P-CCAS interventions ran for about 3–4 months each. This was the time between two consecutive clinical visits. A third difference is that clinicians are also interested in whether results are reliable. So we conducted follow-up studies.

Results from the first P-CCAS study (Yun et al. 2012) showed children that responded to daily text messages had improved lung function and subjective quality of life compared to the control group and children who only received symptom queries. In HCI, this would be considered a successful deployment and researchers would go off to design another system. In psychology a follow-up study would be de rigueur at the very least to show that the positive results were not simply statistical anomalies. Thus, we conducted a second study that replicated the daily text condition and had a single text condition where children were queried about their asthma knowledge. We also tested the effectiveness of P-CCAS for children with different socio-economic backgrounds. We included children with private and public health insurance. Results showed that both groups of children had improved lung function when they answered daily text messages (compared to controls, Yun and Arriaga 2013). Also, children with public insurance, unlike controls or children with private insurance, showed physiological benefits even with a single text message every other day (Yun and Arriaga 2016).

In this section, we saw that a productive collaboration between HCI researchers and behavioral scientists was achieved by combining methods to reach a mutual goal. Along the way there were many bumps. Most notable was the fact that the first P-CCAS paper was rejected by the top Ubicomp conference because the technology was not considered novel enough. Notwithstanding the difficulty in publishing the first paper, the collaboration did lead to a variety of deliverables, including a robust system that improved children's health, a doctoral thesis, and several publications. The latter included an award, at the preeminent HCI conference, for conducting a replication study (Yun and Arriaga 2013) which is a rare practice among computer scientists!

5.2.4   How Theory Improves Design

Having designed P-CCAS using the HBM afforded us another opportunity. This was to test the notion that the system was generalizable and applicable beyond asthma. This is in sharp contrast to an HCI approach where the systems we build are considered useful and usable only to the target user. We adapted the P-CCAS to test the hypothesis that children with type 1 diabetes would benefit from the text message intervention. We kept the technical specifications the same (see Fig. 5.4) and worked with a group of pediatric endocrinologists to adapt the "symptom" and "knowledge" questions. This system was then deployed in a clinical setting. Here too, children who received daily text messages (between two scheduled doctor visits) were found to have improved quality of life compared to a control group (Han et al. 2015).

In our P-CCAS interventions we were able to bridge the HCI and behavioral science space. It met HCI standards in that we showed that it was useful and usable. Children had a very high response rate of nearly 90% across all deployments. P-CCAS was valuable to behavioral scientists because it was shown to improve health outcomes in children with type 1 diabetes and asthma. In using a theoretically driven computational system, we were also able to meet two important gaps in chronic care management: patient engagement and assessment within the "gaps" of care. It improved patient awareness about their own symptoms between doctor's visits; it also provided communication support tools for clinicians. We have also proposed a way that employing a psychology theory can close the third gap of chronic care management, computational models of disease exacerbation.

The second theory that has been central to our collaboration is Bronfenbrenner's Ecological System Theory (EST). The EST emphasizes the need to understand an individual and their interactions, in time (chronosystem) and space, with other individuals (Trudge 2009). The latter is exemplified by a set of four nested layers that envelop the individual. The idea of studying the individual in context is one that is central to User-Centered Design. So too is the idea that we consider how stakeholders (both individuals and organizations) will be affected by the system we build. The novel angle is that we propose that the

EST can provide computer scientists a systematic manner to visualize how they can develop artifacts at the intersection of the various layers. We have simplified the EST to include the individual layer, family layer, community layer, society layer, and environment layer (Jeong and Arriaga 2009; Arriaga 2017). We propose that HCI researchers can design technology at each layer and Ubicomp researchers can use the EST to develop better computational models of disease exacerbation by thinking about what kind of sensors can collect meaningful data at the various ecological layers.

In our view, coupling psychosocial theory and computer science has synergistic advantages for cross-disciplinary collaboration. It helps both the computer scientist and the clinician to visualize how technology can be situated throughout the patient's ecosystem. This can be done, for example, to better understand the likelihood of relapse, exacerbation, or recovery. From a Ubicomp perspective, we can use a "shroud" of sensors to collect a variety of information about the individual at the different layers. We can also think about using the "crowd" (other people around them) to provide information about how they think the patient is doing. This is relevant because caregivers are usually tuned to the patient's health but one single person is not with the patient all of the time. Thus, we can also imagine that a network of caregivers may be able to provide relevant information about the patient. In the case of a child with asthma, a simple text message from a teacher or sports coach could inform us about a child's coughing fit at school. We can imagine that we can use a child's phone to capture location-based information that could tell us if a child has missed school. Finally, we can upload all the data that is streamed from the various ecological layers to the "cloud" to build better predictive models. These are deemed to be better because they integrate objective (e.g., environmental, physiological, biological) triggers and subjective variables (e.g., patient symptom reports).

In our lab, we have used the EST to understand the asthma design space (Jeung and Arriaga), to map new research opportunities in technology for autism (see Arriaga 2017) and also to propose collaborations in novel health domains. Figure 5.5

shows how we conceptualize data collection to better understand the variables that can predict PTSD recovery. We can leverage the sensors on their phones to collect physiological data. Also, to collect information about their location and perhaps how these two types of data are correlated to anxiety causing spaces. We can ask the individual how he is doing but we can also ask other people who he trusts for feedback (e.g., spouse, parent or coworker). Further, with the rise of social computing tools, we understand that clues to the individual's mental health may not only be available in the way he behaves in the physical world but also in the way he behaves in the digital world (posts on Facebook or Instagram). We can also collect a wide range of environmental data (ambient sound, air quality) since these factors are also known to be associated with triggers. Finally, our long-term goal is to use the data to build computational models to understand therapeutic efficacy. Schertz et al. (2019), provide an example of how we applied User-Centered Design (UCD) to explore the needs of clinicians that treat people with PTSD.

To summarize, our theoretical approach allows us to bridge important gaps in chronic care management. While the EST informs our approach to design technology and build computational models of exacerbation, the HBM improves our ability to get the individual to engage in behavior that will lead to improved health management.

5.3 Integrating Behavioral Science and Computer Science: Heuristics for Successful Collaborations

In this section, we will zoom out and consider how our experience as a psychologist and Ubicomp researcher can be mined to foment interactions between behavioral scientists (e.g., psychologists, clinicians, public health researchers) and computer scientists. We will do so in the context of health research, which is where we derive our experience. Computer science research is most fruitful when it is paired with a community of practice. In this sense, computer scientists are

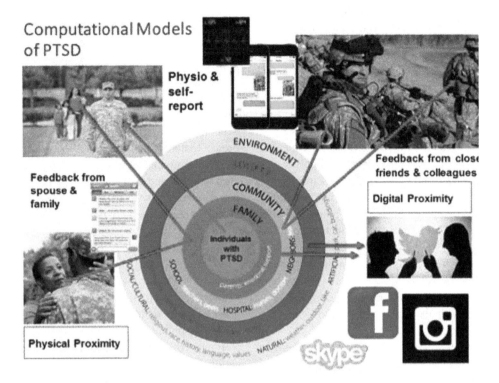

Fig. 5.5 The PTSD P-CCAS

often looking for meaningful interactions with experts from other fields. Behavioral scientists that are concerned with improving health and wellness outcomes understand that interventions need to be contextualized in mediums that are relevant to their patients. This makes mobile devices important tools for chronic care management.

We have found that the key to forming cross-field teams is to leverage the disciplinary strength of the various team members to address a mutually interesting problem. Universities understand that this research activity can drive real impact. Thus, they are partnering with local and regional hospitals to promote seed grants that encourage the formation of these cross-field teams. These seed grants allow both the computer scientists and behavioral scientist to develop concrete projects that harness mutual research goals.

Understanding what constitutes a reasonable deliverable for a computer scientist is imperative for a successful multidisciplinary team. We have had plenty of clinicians come to us and ask that we build the next "App for X." This is an unreal-

istic goal for a deliverable. In order for HCI researchers to do their best work, it is necessary for them to follow the User-Centered Design (UCD) paradigm. This means that one of the greatest assets that behavioral scientist brings to the table is their ability to grant the HCI research access to the real-world setting. This allows the HCI researcher (who could be a graduate student) to engage in the Requirements Gathering step of the UCD. We have often had our clinical partners tell us that this exercise has led them to some insights about their workflow and their patients' needs. The HCI researcher can move on to complete the next step in the UCD and then deliver a set of design alternatives to the behavioral scientists. This process would have taken from 1 to 3 months and the behavioral scientist can now be at a point to decide if they want to move forward with the collaboration. This would require completing an institutional review board (IRB) protocol that would allow the computer scientist and her students to directly interact with the patients.

In computer science, as in most sciences, research is highly dependent on the work of students, both graduate and undergraduate. This means that progress is tied to the student's academic calendar. We can often get a group of talented undergraduates to prototype rudimentary systems (based on the needs that were identified during the requirement gathering phase), whether these are mobile apps or simple devices. This process can often be incorporated into a course project or an individual student's semester-long research experience. At this point we can imagine that the collaboration is coming up on 6 months. With the IRB in place the graduate student can now go back to the clinical setting and evaluate the design. There may now be sufficient data for a conference submission. At this point the team also has enough data to decide if they will move forward with the collaboration and seek some sort of extramural funding.

We have found that there is no way to ensure that research collaborations will blossom. However there are ways to extract the most scientific benefit from cross-field collaborations. For example, what is the smallest meaningful nugget of data that can be gained by the collaboration? How much commitment will it take by both parties? Computer scientists are often tethered to the academic year as this is when students are around to help do the "heavy lifting." However, most students will only work on a project for one semester. This means that it is now the job of the computer scientist to understand how to break the computational problem into chunks that can be addressed by multiple student teams. On the behavioral scientist side, it is important to understand that if real progress is to be made, there are aspects related to theory, IRB etc. that are best handled by them. Also, realistically how much time can they spend on this project? All of the projects that we have worked on take at least 3–4 semesters.

Behavioral scientist can be found in many fields. While most of this chapter has focused on the healthcare domain, governmental and community organizations can be a rich source of important collaboration. We have found that these entities take the long view to exploring problems. The latter has allowed us to make steady progress that has real world impact. Such

is the case with our collaboration with public health experts from the CDC's Learn the Signs Act Early Campaign. Most of our effort has been to investigate the role that technology can play in educating the public about the importance of tracking children's developmental milestones. This project initially started with a master's student who conducted a User-Centered Design project to understand the values that parents have for accessing medical information for their children (Muñoz and Arriaga 2014). This was done in collaboration with the Department of Public Health of our home state. We later took this information and engaged a group of students in a Mobile and Ubiquitous Computing course to design the general specification of the mobile application. Along the way we applied for and received a grant that (among other things) allowed us to building a robust version of the Android application. Another master's student worked on the evaluation component of the application (Armenta et al. 2019). Finally, we were able to handover the robust version of the mobile app to the CDC who in turn had the application revamped to meet their stringent technical requirements. The app finally went live in spring of 2017. The whole process took about 5 years. It should also be noted that along the way we worked on a number of other projects with the CDC that were not as fruitful.

5.4   Conclusion

The rapid proliferation of new technologies and interfaces has created new opportunities for delivering and evaluating health behavior interventions. In this chapter we introduced behavioral scientists to two relevant fields in computer science: ubiquitous computing and HCI. Also, to the primary approach that is used in these fields to develop new interfaces, User-Centered Design (UCD). We then highlighted our collaborative approach of coupling UCD to two psychosocial theories, the Health Belief Model and the Ecological Systems Theory. We showed that in doing so we were able to address fundamental questions at the intersection of chronic care management and technology development. We described how this approach led to the design of futuristic technologies as well as robust applications that have actually improved pediatric patients' psychological and physiological outcomes. Our hope is that in sharing the lessons learned from our decade-long research partnership others will be encouraged to seek out new cross-team collaborations. And that this will usher a new era of health and wellness.

References

Abowd GD. Beyond Weiser: from ubiquitous to collective computing. IEEE Comp. 2016;49:17–23. https://doi.org/10.1109/MC.2016.22.

Armenta A, Warrel L, Nazneen N, Escobedo L, Arriaga RI. ActEarly: a bi-national evaluation study of a mobile application for tracking developmental milestones. IX Latin American Conference on Human Computer Interaction, CLIHC 2019.

Arriaga RI. Using an ecological systems approach to target technology for autism and beyond. In: Casanova MF, El-Baz A, Suri JS, editors. Autism imaging and devices. Boca Raton, FL: CRC Press; 2017. p. 419–36.

Bronfenbrenner U. Toward an experimental ecology of human development. Am Psychol. 1977;32:515–31.

Bronfenbrenner U. The ecology of human development: experiments by nature and by design. Cambridge: Harvard University Press; 1979.

Dix I, Finlay J, Abowd GD, Beale R. Human- computer interaction. 3rd ed. Englewood Cliffs, NJ: Prentice Hall; 2004.

Han Y, Faulkner MS, Fritz H, Fadoju D, Muir A, Abowd GD, Head L, Arriaga RI. A pilot randomized trial of text-messaging for symptom awareness and diabetes knowledge in adolescents with type 1 diabetes. J Pediatr Nurs. 2015;30(6):850–61. https://doi.org/10.1016/j.pedn.2015.02.002.

Hong H, Kim J, Abowd GD, Arriaga RI. Designing a social network to support the independence of young adults with autism. In: Proceedings of the ACM 2012 Conference on Computer Supported Cooperative Work (CSCW'12). New York, NY: ACM; 2012. p. 627–36. https://doi.org/10.1145/2145204.2145300.

Hong H, Yarosh S, Kim J, Abowd GD, Arriaga RI. Investigating the use of circles in social networks to support Independence of individuals with autism. In: Proceedings of the ACM Conference on Human Factors in Computing Systems (CHI). New York, NY: ACM; 2013. p. 3207–16.

Jeong HY, Arriaga RI Using an ecological framework to design mobile technologies for pediatric asthma management. Proceedings of the 11th International Conference on Human-Computer Interaction with Mobile Devices and Services. 2009. https://doi.org/10.1145/1613858.1613880.

Jeong HY, Hayes GR, Yun TJ, Sung JY, Arriaga RI. Act collectively: opportunities for technologies to support low-income children with asthma. Proceedings of the 25th BCS Conference of Human-Computer Interaction. 2011. pp. 413–420.

Muñoz D, Arriaga RI. Low income parents' values involving the use of technology for accessing health information. In: Abascal J, Barbosa S, Fetter M, Gross T, Palanque P, Winckler M, editors. Human-computer interaction—INTERACT 2015. Lecture notes in computer science, vol. 9298. Cham: Springer; 2014.

Norman D. The design of everyday things. Philadelphia, PA: Basic Books; 2013. Revised and Expanded Edition.

Preece J, Rogers Y, Sharp H. Interaction design: beyond human computer interaction. 3rd ed. Chichester: Wiley; 2015.

Rogers Y. HCI theory: classical, modern and contemporary. Synthesis Lectures on Human-Centered Informatics,. 1st ed. 2012;5:1.

Rosenstock I. The health belief model and preventative health behavior. Health Educ Behav. 1974;4(2):354–86. https://doi.org/10.1177/109019817400200405.

Schertz E, Watson H, Krishna A, Evans H, Sherrill A, Arriaga RI. Bridging the gap: creating a clinician-facing dashboard for PTSD. The 17th IFIP TC.13 International Conference on Human-Computer Interaction – INTERACT 2019.

Trudge JRH. Social contextual theories. In: Shweder RA, Bidell TR, Dailey AC, Dixon SD, Miller PJ, Modell J, editors. The child: an encyclopedic companion. Chicago: University of Chicago Press; 2009. p. 268–71.

Weiser M. The computer for the 21st century. Sci Am. 1991;265(3):78–89.

Yun T-J, Jeong HY, Hill TD, Lesnick B, Brown R, Abowd GD, Arriaga RI. Using SMS to provide continuous assessment and improve health outcomes for children with asthma. In: Proceedings of the 2nd ACM SIGHIT International Health Informatics Symposium (IHI '12). New York, NY: ACM; 2012. p. 621–30. https://doi.org/10.1145/2110363.2110432.

Yun T-J, Arriaga RI. A text message a day keeps the pulmonologist away. In: Proceedings of the SIGCHI Conference on Human Factors in Computing Systems (CHI '13). New York, NY: ACM; 2013. p. 1769–78. https://doi.org/10.1145/2470654.2466233.

Yun T-J, Arriaga RI. SMS is my BFF: positive impact of a texting intervention on low-income children with asthma. In: Proceedings of the 10th EAI International Conference on Pervasive Computing Technologies for Healthcare (PervasiveHealth '16). ICST (Institute for Computer Sciences, Social-informatics and Telecommunications Engineering). Brussels, Belgium: ICST; 2016. p. 53–60.

Research Spanning Animal and Human Models: The Role of Serendipity, Competition, and Strategic Actions in Advancing Stroke Research

Patricia D. Hurn and Richard J. Traystman

Contents

Over the past 50 years, the complexity and scale of scientific research in essentially all fields has increased exponentially. The ever-increasing scale and scope of science have been accompanied over these decades by a clear shift toward collaborative research, also referred to as "team science, interdisciplinary research, or interprofessional research." While there are many definitions for these terms, this chapter revolves around our experiences with research that combines two or more disciplines to carry out discovery in a way that creates something new through innovation and by acting across existing professional or cultural boundaries. By innovation, we are referring to creativity with a purpose (Appelros et al. 2010).

This chapter offers a set of stories, written as voices from the field that will be helpful to others who are building, or sustaining, team science in any venue. The first story centers on what the authors label as "team innovation," that is, an activity that occurs in circumstances where innovation and surprising outcomes would not be possible without a team. The story also emphasizes how team members (or even leaders) may ask unschooled questions, which in an almost serendipitous way can lead to new and novel science. These examples arise from our experiences as National Institutes of Health (NIH)-funded stroke researchers who frequently use cell and animal models to investigate cellular and molecular mechanisms of ischemic brain injury. Next, we hypothesize that not only is team science greatly advantaged to be innovative and seek out novel science, this approach can lead to high productivity and effective competition in procuring funding and resources. Lastly, a final story emphasizes how strategic institutional actions and commitments can facilitate cross-disciplinary team science and assure that infrastructures are aligned to assure innovation.

Team innovation is especially powerful. One reason for this power is that teams can work in

P. D. Hurn (✉)
School of Nursing, University of Michigan, Ann Arbor, MI, USA
e-mail: phurn@med.umich.edu

R. J. Traystman
University of Colorado Denver Anschutz Medical Campus, Aurora, CO, USA

© Springer Nature Switzerland AG 2019
K. L. Hall et al. (eds.), *Strategies for Team Science Success*,
https://doi.org/10.1007/978-3-030-20992-6_6

ways that yield novel, and sometimes unexpected, scientific findings. Cross-disciplinary teams drive innovation, a purposeful discovery behavior that exploits the unexpected, utilizes imagination, and provides one avenue of new solutions to complex health problems (Appelros et al. 2010). We see innovation shining through when generating a new hypothesis, or advancing a non-ordinary experimental approach, or developing a previously unimagined technology that is adopted by others. And in today's world, innovation is highly valued as a kind of panacea to solve complex problems, and is not necessarily dependent on intellectual brilliance or technical capability.

6.1 Team Innovation: Sex Matters in Stroke

It has been recognized for many years that stroke rates are higher in men versus women across the globe, and that this sexually dimorphic epidemiology persists until ages well beyond the menopausal years (Bushnell et al. 2014). Although childhood stroke is relatively rare, boys have higher stroke risk than girls, observed well before the onset of puberty (Fullerton et al. 2003). Despite these epidemiological data, stroke researchers have studied male animals almost exclusively, and commonly employ "mixed sex" cell culture systems in order to evaluate molecular mechanisms. This practice persists today despite our growing knowledge of sexually dimorphic brain structures, sex-specific chemical methods of neural transmission, and hormonally dependent cerebral vascular behavior in both animals and humans. For example, there are extremely striking differences in the structural "wiring" of the brain between the sexes. Males have greater within-brain hemisphere neural connectivity, as compared to greater between-hemisphere connectivity in women (Gall et al. 2012). One implication of these findings is that male brains are structured for greater connectivity between areas controlling perception and motor function, while female brains are better connected for communication (Gall et al. 2012). These structural differences have clear implica-

tions for brain injury, that is, the deficits in function that occur post-injury and the likelihood of reconnecting neural pathways from damaged to undamaged brain areas. Despite this emerging knowledge, our field persisted in "unisex" models in the laboratory.

As experienced principal investigators, arising from both basic science (physiology, neuroscience) and clinical departments (anesthesiology), the authors questioned if this practice of conducting experiments in animals of a single sex or in cell preparations that have not been stratified by sex might be obscuring important findings. Given the high failure rate of experimental neuroprotective therapies to move forward to patients of either sex, a move toward understanding and capitalizing on any sex specificity of cell death mechanisms could be a valuable first step toward "precision medicine." And while the epidemiology of stroke incidence is favorable to females versus males until advanced age, outcomes from stroke in women remain poor. Once stroke occurs, women sustain severe damage with high short-term mortality relative to men, and experience considerable loss of quality of life (Herson et al. 2013; Hurn and Macrae 2000; Ingalhalikar et al. 2014). So much might be gained by understanding the details of sex-specific pathobiology in stroke.

How deeply could sex differences penetrate into molecular mechanisms of cell death? Was our field correct to assume that both female (XX) and male (XY) cells would act identically in life or death? To answer these questions, the authors gathered collaborators who were specialists in clinical and experimental stroke, plus endocrinologists, pathologists, geneticists, veterinarians, and cell biologists. To act as a team and move forward, we spent early efforts to assure that we understood each other's language and expertise and to design new ways of conducting experiments.

Our team adapted standard brain injury animal models studies of both sexes and learned quickly that favorable tissue and behavioral outcomes occurred more frequently in females than in males, even in the presence of comorbidities, for example, diabetes and hypertension (Liu et al. 2007; Ness 2012; Offner and Hurn 2012). These data were so compelling that team members who typically worked with in vitro culture systems created innovative sex-stratified, in vitro cell systems despite considerable technical demands and test the long-held assumption that the mechanisms and outcomes of injury are independent of the sex of the cells. Primary cell cultures (i.e., cells obtained from sexed rodent embryos and grown in the absence of sex steroids in the culture media) were used to track the relative sensitivities of XX and XY cells to injury. For example, XX cells tolerate exposure to oxygen-glucose deprivation to a greater extent than do XY cells (Offner et al. 2006) by using a different molecular rescue system.

As our team reported the new approaches, others used and modified them to test their own hypotheses. It became possible for the first time to understand how XX vs. XY cells might rely on differing ischemic cell death molecular signaling or engage differing protective molecules in the face of injury. Such molecules include apoptosis-inducing factor (AIF), caspase 3, glutathione, the neuronal and inducible isoforms of nitric oxide synthase, poly-ADP ribose polymerase (PARP), P450 aromatase, superoxide dismutase and others (Liu et al. 2007). Many sexually dimorphic molecules have been subsequently identified through the use of knockout mice as the practice of using all male animals has become less common. And recent recommendations from the NIH that require sex as a variable of study in preclinical studies will assure growth and innovation in this important area.

A further vignette emphasizes how a serendipitous question arising from a team that operates in a culture of innovation can initiate a wholly new and successful line of investigation. In this context, serendipity is defined not as "luck" per se, but as "chance," that is, the chance that a team member will pose an out-of-the blue question that no one ever thought of before. And the chance that the question can be operationalized to turn a scientific field on its head. For example, in 2005, one of the authors (Hurn) had assembled a large, NIH funded team at Oregon Health and Science University to study estrogen's neuroprotective mechanisms in experimental central nervous system pathology relevant to women (stroke and multiple sclerosis). The team was highly cross-disciplinary, including basic neuroscientists and immunologists, plus a variety of clinician scientists from neurology, anesthesiology, endocrinology, and obstetrics/gynecology.

Early on, the team was heavily engaged in understanding each other's experimental models and techniques that would be used during the extensive collaboration. Mouse models were used to study biological mechanisms by which estrogen might work in the brain, but these models were employed quite differently in experimental stroke and multiple sclerosis. In one data-sharing conference, a senior immunologist and project leader asked a brilliantly naïve question. What happened to the animal's spleen and thymus, the home of many immunological cell types, during evolving stroke in the distant brain where all the action was supposed to be happening? The stroke researchers in the room were quietly uncertain as to how to even locate these tiny organs in mice, much less address the question. Immediately, a small subset of the whole team set out to develop techniques to harvest the organs from animals with stroke and begin studies of the peripheral immune system. In so doing, we found that experimental stroke induced massive early activation, then destruction, of the spleen, its constituent B and T lymphocytes and other highly important immune-competent cell types, leading to compromised systemic immune defenses. These observations (Sacco et al. 1998), and many subsequent mechanistic studies (Vahidy et al. 2016), set out a new concept and overarching hypothesis that has impacted not only the basic science of stroke research but clinical studies in humans. We now understand that ischemic brain injury precipitates extensive effects on anatomically distant immune organs and sets up a deleterious and highly selective cell cycling between immune organs and the brain. And early investigations in stroke patients suggest that the poststroke spleen undergoes similar changes (Vannucci et al. 2001), potentially explaining the long recognized observation that stroke patients are highly susceptible to urinary tract infections, pneumonia and the like. Serendipity and cross-fertilization of scientific experts certainly played a role in this example.

However, only a strong innovative team could have operationalized that question to such a large degree and with such swiftness.

These examples emphasize that success in team innovation is most likely if the investigators have a natural affinity for this kind of approach, that is, it is integral to how they think about science. There can be great excitement when individuals from completely different scientific backgrounds all participate scientifically, work on a shared project, yet see that project from different perspectives. There is always a sense that everyone has something important to contribute, and the contributions make the project stronger, more exciting, and potentially higher impact. One can never predict from whom the ideas will come and sometimes the ideas are so voluminous, it becomes unclear which ideas came from whom. The team programmatic approach results in far more ideas than the single discipline, single investigator approach could provide. And ultimately, the output is always far greater than a sum of its parts.

6.2   Team Resources: Collaborate to Compete

In addition to cross-disciplinary team science's high potential for innovation and novelty, a team has great capability to effectively compete for research funding. And in current tight research times, successful grantsmanship in a highly competitive environment frequently depends on strong, sustained collaboration between or among investigators of differing capabilities and talents. In other words, one recommendation that emerges from the authors' experiences is to collaborate if one wants to be competitive for resources.

A good example arises with programmatic research when teams collaborate in structured ways to take on large research questions. The authors' experiences with programmatic research began early in 1983 at Johns Hopkins Medical Institutions and extended over time to other programs (Traystman at University of Colorado Denver; Hurn at the University of Texas System), as we moved into new phases and locations of our

careers. In 1983, a multigenerational program project grant (PPG) was born (Traystman as principal investigator), at a time when programmatic research was still highly underutilized. This PPG was successfully renewed five times over the next 25 years. The overall objective of this program was a big one, to define the mechanisms of regulation of brain blood flow and metabolism. There were 14 major clinical and basic science investigators involved in the PPG, as well as a host of pre- and post-doctoral students. Five major clinical and science departments were involved (Anesthesiology and Critical Care Medicine, Biostatistics, Medicine (Cardiology and Pulmonary), Neurology, and Pediatrics (Neonatology)). Each new cycle of the grant funding brought in new departments (Biomedical Engineering, Pathology), and new investigators at various levels of scientific maturity.

Despite geographic distances and despite demanding schedules for research and patient care activities, the participants stayed in close daily contact and remained closely involved with each other's projects. We quantified that "connectome" among team members through their peer-reviewed and abstract publications (Fig. 6.1). The visualization of a team through the "connectome" is a useful technique in analyzing relationships among the members. The metric being visualized in Fig. 6.1 is shared peer-reviewed publications; we chose that metric because it is readily trackable and generally accepted as one measure of research productivity. But other forms of output can be analyzed, that is, shared trainees, grant applications, and the like. The team continued their careers as independent investigators, as well as using team science approaches. Many of these individuals have become highly respected leaders in their individual fields, but continue to practice programmatic team science.

Another demonstration of our "collaborate to compete" theme involves the development and successful implementation of a research center grant. This highly desirable grant mechanism allows multidisciplinary collaborators to compete for extramural funding and institutional resources in an effective manner. Center grants allow the mixing of basic science and clinical research

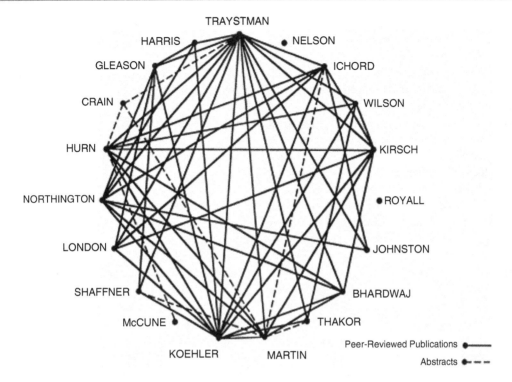

Fig. 6.1 "Connectome" of a National Institutes of Health-funded Research Team. Each node is a member of the team, with connecting lines showing shared publications as a metric for team success

projects, as well as fellowship training activities, all linked by a similar theme. And such grants, and the entities that are subsequently funded, allow for innovative approaches to research that might not happen under other circumstances. In 2014, one of the authors (Traystman) received an award from the American Stroke Association in collaboration with the Bugher Foundation to create a Stroke Collaborative Research Center at the University of Colorado Denver Anschutz Medical Campus. The goal of the grant is to determine mechanisms of injury, protection, and repair of brain following stroke in children and in juvenile animal models, plus to train new pediatric stroke clinicians and researchers. Stroke in children is particularly important, because of the devastating consequences of stroke in young children with years of life ahead. Clinical aspects of pediatric stroke, mechanisms of injury to the brain, protection of the brain, and recovery and repair of brain tissue (plasticity) are different in children versus adults. So it is vital that we understand how children recover from stroke.

To accomplish the goals, a large team was assembled, involving 14 principal investigators (clinicians and basic scientists) and other individuals from 7 different departments: Anesthesiology, Biostatistics, Cell and Developmental Biology, Neurology, Pediatrics, Pharmacology, and Radiology. The center contains a central neuroplasticity theme throughout the program, a Fellowship training component, one clinical project, and two basic science projects. Once we understand more about neuroplasticity in the young, we can then work to restore function as well as understand the remarkable brain plasticity that is lost with age. Only a multidisciplinary team can accomplish such a feat.

6.3   Building Infrastructure for Team Science

Strategic institutional actions and commitments are frequently forgotten as a critical factor to the success of cross-disciplinary team science within that institution or higher education system. One example of how that works is the mindful design of research infrastructure.

All research-intensive universities and academic health centers share a vision that team science should engage research teams that are innovative and have a competitive edge in acquiring extramural funding. However, to make that vision operational, institutions must optimize local conditions so that collaborators can conveniently share space, operations, and equipment as needed. And frequently, infrastructure is the most difficult aspect for universities to manage in a way that augments cross-disciplinarity and collaborations that grow organically into innovative team science.

At the University of Texas (U.T.) System, one of the authors (Hurn) catalyzed investment in structures that are likely to enhance research success of all kinds. U.T. System is the second largest university system in the country, composed of 8 universities and 6 academic health campuses, with 212,000 students and 19,800 faculty, and total research expenditures of approximately $2.5 billion. While each member institution has its own individual research portfolios and priorities, the challenges and pressures for researchers and research trainees across the system share many commonalities. From those commonalities, priorities for action readily emerge. The following two examples, drawn from our many experiences, illustrate how structures can enhance cross-disciplinary teams and collaborations.

Due to the complexity of our 14 institutions and the distributed nature of campus information, it has been challenging for researchers to find the collaborators that are necessary to advance their teams. Accordingly, we have built a data warehouse of research assets and capabilities-in-the-pipeline with analytics drawing from these data as needed by various audiences. The data warehouse (branded as Influuent) holds useful information such as faculty research holdings (grants, public/private partnerships, etc.), faculty areas of expertise, honorifics, and the like. In the late phases of full implementation, Influuent will allow faculty, industry, and other interested stakeholders to search for U.T. research experts, and drive collaboration across disciplines, across campuses, and throughout the world.

A second example involves creating shared technological facilities that can serve multisite health research teams. Building on the collaborative potential of our many campuses, a research core laboratory network has been assembled that widens the service net to faculty and students located at any of our institutions or outside collaborators. Research core laboratories are centralized, shared resources that provide access to instrumentation, technologies, services, and expert consultation on the use of such technologies. The availability of research cores is critical to success in obtaining research funding, in jump-starting students and young faculty without extensive facilities of their own, and in building collaborations of all kinds. Frequently expensive to build and maintain, the use of such facilities often is limited to local researchers within a department, institute, school, or institution. As a result, many efficiencies based on scale are lost, redundancies in equipment purchases occur and useful scientific interactions between users are diminished. The new voluntary network of existing research cores across our institutions uses common laboratory management software platforms which handle scheduling, billing, data-sharing and the like. So for the first time, researchers from geographically distant sites and from very different local research capabilities can operate as a team, shipping samples to a common location and sharing data among team members in an organized manner.

6.4 Conclusion

Our experiences show that team science is naturally strengthened by cross-disciplinarity. As suggested by the examples offered here, innovation springs quickly when collaborators of very different disciplines learn to speak each other's language. Or when novel, "out-of-the box" questions can rise to the forefront of research. Research institutions and funding organizations can also assist with resources for optimizing infrastructure and support of training of faculty and students in entrepreneurism.

References

Appelros P, Stegmayr B, Terent A. A review on sex differences in stroke treatment and outcome. Acta Neurol Scand. 2010;121:359–69.

Bushnell CD, Reeves MJ, Zhao X, Pan W, Prvu-Bettger J, Zinner L, et al. Sex differences in quality of life after ischemic stroke. Neurology. 2014;82:922–31.

Fullerton HJ, Wu YW, Zhao S, Johnston SC. Risk of stroke in children: ethnic and gender disparities. Neurology. 2003;61:189–94.

Gall SL, Tran PL, Martin K, Blizzard L, Srikanth V. Sex differences in long-term outcomes after stroke: functional outcomes, handicap and quality of life. Stroke. 2012;43:1982–7.

Herson PS, Palmateer J, Hurn PD. Biological sex and mechanisms of ischemic brain injury. Transl Stroke Res. 2013;4:413–9.

Hurn PD, Macrae IM. Estrogen as a neuroprotectant in stroke. J Cereb Blood Flow Metab. 2000;20:631–52.

Ingalhalikar M, Smith A, Parker D, Satterthwaite TD, Elliott MA, Ruparel K, et al. Sex differences in the structural connectome of the human brain. PNAS. 2014;111:823–8.

Liu M, Hurn PD, Roselli CE, Alkayed NJ. Role of P450 aromatase in sex-specific astrocytic cell death. J Cereb Blood Flow Metab. 2007;27:135–41.

Ness RB. Innovation Generation. New York: Oxford University Press; 2012.

Offner H, Hurn PD. A novel hypothesis: regulatory B lymphocytes shape outcome from experimental stroke. Transl Stroke Res. 2012;3:324–30.

Offner H, Subramanian S, Parker SM, Afentoulis ME, Vandenbark AA, Hurn PD. Experimental stroke induces massive, rapid activation of the peripheral immune system. J Cereb Blood Flow Metab. 2006;26:654–65.

Sacco RL, Boden-Albala B, Gan R, Chen X, Kargman DE, Shea S, et al. Stroke incidence among white, black, and Hispanic residents of an urban community: the Northern Manhattan Stroke Study. Am J Epidemiol. 1998;147:259–68.

Vahidy FS, Parsha KN, Rahbar MH, Lee M, Bui TT, Nguyen C, Barreto AD, Bambhroliya AB, Sahota P, Yang B, Aronowski J, Savitz SI. Acute splenic responses in patients with ischemic stroke and intracerebral hemorrhage. J Cereb Blood Flow Metab. 2016;36:1012–21.

Vannucci SJ, Willing LB, Goto S, Alkayed NJ, Brucklacher RM, Wook TL, et al. Experimental stroke in the female diabetic, db/db, mouse. J Cereb Blood Flow Metab. 2001;21:52–60.

Collaborating to Move the Laboratory Findings into Public Health Domains: Maxims for Translational Research

7

Gregory J. Madden, Samuel McClure, and Warren K. Bickel

To raise new questions, new possibilities, to regard old problems from a new angle, requires creative imagination and marks real advance in science.

Albert Einstein

Contents

G. J. Madden (✉)
Department of Psychology, Utah State University,
Logan, UT, USA
e-mail: greg.madden@usu.edu

S. McClure
Department of Psychology, Arizona State University,
Tempe, AZ, USA

Decision Neuroscience Lab, Arizona State University,
Tempe, AZ, USA

W. K. Bickel
Fralin Biomedical Research Institute, Virginia Tech
and Virginia Tech Carilion School of Medicine,
Roanoke, VA, USA

Behavioral Health Research, Virginia Tech and
Virginia Tech Carilion School of Medicine, Roanoke,
VA, USA

Addiction Recovery Research Center, Virginia Tech
and Virginia Tech Carilion School of Medicine,
Roanoke, VA, USA

Center for Transformative Research on Health
Behaviors, Virginia Tech and Virginia Tech Carilion
School of Medicine, Roanoke, VA, USA

Department of Psychology, College of Science,
Virginia Tech and Virginia Tech Carilion School of
Medicine, Roanoke, VA, USA

Department of Psychiatry and Behavioral Medicine,
Virginia Tech and Virginia Tech Carilion School of
Medicine, Roanoke, VA, USA

© Springer Nature Switzerland AG 2019
K. L. Hall et al. (eds.), *Strategies for Team Science Success*,
https://doi.org/10.1007/978-3-030-20992-6_7

We recently had occasion to consider the factors that have contributed thus far to our successes in applying basic laboratory research to understanding the nature of addiction. This opportunity led us to recognize anew how our findings, and those of other researchers have allowed us to examine old problems from a new angle. The new perspective raised new questions and pointed to new possibilities for translating laboratory research findings into innovative approaches to reducing addictions.

In considering these factors, we revisited a classic paper in which B. F. Skinner looked back upon his early research discoveries, gleaning from them several informal maxims that might profitably be followed by others (Skinner 1956). In some cases, we found that Skinner's maxims applied well to our experiences, and these are repeated below. In other cases, new maxims were warranted, particularly as the well of knowledge has deepened considerably since 1956, permitting and inviting interdisciplinary research collaborations.

In what follows, we offer our own case history in translational research. Because this chapter focuses on our temporal discounting research, we begin with a brief overview of that phenomenon.

7.1 Temporal Discounting

A universal for humans and other species is that we do not like to wait. As an illustrative thought experiment, if asked to choose between a 4 oz. cup of coffee now and an 8 oz. cup of coffee obtained only after waiting in line for 35 min, most of us would choose the smaller-sooner over the larger-later cup. While this benign choice might be taken as evidence for good time-management skills, other preferences for immediate outcomes have more insidious effects on our health and well-being. For example, when the smaller-sooner alternative is a jelly doughnut now and the larger-later alternative is the improvement in health that can be realized by adhering to a healthy diet, persistently choosing the doughnut represents an impulsive choice. Similarly, choosing to get high and watch football on the couch now (smaller-

sooner alternative) instead of exercising, studying, or spending time with family (each of which, when part of a temporally extended pattern of behavior, leads to superior larger-later outcomes) represents an impulsive choice.

Basic research on temporal discounting dates back to the 1960s when Chung and Herrnstein (1967) explored how delaying the delivery of a food reinforcer led pigeons to allocate their key-pecking behavior away from that alternative and toward a source that produced food immediately. Relatively brief delays (e.g., 4–8 s) produced large shifts in behavior away from the delayed food source. Subsequent pigeon research by Mazur (1987) confirmed this finding and suggested that delays decrease the value of food rewards according to a hyperbolic decay function. The shape of this decay function has been confirmed in rats (e.g., Richards et al. 1997), monkeys (e.g., Freeman et al. 2009) and humans[1] (e.g., Rachlin et al. 1991).

Figure 7.1 illustrates the shape of this temporal discounting function, with two curves corresponding to different discounting rates. The shallow function (dashed curve) is the result of a low discounting rate. For this case, the discounted value of the larger-later reward (LLR), given by the height of the curve at T1, exceeds the undiscounted value of the immediately available smaller-sooner reward (SSR). All else being equal, the individual will select the alternative with the

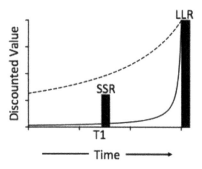

Fig. 7.1 Hyperbolic loss of reward value with increasing delays to reward delivery

[1] See Green and Myerson (2004) for evidence that human choice involving hypothetical delays and rewards deviates systematically from a strict hyperbolic function.

higher subjective value, in this case, the LLR. For the individual whose choices are best described by the steep discounting function (solid curve), the value of the SSR far exceeds the discounted value of the LLR at T1, and the impulsive choice is made. We will return to this analysis below. For now, we consider the maxims that have proven useful in our path from basic research findings to exploring their utility in translation research.

7.2 Maxim 1: Surround Yourself with Smart People and Read Outside Your Research Area

In 1995, Warren Bickel, Nancy Petry, John Roll, and Greg Madden met weekly in a pub in Vermont to share a late dinner and drinks, and to discuss contemporary research articles that were a bit outside our research areas. At the time, our research was focused on substance-abuse treatment and the behavioral economics of demand for drugs of abuse. Recognizing that the ecosystem in which scientific research is conducted (and funded) is constantly changing, we were searching for new adaptations, new methods, novel insights—anything that could spark an adaptive direction for our investigations. Each of the participants in these meetings read the articles before the dinner and took notes that included fledgling ideas for new studies, or variations on old ones. At the meetings, ideas were exchanged freely, wildly even. Like mutations within an ecosystem, most of the ideas went nowhere, but some survived.

Several weeks into these discussions, we read and discussed an article published by Myerson and Green (1995) on temporal discounting. The paper summarized the evidence that nonhumans discount hyperbolically the value of delayed food rewards, and their findings illustrated that the same was true of individual humans choosing between hypothetical smaller-sooner and larger-later monetary rewards. Our group was intrigued by the orderliness of their data, particularly because the hyperbola performed well in describing the data of individual participants. As our discussion ramped up upon the serving of a second round of beers, we began to speculate how

steeply discounting the future consequences of drug use might play a role in substance use disorders. That is, if one steeply discounts the future detrimental effects of drug use, then these consequences would factor little into the decision to abuse illicit drugs.

Borrowing procedures from Rachlin et al. (1991), we set out to test the hypothesis illustrated in Fig. 7.1: that heroin-dependent individuals would more steeply discount delayed monetary rewards than would demographically matched non-drug-using participants. Consistent with that hypothesis, opioid-dependent participant's median discounting rates were substantially higher (0.220) than that of the control group (0.027; Madden et al. 1997). In addition, and consistent with the nonhuman research, a hyperbolic decay function (like those in Fig. 7.1) provided an excellent fit of individual participants' choices (Madden et al. 1999).

Given the size of the difference in temporal discounting between the addicted and control samples, we thereafter largely followed the advice captured in one of Skinner's (1956) maxims:

7.3 Maxim 2: When You Run onto Something Interesting, Drop Everything Else and Study It

This one of Skinner's maxims may sound unrealistic or outdated, and to some extent it is. Where Skinner was describing his own behavior in the 1930s as he tinkered with the operant chamber, the Bickel lab in the late 1990s had obligations to continue work supported by NIH grants, so dropping everything but delay discounting was impossible. That being said, the bulk of our discretionary time was devoted to reading more on delay discounting, designing new discounting studies, and preparing new grants to support this exciting new research line. In part, this redirection of our efforts was fueled by the overwhelmingly positive feedback given when the Madden et al. (1997) data were first presented at the 1997 meeting of the International Study Group Investigating Drugs as Reinforcers. When our first delay discounting grant proposal was funded on the first round, our decision to "drop everything else" was vindicated.

Over the next few years, studies from the Bickel lab replicated the above findings using new methodologies (e.g., Kirby et al. 1999), new delayed outcomes (Odum et al. 2002), and in new populations of substance-dependent individuals such as cigarette smokers (e.g., Bickel et al. 1999) and needle-sharing heroin addicts (Odum et al. 2000). Other laboratories soon extended the general finding that delayed rewards were more steeply discounted among alcohol- (e.g., Vuchinich and Simpson 1998) and stimulant-dependent groups (e.g., Coffey et al. 2003). Approximately, 15 years after our discussion group in the Vermont pub, a meta-analysis of the discounting literature suggested that over 3000 file-drawer studies[2] would have to exist to render nonsignificant the relation between steep temporal discounting and substance use disorders (MacKillop et al. 2011). Extending even further the role that temporal discounting may play in addictive behavior, evidence supports a relation between steep temporal discounting and pathological gambling (e.g., Petry and Casarella 1999) as well as obesity (see meta-analysis by Amlung et al. 2016).

These findings supported the hypothesis that steep temporal discounting is a marker for susceptibility to addictions (Bickel et al. 2014) and might be profitably used as a screening tool for identifying at-risk individuals (Gray and MacKillop 2015). In support of this hypothesis, considerable evidence suggests that discounting is stable over time (e.g., Odum 2011) unless targeted for change by systematic training regimens (e.g., Mazur and Logue 1978). Longitudinal studies suggest that a stable pattern of steep temporal discounting is predictive of subsequent adolescent drug use (e.g., Audrain-McGovern et al. 2009). The same appears to be true in nonhumans. Rodents that steeply discount delayed food rewards are more likely than shallow discounters to acquire low-dose cocaine self-administration (e.g., Perry et al. 2005) and to work harder to

obtain an infusion of cocaine when the price of that commodity increases (Koffarnus and Woods 2013). Steep temporal discounting is correlated with the quantity of drug consumed (e.g., Johnson et al. 2007) and in several studies is predictive of success (shallow discounting) or failure (steep discounting) in substance-abuse treatment (e.g., MacKillop and Kahler 2009).

Given these findings and conceptual analyses, there has been increasing interest in developing methods that might be used to reduce temporal discounting, with the hope that a stable change in discounting could be employed in the prevention and treatment of addictions (Volkow and Baler 2015). Our translational research efforts have led us in this direction, although through circuitous routes explained in the remaining maxims.

7.4   Maxim 3: Serendipity: The Art of Finding One Thing While Looking for Something Else

Our third maxim is another of Skinner's (1956). In the case of our research, we were evaluating the hypothesis that steep hyperbolic delay discounting predicts strength of preference for gambling-like variable delays over non-gambling fixed delays (Madden et al. 2011). In the first phase, we assessed rats' baseline levels of impulsive choice. Next, we asked the rats to choose between variable and fixed delays over >110 sessions, expecting the most impulsive rats to most strongly prefer the variable delays. The evidence supporting the hypothesis was weak, which led us to wonder if delay discounting had changed over these 110 or more sessions. A retest of impulsive choice revealed a significant shift in delay discounting toward less impulsive choice. At the time, we were furious because the original hypothesis could not be evaluated. We should have gone out for drinks with the smartest people we could find, preferably, people who were naïve to our hypothesis. They might have reminded us that to Pavlov the biologist, classical conditioning was a nuisance behavior that disrupted his study of digestion; but to Pavlov the behavioral scientist, the nuisance was a

---

[2] File-drawer studies are those that failed to find the anticipated effect and were filed away rather than published.

serendipitous event that would launch a lifetime of research. But in our teetotaling, frustrated state of hypothesis-myopia, we could only see a failed experiment. Almost a year later, it dawned on us that we may have accidentally discovered a way to reduce impulsivity in rats.

Following maxim #2, we dropped everything else and studied it, providing adolescent rats with extended (4 months) and systematic training earning delayed food rewards. Relative to a group that obtained rewards immediately, delay-exposure training reliably reduced steady-state impulsive choice (Stein et al. 2013, 2015); and this effect has proven robust when reassessed 4-months later, following the rats' participation in other behavioral tasks (Renda and Madden 2016). The potential to translate these serendipitous findings to human preschool classrooms with at-risk children may one day impact the interpersonal, academic, and addiction-related behaviors correlated with steep discounting of delayed outcomes (Audrain-McGovern et al. 2009; Mischel et al. 1989).

7.5 Maxim 4: Embrace New Techniques

In many ways, this maxim is just a restatement of our first maxim. We have always been interested in understanding the nature of drug abuse and measuring delay discounting provided a new technique to probe a construct related to addiction. Given our initial successes, we embraced this new technique. However, with this new maxim, we intend to extend this idea a little further.

Science has always been beholden to engineering new methods to reveal the inner workings of the system under study. For addiction, the system of study is humans and human behavior (rodents serve as model organisms in this sense). Some methodologies include approaches such as behavioral economics that provide new ways to quantify behavior through technologies such as the delay discount function. Other methodologies permit looking into the black box of the human brain to determine what in the mess of neuronal connections gives rise to the behavior we are interested in. To gain a deeper understanding of the temporal discounting phenomena that we were uncovering, it made sense to keep an eye on neuroscience techniques that may permit glimpses at the inner working of the temporal discounting process. Who knows, maybe this would eventually permit us to explain the processes that change when rats (or people) discount progressively less steeply with our experimental manipulations?

To be more explicit, and to keep with our rough timeline of events, we should set the stage by noting that in the early 2000s it was clear that addiction was associated with steep temporal discounting. However, the reasons for these differences were less apparent. Psychologists and behavioral economists had long hypothesized that impulsive choice reflects a conflict between two underlying processes. First, the appeal of immediate reward has strong affective consequences that seem to be related to the tendency to make (often with full knowledge) regrettable choices (Metcalfe and Mischel 1999; Loewenstein 1996). Second, deliberately planning for the future makes us desire superior larger-later consequences. Hyperbolic temporal discounting can be well approximated by positing a conflict between these two motives (Laibson 1997). However, peering into the brain's black box to test this framework as an accurate description of decision-making proved challenging. It made sense to keep our eyes open for advances in neuroscience that would answer this challenge.

The next advance in our thinking came from the emergence of a new technique in neuroscience – functional magnetic resonance imaging (fMRI). fMRI was useful because it allowed for direct noninvasive measurement of human brain activity as they engaged in a temporal discounting task. Additionally, progress in neuroscience provided strong hypothesis about the brain systems that may be associated with the impulsive drive to consume immediate reward and our ability to rationally consider future consequences. The so-called brain reward areas associated with the mesolimbic dopamine system had been shown to be activated by immediate rewards (McClure et al. 2004). The mesolimbic dopamine system has long been associated with drug addiction (Koob and Bloom 1988). Future planning and goal maintenance was also known to be associated with fronto-parietal networks generally implicated in executive functions (Miller and Cohen 2001). Critically, fMRI was the first human neuroimaging method that permitted measuring from both brain reward and executive control regions. Previous available methods, in particular EEG, allowed measurements to be made principally from the cortex, thereby missing the reward system.

In a series of studies, the link between the brain reward system, executive control systems, and delay discounting was established (e.g., McClure et al. 2004, b, 2007; van den Bos et al. 2014). This work suggested ways to experimentally alter temporal discounting. For example, directly manipulating brain function using transcranial magnetic stimulation (TMS) to impair frontal cortex function increases rates of delay discounting (Figner et al. 2010). Likewise, pharmacologically stimulating the mesolimbic dopamine system also increases rates of discounting (Pine et al. 2010). For our purposes, knowledge about the cognitive functions performed by the mesolimbic and executive control system suggested a framework to think about how our manipulations may produce altered discounting and established a causal structure to generate new experimental manipulations. We suspect that advances in animal neuroscience using finer scale brain measurement techniques and genetic manipulations will eventually intersect with our work studying temporal discounting behavior in rats. Regardless, the central insight from this maxim is that remaining open to and embracing new techniques has the potential to transform both the way you study a phenomenon as well as the conceptual framework you use to explain the phenomenon.

The neuroeconomic findings by McClure et al. (2004, b) provided key insights that sparked a new paradigm. McClure found that two different brain regions together determined the extent of delay discounting. Applying that observation to the behavioral data observed with addiction suggested the excessive discounting observed by those with drug dependence resulted from greater relative activity from the mesolimbic regions and relatively less activity in the executive systems. This key insight into the excessive discounting observed among individuals with drug dependence guided the development of a new conceptual model of addiction developed by Bickel and colleagues a few years later. This model is referred to as the "Competing Neurobehavioral Decision Systems" view (Bickel et al. 2007; McClure and Bickel 2014). Specifically, this conceptual model suggested that the impulsive decision system and the executive decision system should be in regulatory balance for those in health. However, for those with addiction, the impulsive decision system exhibits relatively greater control (hyperactive) and the executive decision system exhibits relatively less control (hypoactive) (Bickel et al. 2016a, b). Importantly, temporal discounting provides a behavioral measure of the relative control of these two decision systems. Although many other dual systems have been proposed in psychology, only a few are specifically focused on addiction (Bechara 2005; Bickel et al. 2007). Moreover, the conceptual model of the competing systems has been supported by the results of interventions directed at either increasing the hypoactive executive decision system or decreasing the hyperactive impulsive decision system (for review, see Koffarnus et al. 2013).

7.6 Maxim 5: New Insights Beget New Paradigms

…when paradigms change, the world itself changes with them. …It is rather as if the professional community had been suddenly transported to another planet where familiar objects are seen in a different light and are joined by unfamiliar ones as well.~Thomas S. Kuhn, The Structure of Scientific Revolutions (Kuhn 1962).

7.7 Maxim 6: "If You Want Truly to Understand Something, Try to Change It." Kurt Lewin

While working within the Competing Neurobehavioral Decisions Systems view, several addiction scientists began to concurrently measure delay discounting and drug value. Evidence began to accrue that individuals who exhibited both excessive discounting and high drug value exhibited greater severity of addiction and worse outcomes in treatment. These observations led both Bickel and Epstein (Bickel et al. 2011; Carr et al. 2011) to suggest a new behavioral-economic conceptual model of reinforcer pathology. That model holds that the interaction between discounting of delayed rewards and valuation of substances plays a central role in addictions (Bickel et al. 2011, 2014, 2016a, b). More specifically, delay discounting measures the temporal window over which reinforcers are integrated. Consider the important and often opposing features of drug and prosocial reinforcers. Alcohol delivers a brief, intense reinforcer with immediate and reliable effects. By contrast, prosocial reinforcers (e.g., employment and relationships) function at a lower intensity, are more variable (e.g., one's experience at work are sometimes good, sometimes bad, and often merely okay), and accrue their value over longer temporal windows. At high rates of delay, discounting the temporal window is constricted and prosocial reinforcers are viewed over a short temporal window, with less value than if viewed over a longer duration. Viewed through this constricted temporal window, the relative value of alcohol exceeds that of competing prosocial reinforcers. Moreover, this reinforcer pathology process is self-perpetuating because as prosocial reinforcers are increasingly not selected, they may result in negative outcomes (e.g., job loss) that would further diminish the value of the prosocial option. Importantly, this reinforcer pathology process may permit a novel scientific understanding of how prosocial anhedonia may develop in addiction.

As noted above, several cross-sectional studies have shown that those with high discounting rates and alcohol valuation have greater alcohol problems (e.g., Lemley et al. 2016). However, the greatest empirical evidence in support of reinforcer pathology resulted from interventions such as Episodic Future Thinking (EFT) that targets the executive system (consistent with the Competing Neurobehavioral Decision Systems approach) and alters delay discounting rates. EFT refers to simulating prospective, positive episodes that might occur in one's personal future.

EFT is derived from the science of prospection. Prospection is important for understanding cognitive motivational processing and involves the prefrontal brain regions. Application of EFT in the context of measuring delay discounting not only induces activation in regions previously reported as associated with delay discounting (i.e., lateral prefrontal cortices, anterior cingulate, and parietal cortex), but also increases activity and coupling in regions in the amygdala and hippocampus not usually associated with delay discounting (Peters and Büchel 2010). EFT has previously been shown to decrease delay discounting in individuals with alcohol use disorders (Snider et al. 2016), smokers (Stein et al. 2016), as well as normal weight, overweight, and obese populations (Daniel et al. 2013). Consistent with the reinforcer pathology concept, EFT also reduces demand for hypothetical alcoholic drinks (Snider et al. 2016) and self-administration of cigarettes (Stein et al. 2016). In addition, EFT has been shown to decrease the self-administration of highly palatable snacks in overweight and obese adults and children (Daniel et al. 2013, 2015; O'Neill et al. 2016). Therefore, EFT robustly reduces delay discounting and a variety of reinforcer valuation measures in several populations, as suggested by the notion of reinforcer pathology.

7.8 Recommendations

In considering the development and pathways that have resulted in this translational research program, we think there are several processes that could support the future of translation behavioral research. For researchers, we first acknowledge that statistical chance plays a role in the discovery process and there is little that can be done to program for that, save keeping your eyes open. Some of the greatest discoveries in science owe their origin to serendipity and researchers who hold their favorite theories lightly may be more likely to benefit when the unexpected occurs.

Those researchers who keep eyes and mind open will also be welcoming of new measurement approaches, new statistical methods, and new theoretical models of established findings.

By making time to read and/or attend conferences outside one's primary field, the researcher increases her chances of contacting these approaches, methods, and models. Science leaders and university administrators should support innovative interdisciplinary meetings to enhance such cross-fertilization and perhaps the development of new scientific societies. Distinguishing between skepticism and cynicism, the successful researcher will evaluate fairly the utility of each new approach, method, and model. Those that prove insightful will energize the open-minded researcher but, at the same time, may be resisted by those deriving status, funding, etc. from old ways of understanding the world. Be ready for this and redouble your efforts to evaluate the empirical basis of your thinking. When talking to established researchers is infrequently reinforced, direct your teaching to the next generation of scientists; they have less skin in the game and are open to new ways in which they can contribute to science.

The role of funding agencies and their agenda should not be underemphasized. "Follow the money" has broad applicability and funding agencies should create funding opportunities to induce innovative basic researchers into translational collaborations. Where funding agencies can pair basic and applied researchers who may not be aware of each other's research, they should do so. Again, playing an active role in developing interdisciplinary meetings attended by basic and clinically oriented researchers is important. Funding agencies must also prepare grant reviewers to appreciate the importance of translational and multidisciplinary approaches. One poorly instructed grant reviewer who critiques a proposal on criteria that should not be applied may prevent the proposal from being funded, may keep the researchers from further investing in translational proposal writing, and, when that investigator describes his experience to peers, may derail the efforts of the funding agency. Silos may be the path of least resistance. Dismantling them requires committed, coordinated action; but to best convert taxpayer-funded research into advances that improve public health, the silos must go.

References

Amlung M, Petker T, Jackson J, Balodis I, MacKillop J. Steep discounting of delayed monetary and food rewards in obesity: a meta-analysis. Psychol Med. 2016;46(11):2423.

Audrain-McGovern J, Rodriguez D, Epstein LH, Cuevas J, Rodgers K, Wileyto EP. Does delay discounting play an etiological role in smoking or is it a consequence of smoking? Drug Alcohol Depend. 2009;103:99–106.

Bechara A. Decision making, impulse control and loss of willpower to resist drugs: a neurocognitive perspective. Nat Neurosci. 2005;8(11):1458–63.

Bickel WK, Jarmolowicz DP, Mueller ET, Gatchalian KM. The behavioral economics and neuroeconomics of reinforcer pathologies: implications for etiology and treatment of addiction. Curr Psychiatry Rep. 2011;13(5):406–15.

Bickel WK, Johnson MW, Koffarnus MN, MacKillop J, Murphy JG. The behavioral economics of substance use disorders: reinforcement pathologies and their repair. Ann Rev Clin Psychol. 2014;10:641–77.

Bickel WK, Miller ML, Yi R, Kowal BP, Lindquist DM, Pitcock JA. Behavioral and neuroeconomics of drug addiction: competing neural systems and temporal discounting processes. Drug Alcohol Dependence. 2007;90(Suppl 1):S85–91.

Bickel WK, Odum AL, Madden GJ. Impulsivity and cigarette smoking: delay discounting in current, never, and ex-smokers. Psychopharmacology. 1999;146:447–54.

Bickel WK, Snider SE, Quisenberry AJ, Stein JS. Reinforcer pathology: the behavioral economics of abuse liability testing. Clin Pharmacol Ther. 2016;101:185. https://doi.org/10.1002/cpt.443.

Bickel WK, Snider SE, Quisenberry AJ, Stein JS, Hanlon CA. Competing neurobehavioral decision systems theory of cocaine addiction: from mechanisms to therapeutic opportunities. In: Ekhtiari H, Paulus M, editors. Neuroscience for addiction medicine: from prevention to rehabilitation, vol. 223. 1st ed. Amsterdam: Elsevier; 2016. p. 269–93. https://doi.org/10.1016/bs.pbr.2015.08.002.

Carr KA, Daniel TO, Epstein LH. Reinforcement pathology and obesity. Curr Drug Abuse Rev. 2011;4(3):190–6.

Chung S, Herrnstein RJ. Choice and delay of reinforcement. J Exp Anal Behav. 1967;10:67–74.

Coffey SF, Gudleski GD, Saladin ME, Brady KT. Impulsivity and rapid discounting of delayed hypothetical rewards in cocaine-dependent individuals. Exp Clin Psychopharmacol. 2003;11(1):18.

Daniel TO, Said M, Stanton CM, Epstein LH. Episodic future thinking reduces delay discounting and energy intake in children. Eat Behav. 2015;18:20–4.

Daniel TO, Stanton CM, Epstein LH. The future is now: reducing impulsivity and energy intake using episodic future thinking. Psychol Sci. 2013;24(11):2339–42.

Figner B, Knoch D, Johnson EJ, Krosch A, Lisanby SH, Fehr E, Weber EU. Lateral prefrontal cortex and self-control in intertemporal choice. Nat Neurosci. 2010;13(5):538–9.

Freeman KB, Green L, Myerson J, Woolverton WL. Delay discounting of saccharin in rhesus monkeys. Behav Process. 2009;82:214–8.

Gray JC, MacKillop J. Impulsive delayed reward discounting as a genetically-influenced target for drug abuse prevention: a critical evaluation. Front Psychol. 2015;6:1104.

Green L, Myerson J. A discounting framework for choice with delayed and probabilistic rewards. Psychol Rev. 2004;130:769–92.

Johnson MW, Bickel WK, Baker F. Moderate drug use and delay discounting: a comparison of heavy, light, and never smokers. Exp Clin Psychopharmacol. 2007;15(2):187.

Kirby KN, Petry NM, Bickel WK. Heroin addicts have higher discount rates for delayed rewards than non-drug-using controls. J Exp Psychol Gen. 1999;128(1):78.

Koffarnus MN, Jarmolowicz DP, Mueller ET, Bickel WK. Changing delay discounting in the light of the competing neurobehavioral decision systems theory: a review. J Exp Anal Behav. 2013;99(1):32–57.

Koffarnus MN, Woods JH. Individual differences in discount rate are associated with demand for self-administered cocaine, but not sucrose. Addict Biol. 2013;18(1):8–18.

Koob GF, Bloom FE. Cellular and molecular mechanisms of drug dependence. Science. 1988;242(4879):715–23.

Kuhn TS. The structure of scientific revolutions. 1st ed. Chicago: University of Chicago Press; 1962.

Laibson D. Golden eggs and hyperbolic discounting. Q J Econ. 1997;112(2):443–77.

Lemley SM, Kaplan BA, Reed DD, Darden AC, Jarmolowicz DP. Reinforcer pathologies: predicting alcohol related problems in college drinking men and women. Drug Alcohol Depend. 2016;167:57–66.

Loewenstein G. Out of control: visceral influences on behavior. Organ Behav Hum Decis Process. 1996;65(3):272–92.

MacKillop J, Amlung MT, Few LR, Ray LA, Sweet LH, Munafo MR. Delayed reward discounting and addictive behavior: a meta-analysis. Psychopharmacology. 2011;216:305–21.

MacKillop J, Kahler CW. Delayed reward discounting predicts treatment response for heavy drinkers receiving smoking cessation treatment. Drug Alcohol Depend. 2009;104(3):197–203.

Madden GJ, Bickel WK, Jacobs EA. Discounting of delayed rewards in opioid-dependent outpatients: exponential or hyperbolic discounting functions? Exp Clin Psychopharmacol. 1999;7:284–93.

Madden GJ, Francisco MT, Brewer AT, Stein JS. Delay discounting and gambling. Behav Process. 2011;87:43–9.

Madden GJ, Petry N, Badger GJ, Bickel WK. Impulsive and self-control choices in opiate-dependent patients and non-drug-using control participants: drug and monetary rewards. Exp Clin Psychopharmacol. 1997;5:256–62.

Mazur JE. An adjusting procedure for studying delayed reinforcement. In: Commons ML, Mazur JE, Nevin JA, Rachlin H, editors. Quantitative analysis of behavior, The effect of delay and of intervening events on reinforcement value, vol. 5. Hillsdale, NJ: Erlbaum; 1987. p. 55–73.

Mazur JE, Logue AW. Choice in a "self-control" paradigm: effects of a fading procedure. J Exp Anal Behav. 1978;30(1):11–7.

McClure SM, Bickel WK. A dual systems perspective on addiction: Contributions from neuroimaging and cognitive training. Ann NY Acad Sci. 2014;1327:61–78. https://doi.org/10.1111/nyas.12561.

McClure SM, Ericson KM, Laibson DI, Loewenstein G, Cohen JD. Time discounting for primary rewards. J Neurosci. 2007;27(21):5796–804.

McClure SM, Laibson DI, Loewenstein G, Cohen JD. Separate neural systems value immediate and delayed monetary rewards. Science. 2004;306(5695):503–7.

McClure SM, York MK, Montague PR. The neural substrates of reward processing in humans: the modern role of FMRI. Neuroscientist. 2004;10(3):260–8.

Metcalfe J, Mischel W. A hot/cool-system analysis of delay of gratification: dynamics of willpower. Psychol Rev. 1999;106(1):3–19.

Miller EK, Cohen JD. An integrative theory of prefrontal cortex function. Annu Rev Neurosci. 2001;24(1):167–202.

Mischel W, Shoda Y, Rodriguez ML. Delay of gratification in children. Science. 1989;244:933–8.

Myerson J, Green L. Discounting of delayed rewards: models of individual choice. J Exp Anal Behav. 1995;64:263–76.

O'Neill J, Daniel TO, Epstein LH. Episodic future thinking reduces eating in a food court. Eat Behav. 2016;20:9–13.

Odum AL. Delay discounting: trait variable? Behav Process. 2011;87(1):1–9.

Odum AL, Madden GJ, Badger GJ, Bickel WK. Needle sharing in opioid-dependent outpatients: psychological processes underlying risk. Drug Alcohol Depend. 2000;60:259–66.

Odum AL, Madden GJ, Bickel WK. Discounting of delayed health gains and losses by current, never- and ex-smokers of cigarettes. Nicotine Tob Res. 2002;4(3):295–303.

Perry JL, Larson EB, German JP, Madden GJ, Carroll ME. Impulsivity (delay discounting) as a predictor of acquisition of IV cocaine self-administration in female rats. Psychopharmacology. 2005;178(2–3):193–201.

Peters J, Büchel C. Episodic future thinking reduces reward delay discounting through an enhancement of prefrontal-mediotemporal interactions. Neuron. 2010;66(1):138–48.

Petry NM, Casarella T. Excessive discounting of delayed rewards in substance abusers with gambling problems. Drug Alcohol Depend. 1999;56(1):25–32.

Pine A, Shiner T, Seymour B, Dolan RJ. Dopamine, time, and impulsivity in humans. J Neurosci. 2010;30(26):8888–96.

Rachlin H, Raineri A, Cross D. Subjective probability and delay. J Exp Anal Behav. 1991;55:233–44.

Renda CR, Madden GJ. Impulsive choice and pre-exposure to delays: III. Four-month test-retest outcomes in male Wistar rats. Behav Process. 2016;126:108–12.

Richards JB, Mitchell SH, de Wit H, Seiden LS. Determination of discount functions in rats with an adjusting-amount procedure. J Exp Anal Behav. 1997;67:353–66.

Skinner BF. A case history in scientific method. Am Psychol. 1956;11(5):221.

Snider SE, LaConte SM, Bickel WK. Episodic future thinking: expansion of the temporal window in individuals with alcohol dependence. Alcohol Clin Exp Res. 2016;40(7):1558–66.

Stein JS, Johnson PS, Smits RR, Renda R, Liston KJ, Shahan TS, Madden GJ. Early and prolonged exposure to reward delay: effects on impulsive choice and alcohol self-administration in male rats. Exp Clin Psychopharmacol. 2013;21:172–80.

Stein JS, Renda CR, Hinnenkamp JE, Madden GJ. Impulsive choice, alcohol consumption, and pre-exposure to delayed rewards: II. Potential mechanisms. J Exp Anal Behav. 2015;103(1):33–49.

Stein JS, Wilson AG, Koffarnus MN, Daniel TO, Epstein LH, Bickel WK. Unstuck in time: episodic future thinking reduces delay discounting and cigarette smoking. Psychopharmacology. 2016;233(21–22):3771–8.

van den Bos W, Rodriguez CA, Schweitzer JB, McClure SM. Connectivity strength of dissociable striatal tracts predict individual differences in temporal discounting. J Neurosci. 2014;34(31):10298–310.

Volkow ND, Baler RD. NOW vs LATER brain circuits: implications for obesity and addiction. Trends Neurosci. 2015;38:345–52.

Vuchinich RE, Simpson CA. Hyperbolic temporal discounting in social drinkers and problem drinkers. Exp Clin Psychopharmacol. 1998;6(3):292.

Part III

Approaches for Expanding Engagement in Team Science

Methods for Coproduction of Knowledge Among Diverse Disciplines and Stakeholders

8

Christian Pohl and Gabriela Wuelser

Contents

8.1 Introduction

In order to address complex issues—such as public health, migration, or sustainable development—in an encompassing way, knowledge of different fields is needed. This knowledge is provided, further developed, and transferred to the next generation by universities and their disci-

C. Pohl (✉)
Transdisciplinarity Lab, Institute for Environmental Decisions, ETH Zurich, Switzerland
e-mail: christian.pohl@env.ethz.ch

G. Wuelser
Network for Transdisciplinary Research, Swiss Academies of Arts and Sciences, Bern, Switzerland

plines. Which disciplines should be involved in a project depends on the aims and scope of the project, for example, the scales that should be included in an investigation (e.g., molecules, cells, organs, individuals, specific societal groups, or groups of different nations and cultures). If the aim of research is to have an impact on how an issue is dealt with by society, concerned societal actors have to be involved in the research process, too. This is not only to learn about and take into account their stakes and the power relations between them; importantly societal actors might also have relevant expertise on the issue.

Researchers from different disciplines as well as societal actors enter such collaborations with diverse perspectives on the world. In the words of Fleck (1979), they are members of different thought collectives who share a specific thought style, that is, a specific way of looking at and making sense of the world. For instance, regarding the same piece of land, an oil company might see extractable and marketable oil, the First Nation people a sacred place for their gods and ancestors, the engineer a chance to build a new extracting technology, an environmental NGO potential environmental damage, and a law researcher a case to study the rights of First Nation people. All these actors look at the same piece of land. However, as part of their professional or academic training, they have learned to

© Springer Nature Switzerland AG 2019
K. L. Hall et al. (eds.), *Strategies for Team Science Success*,
https://doi.org/10.1007/978-3-030-20992-6_8

focus on specific aspects of the land and to fade out other aspects. On the one hand, this specialization has provided us with an enormous amount of knowledge, technologies, and societal practices. On the other hand, it also bears the risk that complex issues are framed, analyzed, and solved using only one specific thought style, for instance, the most powerful one. Such a reduction of complexity does not only create tensions with the thought collectives that are less powerful but also runs the risk of providing partial solutions. Partial solutions solve some aspects of the issue (for instance, oil extraction) and, at the same time, create negative side effects (for instance, the destruction of sacred lands).

Scientific attempts to deal with societal issues in an encompassing way are labeled interdisciplinary or transdisciplinary. The call for such approaches has a long tradition (Winch 1947; Anonymous 1966; Jantsch 1970), often at a low level of intensity but with phases of higher interest (cf. Apostel 1972). For more than two decades, there has been continuous and steadily growing interest in interdisciplinary and transdisciplinary research (Klein 1996; Klein et al. 2001; NAS/ NAE/IOM 2005; Hirsch Hadorn et al. 2008; Frodeman et al. 2010). In the field of health, the question of how to collaborate in teams has led to a completely new field of research: the Science of Team Science (Stokols et al. 2008; Falk-Krzesinski et al. 2011; National Research Council 2015).

A key question of interdisciplinarity and transdisciplinarity is how different thought collectives collaborate and integrate their thought styles. If members of different thought collectives collaborate on an issue, they can no longer perform their analysis in isolation. Integration means that the way in which they frame the issue, identify the main research questions, analyze the questions, and try to have an impact is discussed and deliberated among those who participate in the project team. This collaborative effort is called coproduction of knowledge (Lemos and Morehouse 2005; Robinson and Tansey 2006; Polk 2015). The prefix "co-" is used to denote that the production of knowledge is no longer done independently of other thought collectives and that it is influenced by them.

A number of scholars have recently started to develop and collect tools and methods that support team science or the coproduction of knowledge (McDonald et al. 2009; Bergmann et al. 2012; Vogel et al. 2013). They have also compiled online toolboxes, such as the Team Science Toolkit,[1] Integration and Implementation Sciences tools,[2] or td-net's toolbox for coproducing knowledge.[3] In the following sections, we introduce some of the specific challenges of coproduction and give examples of how the tools can help overcome them. For that purpose, we elaborate on td-net's toolbox for coproducing knowledge, which we have been editing. First, we present a background on the main challenges that the toolbox addresses. We then give a short overview of the methods included in the toolbox and present three tools in more detail.

8.2 Brokering Images of Knowledge

Knowledge coproduction is a particular description of a collaborative research process. In the "continuing discussion about whether TD [transdisciplinarity] is descriptive of a research process or whether it best describes the research outcomes that eventually emerge from projects that may include some blend of MD [multidisciplinary], ID [interdisciplinary], and TD processes" (Stokols et al. 2013, p. 5), coproduction stands for first position. It describes the transdisciplinary *process* of framing and analyzing an issue and, when needed, to develop measures and an action plan.

In terms of knowledge, coproduction is an approach aimed at overcoming the "symmetry of ignorance" (Rittel 1984, p. 325). Each of the thought collectives of researchers (with their specialized disciplinary knowledge) and societal actors (with their expertise as members of civil society and the private and public sectors) provides only part of the knowledge that is needed to

---

[1] www.teamsciencetoolkit.cancer.gov

[2] www.i2s.anu.edu.au/category/resource-type/tools

[3] www.transdisciplinarity.ch/toolbox

come to a comprehensive understanding and management of an issue. The knowledge generated by each thought collective is embedded in a particular thought style, a certain way of perceiving an issue. If the thought styles that coproduce knowledge differ in how they perceive an issue, a feeling of misunderstanding each other and the need to clarify terms might evolve. This is because members of a thought collective do not only share a specific way of perceiving an issue; they also share basic assumptions about, for instance, what the right concepts for describing an issue are or what makes arguments about the issue trustworthy. In the words of Elkana (1979), this is because thought styles consist of both a body of knowledge (the knowledge itself) and an image of knowledge (ideas about what constitutes "good" knowledge and how it should be produced). Therefore, what in coproduction might first seem like a question of language and

terminology might turn out be a question of the underlying images of knowledge. Moreover, what seems to require honest knowledge brokering (Pielke 2007) between thought collectives in fact requires the honest brokering of images of knowledge (Pohl 2011).

8.3 Td-net's Toolbox for Coproducing Knowledge

Td-net's toolbox for coproducing knowledge currently compiles 14 tools that support brokering images of knowledge, that is, clarifying the assumptions and expectations underlying different thought styles (see Table 8.1). The main part of the toolbox is a brief description of each method using a standard set of questions (Why should it be applied? When should it be applied? How does it work? etc.). For each tool, further

Table 8.1 td-net's toolbox for coproducing knowledge compiles 14 tools that help clarify implicit assumptions held by members of collaborating thought collectives (www.transdisciplinarity.ch/toolbox)

Tool	Description
Actor constellation	A role-play for jointly sorting out the relevance of various actors involved in tackling a specific research question
Delphi	A poll for consolidating expert views on an issue using ratings and arguments
Emancipatory boundary critique	A set of questions supporting nonexperts in critically challenging an expert's suggested solution to a problem and the solution's underlying assumptions
Give-and-take matrix	A tool for identifying pieces of knowledge to be shared between the subparts of interdisciplinary and transdisciplinary projects
Most significant change	A story-based qualitative method for uncovering most significant project impacts experienced by individuals
Multi-stakeholder discussion group	An approach that allows for expressing tacit knowledge, values, and practices within a group of actors and stakeholders involved in a research project
Nomadic concepts	A heuristic tool for exchanging understandings of concepts across disciplinary, professional, and cultural boundaries
Research marketplace	A tool used to initiate bilateral and small group exchanges between (sub) projects that need to be linked
Scenario integration	Using scenario planning, this tool allows for collectively drafting possible future developments of a societal challenge
Soft systems methodology	A systems thinking-based tool for creating shared understandings of a problem situation, working out possible improvements, and implementing them
Storywall	A story-based, qualitative method for retrospectively assembling crucial events in a collective process
Three types of knowledge tool	A tool for tailoring research questions to (societal) knowledge demands
Toolbox dialog initiative	A tool to uncover implicit assumptions and shared understandings of scientific disciplines
Venn diagram tool	A diagram for forming groups around joint topics based on participants' background, expertise, and interest

reading and, whenever possible, the original literature are made available. For some methods, a short report provides practical experiences and discusses the challenges of applying them. Furthermore, ten related online toolboxes are briefly portrayed and linked. The toolbox is available online and in open access on the webpage of the Swiss Academy of Sciences.

The collection of tools is eclectic in the sense that it is not based on a broad survey aimed at finding the best tools available. Rather, we select tools with which we are familiar or have experimented. Our main inclusion criteria for a tool are as follows: (1) it is easy to handle and does not require specific equipment (although it might be intellectually challenging); (2) it mainly uses everyday language; (3) it helps develop a shared understanding or identify consensus or dissent; and (4) it allows the joint production of knowledge among a group of people belonging to different thought collectives.

In what follows, we briefly present three tools in more detail. First, we introduce the tool and its aim. Second, we describe how the tool works. Third, we discuss how it supports the coproduction of knowledge of different thought collectives.

8.4   Actor Constellation

An actor constellation is a role-play in which one participant plays the research question, and all other participants play one of the thought collectives involved in the project. The thought collectives are placed around the research question, and the distance to the question signals how important they are for the success of the project. The aim of the constellation is to start a discussion on how the different project participants perceive the relevance of the different thought collectives. The idea is taken from family therapy, where a family member positions his or her relatives in a room according to how close/distant he or she feels to/from them. An actor constellation is typically done early in the project. The procedure is as follows:

1. "The project leader writes the project's overall research question on a label. He or she considers a maximum of ten most important actors (who represent various disciplines and are stakeholders from civil society, the private and the public sectors) who can answer the overall research question. The project leader then notes their names on labels.
2. The moderator finds participants to play the respective roles of the actors and labels each accordingly. If a role is not sufficiently clear to a participant (e.g., the general public, the decision makers), the moderator asks the project leader for clarification.
3. The project leader places the research question in the middle of the room and positions the actors around the research question according to the rules described above. The project leader explains to the participants why each actor is standing in a specific position and what the actor will provide to answer the overall research question (e.g., information, institutional support). Arrows can be used to describe how the project leader plans to interact with the actors.
4. Once the actors are in their respective places, they react to the constellation. The moderator asks (a) whether particular actors are missing and (b) whether an actor believes that he or she is in the wrong position, what would be the right position, and why. Through the discussion, the actor constellation changes.

The moderator closes the discussion, for example, by summarizing the main changes in the constellation that have occurred during the discussion."

For the overall purpose of the project, members of different thought collectives perceive the relevance of each thought collective differently. Usually, the perception of each other's relevance is not discussed. It is, however, implicitly expressed, for instance, in the attention that is given to contributions of different thought collectives. An actor constellation triggers an explicit exchange and a critical reflection of the relevance of each thought collective. To begin that discussion, one member has to make her or his perception visible by placing the thought collectives in a room. The discussion evolves around thought collectives that, from the perception of other participants, are in the wrong place. Typically, the positions of some of the thought collectives change after such a discussion. As participants collectively discuss whether and how the constellation should be changed, they challenge the original constellation to make it more acceptable for the collective.

8.5 Give-and-Take Matrix

The give-and-take matrix is a tool used to structure the exchange between subprojects that collaborate within a larger project. The aim of the give-and-take matrix is to clarify what each subproject expects to get from other subprojects and what each subproject intends to provide to the other subprojects. This can be data, methods, theories, models, case studies, or specific results. Ideally, the give-and-take matrix is used early in the project. The procedure is as follows:

"The tool is organized with one core matrix (give-and-take matrix) and proceeds as a group workshop of at least 3 h, along the following steps:

1. Each subproject individually prepares answers to the following questions:
   (a) TAKE: what would you like to get from each of the other subprojects ("desired TAKEs")?
   (b) GIVE: what can you offer to each of the other subprojects ("proposed GIVEs")?
2. Mixed groups of two or three subprojects (depending on the number of the subprojects and/or team members, these steps can be followed in one or several groups) perform the following tasks:
   (a) The first subproject starts by presenting its "desired TAKEs" and "proposed GIVEs."
   (b) The other subproject(s) react(s) by showing its (their) "desired TAKEs" and "proposed GIVEs."

(c) The discussion of interfaces should fit as many "desired TAKEs" and "proposed GIVEs" as possible.
3. They meet again in the subprojects to undertake the following tasks:
   (a) Share what they have learned in the mixed group(s).
   (b) Discuss how feasible it is to secure the "proposed GIVES" for the other subprojects in the research process.
   (c) Define the necessary adaptations in their research design.
4. The plenary session covers the following agenda items:
   (a) All subprojects summarize their proposed GIVEs to the other subprojects, using the give-and-take-matrix.
   (b) All presented GIVE elements are acknowledged.
5. Concrete follow-up actions may be defined, detailing necessary adaptations in the different subprojects in response to the GIVEs promised and the TAKEs received. Some sort of (binding) agreement to follow the mutually discussed "give-and-take matrix" can be helpful."

Unrealistic expectations about how one subproject's contribution will be used by other subprojects and how the other subprojects' outputs will be used in their project can engender frustration and confusion in collaborative projects. The give-and-take matrix helps to clarify and adapt these expectations before close collaboration begins. By going through the exercise, the members of the subprojects will realize what changes in the framing of their research would be needed to enable other subprojects to take up their results. Other participants might realize that the results they plan to provide would come too late in the process or might be on the wrong scale. However, some subprojects might become aware of the results of other subprojects and start to think about how they could improve their research by building on those results.

8.6 Storywall

The storywall (Smit 2005) is a tool used to visualize how members of different thought collectives, who have undergone the same process of coproducing knowledge, have experienced this process. For that purpose, the members retrospectively assemble what they see as important process events on a timeline. The individual perspectives are collected by using a storytelling approach and are drawn on a large sheet of paper in form of a timeline. The storywall is ideally applied after a process or a step is completed. The procedure is as follows:

1. "As a starting point, a simple timeline indicating the start and the end dates of the joint process or story is provided.
2. The group members collectively discuss whether to further structure the paper's timeline, for example, into project parts, organizational levels, or main process phases.
3. The actors individually identify key events or dominant influences. They may also want to identify those that have either supported or hindered the process, as well as other relevant story elements with respect to reflection and exchange.
4. Based on the individual elements, the actors jointly create a storywall picture of their process, representing their group's collective understanding of it. This is the main step because different perceptions and experiences are shared, and the process elements are discussed.
5. In case the storywalls are made in subgroups, they can subsequently be presented to the full group.
6. In addition to the reported stories with their elements, the main lessons learned can be selected and used to create an ideal storywall."

The storywall is a qualitative process evaluation tool. It exploits the fact that members of different thought collectives may, at least partly, experience a process in diverse ways and that they might stress the importance of various elements.

Considering individual experiences on an equal footing uncovers crucial success or hindering factors of a process that might not have been noticed by everyone. By explaining to each other how the process or its various stages have been experienced, participants contrast their different perspectives and learn from each other. This learning experience enables members of different thought collectives to become aware of how similar or different their own perspective is compared to that of others. This learning experience prepares them to enter the subsequent process of coproduction in a more reflective manner. The tool can also be used to retrospectively identify the shared factors of success or failure perceived by the project group (Pohl et al. 2015).

8.7 Conclusion

For more than a decade, we have been using and exploring these tools in various settings. We use them to structure shorter meetings, or we combine several tools for two-day workshops; we use them to support the coproduction of knowledge between researchers of different disciplines or between researchers and societal actors; we use them to facilitate collaboration in ongoing research projects together with all participants or to reflect proactively on who to involve, when, and how with the project leaders only. From the feedback we get, we conclude that, in collaborative projects, underlying assumptions and expectations usually remain implicit and are not discussed. If this is the case, the participants usually assume that the other thought collectives are based on the same assumptions and expectations as their own collective. Learning that this is not the case then takes place at various stages during the project, for instance, when after 2 years of collaboration, the participants realize that central concepts—such as a model—have different meanings or that the results of subprojects are incompatible. Using the tools does not guarantee that results will be compatible and that there will be one shared definition of central concepts. Rather, the tools highlight all the conceptual and practical challenges that have to be dealt with in the coproduction of knowledge. They point to all the tasks that accompany the aim of integrating the knowledge of different thought collectives in order to address an issue in an encompassing way.

References

Anonymous. New job for psychiatry. Sci News. 1966;89(22):426.

Apostel L. Interdisciplinarity; problems of teaching and research in universities. Paris: Organisation for Economic Co-operation and Development; 1972.

Bergmann M, Jahn T, Knobloch T, Krohn W, Pohl C, Schramm E. Methods for transdisciplinary research: a primer for practice. Frankfurt/Main: Campus Verlag; 2012.

Elkana Y. Science as a cultural system: an anthropological approach. In: Bonetti N, editor. Scientific culture in the contemporary world, Special Volume published in Collaboration with UNESCO. Milano: SCIENTIA – International Review of Scientific Synthesis; 1979. p. 269–90.

Falk-Krzesinski HJ, Contractor N, Fiore SM, Hall KL, Kane C, Keyton J, Klein JT, Spring B, Stokols D, Trochim W. Mapping a research agenda for the science of team science. Res Eval. 2011;20(2):145–58.

Fleck L. Genesis and development of a scientific fact. Chicago: The University of Chicago Press; 1979.

Frodeman R, Thompson Klein J, Mitcham C, editors. The Oxford Handbook of Interdisciplinarity. Oxford: Oxford University Press; 2010.

Hirsch Hadorn G, Hoffmann-Riem H, Biber-Klemm S, Grossenbacher-Mansuy W, Joye D, Pohl C, Wiesmann U, Zemp E, editors. Handbook of transdisciplinary research. Dordrecht: Springer; 2008.

Jantsch E. Inter- and transdisciplinary university: a systems approach to education and innovation. Policy Sci. 1970;1(4):403–28.

Klein JT. Crossing boundaries. Knowledge, disciplinarities, and interdisciplinarities. Charlottesville: University Press of Virginia; 1996.

Klein JT, Grossenbacher-Mansuy W, Häberli R, Bill A, Scholz RW, Welti M, editors. Transdisciplinarity: joint problem solving among science, technology, and society. Basel: Birkhäuser Verlag; 2001.

Lemos MC, Morehouse BJ. The co-production of science and policy in integrated climate assessments. Glob Environ Change. 2005;15(1):57–68.

McDonald D, Bammer G, Dean P. Research integration using dialogue methods. Canberra: ANU E Press, The Australian National University; 2009.

NAS/NAE/IOM. Facilitating interdisciplinary research. Washington: National Academy of Sciences, National Academy of Engineering, Institute of Medicine, The National Academies Press; 2005.

National Research Council. Enhancing the effectiveness of team science. Washington, DC: The National Academies Press; 2015.

Pielke RA Jr. The honest broker making sense of science in policy and politics. Cambridge: Cambridge University Press; 2007.

Pohl C. What is progress in transdisciplinary research? Futures. 2011;43(6):618–26.

Pohl C, Wuelser G, Bebi P, Bugmann H, Buttler A, Elkin C, Grêt-Regamey A, Hirschi C, Le QB, Peringer A, Rigling A, Seidl R, Huber R. How to successfully publish interdisciplinary research: learning from an ecology and society special feature. Ecol Soc. 2015;20(2):23.

Polk M. Transdisciplinary co-production: designing and testing a transdisciplinary research framework for societal problem solving. Futures. 2015;65:110–22.

Rittel HWJ. Second-generation design methods. In: Cross N, editor. Developments in design methodology. Chichester: Wiley; 1984. p. 317–27.

Robinson J, Tansey J. Co-production, emergent properties and strong interactive social research: the Georgia Basin futures project. Sci Public Policy. 2006;33(2):151–60.

Smit A. The facilitator's toolkit, vol. 45. Stellenbosch: Centre for Business in Society, University of Stellenbosch; 2005.

Stokols D, Hall KL, Taylor BK, Moser RP. The science of team science: overview of the field and introduction to the supplement. Am J Prev Med. 2008;35(2 Suppl):S77–89.

Stokols D, Hall KL, Vogel AL. Defining transdisciplinary research and education. In: Haire-Joshu D, McBride TD, editors. Transdisciplinary public health: research, education, and practice. San Francisco: Jossey-Bass; 2013. p. 3–30.

Vogel AL, Hall KL, Fiore SM, Klein JT, Michelle Bennett L, Gadlin H, Stokols D, Nebeling LC, Wuchty S, Patrick K, Spotts EL, Pohl C, Riley WT, Falk-Krzesinski HJ. The team science toolkit: enhancing research collaboration through online knowledge sharing. Am J Prev Med. 2013;45(6):787–9.

Winch RF. Heuristic and empirical typologies: a job for factor analysis. Am Sociol Rev. 1947;12(1):68–75.

Engaging the Community: Community-Based Participatory Research and Team Science

9

Nina Wallerstein, Karen Calhoun, Milton Eder,
Julie Kaplow, and Consuelo Hopkins Wilkins

Contents

1

9.1 Introduction

With the intractability of health inequities in communities of color and other marginalized communities across the nation, there has been an increased recognition and growth of cross-disciplinary team science to comprehensively address structural conditions, and other social, cultural, behavioral, and biological factors that contribute to these disparities. Recent investments in NIH-funded transdisciplinary population health centers and multi- and interdisciplinary disparities initiatives have reinforced this research paradigm to not only assess inequities but to design multilevel interventions to reduce inequities within diverse communities (Stokols et al. 2008; Holmes et al. 2008;

The original version of this chapter was revised.
The correction to this chapter is available at
https://doi.org/10.1007/978-3-030-20992-6_46

N. Wallerstein (✉)
College of Population Health, University of
New Mexico, Albuquerque, NM, USA

Center for Participatory Research, Health Sciences
Center, University of New Mexico, Albuquerque,
NM, USA
e-mail: NWallerstein@salud.unm.edu

K. Calhoun
Michigan Institute for Clinical & Health Research,
University of Michigan, Ann Arbor, MI, USA

M. Eder
Department of Family Medicine and Community
Health, Office of Community Engagement
to Advance Research and Community Health,
Clinical and Translational Science Institute,
University of Minnesota, Minneapolis, MN, USA

J. Kaplow
The Trauma and Grief Center, Texas Children's
Hospital, Baylor College of Medicine,
Houston, TX, USA

C. H. Wilkins
Department of Medicine, Vanderbilt University
Medical Center, Nashville, TN, USA

© Springer Nature Switzerland AG 2019
K. L. Hall et al. (eds.), *Strategies for Team Science Success*,
https://doi.org/10.1007/978-3-030-20992-6_9

Gambescia et al. 2006; Abrams 2016; Wallerstein et al. 2011; Cooper et al. 2015; Jernigan et al. 2015). A major challenge, however, for team science is that it has been primarily understood as academics working across multiple disciplines.

The idea of collaboratively engaging community partners in creating, implementing, evaluating, and disseminating disparities research is only starting to gain broader recognition. In the U.S., Stokols (2006) introduced the framework of "transdisciplinary action research" to promote a team science that incorporates community members and leaders to strengthen diversity of the science, problem-solving approaches, and capacity to apply research findings to community change. European literature has reinforced this call for a "transdisciplinary science" that incorporates practitioners and external stakeholders into the academic team as essential for addressing real-world problems (Hadorn et al. 2008). One challenge for academic researchers to extend their teams to community members is their lack of experience and unfamiliarity with engaging community stakeholders in cross-disciplinary team science. Adding to the complexity is uncertainty differentiating cross-disciplinary team approaches and unidisciplinary teams, with individual scholarly contributions depending on the methodologies used (Hall et al. 2008; Borner et al. 2010).

In this manuscript, we use the term "cross-disciplinary" team science to integrate the range of inter-, multi-, and transdisciplinary team science with the participatory values and practice of community based participatory research (CBPR) and community-engaged research (CEnR). We describe the potential for incorporating community–partner perspectives into contemporary team science by recounting contributions made by community–researcher partnerships characteristic of CBPR. These CBPR partnerships look similar to cross-disciplinary academic teams in their histories and imperatives to create shared leadership, mutual benefit, and multidirectional trust and respect.

First, we define and then situate CBPR within the range of community-engaged research practices, and discuss the opportunities as well as challenges for CBPR and CEnR to become established within Academic Health Science centers and clinical translational science award (CTSA) infrastructures. We will share summary results of CTSA surveys about community engagement: from the academic perspective and from community perspectives on barriers they continue to face. An in-depth example will be shared of a successful community–academic partnership that grew from a pilot study to a large-scale clinical and population intervention center. We will end with a CBPR conceptual model that showcases how cross-disciplinary teams are needed to describe the richness of contexts in which research take place, to frame the development and use of measures and metrics to evaluate partnerships, and to identify promising participatory practices associated with research and health outcomes. Recommendations are provided for engagement of community partners within the cross-disciplinary team science enterprise (Fig. 9.1).

9.2   Background to Community-Based Participatory Research (CBPR)

Community engagement in research has been on the rise in the last few decades (Eder et al. 2017). As the most recognized form of community-engaged research, CBPR is defined as an orientation to research that emphasizes "equitable" participation of partners for "combining knowledge and action for social change to improve community health and eliminate health disparities" (Wallerstein et al. 2018, p. 3). CBPR involves authentic engagement of community members and stakeholders in all aspects of the research process, from problem definition through data collection, analysis, and dissemination and use of findings to affect program, practice, and policy changes (Israel et al. 2013). CBPR partnerships working on policy are increasingly seen as critical for taking work to scale to eliminate health disparities (Cacari-Stone et al. 2014; Minkler et al. 2012).

Based on histories of "maximum feasible participation" from the 1960s' War on Poverty and

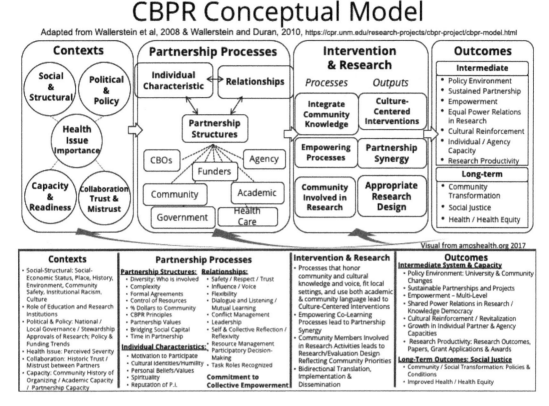

Fig. 9.1 CBPR conceptual model

funding from the Centers for Disease Control and Prevention (CDC) for community participation in public health programs, the National Institute of Environmental Health Sciences launched the first National Institutes of Health (NIH) funding for CBPR in 1995. Increased pressure from community stakeholder groups supported continued CBPR and community-engaged funding from multiple NIH Institutes, most notably the National Center (later Institute) for Minority Health and Health Disparities, as well as from the CDC, private foundations, and newer initiatives such as Patient-Centered Outcomes Research Institute (PCORI) which has promoted patient engagement in research (Eder et al. 2018). Native American Research Centers for Health (NARCH) funding, started as a partnership between the Indian Health Service and NIH, offered a structural first in the creation of authentic community–academic partnerships. Under NARCH, tribes or tribal entities were

mandated to be Principal Investigators of new research centers, receiving a required 30% of the budget, with research projects then conducted with research-intensive (mostly University) partners (NARCH Grants 2008). NARCH's goals were to reduce some of the worst health disparities in the nation through building CBPR partnerships and tribally led research that could decrease research mistrust, and support a pipeline for American Indian/Alaska Native scholars.

CBPR has specifically sought to counter historic research abuses in communities of color and other marginalized communities through recognizing the need to create committed partnerships that challenge histories of research mistrust and build from the core principles of starting from community priorities and strengths (Israel et al, 1998; Israel et al. 2013; Wallerstein et al. 2018). Public health disparities and equity researchers have increasingly adopted CBPR as they recognize the importance of comprehensive engagement of community partners in order to ensure quality, community relevance, culture-centeredness, sustainability of programs, practices and policies, and commitment to redressing social inequities as a result of the research (Dankwa-Mullan et al. 2010; Wallerstein and Duran 2010; Jagosh et al. 2012; Frerichs et al, 2015). One effective practice that has become identified in CBPR research teams has been the role of bridging social capital or the importance of having some academic team members who share identities (racial/ethnic/gender or other social identity) or core values with community members. This bridging social capital becomes a critical mechanism to challenge power differentials and foster mutual respect for the different sources of knowledge that come from both academic and community cultures (Muhammad et al. 2015). Differential command over social capital may help to explain the still meager attention directed toward the incorporation of patients onto primary care teams engaged in practice transformation (Sharma and Grumbach 2017).

9.3 Clinical Translational Science Award (CTSA) Practices in Community Engagement and Community-Engaged Research

Community engagement received an additional boost in 2006 within U.S. research discourse from the initiation of NIH's clinical translational science awards (CTSAs) to approximately 60 academic health centers. In order "to forge a uniquely transformative, novel and integrative home for clinical and translational research," the first CTSA RFA identified community engagement as one option among key functions to "foster collaborative partnerships and enhance public trust in clinical and translational research, facilitating the recruitment of research participants from the community" (Institutional Clinical and Translational Science Award RFA-RM-06-002 2016; Zerhouni and Alving 2006).

Over the past decade, CTSAs have increasingly worked to address the complexities of translational science through collaboration and engagement strategies, including the involvement of community and stakeholder representation on research teams (CTSA U54 2016). With CBPR already established as a successful approach to aligning research with community interests and including community members on research teams, its critically reflective approach to partnerships and team development was seen by many as a model approach for CTSA community engagement, particularly for later stage translational research. Recent publications from the Institute of Medicine (IOM) have called for community engagement to be used more broadly across the entire T1–T5 research spectrum (IOM 2013; Graham et al. 2015).

The spectrum of community engagement across the CTSA consortium however has been varied. A CTSA publication of a community engagement continuum posits a broad range of definitions, from community outreach through shared leadership (McCloskey et al. 2013). Despite the inclusiveness of this definition, there is a risk of co-opting the value of equitable involvement of partners with unidirectional activities, such as educational outreach, unless the more minimal outreach provides the starting place for greater community involvement. As a caution, Trickett (2011) has raised the concern of only seeing engagement as a utilitarian exercise to fulfill the grant activities, versus the potential for an expansive capacity-building enterprise that promotes shared leadership, or beyond, to community-directed research.

To pursue a more defined strategy for community engagement within the CTSAs, scholars from multiple CTSAs constructed a community engagement logic model for academic health centers, proposing infrastructure characteristics and activities as initial inputs. The model recognized complexities in engaging communities across the span of translational science by acknowledging a range of engagement intensities from simple outreach activities to those projects with shared community–academic leadership responsibilities (Eder et al. 2013). While proposed outputs included changed communities, academic environments, and greater involvement of community members in team science, initial measurements tend to be counts of activities, such as numbers of community trainings or numbers of community members participating in the trainings. The logic model however also calls for evaluating community engagement in terms of trust and synergy, as intermediate results that form the foundation for achieving goals of increased recruitment for research, improved clinical trial design, research implementation and dissemination of findings.

The need to shift evaluation thinking about community participation in the CTSA research enterprise was reinforced by a 2015 study of CTSAs, which revealed shared definitions of community engagement but limited evaluation employing community engagement metrics. The study found a majority of CTSA institutions had established Community Advisory Boards, but these same institutions uniformly acknowledged they had no clear strategy for assessing the contributions of those boards in relation to institutional translational science program goals. While activities continue to be collected for annual reports, CTSAs still lack comprehensive strategies for ensuring community engagement in research, including little focus on public dissemination of research activities and findings (Eder et al. 2018).

9.4 Barriers to Engaging Community Stakeholder Perspectives Within CTSAs

Although the number of community representatives involved with academic health research has increased due to CTSAs, the question remains: in what specifically are they involved? In a 2012 inventory, results showed few community members integrated into specific research teams. Instead, community members often served as advisers or in roles relegated to community engagement cores. CTSAs reported an average of

21 community members involved in formal roles, primarily as members of Community or External Advisory Boards (Wilkins et al. 2013). Less than 10% of CTSAs, however, involved community members in areas critical to research such as ethics and participant and clinical interactions resources. Key barriers to community involvement included perceived power differentials between academic leadership and community representatives, perceptions of being undervalued, and inadequate compensation of community members.

In response to the Institute of Medicine's request for input on CTSAs, an invited panel of community engagement stakeholders provided feedback using a Delphi method (Freeman et al. 2014). In this three-round process, community members and researchers identified and prioritized barriers to meaningful community engagement, as well as strategies to enhance engagement and the use of metrics to measure success. Obstacles identified were community distrust of academia, inequitable treatment of community partners, cultural disconnects between institutions and the community, and little funding for community partners. Stakeholders noted that conventional metrics for research such as grant dollars awarded and manuscripts published were unlikely to indicate the degree to which the research was translational. Respondents recommended new metrics that would assess the level of integration of community members in the research, determine the allocation of funds to community partners, document impact of research, such as policy changes and improvements in health, and assess new and sustained partnerships. The suggested metrics are consistent with principles and practices of CBPR and team science.

A 2014 survey of community members sought to better understand experiences and perspectives about research and researchers (Skinner et al. 2018) within CTSAs. Respondent characteristics included 78% female, median age of 46, 66% with graduate degrees, 12% with less than a college degree, and 75% representing a community organization, with 74% employed by that community organization. In all, 75% considered themselves a research partner and 43% represented the CTSAs advisory board. Community members reported trust of research and researchers as fair to average and only one-third believed that research funds were equitably distributed among community partners and academia. Although community members rated their experience with researchers favorably, there were concerns about researchers' preparedness to engage community. On average, researchers were perceived as "moderately prepared" to conduct research with the community and only 6% were perceived as "very prepared," while 13% were "not at all prepared." The perceived lack of preparedness by researchers likely reflects that engaging community stakeholders is a new concept for many researchers, and the skills typically developed in rigorous research training often do not translate to identifying, recruiting and convening patient and community groups, facilitating the participation of a heterogeneous group, and acting on stakeholder input. These skills are equally critical to academic–community research partnerships and team science, and becoming proficient requires training and hands-on experience, which may take years.

A series of focus groups undertaken by Tufts University of their community partners also identified social determinants as contextual barriers to community members participating in research, such as undocumented legal status, the lack of political power, and basic conditions, such as homelessness and inadequate housing as health concerns that overwhelm people's lives. They recommended CBPR initiatives that address these conditions and barriers as essential for CTSAs to facilitate trust, respect and transformation of the *status quo* (Martinez et al. 2015).

9.5 Example of Community-Partnered Social and Behavioral Team Science

The evolution of the Detroit School-Based Health Collaborative (DSBHC) shows the value of incorporating community stakeholders in a cross-disciplinary team science approach to research. Faced with escalating mental health needs of youth growing up in families and neighborhoods overwhelmed by unhealthy social and environmental conditions, and little to no data to describe this phenomena, the Detroit Public Schools, local health systems, state government and several community-based organizations approached the University of Michigan and City Connect Detroit to create a new collaborative.

Seed money from the State of Michigan in 2010 enabled the new team science coalition of school-based and school-linked health centers, state government, community-based organizations, and academia to begin to develop a research agenda. The DSBHC functioned as a community-based coalition, initiated and co-led by a City Connect Detroit staff member (and consultant with the University of Michigan's Clinical Translational Science Institute, CTSI) and an evaluator from Michigan State University. Representation included a school nurse/health promotion administrator, school-based health clinic supervisors, a Federally Qualified Health Center (FQHC), community-based organizations, and academicians from public health, psychiatry, education and community-engaged evaluation. Starting with focus groups in 2011 with students, parents, healthcare professionals and educators, the DSBHC unveiled startling knowledge on young people's perseverance and coping skills to deal with their exposure to unstable homes and neighborhoods, violence, and death. Further dialogue with behavioral healthcare clinicians revealed a lack of access to valid measures and appropriate training to effectively assess and treat youth's increasing experiences with trauma and bereavement. They also identified the need to strengthen cultural appropriateness of their assessments and treatment protocols. This evidence from over 100 stakeholders mobilized the University of Michigan Institute for Clinical & Health Research, the University's CTSI, and City Connect Detroit to provide seed funding in 2012 to address the community's priorities.

A research project, "The Trauma and Grief Needs Assessment," was invited by the

Collaborative to launch in an expanded partnership with 18 school-based and school-linked health centers and two community mental health organizations. The primary goals of the Trauma and Grief Needs Assessment were to (1) assist partners in developing a trauma- and bereavement- informed approach to identifying high-risk youth; (2) test the feasibility of training school-based and school-linked clinicians in screening/ assessment of posttraumatic stress reactions, maladaptive grief, and depression; (3) examine the content validity of two novel measures of childhood grief (Kaplow et al. 2018; Layne et al. 2014) and posttraumatic stress (Kaplow et al. 2019) to enhance their cultural appropriateness for underserved minority youth; and (4) provide a large-scale needs assessment to each partner organization, determining rates of trauma/loss and associated mental health outcomes among students.

The DSBHC transitioned into a community advisory board and practice-research network, comprised of school-based and school-linked clinicians and leadership from Detroit community organizations and health systems. The CAB utilized CBPR to provide guidance and local expertise with regard to the cultural acceptability of the research, including the assessment tools themselves. The academic side of the partnership provided training and consultation to school-based clinicians as well as needs assessment data. Approximately 100 clinicians were trained to administer trauma and grief assessments to identify high-risk youth in underserved school-based settings (Kaplow et al. 2015; Layne et al. 2018). Additionally, regular focus groups were held with the CAB to obtain feedback regarding the assessment process and cultural appropriateness of the tools. Specifically, the CAB was instrumental in legitimizing and refining the grief measure's item pool to reflect the cultural diversity of urban youth, particularly with regard to grief reactions in relation to violent deaths and to culture-specific rituals of grief and mourning (Kaplow et al. 2012). Input from school-based clinicians ensured both the feasibility and acceptability of utilizing this newly validated grief measure in school settings in particular (Kaplow et al. 2018).

The partnership's needs assessment in the city of Detroit and Wayne County, Michigan documented epic levels of trauma, bereavement, and associated PTSD and maladaptive grief reactions among youth (Kaplow et al. 2015). Of 372 assessments, youth reported an average of two deaths of close loved ones, 17.3% of which were due to murder; and an average of 3.6 traumas in their lifetime, most commonly the death of a loved one (75%) or witnessing neighborhood violence (40.3%). Approximately 21.6% of youth met criteria for Posttraumatic Stress Disorder. These findings prompted further interest in meeting needs of traumatized and grieving youth.

Findings from the 2011 focus groups, assessments, and establishment of a strong community–academic partnership, coupled with clinical and research expertise in childhood trauma and grief, helped the University of Michigan Psychiatry Department successfully receive SAMSHA funding (2012–2016) to create its first Trauma and Grief (TAG) Center for Youth to provide in-house care using trauma and bereavement-informed best practices. The CAB, through its community networks, was also able to help disseminate the model in an expanded partnership with 27 schools and two community mental health organizations in Metropolitan Detroit. Through SAMHSA funding, the TAG Center became a member of the National Child Traumatic Stress Network (NCTSN), offering training, support, and resources, including training in an evidence-based school-based intervention (Saltzman et al. 2018), to providers who work with adolescents exposed to trauma and loss.

The TAG Center, now operated by Texas Children's Hospital/Baylor College of Medicine in Houston due to the PI's relocation to Texas, continues to maintain a satellite TAG Clinic at the University of Michigan, and has expanded its initiatives throughout three different school districts in the Greater Houston area (including 288 schools throughout the Houston Independent School District alone). In 2016, the TAG Center received further SAMHSA funding to become a Category II Treatment and Services Adaptation Center, designed to provide wide-spread dissemination of developmentally and culturally appropriate bereavement-informed best practices. In addition, funding from the New York Life Foundation supported the development of a practice-research network (the Grief-Informed Foundations of Treatment or GIFT Network) of ten national sites (including several of the original Detroit partners) to provide evidence-based assessment and treatment of maladaptive grief reactions among bereaved youth.

The TAG Center case study demonstrates the enormous potential for effective CBPR team science in which community organizations and leaders are engaged in research teams as genuine partners from the initial pilot study stage to its current evolution into a far-reaching network of community–academic partnerships. Development of this successful collaborative initiative was furthered by evaluating both engagement dynamics and clinical research outcomes. While CTSAs have begun to include community leaders and members in their infrastructures, such as Community Advisory Boards, barriers to incorporating community members into academic-community research teams remain critical to address. Community-based participatory research, in its history predating CTSAs, offers a promising set of principles, strategies, and goals for such teams.

9.6   CBPR and Cross-Disciplinary Team Science: Current and Future Promise

In 2009, the National Institute on Minority Health and Health Disparities (NIMHD) convened a major national disparities conference in which CBPR was highlighted as a transformational, translational, and transdisciplinary science (Dankwa-Mullan et al. 2010; Wallerstein and Duran 2010; Minkler 2010). Highlighted principles harkened back to recognizing historic research abuses in order to rebuild research trust, and to honor community strengths, priorities and knowledge as important starting places for creating sustainable academic–community research teams. CBPR and team science were recognized as sharing principles of mutual benefit and

respect, transparency, management of team dynamics, and shared decision-making and leadership.

Principles alone however are insufficient and need to be transformed into collaborative practices that foster trust, synergy, and improved health outcomes. A long-term investigation into CBPR initiated in 2006 has been seeking to do just that: support a science of CBPR and community-engaged research that will identify promising or emerging best practices which are associated with better outcomes, such as fulfillment of grant scope, improved community capacities in research, enhanced university capacities to engage communities, and reduced health inequities. Initial pilot funding from NIMHD facilitated an extensive literature review and the creation of a CBPR conceptual model[1] of research contexts, partnering practices, impact on research design, and outcomes, with measures and metrics for evaluating model constructs (Sandoval et al. 2012; Wallerstein et al. 2008; Kastelic et al. 2018).

As the next step to the research, the Universities of New Mexico and Washington joined with the National Congress of American Indians Policy Research Center (NCAIPRC), as the oldest intertribal organization in the country, to receive NARCH/NIH funding (2009–2013). With an additional Think Tank of community and academic CBPR experts, this academic-community partnership was a CBPR cross-disciplinary team (of multiple disciplines and content areas, but also of multiple racial/ethnicities and life experiences) whose goal was to test the CBPR conceptual model and advance the science. The specific aims were to assess the variability of partnerships nationwide, to assess the specific role of governance (in particular the role of tribal sovereignty, critically important to the NCAIPRC community partner), and to identify associations between partnering practices and research and health outcomes (Kastelic et al. 2018). This mixed methods CBPR study, consisting of internet surveys of 200 federally funded research partnerships; and

---

[1] http://cpr.unm.edu/research-projects/cbpr-project/cbpr-model.html; https://engageforequity.org

seven in-depth case studies (Lucero et al. 2018; Pearson et al, 2015), has produced psychometrically validated scales (Oetzel et al. 2015), with the great majority of these community engagement/CBPR metrics and scales overlapping with or complementing team science metrics. Early results of data analysis identity promising practices associated with outcomes, such as the importance of cultural centeredness (Kagawa-Singer et al. 2012; Wallerstein et al, 2019), governance (Oetzel et al. 2015), trust (Lucero et al. 2018), and involving community members in all research activities and steps (Duran et al. in press). Further structural equation modeling has illuminated two interrelated pathways for practices to influence outcomes, one that is based on relationships and one that builds from structural agreements (Oetzel et al. 2018a).

This first cross-site study, to assess correlations between partnering practices and outcomes nationwide, has been extended through National Institute of Nursing Research funding (2015–2020) for the "Engage for Equity: Advancing Community-Engaged Research" study. As a partnership between the University of New Mexico, five other national and international partners, and the Think Tank of community and academic CBPR practitioners, Engage for Equity has refined partnering measures and metrics, translated scales into Spanish, and created evaluation and reflection tools in order to strengthen academic–community engagement collaborative practices.[2] These refined internet survey measures have been tested on another 179 federally funded community-engaged research projects, and analysis is underway of promising practices from the full complement of close to 400 partnerships (Oetzel et al. 2018b). This research, along with the vast array of individual CBPR research projects and new meta-reviews of community-engaged effectiveness worldwide, provide promise to the calls for incorporating community members directly into transdisciplinary research teams (O'Mara-Eves et al. 2015; Cyril et al. 2015; Rifkin 2014; De Las Nueces et al. 2012).

Ultimately, the opportunity is great for team science metrics and CBPR metrics to reinforce each other, as they share the goals of establishing mutually beneficial and respectful group processes that enhance usefulness of knowledge and research outcomes.

9.7 Conclusion

In summary, there is a range of community engagement and community participation within academic–community research teams being implemented across the country. CTSA awards, along with other hubs, such as Clinical Trial Networks, NIH-funded Disparities Centers, PCORI partnership grants, and CDC Prevention Centers, among others, have provided institutional opportunities for academic health centers to develop infrastructures that will more efficiently benefit from community member input across the translational research spectrum. CBPR offers a unique contribution with its focus on community social determinants, recognition of the barriers of power differentials and community distrust, the capacity to incorporate cultural diversity and knowledge into research, and the commitment to social change and transformation as core values for engaging community partners in academic–community research teams. With the ultimate goal of these partnerships to impact policies, programs and practices that improve health and reduce inequities, we need to rethink our perspective on community members so they become active partners in research, from conceptualization through implementation, dissemination, and translation of research results.

To their credit, academic health centers, through CTSAs and other mechanisms, have drawn upon CBPR principles in developing community advisory boards or community cores, and in organizing some community-engaged research. They have not, however, sufficiently incorporated community leaders, organizations, and members into cross-disciplinary research teams. These efforts need to reconceptualize community members and organizations as research *partners*

---

[2] http://cpr.unm.edu/research-projects/cbpr-project/cbpr-e2.html

within their research teams, with appropriate measures and metrics of the benefits of community engagement. With active involvement of communities as colleagues, CEnR and CBPR can build participatory research competencies of both universities and communities, and can encourage long-lasting sustainability of relationships for team science and for research more relevant and responsive to community priorities and needs.

References

Abrams DB. Applying transdisciplinary research strategies to understanding and eliminating health disparities. Health Educ Behav. 2016;33(4):515–31.

Borner K, Contractor N, Falk-Krzesinski HJ, Fiore S, Hall K, Keyton J, Spring B, Stokols D, Trochim W, Uzzi B. A multi-level systems perspective for the science of team science. Commentary Team Science. Sci Transl Med. 2010;2(49):49cm24. https://doi.org/10.1126/scitranslmed.3001399.

Cacari-Stone L, Wallerstein N, Garcia A, Minkler M. The Promise of Community Based Participatory Research for Health Equity: A Conceptual Model for Bridging Evidence with Policy, American Journal of Public Health 2014;104(9):1615–23.

Cooper LA, Ortega AN, Ammerman AS, Buchwald D, Paskett ED, Powell LH, Thompson B, Tucker KL, Warnecke RB, McCarthy WJ, Viswanath KV, Henderson JA, Calhoun EA, Williams DR. Calling for a bold new vision of health disparities intervention research. Am J Public Health. 2015;105(Suppl 3):S374–6.

CTSA U54, Clinical and Translational Science Award U54. 2016. http://grants.nih.gov/grants/guide/pa-files/PAR-15-304.html. Accessed 2 April 2016.

Cyril S, Smith BJ, Possamai-Inesedy A, Renzaho AMN. Exploring the role of community engagement in improving the health of disadvantaged populations: a systematic review. Glob Health Action. 2015;8:29842. https://doi.org/10.3402/gha.v8.29842.

Dankwa-Mullan I, Rhee KB, Stoff DM, Pohlhaus JR, Sy FS, Stinson N, Ruffin J. Moving toward paradigm-shifting research in health disparities through translational, transformational, and transdisciplinary approaches. Am J Public Health. 2010;100(S1):S19.

De Las Nueces D, Hacker K, DiGirolamo A, Hicks LS. A systematic review of community-based participatory research to enhance clinical trials in racial and ethnic minority groups. Health Serv Res., in Measuring and Analyzing Health Care Disparities. 2012;47:1363. https://doi.org/10.1111/j.1475-6773.2012.01386.x.

Duran B, Oetzel J, Pearson C, Magarati M, Zhou C, Villegas M, Muhammad M, Belone L, Wallerstein N. Promising practices and outcomes: learnings from a CBPR cross-site national study, Prog Community Health Partnersh. in press.

Eder M, Carter-Edwards L, Hurd T, Rumala B, Wallerstein N. A logic model for community engagement within the CTSA consortium: can we measure what we model? Acad Med. 2013;88(10):1430–6.

Eder M, Evans E, Funes M, Hong H, Reuter K, Ahmed S, Calhoun K, Corbie-Smith G, Dave G, DeFino M, Harwood E, Kissack A, Kleinman LC, Wallerstein N. Defining and measuring community engagement and community-engaged research: CTSA Institutional Practices. Prog Community Health Partnersh. 2018;12(2):145–56.

Eder MM, Holzer J, Calhoun K, Strong LL. A retrospective on the vision for Progress in community health partnerships: research, education, and action. Prog Community Health Partnersh. 2017;11(1):1–11. https://doi.org/10.1353/cpr.2017.0001.

Freeman ER, Seifer SD, Stupak M, Sprague Martinez LS. Community engagement in the CTSA program: stakeholder responses from a National Delphi Process. Clin Transl Sci. 2014;7(3):191–5.

Frerichs L, Hassmiller Lich K, Dave G, Corbie-Smith G. Integrating systems science and community-based participatory research to achieve health equity. Am J Public Health. 2015;106:215. https://doi.org/10.2105/AJPH.2015.302944.

Gambescia SF, Woodhouse LD, Auld ME, Green BL, Quinn SC, Airhihenbuwa CO. Framing a transdisciplinary research agenda in health education to address health disparities and social inequities: a road map for SOPHE action. Health Educ Behav. 2006;33(4):531–7.

Graham PW, et al. What is the role of culture, diversity, and community engagement in transdisciplinary translational science? Transl Behav Med. 2015;6:1–10.

Hadorn GH, Hoffmann-Riem H, Biber-Klemm S, Grossenbacher-Mansuy W, Joye D, Pohl C, Wiesmann U, Zemp E, editors. Handbook of transdisciplinary science. Dordrecht: Springer; 2008.

Hall KL, Feng AX, Moser RP, Stokols D, Taylor BK. Moving the science of team science forward: collaboration and creativity. Am J Prev Med. 2008;35(2):S243–9.

Holmes J, Lehman A, Hade R, et al. Challenges for multilevel health disparities research in a transdisciplinary environment. Am J Prev Med. 2008;35(2):S182–92.

Institutional Clinical and Translational Science Award. 2016. https://grants.nih.gov/grants/guide/rfa-files/RFA-RM-06-002.html. Accessed 2 July 2016.

IOM, (2013 Institute of Medicine). The CTSA program at NIH: opportunities for advancing clinical and translational research. Washington, DC: Institute of Medicine; 2013.

Israel BA, Eng E, Schulz AJ, Parker EA. Methods in community based participatory research for health. 2nd ed. San Francisco, CA: Jossey-Bass; 2013.

Israel BA, Schulz AJ, Parker EA, Becker AB. Review of community-based research: assessing partnership approaches to improve public health. Annu Rev Public Health. 1998;19:173–202.

Jagosh J, Macaulay AC, Pluye P, et al. Uncovering the benefits of participatory research: implications of a realist review for health research and practice. Milbank Q. 2012;90(2):311–46.

Jernigan V, Peercy M, Branam D, Saunkeah B, Wharton D, Winkleby M, Lowe J, Salvatore A, Dickerson D, Belcourt A, D'Amico E, Patten CA, Parker M, Duran B, Harris R, Buchwald D. Beyond health equity: achieving wellness within American Indian and Alaska native communities. Am J Public Health. 2015;105:S3.

Kagawa-Singer M, Dressler WW, George SM, Elwood WN. The cultural framework for health: an integrative approach for research and program design and evaluation. In: Office of Behavioral and Social Science. Bethesda, MD: National Institutes of Health; 2012.

Kaplow JB, Calhoun K, Porter Howard L, Follebout M. Implementing trauma- and grief-informed assessment in underserved communities: towards a best practice assessment model. School-community Health Alliance of Michigan Conference, Grand Rapids, MI. 2015.

Kaplow JB, Layne CM, Oosterhoff B, Goldenthal H, Howell KH, Wamser-Nanney R, Burnside A, Calhoun K, Pynoos R, et al. Validation of the persistent complex bereavement disorder (PCBD) checklist: a developmentally-informed assessment tool for bereaved youth. J Trauma Stress. 2018;31(2):244–54.

Kaplow JB, Layne CM, Pynoos RS, Cohen J, Lieberman A. DSM-V diagnostic criteria for bereavement-related disorders in children and adolescents: developmental considerations. Psychiatry. 2012;75(3):242–65.

Kaplow JB, Rolon-Arroyo B, Layne CM, Rooney E, Oosterhoff B, Hill R, Steinberg A, Lotterman J, Gallagher K, & Pynoos RS. Validation of the UCLA PTSD Reaction Index for DSM-5 (RI-5): A developmentally-informed assessment tool for trauma-exposed youth. Journal of the American Academy of Child and Adolescent Psychiatry; 2019. https://doi.org/10.1016/j.jaac.2018.10.019

Kastelic S, Wallerstein N, Duran B, Oetzel J. Socioecologic framework for CBPR: development and testing of a model. In: Wallerstein N, Duran B, Oetzel J, Minkler M, editors. Community-based participatory research for health: advancing social and health equity. 3rd ed. San Francisco: Jossey-Bass; 2018. p. 77–94.

Layne CM, Kaplow JB, Pynoos RS. Persistent Complex Bereavement Disorder (PCBD) Checklist – Youth Version 1.0. and Test Administration Manual. Los Angeles: University of California; 2014. http://oip.ucla.edu/sites/default/files/1-Pager_PCBD_Checklist.pdf

Layne CM, Kaplow JB, Youngstrom E. Evidence-based assessment of childhood trauma and bereavement: concepts, principles, and practices. In: Cloitre M, Landolt M, Schnyder U, editors. Evidence-based treatments for trauma-related disorders in children and adolescents. New York: Springer Publications; 2018.

Lucero J, Wallerstein N, Duran B, Alegria M, Greene-Moton E, Israel B, Kastelic S, Magarati M, Oetzel J, Pearson C, Schulz A, Villegas M, White Hat E. Development of a mixed methods investigation of process and outcomes of community based participatory research. J Mix Methods Res. 2018;12:55. https://doi.org/10.1177/1558689816633309.

Martinez L, et al. Community conceptualizations of health: implications for transdisciplinary team science. Clin Transl Sci. 2015;4(3):163–7.

McCloskey DJ, et al. Clinical and translational science awards community engagement key function committee task force on the principles of community engagement. In: Principles of community engagement, vol. 2011. 2nd ed. Bethesda, MD: National Institutes of Health; 2013.

Minkler M. Linking science and policy through community-based participatory research to study and address health disparities. Am J Public Health. 2010;100(Suppl 1):S81–7.

Minkler M, Garcia A, Rubin V, Wallerstein N. Community-based participatory research: a strategy for building healthy communities and promoting health through policy change. In: A report to the California endowment. Oakland, CA: PolicyLink; 2012.

Muhammad M, Wallerstein N, Sussman A, Avila M, Belone L. Reflections on researcher identity and power: the impact of positionality on community based participatory research (CBPR) processes and outcomes. Crit Sociol. 2015;41:1045. https://doi.org/10.1177/0896920513516025.

NARCH Grants, Federal Register. A Notice by the Indian Health Service on 12/22/2008. 2008. https://www.federalregister.gov/articles/2008/12/22/E8-30300/native-american-research-centers-for-health-narch-grants#h-5. Accessed 28 Feb 2016.

O'Mara-Eves A, Brunton G, Oliver S, Kavanagh J, Jamal F, Thomas J. The effectiveness of community engagement in public health interventions for disadvantaged groups: a meta-analysis. BMC Public Health. 2015;15:129. https://doi.org/10.1186/s12889-015-1352-y.

Oetzel J, Wallerstein N, Duran B, Sanchez-Youngman S, Nguyen T, Woo K, Wang J, Schulz AM, Kaholokula JK, Israel BA, Alegria M. Impact of Participatory Health Research: A Test of the CBPR Conceptual Model: Pathways to Outcomes within Community-Academic Partnerships, Biomedical Research International, Article ID; 2018a, 7281405, https://doi.org/10.1155/2018/7281405.

Oetzel JG, Duran B, Sussman A, Magarati M, Khodyakov D, Wallerstein N. Evaluation of CBPR partnerships and outcomes: lessons and tools from the research for improved health study. In: Wallerstein N, Duran B, Oetzel J, Minkler M, editors. Community-based participatory research for health: advancing social and health equity. 3rd ed. San Francisco: Jossey-Bass; 2018b. p. 237–50.

Oetzel J, Villegas M, White Hat E, Duran B, Wallerstein N. Governance of community-engaged research: exploring the associations of final approval with processes and outcomes. Am J Public Health. 2015;105(6):1161–7.

Oetzel JG, Zhou C, Duran B, et al. Establishing the psychometric properties of constructs in a community-based participatory research conceptual model. Am J Health Promot. 2015;29(5):e188–202.

Pearson CR, Duran B, Magarati M, Oetzel J, Zhou C, Lucero J, Villegas M, Wallerstein N. Research for improved health: variability and impact of structural characteristics in federally-funded community engaged research studies. Prog Community Health Partnersh. 2015;9(1):17–29.

Rifkin S. Examining the links between community participation and health outcomes: a review of the literature. Health Policy Plan. 2014;29:ii98–ii106.

Saltzman W, Layne CM, Pynoos RS, Olafson E, Kaplow JB, Boat B. Trauma and grief component therapy for adolescents: a modular approach to treating traumatized and bereaved youth. Cambridge: Cambridge University Press; 2018.

Sandoval JA, Lucero J, Oetzel J, Avila M, Belone L, Mau M, Pearson C, Tafoya G, Duran B, Rios LI, Wallerstein N. Process and outcome constructs for evaluating community-based participatory research projects: a matrix of existing measures. Health Educ Res. 2012;27(4):680–90.

Sharma AE, Grumbach K. Engaging patients in primary care practice transformation: theory, evidence and practice. Fam Pract. 2017;34(3):262–7. https://doi.org/10.1093/fampra/cmw128.

Skinner JS, Williams NA, Richmond A, Brown J, Strelnick AH, Calhoun K, De Loney EH, Allen S, Pirie A, Wilkins CH. Community experiences and perceptions of clinical and translational research and researchers. Prog Community Health Partnersh. 2018;12(3):263–71.

Stokols D. Toward a science of transdisciplinary action research. Am J Community Psychol. 2006;38:63–77.

Stokols D, Hall KL, Taylor BK, Moser RP. The science of team science: overview of the field and introduction to the supplement. Am J Prevent Med. 2008;35(2 Suppl):S77–89.

Trickett EJ. Community-based participatory research as worldview or instrumental strategy: is it lost in translation(al) research? Am J Public Health. 2011;101(8):1353–5.

Wallerstein N, Duran B. Community-based participatory research contributions to intervention research: the intersection of science and practice to improve health equity. Am J Public Health. 2010;100(S1): S40–6.

Wallerstein N, Duran B, Oetzel J, Minkler M. Community-based participatory research for health: advancing social and health equity. 3rd ed. San Francisco: Jossey-Bass; 2018.

Wallerstein N, Oetzel J, Duran B, Magarati M, Pearson C, Belone L, Davis J, Dewindt L, Lucero J, Ruddock C, Sutter E, Villegas M, Dutta, M. Culture-Centeredness in Community Based Participatory Research: Its Impact on Health Intervention Research, Health Education Research, 2019. https://doi.org/10.1093/her/cyz021.

Wallerstein N, Oetzel J, Duran B, Tafoya G, Belone L, Rae R. What predicts outcomes in CBPR? In: Minkler M, Wallerstein N, editors. Community based participatory research for health: process to outcomes. 2nd ed. San Francisco: Jossey Bass; 2008. p. 371–92.

Wallerstein N, Yen I, Syme L. Integrating social epidemiology and community-engaged interventions to improve health equity. Am J Public Health. 2011;101(5):822–30.

Wilkins CH, Spofford M, Williams N, Mckeever C, Allen S, Brown J, et al.' Community representatives' involvement in clinical and translational science awardee activities. Clin Transl Sci. 2013;6(4):292–96.

Zerhouni EA, Alving B. Clinical and translational science awards: a framework for a national research agenda. Trans Res. 2006;148(1):4–5.

Engaging the Patient: Patient-Centered Research

Lorraine B. Johnson and Jaye Bea Smalley

The primary goal of medicine … is to "[improve] health by providing beneficial care to patients."Institute of Medicine (2009)

Contents

L. B. Johnson (✉)
LymeDisease.org, San Ramon, CA, USA
e-mail: lorrainejohnson@outlook.com

J. B. Smalley
Global I & I Patient Advocacy and Life Cycle
Management, Celgene Corporation,
Summit, NJ, USA

10.1 The Growing Mandate for Patient Engagement in Research

There is a growing mandate for patients to play a role in the design and conduct of research to develop and assess drugs, devices, the healthcare system, and other health services and interventions. Often, patient engagement is conceived narrowly as the patient's willingness and ability to participate in his or her care through patient engagement interventions that encourage patient participation. However, since most drugs, devices, and the healthcare system more broadly have not traditionally been developed with the patient perspective in mind, there is a growing consensus that patients should play a more active role on research teams to ensure that the perspective of the patient is represented and understood. To realize the promise of a patient-centered healthcare system, outcomes important to patients must be foundational. Accordingly, those outcomes should inform research to ensure that the technologies, interventions, and healthcare evidence are implemented into guidelines, policy, and ultimately care. This promise could potentially be realized if patients are centrally involved in research as part of the research teams and recognized as uniquely situated to provide the expertise of lived experience.

© Springer Nature Switzerland AG 2019
K. L. Hall et al. (eds.), *Strategies for Team Science Success*,
https://doi.org/10.1007/978-3-030-20992-6_10

Historically, the patient has had a minimal role in the planning for and conduct of research including research used to develop drugs, devices, and secure regulatory approval by the Food and Drug Administration (FDA). Instead, the most influential roles in determining choices available to patients are held by other key stakeholders such as pharmaceutical companies, third-party payers (employers and insurers), guideline developers, and healthcare providers. The actions of healthcare stakeholders are generally based on commercial incentives or the regulatory interests of their organizations, which are primarily accountable for advancing shareholder interests or working within budgetary restrictions.

Various stakeholders value the benefits and risks of healthcare differently (Stakeholder Perspectives on Value, Institute of Medicine 2010). Patients value healthcare services that help them obtain optimal health. While other stakeholders may embrace this value, it may compete with other organizational incentives, including those related to payer cost control, healthcare provider volume-based profit, and pharmaceutical market-size profits (IOM 2016). It may be tempting to believe that the patient interest can be effectively represented by other key stakeholders in health care. However, this assumption is not correct. For example, a study by Devereaux et al. (2001) found that patients and physicians assign different outcome values to stroke versus adverse side effects of treatment.

In addition, the role of the patient in assessing or insuring healthcare value and in holding other key players accountable has been negligible. In part, this is inherent in a third-party payer system, the complexity of the provider–patient relationship, the imbalance of knowledge between experts and lay stakeholders in health care, and patient vulnerability (Stakeholder Perspectives on Value, Institute of Medicine 2010). By the time healthcare decisions trickle down to patients and consumers, all of the important decisions, including what research to conduct, the outcomes measured, how to analyze the results, and the formulation of that research into research guidelines, may have already been made. Ezekiel Emanuel (1999) explains that because the inter-ests of different stakeholders conflict in health care, when someone else speaks for you, "there is a high chance that individuals will be prevented from realizing their interests or their interest will be sacrificed to someone else's interest."

Because of the remarkable power imbalance between patients and other stakeholders, the ability of the market place to self-correct is not present. For example, consumers typically shop for the best quality and price in consumer goods and producers of those goods prioritize the needs of the consumers since they drive the market. In contrast, the options available to a patient are typically predetermined by providers and payers. In health care, the goal—namely improving healthcare outcomes that are important to patients—cannot hold. Recent calls for "patient-centered health care" seek to realign health care by putting the patient interest at the center through initiatives such as patient participation in research, drug approvals, and guideline development processes. These reforms have brought to center stage the notion that it is imperative to bring patient and family voices to decisions about care, to healthcare organizational design and governance, and to public policy (Carman et al. 2013).

Patient-centered outcomes research (PCOR) has evolved to address the decisional dilemmas patients and other healthcare stakeholders face due to a dearth of evidence about the effectiveness of diagnostic and treatment options given the heterogeneity of patient characteristics and individual preferences. The Patient-Centered Outcomes Research Institute (PCORI) was established through the Patient Protection and Affordable Care Act (PPACA) in 2010. Its mission is to help people make informed healthcare decisions and to improve healthcare delivery and outcomes by producing and promoting high integrity, evidence-based information that comes from research guided by patients, caregivers, and the broader healthcare community (PCORI Methodology Committee 2013).

The essence of the PCORI's definition of PCOR is the evaluation of questions and outcomes meaningful and important to patients and caregivers. This definition acknowledges the

PCORI Engagement Rubric

Planning the Study	Conducting the Study	Disseminating the Study Results
Potential Activities		
• Developing research questions and relevant outcomes • Defining characteristics of study participants • Designing the study to minimize disruption to patient and stakeholder study participants	• Drafting or revising study materials and protocols • Participating in study recruitment • Participating in data collection and analysis • Participating in the evaluation of patient and stakeholder engagement • Serving as a patient representative on a data safety monitoring board (DSMB)	• Identifying partner organizations for dissemination • Planning dissemination from the beginning • Participating in dissemination efforts (e.g., manuscripts, presentations) • Identifying opportunities to present or share information about the study
Promising Examples from PCORI-Funded Projects		
• **Comparison of surgery to antibiotic therapy study:** Patients were surveyed about their preferences for these treatment options and that input was used to shape the research proposal. Clinician input changed the study inclusion criteria, logistics, and definition of the outcome "failure". • **Stroke study:** Stroke survivors identified the number of days living at home and not in an institution or the hospital as an important outcome to measure.	• **Chronic pain study:** Patient research partners follow study participants through all aspects of the data collection and intervention to provide guidance on how to make the study processes more patient-centered. • **Asthma study:** To streamline care processes, clinicians and patients provided guidance on who should deliver the intervention, when it should be delivered during the process of care, and how it should be delivered.	• **Comparison of surgery to antibiotic therapy study:** Payers, employers, and policymakers wrote letters of support for the study and agreed to disseminate the study results to peer organizations in their professional networks. • **Neurology study:** The research team (including patient partners) presented information about the study at a neurology patient advocacy conference and alerted those attending about when to expect the results of the study.

Fig. 10.1 PCORI engagement rubric

unique perspectives of patients and caregivers and the impact of their role in better refining and improving the relevance of clinical research questions. The inclusion of patients as stakeholders by PCORI reflects the growing influence of patient advocacy groups in biomedical research and healthcare practice (National Research Council 2015).

PCORI's authorizing legislation requires the institute to develop processes to receive feedback from patients and caregivers in a range of activities to ensure that they have trustworthy, evidence-based information in order to make decisions that reflect their desired outcomes. In order to ensure that PCORI's research is patient centered, the organization engages a broad range of patients and caregivers in the work of the institute, and requires engagement in the research it funds. The alignment of funding opportunities with PCOR provides a powerful incentive for researchers that can help drive cultural change.

This chapter will describe the importance of bringing patients as experts on cross-disciplinary, and multistakeholder research teams to ensure the patient voice is present and considered. It should be noted that caregivers provide and, in certain instances, must provide the perspective of the lived experience of a family member. For simplicity and consistency, we use the term patient throughout this chapter; however, the reader should recognize that a caregiver can also play the same role in research and on research teams. Key learnings and examples from guideline development and the PCORI engagement of patients in research and research governance will be used to illustrate principles of effective patient engagement (Fig. 10.1).

10.2 The Growing Mandate for Patient-Centered Health Care

A number of government-instituted reforms aimed at increasing the engagement of patients in health care have been adopted either through legislative mandate or recommendations by public–private partnerships and government and nongovernmental organizations, such as the National Academy of Medicine (NAM) (formerly the Institute of Medicine [IOM]), the Agency for Healthcare Research and Quality (AHRQ), and the Patient-Centered Outcomes Research Institute (PCORI).

Both PCORI, which funds patient-centered comparative effectiveness research (CER), and the FDA have legislative mandates requiring greater patient centeredness. The FDA mandate for patient engagement arises under Title I of the Food and Drug Administration Safety and Innovation Act (FDASIA) and the Prescription Drug User Fee Act (PDUFA), which requires the agency to "develop and implement strategies to solicit the views of patients during the medical product development process and consider the perspectives of patients during regulatory discussions" (FDASIA, P.L. 112–144). The mandate for PCORI arises under PPACA, which requires that PCORI "provide support and resources to help patient and consumer representatives effectively participate on the board and expert advisory panels" (PCORI Methodology Committee 2013).

The NAM has played a central role in defining and recommending patient engagement in a learning healthcare system and in guidelines development. In 2001, the NAM defined patient-centered care as care that is respectful of and responsive to individual patient preferences, needs, and values and that ensures patient values guide all clinical decisions (IOM 2001). More recently, the NAM has recommended greater engagement of patient in guidelines to ensure (a) greater transparency, (b) the patient perspective and ability to focus attention onto "those individuals most deeply affected by guidelines," (c) the patient context for determining "what matters most to those living with disease regarding the balance of benefits and harms as well as gaps in scientific evidence," and (d) as "a safeguard against conflicts of interest that may skew judgment of clinical and scientific experts" (IOM 2011).

Among the visions for change is the advancement of the model of health care as a learning

system where the emphasis is on continuous improvement of healthcare quality through a collaborative approach that shares data and insights across boundaries between research, healthcare practice, and patient outcomes. In this context, the NAM emphasized the centrality of patient involvement in a learning healthcare system because patients are the ultimate end user of healthcare research findings and the most important stakeholder: "There is a growing appreciation for the centrality of patient involvement as a contributor to positive healthcare outcomes, and as a catalyst for change … [I]n a truly learning healthcare system, learning is bidirectional [and] works not only to better inform patients but also to ensure that patient preference is incorporated into 'best care'" (IOM 2007).

More recently, the IOM has recognized the importance of the patient's voice as an ethical mandate for representation in healthcare policy generally and to insure process integrity to keep other stakeholder interests in check (IOM 2011).

As a result of the FDA and PCORI legislative mandates and the IOM recommendations on creating trustworthy guidelines, patients now have an emerging voice in research enterprise. While the evidence base for patient engagement in research is still evolving, the ethical rationale and principles have been established in community-based participatory research (CBPR). CBPR provides a framework to respond to health issues within a social and historical context while reducing mistrust of the people being studied, through collaboration and partnership between the researcher and community. The ultimate goal is for the community to own the results and use them to improve health outcomes and quality of life (Macaulay et al. 1999).

The remaining sections in the chapter will take a closer look at PCORI and the principles of patient engagement. Finally, a use case applying the engagement principles to PCORnet, PCORI's big data project, will explore one approach to addressing the challenges that arise in ensuring that patient engagement is meaningful.

10.3 PCORI and Patient Engagement in the Institute's Research

"PCORI funds research based on the belief that incorporating the patient perspective into health care research is inherently valuable and that including the end user of research in the research process enhances usefulness and speeds the uptake of research into practice" (Frank et al. 2014).

At the organizational level, there are numerous opportunities to involve patient and stakeholders in the work of the institute. In addition to PCORI's Board of Governors, which includes members representing patients and caregivers, PCORI's authorizing legislation called for the establishment of advisory panels to provide recommendations and advice to the staff, board, and methodology committee. These panels help review and prioritize research questions, provide technical and scientific expertise, and provide other guidance around issues that may arise and are relevant to PCORI's mission and vision. All panels have members from the patient and caregiver community. Although it was not required by the legislation, PCORI established an advisory panel on patient engagement whose charge is to ensure the highest patient engagement standards and a culture of patient-centeredness in all aspects of PCORI's work.

In addition to ensuring patient involvement at the organizational level, PCORI requires meaningful patient engagement in the research it funds. PCORI has established a merit review process that incorporates criteria for patient-centeredness and engagement. Each merit review panel is represented by multiple stakeholders including patients and caregivers to provide the unique perspectives to ensure that the research meets our five funding criteria, which include patient centeredness and patient and stakeholder engagement. Reviewers are given equal weight in the final review score, even when patients and caregivers only score for select funding criteria. PCORI works with reviewers to make sure all patients, caregivers, and other stakeholders have the appropriate training to meaningfully participate in the merit review process and mentorship from peers.

Patient centeredness is the goal that PCOR aims to achieve by ensuring the relevance and quality of the research question and outcomes assessed. Patient engagement is a process of involving patients and caregivers in the research process as partners, not research subjects or participants, to ensure patient centeredness. This partnership, distinct from research participation as subjects and characterized by active and meaningful engagement between scientists, patients, caregivers, and other healthcare stakeholders, reflects the PCOR principles of partnership, colearning, reciprocal relationships, and trust, transparency, and honesty. Patient engagement in research requires a thorough plan that may build upon existing partnerships.

10.4 PCORI's Framework for Patient Engagement: The PCORI Engagement Rubric

When the institute started to fund research, there were many questions about how and when to engage patients and caregivers in research. While there is literature that establishes the need for community engagement in CBPR and additional resources, such as the Team Science Toolkit developed by the National Cancer Institute provide significant resources in this area, patient and caregiver engagement is considered novel. In an effort to better understand how and where engagement was occurring, PCORI staff conducted a targeted review of all 150 funded research project applications from PCORI's first 3 award cycles to identify applications with novel and promising engagement activities that could potentially direct the study to be more patient centered (Sheridan et al. 2017). Three distinct areas emerged that reflect engagement throughout the research continuum: definition of the research question, conduct of the study, and plans for dissemination. These three areas lead to the development of the PCORI Engagement Rubric, PCORI's framework for engagement (PCORI

2016). The PCORI Engagement Rubric is the foundation of PCORI's approach to engagement in research. The rubric identifies opportunities and potential activities for engagement in research, shares real-world examples of promising practices from PCORI-funded research, and provides guidance to a range of stakeholders, including to applicants on the development of engagement plans for research proposals, to merit reviewers for evaluating proposals, and to PCORI staff for reference in evaluating applications and monitoring funded projects (PCORI 2014).

10.4.1 Understanding Patient Engagement in Research and Evaluating Impact

PCORI aims to better understand the relationship between levels of involvement and changes to the research process, such as changes to study design and recruitment rates. To this end, PCORI developed tools to collect information from awardees and partners on engagement in research (PCORI 2017). PCORI uses an annual engagement report completed by the principal investigator of PCORI-funded studies and patient/stakeholder partners nominated by the principal investigators. Key evaluation domains include:

- Who is involved, when they are involved, how they are involved, and what is the level of involvement (information, consultation, collaboration, and patient/stakeholder direction).
- Influence of patient and stakeholder partners.
- Impact of patient involvement

The evaluation provides free text space for respondents to describe impact.

As an example of such impact, PCORI conducted an evaluation of patient involvement from the PCORI Pilot Projects. PCORI funded their first 50 research projects through the Pilot Projects to collect as much information as possible about engagement with these first awardees in a timely fashion. Data were collected at 6 and 12 months through a self-report tool that

captured barriers and facilitators to engagement, contributions and lessons learned. There was a 94% response rate. Most respondents reported engaging more than one stakeholder and common areas for engagement included question solicitation, study design, and data collection. The most common barrier reported was lack of time. Key facilitators included shared leadership and communication. Early lessons learned included the importance of continuous and genuine partnerships, strategic selection of stakeholders, and accommodation of stakeholders' practical needs (Forsythe et al. 2015).

10.5 Opportunities for Patient Engagement in the Research Process

Patients can engage in research in a number of ways, including any of the following:

- Being involved in defining the research question and selecting the outcomes.
- Being a coapplicant in a research proposal.
- Working with funders to review patient-focused section of applications.
- Being an active member of a steering group for a research study.
- Providing input into a study's conception and design.
- Assisting with patient recruitment.
- Coauthoring a research study.
- Assisting in the dissemination of research results (O'Connor 2016).

Whatever aspect of research patients are involved in, it is critical that patients be involved early enough to affect the decision. For example, decisions about how an issue is framed may essentially determine the outcome of a process. Similarly, bringing patients in for comment after the decisions have been made by another group is usually too late for patients to be able to meaningfully affect the decision-making process. The IOM recognizes the importance of early patient engagement in its standards on creating

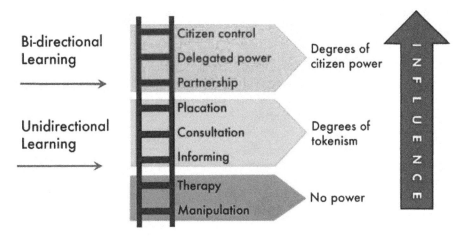

Fig. 10.2 Arnstein's ladder of public participation

trustworthy guidelines by requiring that patients be involved at the time the questions are framed (IOM 2011).

10.6 How to Determine if Patient Engagement Is Meaningful

One well-known assessment tool for public participation may be considered to gauge the effectiveness of patient engagement is the extent to which patients can actually influence decision-making. The model most commonly used as a framework for meaningful participation is Arnstein's ladder of public participation, where the bottom rungs represent either illusory participation or tokenism (Arnstein 1969). More meaningful participation gives patients the ability to influence decision-making through dialogue—an exchange of ideas. This is known as bidirectional learning. For example, focus groups are efficient and give patients voice, but because they provide patients with input only they can be a form of token participation.

To apply Arnstein's ladder, meaningful engagement must not only provide voice, but it must also provide patients with the ability to influence decision-making. There are four essential components to meaningful patient engagement (Fig. 10.2):

- The patient voice must be representative of the affected population.
- Patients must be both sufficiently informed and prepared to engage in meaningful deliberation about the issues.
- Patients must be involved early enough to affect the decision.
- Patients must have the ability to actually influence the decision (Renn et al. 1995).

Similarly, a meta-analysis by Garces of 34 studies about patient engagement identified four common iterative steps (Garces and Lopez 2016). These included patient selection, building a reciprocal relationship, colearning, and feedback and reassessment. The feedback and assessment steps aim to evaluating the engagement as a whole to improve the engagement process and foster further empowerment of the patient. Garces describes patient engagement as occurring along a spectrum that ranges from a passive role to the most engaged role—"from study subject, to collaborator, to a researcher." Engagement activities also occur along a spectrum, including preparation, execution, and translation.

10.7   Patient Selection and Representation

Selecting the patient or surrogate is a threshold issue. Since everyone is a patient at one time or another, does patient selection matter? Of course, representation is a fundamental principle in a pluralistic democracy, but calls to democratize healthcare policy often depend on context. For example, treatment guidelines, while not regulatory, can carry considerable weight and may be essential determinants of access to care for patients. Hence, the NAM recognizes the need for representation in its standards on creating trustworthy guidelines when it specifies "those affected" by the decision be represented in guideline development (IOM 2010).

Those calling for the democratization of research in particular introduce a different perspective—the need to "put the very people it is meant for to serve at the center" as a means of improving innovation and ensuring that research funded addresses issue important to patients (Anderson 2017). At one end of the continuum lies patient-driven registries and research platforms run by patient advocacy organizations, where patient representation may be an integral part of the process. At the other end lies research funded with public monies, where patient representation may be patched onto an existing grant review process. Patient engagement in research funded by pharma may contain a commercial element— that is, a market research perspective (making sure that drugs address the needs of the end consumer) and a marketing perspective (obtaining consumer buy-in.).

Whatever the context, however, there is still a need to authentically reflect the patient voice. There is also the need for engagement to be meaningful rather than token. Hence, one consideration is whether the patient is actually a representative of a disease community that is empowered to speak for the community with some form of accountability to the community (e.g., through loss of organizational membership). In other situations, an independent patient or caregiver with lived experience of the disease might be an appropriate selection, bearing in mind that independent patients do not speak for a community because individual patients may differ in viewpoints. A good rule of thumb might be to aim for a patient who represents a community when there is a community charged with representing the interests of those with the particular condition. Hence, it would be inappropriate to select a consumer with no lived experience of HIV/AIDS to represent the concerns, values, and preferences, and characteristics of that community. On the other hand, acute conditions like the common cold have no such community and the concept of representation does not carry the same weight.

At the same time, a science of the methods for patient engagement in research is evolving. PCORI has established methodology standards for patient centeredness in research, which requires that patients or caregivers involved have "lived experience" with the disease (PCORI Methodology Committee 2013). PCORI methodology standards also emphasize the importance of sufficient representation: "Engage people representing the population of interest and other relevant stakeholders in ways that are appropriate and necessary in a given research context" (PCORI Methodology Committee 2013). The NAM calls for "a current or former patient, as well as a patient advocate or patient/consumer organization representative." This requirement is intended to cover both the concepts of lived experience with the disease and the centrality of recognizing true representation where patient organizations exist (IOM 2011).

Another factor important for representation is the ability of the patient to *effectively* represent the interests of the community. To do this, the patient must be sufficiently involved with the disease to be able to speak knowledgeably about the issues—not as experts, but from the patient perspective. Patients must also be sufficiently versed in the nature and methods of the deliberative process that they will be involved in. For example, research grant application assessment may be rigorous, and patients involved in these processes should have sufficient training to contribute effectively.

Other challenges arise due to inherent power imbalances between patients and other stakeholders. Individual patients may need support to hold their own on a panel of experts. A common complaint heard regarding patients is that they may be intimidated by their lack of expertise and remain quiet. Patients have often been in a position of being the sole representative on panels or advisory groups. Therefore, it is important to consider including more than one patient in any forum for patients to effectively hold their own among a panel of scientific experts. It is also important to bear in mind that this is not a numbers game. The essential issue is whether the patient has the actual ability to influence outcomes.

A single patient on a panel may be insufficient to effectively represent the patient interest even where other stakeholders are also allotted a single seat at the table. For example, others at the table frequently have powerful trade associations such as the Pharmaceutical Manufacturers of America (PHRMA) to lobby for their interests. While patients have advocacy groups that do lobby on specific issue affecting their community, there is no correspondingly centralized powerful lobbying force for patients.

10.7.1 Reciprocal Relationships

Whether patient engagement actually can influence a decision also depends upon fostering reciprocal relationships. The ability to merely comment, for example, may not actually influence a decision as the comments may be ignored, no discourse is involved, and the give and take of bidirectional learning is not at play.

The importance of bidirectional learning or colearning is well recognized in patient engagement models in health care. Effective patient engagement requires reciprocal relationships of respect with a collaborative exchange of ideas. It is essential to realize the full potential and promise of patient-centered processes.

Realizing the full potential of reciprocal relationships involves overcoming cultural barriers in the research culture. The culture of research is expertise driven and hierarchical. Patients injected into this culture struggle to have standing because their lay expertise is not recognized in research historically. This disparity can create a power imbalance that is difficult for patients to overcome, particularly when the patient representation constitutes a minority of a larger group of researchers. Denning describes culture change as one of the most difficult challenges and points out that an organization's culture comprises an interlocking set of goals, roles, processes, values, communications practices, attitudes, and assumptions (Denning 2016).

Overcoming these barriers requires targeted efforts to address cultural barriers on the part of all participants. For their part, patients need to recognize the obligation to their respective community to speak up and provide input even when they are feeling uncomfortable. Moderators need to help bridge the cultural chasm by both encouraging patient participation and creating space for the patient voice. They can do this by actively calling on patients and inviting their comments. The importance of patient training was noted previously, however, equally important may be training of researchers and particularly training of the moderator.

10.7.2 Patient Engagement and Value Added

A common perception among researchers is that patient engagement will inherently slow down the research process. For example, patients may require training and dialogue may be more extended to reflect the patient voice. Time schedules may not reflect that increase in the amount of time required to fully incorporate patient input.

On the other hand, patient engagement may make certain aspects of research and health care more efficient in the long run by ensuring that questions important to patients are adequately addressed and by accelerating research recruitment and dissemination of research findings.

In addition, patient compensation needs to be considered to encourage and allow for patient involvement. For many healthcare stakeholders, involvement in advisory panels or other convening events for input on healthcare sector issues are part of their job responsibilities. This means these participants are inherently compensated for the time spent to prepare and participate as well as any travel expenses that may be incurred. Patients often have to take time away from work or other responsibilities to participate. Consideration of compensation and expenses for their involvement needs to be taken into account. PCORI has developed a framework to consider compensation and recommends in their public funding announcements that budgets for all funded projects plan for these expenses (PCORI 2015).

There are a number of additional reasons that patient compensation is recommended. These include rectifying a power imbalance, acknowledging the value of patient contributions (such as easing recruitment and assisting in research dissemination), and avoiding relegating patient participation to the "luxury class" hobby sport where only those who can pay can play.

Researchers should address these challenges of time and money required for patient engagement upfront by incorporating enough time in the research project for engagement in their research grant applications.

10.8 PCORnet: A Use Case for Assessing and Improving Patient Engagement

As mentioned previously, PCORnet is PCORI's signature infrastructure initiative, which leverages big data for research. PCORI funded 29 research networks to begin designing and building a national research infrastructure based on electronic health record data and other healthcare data sources. PCORnet is a network of networks. In the Phase I PCORnet initiative, PCORI funded 18 patient-powered research networks (PPRNs); groups of patients, patient organizations, or researchers partnered with patients around a specific health condition. In addition, 11 Clinical Data Research Networks (CDRNs) were funded. These were primarily rooted in large health systems that have large representative populations.

One of the primary goals of Phase I was to establish the governance structure and policies that would apply to the members of its network. Institutions set their sites for patient engagement at different levels, but PCORI sets a high bar—a true collaborative partnership with patients actively involved in decisions. PCORnet aimed to allow for meaningful patient participation in the establishment of policies for the network from the patient perspective. Under Arnstein's ladder, this would require that:

- Patient representatives have the ability to influence change.
- Patient representatives be brought in early enough to make a difference.
- The relationship between the patient representatives and other stakeholders be reciprocal, and learning be bidirectional.
- Patient representatives be sufficiently prepared and informed to effectively represent patient concerns.

PCORnet's governance structure evolved substantially in an effort to best involve patients and stakeholders. During the Phase I, the governance structure consisted of a *steering committee*, which voted on central issues, and an *executive committee*, which developed strategic goals and determined topics that would be submitted to the steering committee for vote. In addition, there were a number of task forces established that were dedicated to addressing specific issues that may accelerate or impede the research enterprise, such as the standards for privacy and data security. These task forces made recommendations to the executive committee, which approved policies for a vote. Behind all of the governance stood PCORI and its interest in advancing patient-centered processes as its "true north" in all of its projects. PCORI, itself, approved policies before they were adopted or implemented under the Phase I governance structure.

The steering committee included one representative from each of the participating 29 networks so each network had one voting member. Since 18 of the 29 networks were patient-powered research networks, it was originally thought that the patient voice would be adequately represented. However, each network was required to select only one person to serve on the steering committee and many PPRNs selected the principle investigator who was often a researcher. Because of this, as initially constituted, the steering committee had no meaningful patient voice.

For example, on a simple vote the patient representative on the steering committee would be outnumbered 28 researchers to 1 patient. In addition, to be influential, patient engagement should be at the time the issues are developed for consideration by the steering committee because the framing of issues may determine the outcome. This is consistent with guidance from the NAM and PCORI that recognizes the need for patients to be involved in guidelines when the questions are initially framed.

The first solution proposed to address the lack of patient participation was to add a patient representative to both the steering committee and to the executive committee. The patient representative selected, the lead author of this chapter, was the Co-Chair of Consumers United for Evidence Based Healthcare (CUE), a national coalition of evidence-based consumers and patients. Hence, the representative was arguably informed and empowered. The degree of empowerment must, however, be viewed in the context that the committee itself was comprised of some of the most influential and powerful members involved in the health services research enterprise.

In addition to sitting on the steering committee, the patient representative was also given seat on the executive committee. Although here again in a simple vote, the patient voice was clearly outnumbered six researchers to one patient. Even on the executive committee, the patient voice was not involved early enough to help frame the policies as these were often developed by the task forces through separate processes and had membership largely comprised of researcher and healthcare provider expertise.

Once the structural challenges of incorporating the patient voice became clear, it was decided that a patient council would be established that would weigh in on matters central to patients. In Phase I, these matters were in the development of

policies with provisions for patient consent, autonomy, privacy, and data security. The patient council consisted of six experienced patients who represented diverse disease organizations and the PCORI director of patient engagement.

The patient council was empowered to identify the concerns of patients and deliberate on these issues so as to make policy recommendations to PCORI. This direct relationship to PCORI, which as the funder, held ultimate veto power over all of PCORnet's activities, was to correct the structural power imbalance on the steering and executive committees. Hence, the patient council took on an advisory role to PCORI in addition to having a representative on the steering and executive committees.

Once the structural imbalance issue was addressed, the patient council assessed its ability to effectively represent the patient voice on highly complex ethical and technical topics key to assessing privacy and data security and found itself lacking. To remedy this short fall, over a 6-month period, the council began a program of reading and discussing key ethics papers on a weekly basis. It also invited and interviewed ethics and research ethics experts to present on these key topics. To encourage bidirectional learning and reciprocal relationship, the chair of the patient council also engaged in weekly calls with PCORnet program director to discuss its progress, the results of its deliberations, and ultimately to advise PCORI. Although there were a number of twists and turns along the way, the council members felt that they had reached the type of process integrity advanced by Arnstein's ladder as a result of the structural and process readjustment.

10.9 Conclusion

In summary, patients serve a unique and important role on cross-disciplinary research teams. While the field of team science traditionally considers diversity of discipline, the lived expertise that patients bring to cross-disciplinary team should be conceptualized as its own discipline that has the potential to bring equal and additional value. Cross-disciplinary research teams can continue to look to PCORI for guidance and promising practices. While the institute has advanced a framework and the undertaking of systematic evaluation of patient engagement in research, many learnings will be forthcoming as PCORI's portfolio and evaluation efforts mature.

While further evidence of promising practices for how to engage patients and the effects of patient engagement is needed, the Arnstein's ladder of public participation offers a potential model for evaluating the success of patient engagement on a continuum. The National Institute of Health (NIH) *Collaboration and Team Science: A Field Guide* suggests that scientific research team can also be considered as a continuum of levels of interaction and integration suggesting that the ideal teams have the highest levels of interaction and integration of shared leadership and decision-making. As such, Arnstein's ladder could be considered as a framework for measuring the extent to which patients are involved in all stages of the process from inception to end, the extent to which they can influence outcomes, the representativeness of the patient participants, and the bidirectional quality of the patient engagement. To the extent that any team initiative can achieve these four goals, patient engagement will likely be more robust and more meaningful.

The science of team science has already embraced many important principles such as trust that are also foundational to patient engagement in research (Bennett et al. 2010). The field will benefit from further work that describes the role of patients on multistakeholder teams, in the form of publication and case studies. Existing guidance on the science of team science should also be shared with patients to help provide training and education on the best practices for the domain of team science and collaboration. Additionally, members of cross-disciplinary teams that have not traditionally incorporated patients or other lay stakeholders may also need further training and resources to better understand the unique expertise that these team members bring to a research project. Incorporating patient stakeholders into research teams consis-

tently will require culture change. Fortunately, there are several efforts already underway to facilitate this change in the medical and health research enterprise. Cross-disciplinary team science will benefit from these existing efforts and is well positioned to further enhance the role of patients in health research.

The views presented here are solely the responsibility of the authors and do not necessarily represent the official views of the National Institutes of Health or of the Patient-Centered Outcomes Research Institute (PCORI), its Board of Governors or Methodology Committee, or other participants in the National Patient-Centered Clinical Research Network (PCORnet).

References

Anderson M. Rx for innovation: a path forward for us all. Sci Transl Med. 2017;9:379.

Arnstein SR. A ladder of citizen participation. J Am Inst Planners. 1969;35(4):216–24.

Bennett LM, Gadlin H, Levine-Finley S. Collaboration and team science: a field guide. In: Collaboration and team science: a field guide—team science toolkit. Washington, DC: National Institutes of Health; 2010.

Carman KL, Dardess P, Maurer M, Sofaer S, Adams K, Bechtel C, Sweeney J. Patient and family engagement: a framework for understanding the elements and developing interventions and policies. Health Aff. 2013;32(2):223–31.. Web. 30 May 2016.

Denning S. How do you change an organizational culture. Forbes Magazine. 2016.

Devereaux PJ, Anderson DR, Gardner MJ, Putnam W, Flowerdew GJ, Brownell BF, Nagpal S, Cox JL. Differences between perspectives of physicians and patients on anticoagulation in patients with atrial fibrillation: observational study. Br Med J. 2001;323(7323):1218–21.

Emanuel EJ. Choice and representation in health care. Med Care Res Rev. 1999;56(1):113–40.

Forsythe LP, Ellis LE, Edmundson L, Sabharwal R, Rein A, Konopka K, Frank L. Patient and stakeholder engagement in the PCORI pilot projects: description and lessons learned. J Gen Intern Med. 2015;31(1):13–21.

Frank L, Basch E, Selby JV. The PCORI perspective on patient-centered outcomes research. JAMA. 2014;312(15):1513.

Garces JP, Lopez GP. Eliciting patient perspective in patient-centered outcomes research: a meta narrative systematic review. PCORI. 2016;. http://www.pcori.org/sites/default/files/Eliciting-Patient-Perspective-in-Patient-Centered-Outcomes-Research-A-Meta-Narrative-Systematic-Review1.pdf

Institute of Medicine (Committee on Quality of Health Care in America). Crossing the Quality Chasm: A New Health System for the 21st Century. Washington, DC: National Academies Press; 2001. Available from: http://www.nap.edu/openbook.php?isbn=0309072808

Institute of Medicine (IOM). The learning healthcare system: workshop summary. Washington, DC: The National Academies Press; 2007.

Institute of Medicine (Committee on Conflict of Interest in Medical Research E and Practice) Conflict of interest in medical research, education, and practice. Washington, DC: National Academies Press; 2009.

Institute of Medicine (US) Roundtable on Value & Science-Driven Health Care; Yong PL, Olsen LA, McGinnis JM, editors. Value in Health Care: Accounting for Cost, Quality, Safety, Outcomes, and Innovation. Washington (DC): National Academies Press (US); 2010. 2, Stakeholder Perspectives on Value. Available from:https://www.ncbi.nlm.nih.gov/books/NBK50926/

Institute of Medicine. Clinical Practice Guidelines We Can Trust. Washington, DC: National Academies Press; 2011. Available from: http://books.nap.edu/openbook.php?record_id=13058

Institute of Medicine (US) Roundtable on Value & Science-Driven Health Care. Roundtable on value & science-driven health care. Institute of medicine: roundtable on value & science-driven health care: charter and vision statement. U.S. National Library of Medicine; 2016. http://www.ncbi.nlm.nih.gov/books/NBK50934/

Macaulay AC, Commanda LE, Freeman WL, Gibson N, Mccabe ML, Robbins CM, Twohig PL. Participatory research maximises community and lay involvement. BMJ. 1999;319(7212):774–8.

National Research Council. Enhancing the effectiveness of team science. In: Cooke NJ, Hilton ML, Committee on the Science of Team Science, Board on Behavioral, Cognitive, and Sensory Sciences, Division of Behavioral and Social Sciences and Education, editors, vol. 208. Washington, DC: The National Academies Press; 2015.

O'Connor M. Nothing about us without us: patient involvement in research. 2016.

PCORI Methodology Committee, The PCORI Methodology Report; 2013. Available from: https://www.pcori.org/sites/default/files/PCORI-Methodology-Report-November2013.pdf

PCORI. Financial compensation of patients, caregivers, and patient/caregiver organizations engaged. In: PCORI-funded research as engaged research partners. PCORI. 2015.

PCORI.Howweevaluatekeyaspectsofourwork.2017.http://www.pcori.org/research-results/evaluating-our-work/how-we-evaluate-key-aspects-our-work.

PCORI Engagement Rubric. PCORI (Patient-Centered Outcomes Research Institute) website. 2014. http://www.pcori.org/sites/default/files/Engagement-Rubric.pdf. Updated October 13, 2015.

PCORI Methodology Standards. PCORI (Patient-Centered Outcomes Research Institute). 2016.

Renn O, Webler T, Wiedemann PM. Fairness and competence in citizen participation: evaluating models for environmental discourse. Dordrecht: Kluwer Academic; 1995.

Sheridan S, Schrandt S, Forsythe L, Hilliard TS, Paez KA. The PCORI engagement rubric: promising practices for partnering in research. Ann Fam Med. 2017;15(2):165–70.

Engaging the Practitioner: "But Wait, That's Not All!"— Collaborations with Practitioners and Extending the Reasons You Started Doing Research in the First Place

11

Marc T. Kiviniemi

Contents

As the existence of this volume shows, there is a growing movement toward encouraging transdisciplinary team science approaches to address both "basic" research questions and "applied"

M. T. Kiviniemi (✉)
Department of Health, Behavior and Society,
University of Kentucky, Lexington, KY, USA
e-mail: Marc.Kiviniemi@uky.edu

approaches toward alleviating real-world problems. The call for basic-applied collaborations isn't new (Kessel and Rosenfield 2008). Kurt Lewin (1951), the acknowledged founder of my home academic discipline of social psychology, is probably most famous beyond the discipline for his assertion that "there is nothing so practical as a good theory...." What is sometimes missing from discussions of this assertion is that it was made as part of an argument for the importance of close connections between basic behavioral sciences research and applied work. My current academic home in public health has, throughout its history, involved transdisciplinary approaches to address the complex, multilevel problems that are characteristic of public health issues.

If this isn't a new conversation, why do we still need to put forth the call for both researchers and clinicians to consider taking part in team science approaches to inquiry and application? Team science requires team members. For many researchers and practitioners, working individually versus working as part of teams is a voluntary act. Although the broader social and cultural context is shifting in ways more amenable to team science approaches (Stokols et al. 2008), the nature of the research environment is still that there is still an inherent element of individual decision-making and individual choice in whether and how one involves oneself in team science.

Given this, encouraging researchers to become involved in team science approaches will require not only selling its value for the field (a point made in several of the other chapters in this book) but also making clear why team science can be tremendously advantageous for the individual researcher or practitioner. This chapter provides a framework for thinking about motivations for individuals to engage in team science and ways in which researchers interested in team science collaborations can move forward with developing collaborations in ways that satisfy those motivations.

The primary focus will be on elucidating reasons why team science approaches are beneficial to the individual investigator and should be considered. A common theme in conversations on transdisciplinary work and team science approaches is to focus on the impediments to doing team science and to doing it well. However, a mainstay of our understanding of human behavior is that people do things for a reason—they engage in actions when they perceive a personally relevant benefit or benefits to doing so (e.g., Edwards 1954; Kreuter et al. 1999). This understanding and focus on personally relevant benefits is especially key for behaviors which are effortful but voluntary (Stukas et al. 2008).

Given that taking part in team science collaborations is typically voluntary and definitely effortful, building a compelling case for why team sciences offer motivationally important benefits for both the basic scientist and the clinician is a key first step. The hurdles should not be understated, but there are known ways to overcome them and those ways are ably covered both in other chapters in this book and in other places (e.g., Bennett et al. 2010). Thus, approaching both the chapter and considerations about engaging in team science through the lens of considering *why* it is worth doing team science and doing it well and how doing so can actually advance your individual motives as either a basic scientist or a clinician provides an important route toward motivating greater engagement in team science approaches.

11.1 My Journey to Team Science

Through the remainder of the chapter, I'll give some specific examples of team science projects I have worked on and observations about outcomes that have accrued from them. In the traditional "basic" versus "applied" or "researcher" versus "clinician" dichotomies, I fall squarely in the domain of a basic social and behavioral sciences researcher, with formal training in social psychology. I began my career focused on understanding basic social cognitive processes relevant to understanding how individuals maintain a positive sense of self in the face of potentially threatening information. Even when working on studies relevant to health psychology, my primary focus and professional identity was as a social psychologist doing basic process work to understand human judgment and decision-making, with health serving only as a useful content domain in which to study those processes.

As my career progressed, I developed what has become my primary research program, examining how individuals integrate social cognitive determinants of decision-making with affective determinants, in particular, the feelings and emotions individuals associate with particular behaviors. I continued to pursue this work in the health domain, looking at decision-making about behaviors like physical activity, fruit and vegetable consumption, and cancer screening. In the course of doing this, I gradually shifted my focus and professional identity to one where I framed my interests as being at the intersection of basic behavioral sciences and applications in the health domain—to "use inspired basic research" in Pasteur's quadrant terms (Stokes 1997).

During this period in my career, I also made my first forays into team science. I worked with health educators at the local health department on designing effective communications to encourage walking behavior in sedentary adults. I also worked with a physician on developing assessments on decision-making determinants of dietary and diabetes management behaviors for Native American communities. These team approaches, in particular meshing my background in the basic social and behavioral sciences with the expertise of practitioners in the field, gave me insight into the value of and ways of going about doing team science.

Since that time, I have continued to develop team science, researcher–practitioner collaborations to the point where they are now a hallmark of the majority of my research activity. I have worked with cancer outreach and health disparities specialists on work advancing colorectal cancer screening and participation biobanking research protocols (Erwin et al. 2013; Kiviniemi et al. 2013, 2014), a physician on work on understanding H1N1 precautionary behaviors (Kozlowski et al. 2010, 2011), nurse scientists on decision-making for breast and colorectal cancer screening (Othman et al. 2012; Underhill and Kiviniemi 2012; Underhill et al. 2012), and a community-based HIV prevention and treatment center on health literacy assessments for client management cases (Kiviniemi et al. 2011; Rintamaki et al. 2011).

This engagement in team science has had a strong influence on the shape and trajectory of my programs of research. I continue work on the interrelation of cognition and affect in health decision-making. In addition to studies that are basic behavioral sciences, laboratory studies to elucidate decision-making mechanisms, this line of work has expanded to include the development and testing of community-based interventions framed around my decision-making models (Erwin et al. 2013; Kiviniemi et al. 2013); this expanded focus is a direct result of team science partnerships with interventionists and clinicians. In addition, my portfolio also includes work on a phenomenon with multiple applied implications—what happens when people don't know their risk for a health problem (Hay et al. 2015; Waters et al. 2013)? Finally, I have developed work in an applied area—cancer screening—examining a range of determinants of engagement in colorectal and breast cancer screening behaviors (Kiviniemi and Hay 2012; Kiviniemi et al. 2014; Underhill et al. 2012).

So, my expertise and habits of thought are still very much grounded in the basic social and behavioral sciences. However, I have shifted my work to be use-inspired, health problem focused, more amenable to considering and incorporating outcomes for interventions, and transdisciplinary team science. This transformation has taken place through collaborations with a variety of applied researchers, clinicians, and other field-based practitioners. It has also involved an important reframing of how I consider the research questions I ask. Considering the nature of this reframing and how it can be used to consider the motivations driving engagement in team science may have value for both characterizing why individuals engage in team science and for motivating greater engagement from individuals who are not currently doing team science.

11.2 Conceptualizing Researcher–Practitioner Collaborations: Useful Reframing

A relatively subtle but critically important reshaping of our typical framing of types of research can be tremendously valuable in both helping individual contributors see the potential benefits of collaborations across disciplines and broader fields and in making such collaborations seem more achievable. We often divide the research world into "basic" versus "applied" research and the domain of individuals involved in health research into "researchers" versus "practitioners."

Although these distinctions can be useful, they can also artificially inhibit desires to engage in team science. Often times when one hears about collaborations, both between basic scientists and applied researchers and between researchers and clinicians, they are described using metaphors like bridging a wide gap between fields or managing cross-cultural encounters. These metaphors frame the two fields involved as being utterly different from one another, separate and distinct with few commonalities, different more so than similar, non-overlapping cultures, etc.

The framing resulting from these metaphors makes the challenges involved in pursuing such collaborations seem massive and suggests that one must be super motivated and perhaps even superhuman in order to overcoming the challenges involved in pursuing team science. There are, of course, moments in almost any collaborative relationship that feel this way. However, I would argue that we do both ourselves and the field a substantial disservice through use of such metaphors. The bridging the gap metaphors come from early conceptualizations of the distinction between basic and applied work that consider the two as separate and distinct, see basic as coming before applied, and don't consider the possible more complex interrelations among the two (for further discussions, see Crow and Dabars 2015; Stokes 1997).

A more fruitful way to frame the relations among fields in research–practitioner collaborations comes through a lens provided by the political scientist and public policy analyst Donald Stokes (1997). Stokes argued that we should move past the traditional dichotomy imposed between basic and applied research. He proposed that, rather than conceptualizing basic and applied work as two separate stopping points on a one-way continuum, a more fruitful conceptualization of the relation between the two is to consider a 2 × 2 grid of primary motivations for conducting research (see Fig. 11.1). One motivation is the desire to contribute to fundamental knowledge and to understand the world (broadly writ) and how it works. Another motivation is the desire to generate understanding that has practical applications for addressing an issue or solving a problem. Stokes argues that all research programs can be classified into the quadrants generated by this grid.

Importantly for understanding the potential value added by team science, a given individual study or program of research can be designed to address *both* the desire for basic understanding *and* the desire to contribute to applications or to solve the world's problems. Stokes labeled this point of intersection "Pasteur's quadrant" after

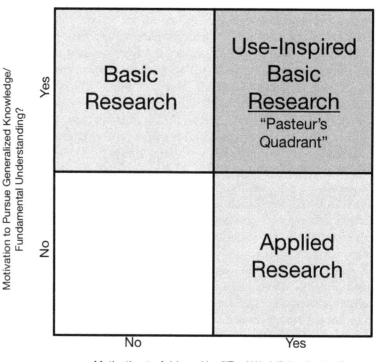

Fig. 11.1 Reframing the motivations for engaging in research—Pasteur's quadrant

Louis Pasteur, who conducted research that both advanced the basic science of microbiology and simultaneously led to important applied advances in food safety.

Conceptualizing the landscape of motivations for conducting research using Stokes' 2 × 2 grid and considering the quadrants created is a useful exercise. Doing so leads one to very different images of where the basic/researcher and the applied/practitioner camps sit relative to one another. This framing leads to different images and metaphors which, I think, make the challenge of team science less daunting and the benefits more apparent.

A similar motivational analysis can help us consider the "primary researcher" versus "primary clinician" divide. Add in for the clinician the motivation to provide care and improve health for a specific group of people (as opposed to the quite possibly more hypothetical or more diffuse "help the world" or "address this societal problem" motivation for the applied researcher) and Stokes' quadrant framework for motivation is equally applicable to the researcher–practitioner intersection.

For readers considering collaborations that bridge past their traditional areas of work, consider the quadrant approach for thinking about and addressing motivations. Relative to the "bridging the divide" metaphor, a quadrant approach doesn't involve leaving behind or even short-changing one's professional identity as a basic or applied researcher. Rather, one is simply shifting and expanding one's existing motivations and focus for selecting projects to selecting and embracing projects and research questions that satisfy both research and practitioners goals—there's no inherent "giving up" of one's motivations for working involved.

This motivational approach also highlights ways to communicate about the value of team science collaborations in ways that will more effectively encourage engagement. As I mentioned earlier, my own primary intellectual focus is on basic social/behavioral science—I like figuring out how people's minds work and how the workings of those minds translate into behavioral actions. There are two key reasons for my involvement in team science collaborations that bridge basic and applied and bridge research and clinical. First, such collaborations are tremendously intellectually engaging—pushing one's thinking to consider how one's work fits in applied arenas or how it might explain a single clinical case is, simply put, a lot of fun. Second, and ultimately more importantly, I am firmly convinced that I do better basic science because I engage in applied and clinical collaborations. The latter is, I believe, the strength of doing work in Pasteur's quadrant, addressing practical use goals while still answering fundamental questions. The former is, in my own personal experience, how you convince a "basic" researcher (or, for that matter, an "applied" researcher or practitioner) to do team science. Highlighting how shifting from either the "purely basic" or "purely applied" quadrants into Pasteur's quadrant is to highlight the ways that being in that space strengthens the basic or applied research goals that motivated the individuals to work in science in the first place.

11.3 What Do You Get? Motivational Outcomes for the Basic Research Scientist Collaborating with Practitioners

If we take as a starting point that people will be more likely to engage in team science collaborations when they perceive those collaborations as helping them meet their own individual research motivations, why would a basic research scientist want to engage in collaborations with applied researchers and/or with practitioners? Based on my collaborative experiences, team science enhances the "basic" science outcomes of my work. There are several reasons for this enhancement.

First, the kinds of problems encountered in practitioner/clinical settings become very rich fodder for developing theories. The goal for the basic sciences researcher is to explain, describe, predict, and understand reality. A (hopefully) obvious but often overlooked point is that the applied domains encountered by practitioners and clinicians *are* the reality we're trying to explain, describe, predict, and understand.

Most of the interesting phenomena in the social and behavioral sciences, including my own focus on health behaviors, are complex, multifaceted, and multidetermined. Understanding such phenomena requires theoretical perspectives that adequately address that complexity. However, starting from a purely abstract understanding of reality often doesn't get you as far in terms of expanding the understanding of that reality as does the "real-world" context. Solving the kinds of problems that applied researchers and practitioners face—the very definition of use inspired research—allows the basic scientist access to problems that demand the best that basic science has to offer. The applied/practice realm is replete with rich observations about people and their behavior; those observations become fodder for developing and refining theories.

As a concrete example of this, my own work on colorectal cancer screening was very much informed by set of conversations that I had with gastroenterologists about their experiences with patients. One gastroenterologist told me about patients who do all the work and pay all the money to come to a colorectal cancer screening but don't actually follow through on the prep procedure, leaving the test more or less useless (a not uncommon occurrence; Ness et al. 2001). Another told me about patients who come for the screening test but then leave from the waiting room leaving the test undone.

These clinical encounter stories gave me a powerful set of observations to try to account for with my decision-making models, which led to development of some of the hypotheses we're currently testing in work on colorectal cancer screening decisions. This real-world, practitioner-based context raises strong questions about the competing motivations that push individuals toward and away from behavioral engagement—in both of these illustrations there are clearly factors that are motivating the individuals to engage in screening behavior but equally compelling factors that are pushing them away from the behavior. Understanding those tensions and how they resolve is a fascinating question for a

basic decision-making researcher to grapple with to understand the interplay of different determinants of behavioral practice. For examples of other ways that applied/clinical contexts can improve the operation of basic sciences, see Dugan and Gabriel (2013).

Second, collaborations involving work in the applied context or clinical context, and particularly interventions developed within that context, provide remarkably rich tests of our theories (Rothman 2004, 2009). Much of the social and behavioral sciences, especially in the purely basic context, largely relies on studies done in artificial settings (and, at least in my home discipline of social psychology, often involving college students as participants) and observational tests. There's nothing inherently wrong with this approach—indeed, as a starting point for progressing particular areas of work it can be quite valuable. However, without moving on into the complexity of testing interventions, especially real-world interventions in applied settings, we miss much of the richness that the "real-world" environment has to offer. Much of my own work has been developed and refined through such clinical observation.

There's a distinction made in both the drug trials and the program evaluation literature (Glasgow et al. 1999; Green and Kreuter 2004) about efficacy versus effectiveness. Efficacy is the effect of a given treatment under ideal, laboratory, controlled conditions (i.e., how well does this work in the cleanest, best case scenario) whereas effectiveness is the effect of a given treatment under real world, uncontrolled conditions with multiple influences on the outcome, potentially subpar adherence to the regimen, etc. The argument made in both is that although efficacy is an important precondition to effectiveness (given that real world, multiple influences will usually lead to effectiveness being lower than efficacy), for a treatment to have real-world impact it must have "real-world" effectiveness.

A similar analogy can be used to argue for why a basic scientist should pursue collaborations with applied researchers and practitioners. Many basic science tests of theories are arguably under efficacy rather than effectiveness conditions, especially when these tests take place in behavioral sciences laboratories or are observational, questionnaire studies under fully artificial conditions. By contrast, seeing if a theory-based prediction obtains when an experimental manipulation takes place in a real-world, applied setting (e.g., a clinical trial of a behavioral sciences intervention) is a much higher bar and pushes toward effectiveness rather than efficacy.

At a surface level, one could make the basic argument that, if a theory really does describe the "real world," it will predict an outcome under effectiveness, real-world conditions, and not just under artificial, behavioral sciences laboratory conditions. At a deeper level, if there is a disparity between efficacy (behavioral sciences controlled laboratory) and effectiveness (real world) outcomes, the questions that the basic scientist can and should grapple with become deeper, more complex, and arguably more interesting—why is a given theory-based prediction obtained in one situation but not the other; what are the setting-based and other contextual characteristics that shift from one setting to the other and why might they matter? For more on this line of argument, see Rothman (2009).

Even if one doesn't take the full-fledged approach of ensuring that one's theory can stand up to "real-world" complexities, there can still be considerable value in using the applied realm as a way of creating "experimental analogues"—identifying the key real-world features that impact a phenomena and then designing laboratory approaches that approximate those real-world features (Brewer 1985).

Third, in addition to these factors, collaborations with applied researchers and practitioners advance basic science because such collaborations can often provide access to populations of interest that would be nearly impossible, or at least substantially more challenging, for a basic scientist to obtain without such collaborative relationships. This kind of population access can both allow answering new and different research questions and allow for testing hypotheses that might not otherwise be testable.

For example, in my early work on affect and health decision-making (Kiviniemi et al. 2007), I was able to get a broad community sample because I created a collaborative relationship with a local health department who, in turn, had access to county-funded community centers with populations substantially more diverse than the college student populations I was able to access on my own. As another example, my current work on community-based intervention testing for colorectal cancer screening is made feasible by my partnership with cancer health educators at my local comprehensive cancer center who have ties to community groups. Such ties have allowed me to enrich the work I do, especially in terms of considering the impact of race/ethnicity, socioeconomic status, and other characteristics on outcomes.

11.4 Satisfying the Motives for the Applied Researcher or Practitioner

Because of my background and focus in the social and behavioral sciences, the perspective outlined above is centered on how Pasteur's quadrant enhances the goals of "basic" research. I would argue, though, that a similar enhancement of intrinsic research motivations will occur for the applied researcher or practitioner when pursuing team science collaborations with basic scientists.

As a starting point, take the frequent motive of the applied researchers in the social and behavioral sciences of developing the most efficacious interventions approaches to change behavior and health outcomes. For practitioners, the slight variant on that motive is to utilize the most efficacious treatment strategies for the patient under their care.

There is a strong argument to be made that knowledge of the underlying basic processes involved in a system (e.g., how behavioral decision-making and self-regulation works) enables creation of stronger, higher quality intervention approaches to address problems with that system (Baranowski 2006; Glanz and Bishop 2010; Rothman and Kiviniemi 1999). It has also been observed that there is a substantial paucity of such cutting edge work in many interventions

(Onken et al. 2014). Thus, the applied research and the clinician stand to improve the intervention and treatment outcomes that serve as a primary motivator by addressing basic behavioral sciences issues in their work.

11.5   Advice for Getting Started: Points to Consider in Team Science Collaborations and How to Build Collaborative Relationships

So if one is convinced of the merits of doing team science, how should one move forward? On this question, I have three pieces of conceptual advice as well as three practical strategies for beginning. First, the team science approach means, by definition, that different team members will come to the collaboration with different areas of expertise and, since no one knows everything, different areas of profound ignorance. This necessary fact is important to acknowledge and to address in forming and performing in team science work. It is quite easy to undervalue what one knows and can bring to the table if one focuses on expertise that other collaborators possess but that oneself lacks. It is equally easy, because of our human tendency to over assume that people should know what we know, to make unwarranted negative assumptions about the abilities of one's collaborators if they lack what one sees as basic, universal knowledge.

Second, very much related to the first point, taking a team science approach will involve the need to both educate and to be educated. Although the beauty of a team science approach is that the range of expertise around the table strengthens the final research product, for that product to be an intricately woven, transdisciplinary melding and not a tacked together, patchwork of different perspectives without integration, all of the team members need to be willing and able to provide basic education in the key points of their own disciplinary perspective. Likewise, all of the team members need to be willing and able to receive basic education in the key points of the other disciplinary perspectives at the table.

Third, a team science collaborator needs to always be mindful of the power of and limitations of disciplinary lenses. We know that each discipline's separate paradigms and default assumptions shape virtually all aspects of the research process, including those that shape choices of questions methodologies for addressing those questions, and ways of interpreting and utilizing data (Gholson and Barker 1985; Kuhn 1975). Because team sciences involve a very intentional intersection of these different disciplinary paradigms, the issues raised when paradigms meet and shift are inherent in transdisciplinary work. Handled well, this can be a true core strength of a team science approach—working through the conflicts and seeming contradictions of different perspectives can result in a stronger intellectual product. However, the "handled well" caveat is key. In order to make the meshing of disciplinary perspectives a net positive for the collaboration and not a source of debilitating tension, the team must remain mindful of the differing disciplinary lenses for viewing the world and, when issues arise, address them head on.

On the more practical side, if one is a researcher who is interested in pursuing team science collaborations, how would one start? First, know where to look. For the basic social/behavioral scientist looking to do work in an applied arena, identifying where to find practitioners and applied researchers with whom to build collaborative connections is the first challenge. Within the university setting, there are a number of places to look. For health-related applications, schools of medicine, public health, dentistry, nursing, pharmacy, and so on are good places to start, but so are programs addressing health education and community health, which are often housed in schools of education. More broadly, schools of education do a variety of work that could involve "Pasteur's quadrant collaborations" with basic social and behavioral sciences, such as ways that cognitive science could inform curriculum design, or how principles of intergroup relations impact programs to address diversity issues in higher education. Finally, for individuals associated with land grant institutions, agricultural extension services often are involved in a wide array of practical, use inspired projects in a variety of domains.

Second, having identified potential focal areas and individuals to collaborate with, how does one approach the topic with a potential collaborator? Here, returning to the motivational analysis discussed earlier in the chapter is helpful. A successful collaboration will be one that allows each of the parties in the relationship to meeting their individual motivations for pursuing the research topic. Starting the conversation with an eye toward how, within the topic domain being discussed, a collaboration can satisfy the motivations of each individual player, as well as how the broaden of perspectives provided by the collaboration would further the development of the research domain, can be a strong beginning. Then, return to this conversation at various points along the way—check in to ensure that the research design allows for answer questions from both the basic and the applied sides of the collaboration and that the questions being asked by each are informed by the other.

Third, consider that relationship building and collaboration building takes time and may not be successful on the first go. Cast your net broadly. Be proactive about introducing yourself to potential collaborators. Don't assume that one introduction will be sufficient to achieve an agreement to collaborate. Don't worry (too much!) when a seemingly promising prospect doesn't work out, but go back to the previous steps and continue trying. Much like dating, career development, and other important life tasks, collaboration building is neither a simple nor a linear process, but it is one well worth the effort.

11.6 Conclusions

Team science has numerous benefits for the field—complex and multilayered problems require complex and multidisciplinary teams to solve them. This chapter has hopefully made the important point that team science also has numerous benefits for the individual researchers and practitioners who make up the "teams" in team science. Strong team science, pursued with a strong and well-functioning team, can satisfy the motives that led the basic researcher, the applied interventionist, and the practitioner to pursue their work in ways that individual action on these problems cannot. From the perspective of convincing individuals to take part in team science collaborations, such a motivational focus can be an effective tool for motivating engagement. From the perspective of doing high-quality science, considering the ways in which well-structured team science projects can synergistically enhance both the basic and applied goals of the work can advance the field. Ultimately, this focus on motivational underpinnings of scientific inquiry and field-based application can enhance both the individual and the collective outcomes of team science.

References

Baranowski T. Advances in basic behavioral research will make the most important contributions to effective dietary change programs at this time. J Am Diet Assoc. 2006;106(6):808–11.

Bennett LM, Gadlin H, Levine-Finley S. Collaboration and team science: a field guide. Bethesda, MD: National Institutes of Health; 2010.

Brewer MB. Experimental research and social policy: must it be rigor versus relevance? J Soc Issues. 1985;41(4):159–76. https://doi.org/10.1111/j.1540-4560.1985.tb01149.x.

Crow MM, Dabars WB. Designing the new American University. Baltimore: JHU Press; 2015.

Dugan RE, Gabriel KJ. "Special forces" innovation: how DARPA attacks problems. Harv Bus Rev. 2013;91(10):74–84.

Edwards W. The theory of decision making. Psychol Bull. 1954;51(4):380–417.

Erwin DO, Moysich K, Kiviniemi MT, Saad-Harfouche FG, Davis W, Clark-Hargrave N, et al. Community-based partnership to identify keys to biospecimen research participation. J Cancer Educ. 2013;28(1):43–51. https://doi.org/10.1007/s13187-012-0421-5.

Gholson B, Barker P. Kuhn, Lakatos, and Laudan: applications in the history of physics and psychology. Am Psychol. 1985;40(7):755–69.

Glanz K, Bishop DB. The role of behavioral science theory in development and implementation of public health interventions. Annu Rev Public Health. 2010;31:399–418.

Glasgow RE, Vogt TM, Boles SM. Evaluating the public health impact of health promotion interventions: the RE-AIM framework. Am J Public Health. 1999;89(9):1322–7.

Green LW, Kreuter MW. Health promotion planning: an educational and ecological approach. 4th ed. Boston, MA: McGraw-Hill; 2004.

Hay JL, Orom H, Kiviniemi MT, Waters EA. "I don't know" My cancer risk: exploring deficits in cancer knowledge and information-seeking skills to explain an often-overlooked participant response. Med Decis Mak. 2015;35(4):436–45. https://doi.org/10.1177/027 2989x15572827.

Kessel F, Rosenfield PL. Toward transdisciplinary research: historical and contemporary perspectives. Am J Prev Med. 2008;35(2 Suppl):S225–34. https://doi.org/10.1016/j.amepre.2008.05.005.

Kiviniemi MT, Hay JL. Awareness of the 2009 US preventive services task force recommended changes in mammography screening guidelines, accuracy of awareness, sources of knowledge about recommendations, and attitudes about updated screening guidelines in women ages 40--49 and 50+. BMC Public Health. 2012;12(1):899. https://doi.org/10.1186/1471-2458-12-899.

Kiviniemi MT, Jandorf L, Erwin DO. Disgusted, embarrassed, afraid: affective associations relate to uptake of colonoscopy screening in an urban, African American population. Ann Behav Med. 2014;48:112–9.

Kiviniemi MT, Ram PK, Kozlowski LT, Smith KM. Perceptions of and willingness to engage in public health precautions to prevent 2009 H1N1 influenza transmission. BMC Public Health. 2011;11(1):152.

Kiviniemi MT, Rintamaki LS, Smith KM. Low levels of health and general literacy are associated with less optimal psychosocial functioning. Paper Presented at the Health Literacy Research Conference, Chicago, IL; 2011

Kiviniemi MT, Saad-Harfouche FG, Ciupak GL, Davis W, Moysich K, Hargrave NC, et al. Pilot intervention outcomes of an educational program for biospecimen research participation. J Cancer Educ. 2013;28(1):52–9. https://doi.org/10.1007/s13187-012-0434-0.

Kiviniemi MT, Voss-Humke AM, Seifert AL. How do I feel about the behavior? The interplay of affective associations with behaviors and cognitive beliefs as influences on physical activity behavior. Health Psychol. 2007;26(2):152–8.

Kozlowski LT, Kiviniemi MT, Ram PK. Easier said than done: behavioral conflicts in following social-distancing recommendations for influenza prevention. Public Health Rep. 2010;125:789–92.

Kreuter MW, Strecher VJ, Glassman B. One size does not fit all: the case for tailoring print materials. Ann Behav Med. 1999;21(4):276–83. https://doi.org/10.1007/bf02895958.

Kuhn TS. The structure of scientific revolutions. 2nd ed. Chicago, IL: University of Chicago; 1975.

Lewin K. Field theory in social science: selected theoretical papers (Edited by Dorwin Cartwright). Harpers: Oxford; 1951.

Ness RM, Manam R, Hoen H, Chalasani N. Predictors of inadequate bowel preparation for colonoscopy. Am J Gastroenterol. 2001;96(6):1797–802.

Onken LS, Carroll KM, Shoham V, Cuthbert BN, Riddle M. Reenvisioning clinical science: unifying the discipline to improve the public health. Clin Psychol Sci. 2014;2(1):22–34. https://doi.org/10.1177/2167702613497932.

Othman AK, Kiviniemi MT, Wu Y-WB, Lally RM. Influence of demographic factors, knowledge, and beliefs on Jordanian women's intention to undergo mammography screening. J Nurs Scholarsh. 2012;44(1):19–26. https://doi.org/10.1111/j.1547-5069.2011.01435.x.

Rintamaki LS, Kiviniemi MT, Smith KM. A head-to-head comparison of basic and health literacy measures. Paper Presented at the Health Literacy Research Conference, Chicago, IL; 2011.

Rothman AJ. "Is there nothing more practical than a good theory?": why innovations and advances in health behavior change will arise if interventions are used to test and refine theory. Int J Behav Nutr Phys Act. 2004;1(1):11. https://doi.org/10.1186/1479-5868-1-11.

Rothman AJ. Capitalizing on opportunities to refine health behavior theories. Health Educ Behav. 2009;36(5 Suppl):150S–5S. https://doi.org/10.1177/1090198109340514.

Rothman AJ, Kiviniemi MT. Treating people with information: an analysis and review of approaches to communicating health risk information. J Natl Cancer Inst Monogr. 1999;1999(25):44–51.

Stokes DE. Pasteur's quadrant: basic science and technological innovation. Washington, DC: Brookings Institution Press; 1997.

Stokols D, Misra S, Moser RP, Hall KL, Taylor BK. The ecology of team science: understanding contextual influences on transdisciplinary collaboration. Am J Prev Med. 2008;35(2. Suppl):S96–115.

Stukas AA, Snyder M, Clary EG. The social marketing of volunteerism: a functional approach. In: Haugtvedt CP, Herr PM, Kardes FR, Haugtvedt CP, Herr PM, Kardes FR, editors. Handbook of consumer psychology, vol. 4. New York, NY: Taylor & Francis Group/ Lawrence Erlbaum Associates; 2008. p. 959–79.

Underhill ML, Kiviniemi MT. The association of perceived provider-patient communication and relationship quality with colorectal cancer screening. Health Educ Behav. 2012;39(5):555–63. https://doi.org/10.1177/1090198111421800.

Underhill ML, Lally RM, Kiviniemi MT, Murekeyisoni C, Dickerson SS. Living my Family's story: identifying the lived experience in healthy women at risk for hereditary breast cancer. Cancer Nurs. 2012;35(6):493–

Waters EA, Hay JL, Orom H, Kiviniemi MT, Drake BF. "Don't know" responses to risk perception measures: implications for underserved populations. Med Decis Mak. 2013;33(2):271–81. https://doi.org/10.1177/027 2989x12464435.

Engaging the Public: Citizen Science

12

Jennifer Couch, Katrina Theisz,
and Elizabeth Gillanders

Contents

J. Couch (✉) · K. Theisz
Division of Cancer Biology, National Cancer
Institute, Bethesda, MD, USA
e-mail: couchj@ctep.nci.nih.gov

E. Gillanders
Division of Cancer Control and Population Sciences,
National Cancer Institute, Bethesda, MD, USA

12.1   Overview

This chapter focuses on citizen science and related methods which aim to involve the public in scientific research. "Citizen Science" can be defined as a collaborative approach to research involving the public, not just as subjects of the research or advisors to the research but as direct collaborators and partners in all aspects the research process itself.

Citizen science is a complex set of methods that includes an ever-expanding lexicon of related terms which are constantly evolving (e.g., participatory action research, public participation in scientific research, etc.). A particular emphasis will be given to community-based participatory research (CBPR) and community-engaged research (CEnR) in Chap. 10 (Johnson et al.). The usefulness of citizen science methods in scientific research and how it has become the ultimate team science will also be highlighted.

12.2   Introduction

The term "Citizen Science" has been used to cover a wide breadth of methods that engage members of the public—including nonexperts or individuals not traditionally associated with the field of inquiry—to join in scientific research. Through direct participation and partnering with

© Springer Nature Switzerland AG 2019
K. L. Hall et al. (eds.), *Strategies for Team Science Success*,
https://doi.org/10.1007/978-3-030-20992-6_12

the public, citizen science opens new opportunities for biomedical research including many aspects of behavioral and social research. Provided the right tools and opportunities, patients and healthy individuals are eager to contribute and can provide unique data, insights, creative solutions and interpretations not possible through conventional research methods.

Citizen science could be considered the ultimate "team science." Collaboration among individuals and groups from varied backgrounds and diverse skill sets necessitates different organizational, technical, and methodological approaches than those used by traditional research teams. In addition, citizen science projects vary greatly in their scope and the numbers of participants or collaborators can be quite large in comparison to traditional scientific teams. Given the innately multidisciplinary nature of citizen science and crowdsourcing, as well as their relatively recent adoption in many areas of scientific research, a need for the science of citizen science is warranted (Bonney et al. 2014).

In the fields of ecology and astronomy, direct and collaborative engagement of the public in scientific research has a long history of use and it is increasingly common for individuals to collect, annotate and analyze scientific data for both educational and research purposes. Projects such as the Audubon Bird Count during which the public has collected information on bird species throughout the country for the past 115 years, have created extensive datasets which would not have been possible without the volunteer efforts of the public. These data are used to track migration, habitat change, and the effects of climate change on species abundance and distribution (Cooper et al. 2014). Furthermore, efforts such as Galaxy Zoo have used internet-enabled microtasking, breaking down large projects into small tasks that can be worked on by a large number of individuals, to make extensive progress with large data annotation or analysis problems.

These projects build on the interest, creativity, pattern recognition skills, and problem-solving capabilities of the public to analyze large datasets through activities such as galaxy classification. These innate abilities and interest of the public

have resulted in scientific advances such as the discovery of a new class of galaxies called Green Pea Galaxies which were first noticed and discussed by the citizen scientist contributors to Galaxy Zoo (Cardamone et al. 2009).

A hallmark of citizen science is the collaboration among amateurs and experts to collect, analyze, and interpret data and information. Along those lines, Shirk et al. (2012) propose five distinct types of projects in which the public participates:

1. *Contractual* projects, where communities ask professional researchers to conduct a specific scientific investigation and report on the results;
2. *Contributory* projects, which are generally designed by scientists and for which members of the public primarily contribute data;
3. *Collaborative* projects, which are generally designed by scientists and for which members of the public contribute data but also help to refine project design, analyze data, and/or disseminate findings;
4. *Co-Created* projects, which are designed by scientists and members of the public working together and for which at least some of the public participants are actively involved in most or all aspects of the research process; and
5. *Collegial* contributions, where noncredentialed individuals conduct research independently with varying degrees of expected recognition by institutionalized science and/or professionals.

While biomedical research has been slower to adopt some "citizen science" practices, there is of course a strong history of Community Based Participatory Research (CBPR) through which community input and community-initiated biomedical research is accomplished. In CBPR, a community may be virtual, united by a common disease or condition, or may be defined by geography, ethnicity, or shared culture. However, historically, the community's interests, needs, values, and questions are often represented by a limited number of people, such as an advocate, community elder, or other official representative.

Fig. 12.1 Venn diagram of converging terms with the common theme of public engagement in research. The types of and terms surrounding public engagement in research are constantly evolving, with new terms and themes entering the space

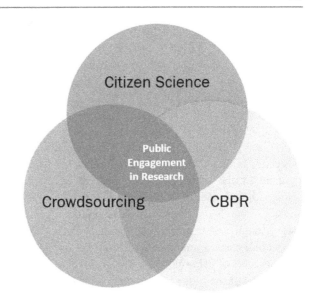

Many have called for a more engaged approach. For example, Pearson et al. (2015) expand on CBPR, in which they define the role of the public participant as reaching a point of equity with traditional researchers, to community-engaged research, which focuses on collaboration between stakeholders and is not necessarily focused on equity. This will be discussed in greater detail in Chap. 11. This expanded view of CBPR would align more closely with "citizen science" which involves members of the public working with professional scientists to jointly lead and complete a research project. Certainly, in biomedical research, the terms CBPR and citizen science are converging as community members take more active roles in research in greater numbers and frequency (see Fig. 12.1).

From a social science perspective, citizen science is a science, which can also assist the needs and concerns of citizens (Kullenberg and Kasperowski 2016). A clear example of this citizen engagement in research prioritization is the Community Partners in Care (CPIC) program (http://www.communitypartnersincare.org/). The CPIC program is a collaborative research project, which engages both community and academic partners to determine the best way to reduce the burden of depression on the communities of South Los Angeles and Hollywood-

Metro LA as well as other under resourced, vulnerable populations. Strikingly, the academic-community partnership found that incorporating the community-network-building approach added value and can help improve people struggling with depression's quality of life and lower the risk of a life crisis (Wells et al. 2013). It also increased participants' physical activity, and decreased risk factors for homelessness by 25%, and behavioral hospitalizations by 50%. Initially, the community and academic partners had planned to focus exclusively on how well each approach improved clients' clinical symptoms of depression. However, from broad input from more than one thousand citizens, they learned that many community members placed equal or greater weight on other issues such as finding and keeping employment, avoiding homelessness, dealing with family issues, and maintaining physical health; therefore, the community and academic partners shifted the focus of the project toward those goals. Traditional research projects that are described as "community-based" may only involve the community as an advisor, or broker, for recruiting subjects without partnering with the community to jointly lead the study. The Community Partners in Care program illustrates clearly that with a fully engaged community–

academic partnership, citizens can provide meaningful direction to the research process.

In parallel, due to technical advances in genomics, other "omics," medical imaging, and wearable technologies that allow for vast datasets to be collected in a cost-effective manner, biomedical research is increasingly becoming a data science. "Big data" impacts and enables all aspects of biomedical research from our understanding of the underlying biological mechanisms of health and disease, to translational and clinical research and decision-making, epidemiology, social and behavioral research, and the impact of the environment on health and disease. Many aspects of data science, software development, and data analysis can be accomplished in a distributed, often microtasked manner with few technical resources, all of which lend themselves to distributed capabilities, virtual collaborations, and collaboration between the general public and researchers. Researchers and funding agencies, such as the NIH and CDC have successfully used crowdsourcing mechanisms such as challenges, hackathons, and game jams which often offer monetary prizes or other rewards to individuals and teams who design algorithms, generate ideas, and develop software tools or engineered solutions to posed questions using open data.

12.3 Crowdsourcing, Microtasking, and Games: The Power of the Crowd in Data Analysis and Annotation

One rapidly emerging method for crowdsourcing, microtasking, and citizen science in the biomedical space is the use of games and game technologies. Games are widespread and popular and the technologies behind them used to render images, share and compile information, and enable both collaborative and competitive play are all aspects that make them useful for research purposes (Zanto et al. 2011). Games have been widely used for educational and outreach purposes and more recently are beginning to be

employed to facilitate scientific research (Cooper et al. 2013). These games employ a variety of methods ranging from highly abstract representations of the science to very direct representations of the scientific question. Many research-focused games strive for a combination of fun, collaborative, competitive game play with enough information about the science or medical rationale to entice players. One example, Foldit, leverages the capabilities of complex algorithms and human ingenuity to elucidate 3D protein structures from amino acid sequence. Using this approach, Foldit players acting on an abstracted version of a partially folded protein structure, have solved a variety of previously unsolved proteins structures (Khatib et al. 2012). Another pivotal game example is EyeWire, which engages over a million players in helping to render neuronal connections in the mouse retina from 2D images (Kim et al. 2014).

When presented with the right tools, people are interested and capable of performing various aspects of scientific research including visual puzzle solving, extracting meaning from text, and adding social/cultural context and insight. Projects such as Mark2Cure have shown that the public is interested and capable of tagging scientific text, such as the text in the abstracts of scientific publications. Li et al. (2016) have shown that the public can help to map concepts embedded in the scientific literature to draw connections or relationships between diseases, genes, and events. In addition, they showed that in aggregate, these nonexperts were as effective as experts in these tasks and that volunteer participation was as effective as paid participation. Recognition is important; research indicates that when users of a particular virtual medium are recognized, they may continue or increase their use of that medium (Hamari and Koivisto 2015).

12.4 Unique Data and Insights Through Direct Contribution

In addition to participating in the scientific process by analyzing data, patients, healthy individuals, and caregivers are also interested in sharing their personal health data, insights, and experience in ways that will enhance and speed biomedical research. Many websites, platforms, and portals have sprung up to offer patients and their advocates a place to share information, stories, resources, and connect with one another. PatientsLikeMe is an example of such a website, which also offers a way for researchers to check in and get real reactions and feedback from patients to get a better and broader sense of the patient experience (patientslikeme.com). An Institute of Medicine Report in 2014 surveying PatientsLikeMe participants showed that individuals are eager to share health information if it will help themselves and others, even when they anticipate that there could be risks involved with sharing (Grajales et al. 2014). Even individuals who do not normally share personal health data are willing to do so through personal fitness apps, but are more likely to have concerns regarding data privacy (Chen et al. 2016). This interest and enthusiasm coupled with the unique insights that patients, healthy people, and caregivers have into the maintenance of health and the development and progression of disease, provide a unique opportunity to enhance the overall research endeavor.

Some of the platforms that enable direct collaboration between the public and academic researchers also include PEER (Platform for Engaging Everyone Responsibly), which gives patients the ability to form online communities around the same diagnoses (https://www.peer-platform.org/). For individuals interested in contributing their data and participating in biomedical research via their iPhone, Apple has created ResearchKit, a way for patients, physicians, and researchers to learn more about disease in a much more immediate way and on a much larger scale than they could before (http://www.apple.com/researchkit/).

Community advocates and organizations, such as those representing communities of individuals with the same disease or geographically or culturally defined communities have engaged researchers directly and have pushed for new sharing and collaboration models. For example, projects such as Free the Data (http://www.free-the-data.org/) create a way for interested and motivated communities to collect and share personal health data. Specifically, the Free the Data project enters BRCA1 or two genetic mutation information into a public database so that associations between gene mutations and breast cancer risk can be discovered, and research can be advanced. Additionally, in the Parkinsons mPower study, individuals diagnosed with Parkinson's disease use a specially designed app which combines sensor data, physical measurements, and questionnaires to track health and symptom progression by utilizing ResearchKit infrastructure. The app provides the participant with a personalized report they can share with their health professionals, as well as the opportunity to share this data freely with individuals who use the data for research. Likewise, community-driven research where a community initiates the research project, often partnering with academic researchers and often participating in or leading much of the data collection and analysis effort. For example, the Gardenroots project participants have gathered and analyzed data on arsenic contamination of vegetables in their community. Their scientifically rigorous methods and results led to increased scientific knowledge, open data, and safe practices guidelines for local gardeners and consumers of locally grown produce in the affected community (Ramírez-Andreotta et al. 2016)

For-profit organizations such as uBiome have also created space in which people who paid, in this case for the sequence of their gut microbiome, to share that information with each other and with researchers. The quantified self-community (quantifiedself.com) have created ad hoc methods for individuals to share personal health data, such as fitness data, diet, and in some cases genome sequence or other molecular data. Though some users of personal fitness apps or mobile or wearable sensors only utilize these tools for a limited amount of time, the motives may be the same at the beginning of use for both long- and short-term users according to Stragier et al. (2016). These motives include social ones (e.g., virtual social interaction, general enjoyment of use or of related activities) and what the authors define as self-regulatory motives, which, in this context, include activities involved in the monitoring, assessment, and regulation of one's personal health. Self-regulatory motives are more commonly found in long-term participants in quantified health.

12.5 The Potential for Citizen Science in Social and Behavioral Research

It is well recognized that human behavior is fundamental in the etiology and management of cancer outcomes and presents several avenues for targeted intervention (Klein et al. 2014). For example, suboptimal patient compliance with treatment regimens is a common problem in medicine. In particular, adherence to self-administered treatments such as oral chemotherapy proves especially challenging for young adults with cancer. This is a critically important challenge to address because although cancer in young adults is relatively rare, it has now become the leading cause of death by disease past infancy among children in the United States (The National Cancer Institute 2014). The "Remission" video game intervention was developed specifically to improve treatment adherence and other behavioral outcomes in adolescent and young adult cancer patients (Kato et al. 2008). The efficacy of the intervention was tested in a randomized controlled trial including adolescents and young adults diagnosed with several cancers including acute leukemia, lymphoma, and soft-tissue sarcoma. Patients within the intervention group received treatment as usual and played the "Remission" video game, which addressed issues of cancer treatment and care for teenagers and young adults. Notably, playing "Remission" significantly improved indicators of cancer-related self-efficacy and treatment adherence in adolescents and young adults who were undergoing cancer therapy. This randomized controlled trial provides evidence for the efficacy of a video-game intervention to alter behavior and given the role of behavioral factors in influencing cancer management more broadly, similar approaches

could potentially be developed to reduce the cancer burden.

Patients and healthy individuals are highly motivated to contribute to the biomedical research endeavor (Grajales et al. 2014). Citizen Science offers the tools and approaches necessary to engage the public and to benefit from their unique insights and creativity. Just as the evolution of interdisciplinary teams in biomedical research benefited from the Science of Team Science, the rapidly emerging world of Citizen Science will also benefit from a Science of Citizen Science. Researchers and the public working together with an increased understanding of which methods and approaches work best for which research questions, will bring these new and complementary approaches to biomedical and behavioral research enabling new discoveries and accelerating research (Chen et al. 2016).

12.6 The Need for the Science of Citizen Science: What Works for What Kinds of Projects, and When?

The Science of Team Science field has laid extensive groundwork for the evaluation of large, multidisciplinary teams. Much can be gleaned by examining lessons learned from the field of the Science of Team Science. Many of the Science of Team Science strategies and methods used to evaluate team science can be utilized to evaluate citizen science. For example, utilizing the Science of Team Science research on how best to increase diversity in a research team, or methods of increasing collaboration and communication across disciplines may prove to be quite relevant to studying the science of citizen science. Just as traditional approaches benefit from evaluation, citizen science and crowdsourcing not only require this level of scrutiny; the community of citizen science practitioners welcomes it (Newman et al. 2011).

However, citizen science poses unique challenges to evaluation, as it includes a broad array of methods and approaches. Just as understanding and effectively evaluating the science of interdisciplinary teams required study, effective use of citizen science in biomedical and behavioral research will require study. Studying the science of citizen science will help practitioners understand when citizen science methods work in conjunction with or better than traditional methods and which of the many different citizen science and crowdsourcing approaches work best for which kinds of biomedical research questions. Literature on the efficacy and accuracy of citizen science continues to expand, and research on how to evaluate and improve data quality have flourished as the popularity and use of citizen science as a method of scientific research continues to grow (Wiggins et al. 2011). Though a recent scientometric meta-analysis of citizen science publications showed the amount of publications to be low in comparison to other older established fields, it reasoned that this was because the field (in some ways) is quite new- and productive (Kullenberg and Kasperowski 2016). The authors found that citizen science publications have been increasing over time in recent years, as has the proliferation of digital collaboration spaces to support these endeavors.

As digital collaboration increases and technology advances, it is easy to assume that many scientific roles can be easily performed by computers, given their immense data processing and storage abilities. Despite recent rapid advances in technology, computers have not taken over the scientific process; there are still many things computers cannot do, that can only be done by humans (Michelucci and Dickinson 2016). Things like pattern recognition, creativity, social/cultural norms, abstraction, and inference are a few key areas where the human mind excels over the computer. Indeed, visual perception is a widely accepted ability used for establishing the identity of a computer end user as a human through the use of CAPTCHA, an established method of asking users to transcribe words, letters, numbers, or images from scanned documents that were not recognized by a computer program. The ReCAPTCHA program leveraged this capability to digitize old books and other documents (von Ahn et al. 2008). Until technology can replicate the innate skills of the human

mind, it will still be more efficient to crowdsource to humans.

Until citizen science is seen universally as a valid research method complementary to existing methods, best practices will need to be evaluated, prior to and after their establishment (Garbarino and Mason 2016) and are not without barriers. Some potential barriers to implementing citizen science methods vary from using different ontologies and lexicons to describe the same or similar things (or the same word to describe vastly different things), to citizen science and citizen scientists not receiving recognition in scholarly papers describing work done entirely or in part by citizen scientists—indeed, in the past some researchers chose not to credit citizen scientists who worked alongside them on their research (Cooper et al. 2014). Now, instead of using the work of citizen scientists without providing them their due credit, many researchers are changing this culture in several different ways. Some, by crediting their citizen scientists in general terms, as the number of volunteers may be too vast to fit in a publication (Kim et al. 2014). Others, by making it known how much work was performed by volunteers, or by making it clear that the citizen scientists (or, "volunteers") were not just contributors to the work but the individuals responsible for a particular breakthrough and thanking them in the acknowledgments, such as the Galaxy Zoo project (Cardamone et al. 2009):

- This publication has been made possible by the participation of more than 200,000 volunteers in the Galaxy Zoo project. Their contributions are individually acknowledged at http://www.galaxyzoo.org/Volunteers.aspx.

One of the very first scholarly papers to acknowledge citizen scientists (in this instance, game players) through authorship who contributed to a scientific breakthrough came out of the Foldit project (Cooper et al. 2010). A more recent example is the RNA puzzle game, EteRNA, which published a paper authored primarily by the EteRNA players, some of whom are listed as first authors (Anderson-Lee et al. 2016).

12.7   Conclusion

As citizen science evolves and gains acceptance in the biomedical, social, and behavioral research communities, perpetual uncovering of the ways in which it works best can only help to increase its efficacy, and catalyzing change in research culture. Citizen science methods offer the tools and approaches necessary to engage the public and thereby benefit from their unique insights and creativity. When community advocates, patients, and caregivers engage directly with researchers, new sharing and collaboration models can flourish. Patients and healthy individuals are highly motivated to contribute to the biomedical research endeavor. But it's not just people powering research; combining the computational power and storage capacity of machines with human strengths like pattern recognition, creativity, social/cultural norms, and abstraction, will help drive research forward. Citizen science could be considered the ultimate "team science."

References

Anderson-Lee J, Fisker E, Kosaraju V, Wu M, Kong J, Lee J, Lee M, Zada M, Treuille A, Das R, EteRNA Players. Principles for predicting RNA secondary structure design difficulty. J Mol Biol. 2016;428(5):748–57. https://doi.org/10.1016/j.jmb.2015.11.013.

Bonney R, Shirk JL, Phillips TB, Wiggins A, Ballard HL, Miller-Rushing AJ, Parish JK. Next steps for citizen science. Science. 2014;343(6178):1436–7.

Cardamone C, Schawinski K, Sarzi M, Bamford SP, Bennert N, Urry CM, Lintott C, Keel WC, Parejko J, Nichol RC, Thomas D, Andreescu D, Murray P, Raddick MJ, Slosar A, Szalay A, VandenBerg J. Galaxy zoo green peas: discovery of a class of compact extremely star-forming galaxies. Mon Not R Astron Soc. 2009;399(3):1191–205.. https://arxiv.org/pdf/0907.4155v1.pdf

Chen J, Bauman A, Allman-Farinelli M. A study to determine the most popular lifestyle smartphone applications and willingness of the public to share their personal data for Health Research. Telemed J E Health. 2016;22(8):655–65. https://doi.org/10.1089/tmj.2015.0159.

Cooper S, Khatib F, Baker D. Increasing public involvement in structural biology. Structure. 2013;21(9):1482–4. https://doi.org/10.1016/j.str.2013.08.009.

Cooper S, Khatib F, Treuille A, Barbero J, Lee J, Beene M, Leaver-Fay A, Baker D, Popovic Z, Foldit Players.

Predicting protein structures with a multiplayer online game. Nature. 2010;466:756–60. https://doi.org/10.1038/nature09304.

Cooper CB, Shirk J, Zuckerberg B. The invisible prevalence of citizen science in global research: migratory birds and climate change. PLoS One. 2014;9(9):e106508. https://doi.org/10.1371/journal.pone.0106508.

Garbarino J, Mason CE. The power of engaging citizen scientists for scientific Progress. J Microbiol Biol Educ. 2016;17(1):7–12. https://doi.org/10.1128/jmbe.v17i1.1052.

Grajales F, Clifford D, Loupos P, Okun S, Quattrone S, Simon M, Wicks P, Henderson D. Social networking sites and the continuously learning health system: a survey, vol. 4. Washington, DC. http://nam.edu/wp-content/uploads/2015/06//SharingHealthData.pdf: Discussion paper, Institute of Medicine; 2014.

Hamari J, Koivisto J. "Working out for likes": an empirical study on social influence in exercise gamification. Comput Hum Behav. 2015;50:333–47. https://doi.org/10.1016/j.chb.2015.04.018.

Kato PM, Cole SW, Bradlyn AS, Pollock BH. A video game improves behavioral outcomes in adolescents and young adults with cancer: a randomized trial. Pediatrics. 2008;122:e305. https://doi.org/10.1542/peds.2007-3134.

Khatib D, DiMaio F, Foldit Contenders Group, Foldit Void Crushers Group, Cooper S, Kazmierczyk M, Gilski M, Krzywda S, Zabranska H, Pichova I, Thompson J, Popovic Z, Jaskolski M, Baker D. Crystal structure of a monomeric retroviral protease solved by protein folding game players. Nat Struct Mol Biol. 2012;19:1175–7. https://doi.org/10.1038/nsmb.2119.

Kim JS, Greene MJ, Zlateski A, Lee K, Richardson M, Turaga SC, Purcaro M, Balkam M, Robinson A, Behabadi BF, Campos M, Denk W, Seung HS, the EyeWirers. Space–time wiring specificity supports direction selectivity in the retina. Nature. 2014;509(7500):331–6. https://doi.org/10.1038/nature13240.

Klein WM, Bloch M, Hesse BW, McDonald PG, Nebeling L, O'Connell ME, Riley WT, Taplin SH, Tesauro G. Behavioral research in cancer prevention and control: a look to the future. Am J Prev Med. 2014;46(3):303–11. https://doi.org/10.1016/j.amepre.2013.10.004.

Kullenberg C, Kasperowski D. What is citizen science?-a Scientometric meta-analysis. PLoS One. 2016;11:e0147152. https://doi.org/10.1371/journal.pone.0147152.

Li TS, Bravo A, Furlong LI, Good BM, Su AI. A crowdsourcing workflow for extracting chemical-induced disease relations from free text. Database. 2016;2016:baw051. https://doi.org/10.1093/database/baw051.

Michelucci P, Dickinson JL. The power of crowds. Science. 2016;351(6268):32–3.

Newman G, Graham J, Crall A, Laituri M. The art and science of multi-scale citizen science support. Eco Inform. 2011;6(3–4):217–27. https://doi.org/10.1016/j.ecoinf.2011.03.002.

Pearson CR, Duran B, Oetzel J, Margarati M, Villegas M, Lucero J, Wallerstein N. Research for improved health: variability and impact of structural characteristics in federally funded community engaged research. Prog Community Health Partnersh. 2015;9(1):17–29. https://doi.org/10.1353/cpr.2015.0010.

Ramírez-Andreotta MD, Brody JG, Lothrop N, Loh M, Beamer PI, Brown P. Improving environmental health literacy and justice through environmental exposure results communication. Int J Environ Res Public Health. 2016;13(7):E690. https://doi.org/10.3390/ijerph13070690.

Shirk JL, Ballard HL, Wilderman CC, Phillips T, Wiggins A, Jordan R, McCallie E, Minarchek M, Lewenstein BV, Krasny ME, Bonney R. Public participation in scientific research: a framework for deliberate design. Ecol Soc. 2012;17(2):29. https://doi.org/10.5751/ES-04705-170229.

Stragier J, Vanden Abeele M, Mechant P, De Marez L. Understanding persistence in the use of online fitness communities: comparing novice and experienced users. Comput Hum Behav. 2016;64:34–42. https://doi.org/10.1016/j.chb.2016.06.013.

The National Cancer Institute. Cancer in children and adolescents. 2014. http://www.cancer.gov/types/childhood-cancers/child-adolescent-cancers-fact-sheet

von Ahn L, Maurer B, McMillen C, Abraham D, Blum M. reCAPTCHA: human-based character recognition via web security measures. Science. 2008;321(5895):1465–8.

Wells KB, Jones L, Chung B, Dixon EL, Tang L, Gilmore J, Sherbourne C, Ngo VK, Ong MK, Stockdale S, Ramos E, Belin TR, Miranda J. Community-partnered cluster-randomized comparative effectiveness trial of community engagement and planning or resources for services to address depression disparities. J Gen Intern Med. 2013;28:1268–78. https://doi.org/10.1007/s11606-013-2484-3.

Wiggins A, Newman G, Stevenson RD, Crowston K. Mechanisms for data quality and validation in citizen science. In: Workshop Proceedings: 7th IEEE International Conference on e-Science. Stockholm: Institute of Electrical and Electronics Engineers; 2011. p. 14–9.

Zanto TP, Rubens MT, Thangavel A, Gazzaley A. Causal role of the prefrontal cortex in top-down modulation of visual processing and working memory. Nat Neurosci. 2011;14:656. https://doi.org/10.1038/nn.2773.

Individual-Level Competencies for Team Collaboration with Cross-Disciplinary Researchers and Stakeholders

13

Paula S. Nurius and Susan P. Kemp

Contents

P. S. Nurius (✉)
School of Social Work, University of Washington,
Seattle, WA, USA
e-mail: nurius@u.washington.edu

S. P. Kemp
School of Social Work, University of Washington,
Seattle, WA, USA

Faculty of Education and Social Work,
University of Auckland, Auckland, New Zealand

13.1   Introduction

Societies worldwide are struggling to address complex social, environmental, and public health problems. Effectively understanding and tackling "wicked" problems (Weber and Khademian 2008) such as climate change, health disparities, and poverty requires the combined knowledge, skills, and innovative capacity of a wide array of disciplines. Increasingly, such collaborative partnerships encompass not only diverse disciplinary scientists but also community, agency, and policy stakeholders. As the chapters in this book make clear, the success of these collaborative research efforts depends on a range of individual, leadership, organizational, funding, and related factors. At the center of this hub lie individual-level factors crucial to team success. This chapter provides an overview of the state of the science on individual-level competencies: the inter-related knowledge, skills, attitudes, values, and "habits of mind" that are critical facilitators to the success of cross-disciplinary scientific collaborations.

Although understandings of collaborative science are coalescing, differences remain in how terminology around various forms of disciplinarity is conceptualized and used. We will draw from the following definitions in this chapter. In *multidisciplinary* projects (Oskam 2009), specialists from different disciplines work

© Springer Nature Switzerland AG 2019
K. L. Hall et al. (eds.), *Strategies for Team Science Success*,
https://doi.org/10.1007/978-3-030-20992-6_13

sequentially or alongside each another, bringing multiple perspectives, content knowledge, and methods to bear on a common issue, yet maintaining their separate disciplinary frameworks and methods. *Interdisciplinarity* is distinguished by a greater degree of communication, collaboration, and integrative work, requiring the capacity and willingness among participants to exchange knowledge, influence one another, and jointly produce (and potentially apply) new knowledge. *Transdisciplinarity* entails even greater integration of knowledge, theory, and methods, transcending disciplinary divisions to create new conceptual frameworks, allow for more complex and generative products, and encompass collaborations between researchers and community stakeholders, who work together to understand and ultimately resolve collectively identified problems (see Gehlert et al. 2008; Hall 2013; Nash 2008; and Stokols 2006 for discussion of definitions). Since team science spans both interdisciplinary and transdisciplinary efforts, in this chapter we use the term cross-disciplinary to encompass both forms of collaborative endeavor.

This chapter provides an overview of individual-level characteristics that have garnered broad-based attention as facilitators to the success of cross-disciplinary scientific collaborations. We first describe growing use of the T-shaped metaphor to convey the individual-level competencies diverse specialists need to engage effectively in deeply collaborative work. Drawing from a robust literature, we articulate four broadly applicable domains of individual competencies (the crossbar of the T) critical to team science innovation, including descriptions of specific skill sets within each domain. In addition to noting the importance of training for and nurturing these boundary-spanning competencies across diverse disciplinary scientists, we emphasize the parallel value of these competencies in engagement with nonscientific stakeholders, who similarly bring their particular world views, languages, knowledge sets, and interpersonal practices to the team science enterprise.

13.2 T-Shaped Collaborators: A Framework for Conceptualizing Boundary-Spanning Competencies

In applied fields such as design, architecture, engineering, technology, medicine, and water (Donofrio et al. 2010; McIntosh and Taylor 2013), as well as in research and academia (Bajada and Trayler 2013; Simpson et al. 2008), the notion of "T-shaped" scientists and professionals is increasingly used to describe individuals with the both/and skill sets needed for collaborative problem solving and innovation. In contrast to the columnar "I" shape of single disciplinary or professional preparation, T-shaped professionals combine depth of disciplinary expertise (the vertical trunk) with boundary-spanning competencies (the horizontal bar) that facilitate engagement with others bringing complementary expertise to research and application efforts. The term meta-competencies is also used to denote competencies that are broadly applicable across team needs (Uhlenbrook and de Jong 2012).

In business and professional settings, the idea of the T-shaped professional captures the skills needed to work deliberately and effectively across the boundaries of organizational units (e.g., departments) or expertise to solve complex problems and generate "out of the box" innovative thinking. Uhlenbrook and de Jong (2012), for example, note the critical importance of water professionals with these skills, given the unprecedented complexity and magnitude of problems associated with global environmental changes. Contemporary water professionals must bridge fields such as hydrology, water chemistry, hydraulics, aquatic ecology, and land-use management, as well as functions such as water governance, environmental policy and law, water transfer, and knowledge related to water applications such as agronomy. The recent water poisoning crisis in Flint, Michigan also underscores the vital importance of values and ethics in collective work on complex public issues, along with the ability to interface competently not only with other disciplines and professions such as public health and emergency response specialists but with the media, activists, and the community (Edwards and Pruden 2016).

Our emphasis on T-shaped competence is not intended to convey a preference for generalists with limited knowledge across many areas. Team science contexts for producing, translating, and applying research *depend* on participants bringing distinctive, in-depth disciplinary knowledge and skills to the tables of collaborative science. The Flint water crisis, for example, demands incisive content knowledge and methodological expertise across multiple domains—including the source of lead, the decision pathways resulting in its transmission, the effects of consuming lead, and flow-on implications for affected individuals and families—necessitating the engagement of very differently trained people with potentially differing priorities. At the same time,

the complexity of knowledge needed to engage problems such as these demands not only advanced disciplinary specialization and even sub-specialization, but also the ability to engage deeply with other similarly trained experts.

As Strober (2006) points out, disciplinary immersion can constrain innovation. The narrowing effect of specialized training can make exchange with others outside one's disciplinary culture challenging. Yet the "tables" of science and problem response are increasingly populated not by others who share similar training and socialization (and, thus, the same language, tools, and perspectives), but by "strangers" (Schnapp et al. 2012) whose expertise is needed, yet foreign. As illustrated in Fig. 13.1, therefore, amassing needed disciplinary expertise is critical, but not in itself sufficient, to team science preparedness.

By definition, the sophisticated knowledge production and translation aims of team science

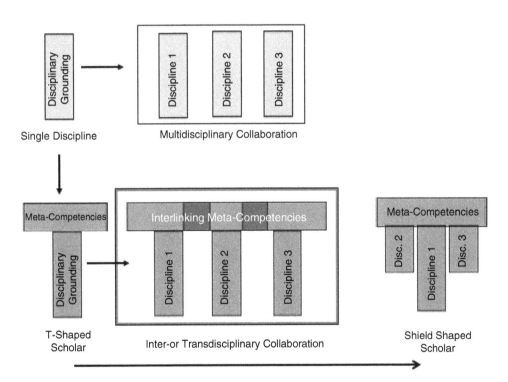

Fig. 13.1 Illustrating "I," "T," and Shield Shaped Readiness for Cross-Disciplinary Collaborations. Adapted from Bosque-Pérez et al. (2016), Oskam (2009), and Uhlenbrook and de Jong (2012). Meta-competencies refer here to the broadly applicable, boundary spanning competencies described in this chapter

require readiness for more intensive cross-disciplinary or cross-field work. A balance of disciplinary coherence combined with the knowledge, values, and functional abilities to work effectively with other professionals (Hall et al. 2016) and with stakeholders important to community or system research engagement and translation (Altman 1995; Ochs-Balcom et al. 2015) is vital. In this chapter, we therefore focus on the T cross-bar: the attitudes, knowledge, and skills that each individual scientist, professional, or community stakeholder ideally brings to the enterprise. Other chapters in this book address the broad range of factors within which cross-disciplinary team science is embedded, unpacking structural, institutional, team formation and functioning, leadership, and characteristics of various problem domains that serve to shape team needs and practicalities.

13.3 Team Science Readiness: Core Domains of Individual-Level Competencies

The past decade has seen growing investment in articulating the individual-level attitudes, knowledge, and skills key to success in cross-disciplinary team science. These efforts, typically framed in terms of transdisciplinary (TD) and translational (TL) dimensions of cross-disciplinary science, have resulted in a number of core thematic areas and recommendations (see, e.g., Begg et al. 2015; Borrego and Newswander 2010; Gamse et al. 2013; Holt 2013; National Research Council 2015), with more or less specificity regarding key elements—reflecting developing but not yet solidified conceptual clarity. There is nonetheless considerable overlap across these specification efforts. The competencies in Table 13.1 build upon the

Table 13.1 Competencies for productive participation in team science

Competency	Examples
Values, attitudes, and beliefs	
Valuing interdisciplinarity or transdisciplinarity collaboration	Attitudes that predispose one to seek and integrate knowledge from varied disciplines and stakeholders Beliefs that such efforts are necessary, that support greater relevance, innovation, impact of outcomes
Contextual and multi-level perspectives	Belief that complex problems should be approached from and appreciative of contexts and multi-level factors
Collaborative orientation	Values that emphasize qualities important to inclusion of multiple and diverse perspectives and team work (e.g., building trust, taking intellectual risks)
Habits of mind	
Curiosity and open-mindedness	Broad intellectual curiosity, maintenance of open-mindedness in light of differences
Nondefensive reflectiveness	Openness to examining assumptions and limitations of one's disciplinary or personal predispositions
Critical thinking	Critical awareness about one's biases in collaborative situations, suspending judgment, deliberately taking into consideration multiple perspectives, re-evaluating in light of new information
Developing confidence	Understanding how one's own expertise adds value to interdisciplinary efforts; balancing assertiveness with patience
Knowledge-based competencies	
Disciplinary grounding	Cultivation of deep knowledge within one's home discipline
Other disciplinary and stakeholder knowledge accrual	Understanding core substantive and conceptual knowledge from selected disciplines and stakeholders relevant to problem focus
Cross-disciplinary synthesis	Personal and interpersonal capacity to make connections across varied concepts, theories, or research methods
Participating in collective integrative processes	Develop shared interdisciplinary vision or models with disciplinary and other partners; joint questions or hypotheses; integrated research protocols and methods; modify work based upon the influence of others

(continued)

Table 13.1 (continued)

Competency	Examples
Interpersonal competencies	
Interdisciplinary communication: understand others	Learn the language and methods of other disciplines sufficiently to work together effectively; actively engage perspectives of other stakeholders
Interdisciplinary communication: be understood by others	Explain one's own work and perspectives in terms understandable to other disciplines and non-academic partners
Interdisciplinary communication: managing differences	Collaborate respectfully and equitably with disciplinary partners and stakeholders; effectively navigate tensions and conflicts
Interdisciplinary communication: social and relational skills	Build effective relationships with diverse partners: self-awareness; sensitivity to cultural and power differences; active engagement with project and other team members

National Research Council (2015) compilation, itself drawn from multiple sources. These are organized in four domains:

1. values, attitudes, and beliefs,
2. habits of mind,
3. knowledge-based competencies, and
4. interpersonal competencies.

We must emphasize at the outset that the focus in this chapter on individual-level attributes is somewhat artificial, given that multiple levels of influences inevitably interact with and shape individual-level capabilities, including team characteristics and processes, conditions of the organizations or institutions within which team science is pursued, characteristics of leadership and other cohering elements of infrastructure, financing factors, and so on (e.g., Stokols et al. 2008; see also related chapters in this book). Similarly, the clusters of competencies we depict in Table 13.1 are not discrete or independent from one another. Characteristics such as curiosity and open-mindedness, for example, shape and are shaped by one's values as well as one's cognitive stance and interactional tendencies.

We have nonetheless pulled out what we see to be well-supported domains, focusing on what Fiore and Bedwell (2011) refer to as *transportable* cross-disciplinary individual-level competencies—those with broad-based applicability. We use competencies or meta-competencies as umbrella terms to refer to clusters of characteristics and abilities. Other chapters in this book address more task-, team-, or context-contingent factors. We conclude this section with a caution

about correctness. Although we describe individual-level competencies with demonstrated utility for team science, factors such as temperament and socialization (within a culture or a discipline) can and do shape individual propensities: people will reasonably have differential capacities and willingness. We thus recognize, and emphasize, the value of each scientist and stakeholder establishing niches and roles in which they can sustainably contribute.

13.4 Values, Attitudes, and Beliefs

The communicative and collaborative success of cross-disciplinary teams is at least partially dependent on the commitments, proclivities, and worldviews that members bring to the table (see, e.g., Winowiecki et al. 2011). Transdisciplinary scholars have been characterized as "inclusive...thinkers, broad gauged and contextually oriented in their theorizing and research, methodologically eclectic,... open-minded and respectful of divergent view points, and adept at promoting good will and cross-discipline tolerance" (Mitrany and Stokols 2005, p. 439). Perhaps most bedrock are the values, attitudes, and beliefs that motivate any given researcher and tend to characterize the collaborative orientations and frameworks they bring to their work. Stokols (2014) refers to these (the first set in Table 13.1) as a *transdisciplinary orientation*. Klein (2004) has similarly described transdisciplinarity as "simultaneously an attitude and an action" (p. 521), encompassing both a mindset and predispositions toward more integrative and diverse perspectives and approaches.

Stokols (2014) identifies values, attitudes, and beliefs that are particularly salient to transdisciplinary (TD) readiness for team science (described below):

- TD Values: aspires to integrity and fairness, tolerance in accepting differences, open-mindedness, an inclusionary or pluralistic stance, and shared responsibility. A desire to promote value-based outcomes such as social justice or environmental equitability or sustainability is also likely to provide part of the motivational core that fuels the effort to build and sustain effective scientific and translational teams.
- TD Attitudes: Closely related to values are attitudes that reflect an individual's general orientation to ideas, people, activities, and types of situations. Positive attitudes that support persistence with boundary-spanning tasks and skill development despite unavoidable challenges are, for example, an important prerequisite to achieving success. Personal qualities that are likely to scaffold such efforts include optimism, tolerance for uncertainty, stamina, and adaptability.
- TD Beliefs: The focus here is on beliefs related to the favorability of cross-disciplinary scientific collaboration; for example, that one will be more productive, that one's work will have greater relevance, innovation, and impact, and that one has the capacity to be successful in these roles. Closely related are ontological and epistemological beliefs regarding, for example, how research questions should be defined, what study designs or forms of evidentiary support are superior, and the role of values in research. Transdisciplinarity also tends to be anchored in beliefs such as the value of diversity and of stakeholder involvement.

Although some of these predispositions may stem from personality or related personal characteristics, they also reflect team members' particular exposures and experiences, including their disciplinary socialization (Strober 2006). Overcoming challenges to collaboration such as linguistic barriers and disciplinary identities and tools of the trade takes considerable patience, trust, and tenacity, as well as practice. Intentional efforts to progressively nurture TD-oriented philosophical, intellectual, and attitudinal capacities have thus been identified as central to sustained engagement and success in team science.

Writing as former NSF IGERT-supported students, for example, Graybill et al. (2006) underscore the point that individual readiness for collaborative cross-disciplinary research is a developmental process, noting that with time and intentional supports, knowledge, interpersonal and team competencies, and scientific skills progressively accumulate and become more integrated and comfortable as an identity, a complex skill set, and a body of work. Drawing on their IGERT experiences, these authors provide a developmental framework and pedagogical recommendations for fostering these and related competencies. Stokols (2014) also describes a social ecology curricula designed to nurture a TD intellectual orientation. Related resources that address development of this competency set include Borrego and Newswander (2010); Kemp and Nurius (2015); Larson et al. (2011); Nash (2008); Vogel et al. (2014); and McGregor (2015).

13.5 Habits of Mind

We use the term habits of mind to encompass a range of "intellectual resources" (Costa and Kallick 2000), including openness and respect for differences, intellectual curiosity, willingness to take intellectual risks, creativity, self-assuredness and non-defensiveness, tolerance for uncertainty, and the capacity to engage rather than retreat from the challenges of working across the differences that cross-disciplinary collaborative teams invariably entail (Nash 2008; Augsburg 2014). Augsburg (2014), citing Godemann (2008), notes for example that scholars drawn to collaborative research evidence "the ability to look beyond one's own disciplinary boundaries, the capacity for disciplined self-reflexivity, the ability to reflect on knowledge integration processes, and the ability to take on new ideas" (p. 238).

Intellectual nimbleness is likewise key, as is the ability to see problems and research reflexively and critically from multiple perspectives and levels of analysis (Stokols 2014). This includes the capacity for systems thinking, the ability to grasp the multiple scales within which a problem or solution is located, and a belief that complex problems will be more successfully and satisfyingly accomplished through incorporation of contextual and multi-level factors. Gehlert (2012, 2013) offers illustrations of these and related competencies in transdisciplinary research related to cancer and other health disparities, describing the importance of multi-level frameworks spanning cellular level (e.g., animal studies of endocrine disruption) to societal level investigations (e.g., economic studies related to state tobacco policies). She also underscores the value of transdisciplinary collaboration to help ensure that translation of findings to health professionals, policymakers, the news media, and the public is consistent and coordinated.

We also include within this set of competencies an orientation toward curiosity, and active openness to differing worldviews and analytic levels, including the capacity to manage discomforts this poses to one's own disciplinary outlook and habits. Indicators suggest that scholars who equip themselves with diverse knowledge coherently drawn from multiple fields, in combination with an *inclination* to integrate multiple levels and bridging mechanisms, are more likely to generate comprehensive, novel, and radical innovations compared to colleagues whose knowledge base or conceptual strategies are more narrowly defined (Piso et al. 2016; Stokols 2014). Misra et al. (2015) similarly report two interrelated yet complementary components of the Transdisciplinary Orientation Scale: collaboration-oriented values, beliefs and attitudes, and the conceptual skills needed to bridge cross-disciplinary theory, methods, and results.

Realistic expectations regarding factors such as complete harmony and cooperation are nonetheless critical (Stokols et al. 2008). Ambiguity of goals and teamwork processes, disagreements, and frustrations are inevitable features of complex teams. Although factors such as attitudes and interpersonal skills are important to managing such challenges, habits of mind such as those reflected here also provide an important for navigating collaborative processes.

Traditional academic contexts tend to foster tendencies toward disciplinary parochialism, stereotyping of other disciplines, prejudice, and rivalry. Preparation for successful team science thus benefits from opportunities to develop habits of mind such as the capacity for non-defensive reflectiveness about the organizing assumptions of one's home discipline and one's own normative operating style. Interviews of investigators and trainees with the Transdisciplinary Research on Energetic and Cancer I Center emphasized that, rather than being fixed traits, curiosity and open-mindedness benefited from regular reminders, encouragement, and self-talk about what one realistically brings to the table: "Just being open to the fact that no one person, including yourself, is going to bring in all the technology or methodology or scientific expertise. I think, being somewhat humble" (Vogel et al. 2014, p. 9). Similarly, purposeful use of critical thinking habits slows down otherwise automatic biases in collaborative situations, enhancing the ability to suspend judgment, reflect on one's organizing assumptions, and more deliberately consider other perspectives. Among recommendations for clinical and translational team research preparation, Begg et al. (2014) emphasize both the value of small group training to foster microskills of learning collaboratively, and the use of assessment metrics to support awareness of engagement habits that may or may not serve the aims of successful team functioning.

Appreciative inquiry strategies can, for example, be useful in countering negative bias toward what is unfamiliar, tendencies toward knee-jerk critique, and disciplinary competitiveness. In its various forms, appreciative inquiry stimulates participants to be aware of and reflect on their value judgments and biases, and seeks to cultivate innovative generativity and intellectual flexibility (Cooperrider et al. 2008). Graybill et al. (2006), for example, point to the value of questions such as "What can I learn from X? How can we help one another?" in contrast to "What are the flaws in Y? How does it compete with Z?" (p. 762). Appreciative inquiry and related tools serve as team reminders, cultivating conscious efforts to hold conflicting epistemologies, theoretical investments, and methodological preferences in abeyance and instead create spaces that allow intellectual curiosity and collectivity to thrive. Capacities such as creative confidence and tolerance for ambiguity—hallmarks of innovative, efficacious researchers—can also be cultivated through structured involvement in design thinking activities derived from applied fields such as architecture and industrial design (Ulibarri et al. 2014; see also Guyotte et al. 2014).

13.6 Knowledge-Based Competencies

Readiness for team science requires that each member come to the table with the disciplinary depth needed to engage the problem or topical area that constitutes the research focus, as well as the capacity to efficiently and accurately locate other disciplinary content as needed (Boix Mansilla and Dawes Duraisingh 2007; Repko 2008). The heads of interdisciplinary IGERT programs have for example repeatedly emphasized the importance of this firm disciplinary grounding, underscoring the need for individuals to bring to team research solid preparation in the language, concepts, theories, methods, and empirical base that coherently define a specific discipline (Borrego and Newswander 2010). Somewhat paralleling the exploratory behaviors of the developing child, a sound disciplinary footing also provides the emerging cross-disciplinary researcher with a secure base from which to confidently explore and engage with other disciplinary domains (Giri 2002).

Increasingly, the collaborative work of cross-disciplinary teams also requires at least some degree of fluency in one or more other disciplines—reflected as cross-disciplinary knowledge acquisition in Table 13.1. This preparation need not reach the level of mastery one might achieve within a home discipline. Training in other disciplines does however need to ade-

quately support meaningful engagement with other disciplinary partners, as well as the ability to "work with" and synthesize diverse bodies of knowledge and to develop shared interdisciplinary models that capably bridge across levels or elements.

To capture the reality that many contemporary scholars and practitioners not only work in teams but have training in more than one discipline, recent conceptualizations expand the T-shaped image to include π-shaped (pi), comb-shaped, or shield-shaped skill sets (see Bosque-Pérez et al. (2016) for a discussion of this conceptualization within a team-based interdisciplinary training program). Extending the prior discussion of T-shaped training focused on collaborative meta-competencies, Fig. 13.1 illustrates pluralistic knowledge competencies (the central plus subsidiary "trunks" indicating the varying degrees of content knowledge that may be needed to function as an effective team member). In general, these conceptualizations aim to convey not a "jack of all trades" competency set but rather an intentional balance between core disciplinary investments and purposeful acquisition of relevant expertise in other fields.

As illustrated by Boh et al. (2014) in a study of innovation at 3M, for example, successful system integrators develop deep expertise in core domains, and then progressively expand this expertise as they understand how domains interact and learn to recombine components in innovative ways. The degree of cross-disciplinary knowledge acquisition also varies considerably by problem area and research aims. Notably, although inventors in the 3M study with deeper expertise achieved more patents and citations, those with balanced depth and breadth were value-added in helping to move innovations into products, the translational dimension.

Shifts in team science models toward active stakeholder involvement—notably in transdisciplinary domains such as sustainability and environmental science (see, e.g., Hauck et al. 2014) but also in social and health research (see, e.g., Martinez et al. 2012)—add additional dimensions to calls for intellectual openness and flexibility. When research teams expand to include community members, knowledge competencies must similarly stretch to include openness to the local knowledge of community members and other constituent groups. At issue here is not mastery of locally acquired contextual and content knowledge but rather the capacity for bridging highly diverse knowledge cultures (Brown et al. 2010): for imaginatively engaging, recognizing, valuing, and including indigenous and local knowledges *not* derived from academic research and scholarship—forms of knowledge frequently excluded from the scientific canon (see, e.g., Chilisa 2017).

Formulations of team science under the rubric of convergence (life science applications) frequently involve stakeholders from industry and governmental or regulatory bodies, adding other dimensions to the range of knowledge and engagement competencies that may be relevant to addressing a particular problem or issue (National Research Council 2014). Skills needed for integration and implementation science, moreover, include not only the capacity to synthesize disciplinary and stakeholder knowledge but also translational or knowledge brokering skills: the capacity to provide policymakers and practitioners with a better understanding of the problem in ways that support them in making decisions and taking action (Bammer 2005, 2013). In Bammer's analysis, the scope of training needed to achieve effective collaboration within densely complex problems as well as an engaged cross-walk between research and its application for change may require commitment to a new Integration to Implementation Science (I2S) specialization or discipline. The shield metaphor aims to capture the balance of breadth and depth at the individual level of knowledge competency seen as facilitating collective processes of knowledge integration at the team level. This goes beyond static knowledge acquisition to include skills in coherent knowledge synthesis. At the individual level, members have to create synthesis within their own mental models (Godemann 2008), preparing them, in turn, for more effective participation in joint construction of hypotheses, research protocols, and ongoing communication, as well as interdisciplinary products; e.g., grants and publications.

The ability to synthesize cross-disciplinary knowledge at the individual level is foundational to coherent *collective* knowledge integration. An in-depth analysis of faculty perspectives among those experienced in interdisciplinary teaching as well as selected students and their written work informed Boix Mansilla and Dawes Duraisingh's (2007) specification of broadly applicable dimensions of the quality of interdisciplinary integration (see Box 13.1). This and related work (e.g., Kemp and Nurius 2015; Morse 2013; Neuhauser et al. 2007; Stokols 2014) provide illustrations of activities that foster interpersonal capacities supportive of theoretical and methodological integration. However, these training initiatives also open an important question: do resultant competencies and skills lead to improved collaborative products or outcomes? In response, a range of assessment tools are being developed to evaluate the attributes of research products emanating from this kind of training and TD-oriented teams and scholars (for a summary, see Misra et al. 2015).

Box 13.1 Indicators of Quality in Interdisciplinary Products (drawn from Boix Mansilla and Dawes Duraisingh 2007)

1. *Disciplinary Grounding Beyond One's Home Discipline*: the degree to which the person's work shows nuanced understanding and appropriate use of selected disciplinary tools or defining constructs such as theories, findings, examples, methods, and forms of communication appropriate to their research topic. Grounding may not achieve the level of mastery but does exhibit understanding consistent with the disciplinary perspective(s), without misconceptions.

2. *Advancing Understanding Through Integration*: the degree to which the work demonstrates that the writer has enriched understanding (his, hers, that of a group) by integrating more than one set of disciplinary lenses. Integrative devices might include conceptual frameworks, graphic representations,

models or metaphors, methodological tools or premises, complex explanations put together, or solution ideas that demonstrate understanding gains through more complex, effective, empirically grounded, or comprehensive accounts or products than could previously been achieved.

3. *Critical Awareness*: The degree to which the work exhibits clarity of purpose, reflectiveness, and self-critique. Are there clear interdisciplinary goals? Is there reflectiveness about choices, judgments, and trade-offs? Awareness of limitations of the underlying interdisciplinary work (e.g., what can and cannot be well addressed) as well as how well the integration "works?"

As Lyall et al. (2015) point out, the ability to fruitfully exchange knowledge and ideas, to stay the course with the aim of effective and innovative knowledge co-production and, in partnership with stakeholders important to translation and sustainability, to potentially develop more "socially robust knowledge" (Nowotny 2006), is fundamentally reliant on well-developed interpersonal skills (Cheruvelil et al. 2014). We thus turn next to interpersonal competencies.

13.7 Interpersonal Competencies

Interpersonal competence, "the ability to motivate, enable, and facilitate collaborative and participatory…research and problem-solving" (Wiek et al. 2011, p. 211), entails an interlocking mix of communication skills, relationship skills, and collaborative skills. Many of the values, attitudes, beliefs, and habits of mind reviewed earlier—such as respect for the roles and contributions of others, the ability to suspend judgment, and to balance advocacy of one's own perspective with the need to develop a team vision—are intertwined with interpersonal skills. Curiosity, open-mindedness, non-defensive

reflectiveness, and willingness to compromise and risk are likewise key ingredients in interpersonal skills that effectively foster engagement and trust.

Communicating one's disciplinary or experiential knowledge clearly to colleagues with different training or backgrounds is a difficult task in itself. Team science adds to this both the complexities involved in eliciting and engaging the diverse perspectives of other team members, including those emerging from different demographic and cultural positionalities, and the communicative challenges entailed in crafting integrative frameworks. Unsurprisingly, therefore, communication competence—the "cognitive and behavioral abilities to construct meaning with others in contextually sensitive ways" (Read et al. 2016, p. 2)—is widely recognized as fundamental to effective team functioning. Interconnected elements of individual communicative competence include: (1) the ability to work across different disciplinary languages; (2) the willingness and ability to unpack disciplinary and worldview differences, including differences in ontological and epistemological assumptions; (3) basic communication and group skills; (4) skills in working across difference/through conflict; and (5) skills in building and maintaining relationships, including with community partners and stakeholders.

Talking across difference: Some of the most time consuming and (often) frustrating team science experiences have to do with the challenges involved in navigating different disciplinary languages (Bracken and Oughton 2006; Nash 2008). As a recent study exploring disciplinary differences in understandings of the term *hypothesis* reveals (Donovan et al. 2015), even constructs around which researchers assume broad agreement may in reality be framed and interpreted quite differently in varying disciplinary contexts. Left unexplored, such differences can have significant implications not only for team functioning but for project outcomes. The ability to talk across disciplinary differences is thus frequently identified as an important marker of preparation for cross-disciplinary work (Borrego and Newswander 2010).

The centrality of language and conceptual framing in team science points to the importance of cultivating habits that allow researchers both to recognize their own "specialized dialects" (Bracken and Oughton 2006, p. 376) and to productively engage and explore those of interdisciplinary colleagues. These skills become even more salient with the inclusion of community stakeholders, requiring researchers in broadly collaborative teams to be adept at communicating effectively with lay people as well as academic colleagues. Language differences—such as those between academic terminology and lay or everyday language—not only create barriers to mutual understanding and engagement, but also reflect, and frequently maintain, power differentials. Typologies of transferable team science competencies thus routinely underscore the importance of the ability to communicate effectively with a broad range of constituents, including the capacity to speak and write in language readily understood by lay as well as academic audiences (see, e.g., Begg et al. 2015).

Engaging diverse worldviews: Connected with and underlying differences in language are differences in worldviews, particularly fundamental ontological and epistemological differences. The ability to engage these differences requires, as Read et al. (2016) note, the "capacity for conversations and dialogue that make visible members' assumptions about what are considered to be researchable questions, appropriate methods, and what constitutes adequate/appropriate answers" (p. 6). Helpful tools for surfacing and openly exploring deep-rooted differences in epistemological and ontological assumptions include The Toolbox Dialogue Method, a structured framework grounded in philosophical principles (Schnapp et al. 2012; Winowiecki et al. 2011). Strategies such as the Toolbox help to scaffold the individual and group communication skills increasingly seen as central to effective cross-discipline and cross-sector partnerships. For an example of use of the Toolbox in concert with other strategies, see Winowiecki et al. (2011), who describe a self-organized, semester-long exploration by a diverse group of post-doctoral scholars at Columbia University's Earth Institute.

Although in the team science literature differences in worldviews and underlying assumptions are typically thought of as primarily rooted in disciplinary socialization, they also derive from members' life experiences, including key aspects of their social, racial, cultural, or class identities. An extensive but mixed body of research documents both positive and negative effects of diversity, on multiple axes including demographic factors such as race, ethnicity, gender, and age, on team processes and outcomes (Joshi and Roh 2009; Woolley et al. 2010). For example, research on "demographic faultlines"—subgroups in teams that form around clusters of intersecting demographic attributes—suggests that these have significant implications for team learning, psychological safety, satisfaction, and expected performance (Lau and Murnighan 2005; see also Bezrukova et al. 2009). As teams become increasingly diverse, therefore, the capacity for interacting with others in culturally sensitive ways, including accepting and respectfully engaging differences beyond those related to disciplinary training, is regarded as vital to successful team processes and outcomes (Cheruvelil et al. 2014). Although the research literature in this area evidences mixed findings, meta-analytic reviews nonetheless indicate that awareness of and sensitivity to the implications of diversity can be cultivated through training (Bezrukova et al. 2012), as can strategies for enhancing the positive value of team diversity and minimizing potential harms and costs of problematic interactions among team members (Joshi and Roh 2009). Fields such as sustainability science, therefore, where collaborative research teams commonly include diverse stakeholders, increasingly underscore the importance of contextual and cultural awareness, self-reflection on one's own background and experiences, and awareness of one's own cultural values, cultural and racial or ethnic identity, and worldview (Quigley 2016).

Navigating conflict: Given the range of differences typically present in cross-disciplinary, cross-sector teams—stemming from divergent world views, different departmental or other affiliations, contrasting and potentially competing theoretical or methodological approaches, and dissimilar cultures or styles of working and inter-acting—conflict and tensions are frequently cited challenges. Differences and disagreements can productively contribute to learning, problem solving, and innovation (Bennett and Gadlin 2012; Piso et al. 2016; Stokols et al. 2008). However, they must also be carefully managed to avoid fostering fragmentation, competing agen-das, or other problems that undermine effective collaboration. At the individual level, skills in effectively anticipating, negotiating, and resolv-ing tensions and conflicts with and among team members are thus a key asset. Regular and in-depth exchange of ideas, conveyance of respect even within difficulties, and ongoing investments in building personal relationships and trust are essential to navigating conflict, as are the ability to manage one's emotional reactivity and to either resolve or put aside difficult disagreements (Stokols et al. 2008).

Active listening, dialogue, and reflexivity: The interpersonal competencies at the heart of these imperatives build from but also extend basic, well-understood communication skills such as active listening: the ability to hear what someone else is saying while suspending one's own point of view. Given valued diversity in cross-disciplinary teams, also important is the "…capacity for meaningful and productive dia-logue" (Giri 2002)—described by Jacobs and Nienbar (2011) as "the mechanism that unlocks the opportunity to understand, co-create and build networks" (p. 673). Giri (2002) notes, importantly, that the capacity for engaging effec-tively in dialogue with other team members has two key dimensions. First, and fundamentally, it requires solid interest and skills in engaging with others. Also important, however—and linking back our earlier points about T-shaped profes-sionals—is firm disciplinary grounding. Being "authentically embedded in one's own disci-pline," Giri asserts (p. 108), affords team mem-bers the confidence in what they bring to the table to be secure in then engaging actively with the contributions of others.

Also key to the "deep listening" described as a key ingredient in building partnerships across

multiple differences (Jacobs and Nienbar 2011, p. 673) is sensitivity to and awareness of the power dynamics invariably present in diverse teams. Attentiveness to power relations is vital to nurturing inclusive, productive conversations and collaborations, but difficult to achieve in practice. Some disciplines, for example, emphasize episte-mological strategies such as objectivity or neu-trality that tend to obscure power differentials. Other disciplinary differences, such as artificial divisions between the "hard" and "soft" sciences, can create assumptions of positional superiority or inferiority. Given historically challenging rela-tionships between universities and local commu-nities, relationships with stakeholders add additional complexities (see, e.g., Klenk et al. 2015).

Navigating these differences requires individ-ual researchers with the capacity for reflexivity about power dynamics in concert with the will-ingness and ability to share power, minimize sta-tus differences, and encourage participation (Foster-Fishman et al. 2001, p. 244). In various forms, reflexivity—the capacity for reflecting on one's own predispositions and assumptions in the context of relationships with others—emerges in the literature as a key dimension of interpersonal competence (Read et al. 2016; Thompson 2009). Bennett and Gadlin (2012), for example, empha-size a combination of self-awareness and "other-awareness"—sometimes conceptualized as the capacity for empathy (Darbellay 2015)—as a necessary base for engaging effectively with oth-ers in team science contexts.

Relational Skills: All of the interpersonal competencies described above are anchored in relationships (Tebes et al. 2014; Read et al. 2016). Team science is an essentially social and rela-tional endeavor. In this regard, Cheruvelil et al. (2014) identify two key dimensions of interper-sonal competence: (a) social sensitivity, and (b) emotional engagement. Underscoring the central importance of relational skills, they define social sensitivity as the "capacity to successfully navi-gate a full range of social relationships and inter-actions" (p. 32)—a capacity that is commonly referred to as having "people skills." Emotional engagement is defined as "the presence and depth of feelings, both personal and professional, toward other team members and the project as a whole" (p. 32). Individual members, in other words, need to be "present": to bring to teamwork an active, commitment not only to the work but also to the people involved in it.

Although leadership abilities are not the focus of the current chapter, they are nonetheless key to ensuring a mutually supportive interplay between the individual competencies we describe here and facilitative team processes such as a productive team climate, cohesion, efficacy, sense of safety, generation of team mental models, and conflict management (National Research Council 2015, Chap. 6). Leadership skills also play a critical role in multi-team systems, which further extend the team support skills needed to achieve the innovation and impact sought through team science (Zaccaro and DeChurch 2012). Salazar et al. (Chap. 24, this volume) argue that leaders with *integrative capabilities* are likely to be better equipped to help disciplinarily diverse teams be successful and overcome challenges of cross-boundary collaboration. They also provide a model and specification of leaders' integrative capabilities, team emergent states, and outcomes that are complementary to the individual team member meta-competencies we describe in Table 13.1.

13.8   Scaffolding the Development of Individual-Level Competencies

The literature repeatedly emphasizes the value of structured opportunities for practicing and enhancing interpersonal skills as one incrementally builds one's cross-disciplinary competencies (Read et al. 2016). As Cheruvelil et al. (2014) note, collaborative skills can be taught and practiced. Boundary-spanning contexts such as course work, seminars and workshops, conference attendance, mentoring (both formal and more informal peer support), integrative groups

(e.g., journal clubs, discussion groups), and cross-discipline research team experiences serve to increase appreciation, expertise, and comfort (e.g., Hall et al. 2008; James et al. 2015; Lawlor et al. 2015; Nash et al. 2003; Stokols et al. 2008).

Larson and Begg (2011), for example, illustrate an interdisciplinary graduate course designed to foster key team science-related competencies. In addition to didactic content through lectures, readings, and case studies, students were required to engage in considerable reflection about their experiences, give and receive feedback, and demonstrate the capacity to modify perspectives and products in response to interactions with interdisciplinary colleagues. A range of assessment and training tools and resources that address technical and behavioral competencies are also available through the online Team Science Toolkit. One practical illustration is guidelines for how to write a collaboration plan (Hall et al. 2014) organized around ten factors central to preparation for effective team functioning. Training guidelines can also be productively borrowed from the team training literature. A meta-analysis by Delise et al. (2010) provides guidelines for the efficacy of team models of training to improve team outcomes in multiple aspects of team task-based and team functioning effectiveness. At the doctoral program level, Kemp and Nurius (2015) describe a developmental approach to advancing team science-related competencies that similarly advocates a mix of didactic and experiential training from entrance into skill preparation through mid-stream training into early career roles. Purposefully structured dialogue and interaction-based learning provide opportunities for communication around energizing and yet challenging questions related to integration, to the give and take of cross-disciplinary critique, to managing differences and to developing norms and habits of responsible engagement. Examples of pedagogical elements designed to support collaboration readiness and communication include: structured activities to communicate about one's personal knowledge frameworks (e.g., the Toolbox Dialogue Method, writing intellectual biographies); content that provides exposure to and critical reflection on disciplinary frameworks and world views; material and discussion illustrating processes of interdisciplinary communication and building integrated models and protocols; and practice activities among peers within and beyond home disciplines to hone communication and collaboration skills (see also Arnold et al. 2013; Nurius and Kemp 2014).

Drawing on the perspectives of early career researchers, Bridle et al. (2013) point to the value of both "cultivation" and "development" interdisciplinary encounters (occurring within 2–7 day targeted meetings) in progressively building team science competencies. Open and effective communication across researchers from different fields was prominent in both "teamwork" (e.g., strengthening appreciative inquiry attitudes and skills) and "task work" (e.g., building disciplinary linguistic fluency and more specific scientific integration capacity). Attending cross-disciplinary conferences and reading (and writing for) journals outside of one's primary fields of training also offer pivotal opportunities for learning and skill development, both getting the lay of the land and developing skills in cross-disciplinary fluency.

It is becoming clear that successful competency-building outcomes do not accrue simply by virtue of bringing motivated and qualified participants together in one place. Rather, facilitated workshops, group discussions or activities, the sharing of experiences through well-crafted presentations as well as informal chats, frequent reflection moments, and the availability of skillful leadership or facilitation all constitute productive ingredients. The central importance of relational development in extending individual-level competencies to achieve collective competence, particularly regarding communication skills, is stressed in Read et al.'s (2016) description of a modular, adaptable network science training framework. Finally, team science collaborations are rapidly spanning national boundaries. This expands consideration of societal, cultural, scientific, training and related differences and the competencies needed to bridge them (Lyall and Meagher 2012; Nurius et al. 2017).

13.9 Conclusion

We conclude by acknowledging what this and many of the other resources cited in this chapter underscore: the interdependent, trust-laden, and interpersonally tangled nature of team science. The boundaries across the topics and capacities represented in this book are porous and interdependent. The focus here on individual team member meta-competencies is by no means wholly comprehensive. Chapters addressing or illustrating field innovations on a range of topics can profitably stretch our focus to include extensions. Pursuit of individual-level competencies for our future scientific workforce will require no small measure of readiness for the messy work of cooperation toward complex and challenging scientific and translational aims.

References

Altman D. Sustaining interventions in community systems: on the relationship between researchers and communities. Health Psychol. 1995;146:526–36.

Arnold LD, Kuhlmann AS, Hipp JA, Budd E. Competencies in transdisciplinary public health education. In: Haire-Joshu D, McBride TD, editors. Transdisciplinary public health: research, education, and practice. San Francisco: Jossey-Bass; 2013. p. 53–76.

Augsburg T. Becoming transdisciplinary: the emergence of the transdisciplinary individual. World Futures. 2014;70:233–47.

Bajada C, Trayler R. Interdisciplinary business education: curriculum through collaboration. Education Training. 2013;55(4/5):385–402.

Bammer G. Integration and implementation sciences: building a new specialization. Ecol Soc. 2005;10(2):95–107.

Bammer G. Disciplining interdisciplinarity: integration and implementation sciences for researching complex real-world problems. Canberra: Australian National University Press; 2013.

Begg MD, Bennett LM, Cicutto L, Gadlin H, Moss M, Tentler J, Schoenbaum E. Graduate education for the future: new models and methods for the clinical and translational workforce. Clin Transl Sci. 2015;8(6):787–92.

Begg MD, Crumley G, Fair AM, Martina CA, McCormack WT, Merchant C, et al. Approaches to preparing young scholars for careers in interdisciplinary team science. J Investig Med. 2014;62(1):14–25.

Bennett LM, Gadlin H. Collaboration and team science: from theory to practice. J Investig Med. 2012;60(5):768–75.

Bezrukova K, Jehn KA, Spell CS. Reviewing diversity training: where have we been and where we should go. Acad Manag Learn Edu. 2012;11(2):207–27.

Bezrukova K, Jehn KA, Zanutto EL, Thatcher SMB. Do workgroup faultlines help or hurt? A moderated model of faultlines, team identification, and group performance. Organ Sci. 2009;20(1):35–50.

Boh WF, Evaristo R, Ouderkirk A. Balancing breadth and depth of expertise for innovation: a 3M story. Res Policy. 2014;43:349–66.

Boix Mansilla V, Dawes Duraisingh E. Targeted assessment of students' interdisciplinary work: an empirically grounded framework proposed. J High Educ. 2007;78(2):215–37.

Borrego M, Newswander LK. Definitions of interdisciplinary research: toward graduate-level interdisciplinary learning outcomes. Rev High Educ. 2010;34(1):61–84.

Bosque-Pérez NA, Klos PZ, Force JE, Waits LP, Cleary K, Rhoades P, et al. A pedagogical model for team-based, problem-focused interdisciplinary doctoral education. Bioscience. 2016;66(6):477–88.

Bracken LJ, Oughton EA. 'What do you mean?': The importance of language in developing interdisciplinary research. Trans Inst Br Geogr. 2006;31:371–82.

Bridle H, Vrieling A, Cardillo M, Araya Y, Hinojosa L. Preparing for an interdisciplinary future: a perspective from early-career researchers. Futures. 2013;53:22–32.

Brown VA, Deane PM, Harris JA, Russell JY. Towards a just and sustainable future. In: Brown VA, Harris JA, Russell JY, editors. Tackling wicked problems through the transdisciplinary imagination. New York: Earthscan; 2010. p. 3–15.

Cheruvelil KS, Soranno PA, Weathers KC, Hanson P, Goring SJ, Filstrup CT, Read EK. Creating and maintaining high-performing collaborative research teams: the importance of diversity and interpersonal skills. Front Ecol Environ. 2014;12(1):31–8.

Chilisa B. Decolonizing transdisciplinary research approaches: an African perspective for enhancing knowledge integration in sustainability science. Sustain Sci. 2017;12:813–27.

Cooperrider DL, Witney D, Stavros JM. Appreciative inquiry handbook. 2nd ed. Brunswick, OH: Crown Custom Publishing; 2008.

Costa AL, Kallick B. Discovering & exploring habits of mind. In: A developmental series, book 1. Alexandria, VA: Association for Supervision and Curriculum Development; 2000.

Darbellay F. The gift of interdisciplinarity: towards an ability to think across disciplines. Int J Talent Dev Creativity. 2015;3(2):201–11.

Delise LA, Allen Gorman C, Brooks AM, Rentsch JR, Steele-Johnson D. The effects of team training on team outcomes: a meta-analysis. Perform Improv Q. 2010;22(4):53–80.

Donofrio N, Sophrer J, Zadeh HS. Research-driven medical education and practice: a case for T-shaped professionals. Med J Aust. 2010. http://www.ceri.msu.edu/wp-content/uploads/2010/06/A-Case-for-T-Shaped-Professionals-20090907-Hossein.pdf

Donovan SM, O'Rourke M, Looney C. Your hypothesis or mine? Terminological and conceptual variation across disciplines. SAGE Open. 2015 May 11;5(2):2158244015586237.

Edwards MA, Pruden A. The Flint water crisis: overturning the research paradigm to advance science and defend public welfare. Environ Sci Technol. 2016;50:8935–6.

Fiore SM, Bedwell W. Team science needs teamwork training. Presented at the Second Annual Science of Team Science Conference; Chicago, IL; 2011.

Foster-Fishman PG, Berkowitz SL, Lounsbury DW, Jacobson S, Allen NA. Building collaborative capacity in community coalitions: a review and integrative framework. Am J Community Psychol. 2001;29(2):241–61.

Gamse BC, Espinosa LL, Roy R. Essential competencies for interdisciplinary graduate training in IGERT: final report. GS-10F-0086K. Bethesda, MD: Abt Associates; 2013.. http://files.eric.ed.gov/fulltext/ED553232.pdf

Gehlert S. Shaping education and training to advance transdisciplinary health research. Transdisciplinary J Eng Sci. 2012;3:1–10.

Gehlert S. Turning disciplinary knowledge into solutions. J Adolesc Health. 2013;52(5):S98–S102.

Gehlert S, Sohmer D, Sacks T, Mininger C, McClintock M, Olopade O. Targeting health disparities: a model linking upstream determinants to downstream interventions. Health Aff. 2008;27(2):339–49.

Giri AL. The calling of creative transdisciplinarity. Futures. 2002;34:103–15.

Godemann J. Knowledge integration: a key challenge for transdisciplinary cooperation. Environ Educ Res. 2008;14(6):625–41.

Graybill JK, Dooling S, Shandas V, Withey J, Greve A, Simon GL. A rough guide to interdisciplinarity: graduate students' perspectives. Bioscience. 2006;56(9):757–63.

Guyotte KW, Sochacka NW, Costantino TE, Walther J, Kellam N. STEAM as social practice: cultivating creativity in transdisciplinary spaces. Art Educ. 2014;67:12–9.

Hall KL. Transdisciplinary research: conceptual and practical issues. Paper Presented at the Transdisciplinary Translation for Prevention of High risk Behaviors Conference. 2013. http://www.ttpr.org/images/2013_Presentation/_Keynote_Hall_2013.pdf

Hall KL, Crowston D, Vogel AL. How to write a collaboration plan. Rockville, MD: NCI Team Science Toolkit; 2014.. https://www.teamsciencetoolkit.cancer.gov/public/TSResourceBiblio.aspx?tid=3&rid=3119

Hall K, Croyle R, Vogel A, editors. Advancing social and behavioral health research through cross-disciplinary team science: principles for success. New York, NY: Springer; 2016.

Hall KL, Feng AX, Moser RP, Stokols D, Taylor BK. Moving the science of team science forward: collaboration and creativity. Am J Prev Med. 2008;35(2):S243–9.

Hauck J, Saarikoski H, Turkelboom F, Keune H. Stakeholder involvement in ecosystem service decision-making and research. In: Potschin M, Jax K, editors. OpenNESS reference book. EC FP7 Grant agreement no. 308428. 2014. www.openness-project.eu/library/reference-book

Holt VC. Graduate education to facilitate interdisciplinary research collaboration: identifying individual competencies and developmental learning activities. Presented at the Science of Team Science Conference Session on Learning and Training for Team Science, June, Evanston, IL; 2013. http://www.scienceofteamscience.org/2013-sessions%2D%2Dlearning-and-training-for-team-science.

Jacobs IM, Nienbar S. Waters without borders: transboundary water governance and the role of the 'transdisciplinary individual' in Southern Africa. Water SA. 2011;37(5):665–78.

James AS, Gehlert S, Bowen DJ, Colditz GA. A framework for training transdisciplinary scholars in cancer prevention and control. J Cancer Educ. 2015;30(4):664–9.

Joshi A, Roh H. The role of context in work team diversity research: a meta-analytic review. Acad Manag J. 2009;52(3):599–627.

Kemp SP, Nurius PS. Preparing emerging doctoral scholars for transdisciplinary research: a developmental approach. J Teach Soc Work. 2015;35:131–50.

Klein JT. Prospects for trandisciplinarity. Futures. 2004;36:515–26.

Klenk NL, Meehan K, Pinel SL, Mendez F, Lima PT, Kammen DM. Stakeholders in climate science: beyond lip service? Science. 2015;350(6262):743–4.

Larson EL, Begg MD. Building interdisciplinary research models: a didactic course to prepare interdisciplinary scholars and faculty. Clin Transl Sci. 2011;4(1):38–41.

Larson EL, Cohen B, Gebbie K, Clock S, Saiman L. Interdisciplinary research training in a school of nursing. Nurs Outlook. 2011;59(1):29–36.

Lau DC, Murnighan JK. Interactions within groups and subgroups: the effects of demographic faultlines. Acad Manag J. 2005;48(4):645–59.

Lawlor EF, Kreuter MW, Sebert-Kuhlmann AK, McBride TD. Methodological innovations in public health education: transdisciplinary problem solving. Am J Public Health. 2015;105(S1):S99–S103.

Lyall C, Meagher LR. A masterclass in interdisciplinarity: research into practice in training the next generation of interdisciplinary researchers. Futures. 2012;44(6):608–17.

Lyall C, Meagher L, Bruce A. A rose by any other name? Transdisciplinarity in the context of UK research policy. Futures. 2015;65:150–62.

Martinez LS, Russell B, Rubin CL, Leslie LK, Brugge D. Clinical and translational research and community engagement: implications for researcher capacity building. Clin Transl Sci. 2012;5(4):329–32.

McGregor SLT. Transdisciplinary knowledge creation. In: Gibbs PT, editor. Transdisciplinary professional learning and practice. New York, NY: Springer; 2015. p. 9–24.

McIntosh BS, Taylor A. Developing T-shaped water professionals: building capacity in collaboration, learning, and leadership to drive innovation. J Contemp Water Res Educ. 2013;150:6–17.

Misra S, Stokols D, Cheng L. The transdisciplinary orientation scale: factor structure and relation to the integrative quality and scope of scientific publications. J Transl Med Epidemiol. 2015;3(2):1042.

Mitrany M, Stokols D. Gauging the transdisciplinary qualities and outcomes of doctoral training programs. J Plan Educ Res. 2005;24(4):437–49.

Morse W. Integration of frameworks and theories across disciplines for effective cross-disciplinary communication. In: O'Rourke M, Crowley S, Eigenbrode SD, Wulfhorst JD, editors. Enhancing communication and collaboration in cross-disciplinary research. Thousand Oaks, CA: SAGE Publications; 2013. p. 244–70.

Nash JM. Transdisciplinary training: key components and prerequisites for success. Am J Prev Med. 2008; 35:S133–40.

Nash JM, Collins BN, Loughlin SE, Solbrig M, Harvey R, KrishnanSarin S, et al. Training the transdisciplinary scientist: a general framework applied to tobacco use behavior. Nicotine Tob Res. 2003;5(Suppl 1):S41–53.

National Research Council. Convergence: Facilitating transdisciplinary integration of life sciences, physical sciences, engineering, and beyond. Washington, DC: The National Academies Press; 2014.

National Research Council. Enhancing the effectiveness of team science. In: Cooke NJ, Hilton ML, editors. Committee on the science of team science, Board on behavioral, cognitive, and sensory sciences, division of behavioral and social sciences and education. Washington, DC: National Academies Press; 2015.

Neuhauser L, Richardson D, Mackenzie S, Minkler M. Advancing transdisciplinary and translational research practice: issues and models of doctoral education in public health. J Res Pract. 2007;3(2):M19.

Nowotny H. Rethinking interdisciplinarity: the potential of transdisciplinarity. Paris: Centre National de la Recherche Scientifique; 2006.. http://www.helga-nowotny.eu/downloads/helga_nowotny_b59.pdf

Nurius PS, Kemp SP. Transdisciplinarity and translation: preparing social work doctoral students for high impact research. Res Soc Work Pract. 2014;24:625–35.

Nurius PS, Kemp SP, Köngeter S, Gehlert S. Next generation social work research education: fostering transdisciplinary readiness. Eur J Soc Work. 2017;20:907–20.

Ochs-Balcom HM, Phillips LS, Nichols HB, Martinez E, Thompson B, Ojeifo J, Rebbeck TR. Building a funded research program in cancer health disparities: considerations for young investigators. Cancer Epidemiol Biomark Prev. 2015;24:882–5.

Oskam IF. T-shaped engineers for interdisciplinary innovation: an attractive perspective for young people as well as a must for innovative organisations.

In: 37th Annual Conference–Attracting Students in Engineering, Rotterdam, The Netherlands (Vol. 14); 2009.

Piso Z, O'Rourke M, Weathers KC. Out of the fog: catalyzing integrative capacity in interdisciplinary research. Stud Hist Phil Sci. 2016;56:84–94.

Quigley D. Building cultural competence in environmental studies and natural resource sciences. Soc Nat Resour. 2016;29(6):725–37.

Read EK, O'Rourke M, Hong GS, Hanson PC, Winslow LA, Crowley S, Brewer CA, Weathers KC. Building the team for team science. Ecosphere. 2016; 73(1):1–9.

Repko AF. Interdisciplinary research: process and theory. Chicago: Sage; 2008.

Schnapp LM, Rotschy L, Hall TE, Crowley S, O'Rourke M. How to talk to strangers: facilitating knowledge sharing within translational health teams with the toolbox dialogue method. Transl Behav Med. 2012;2(4):469–79.

Simpson T, Barton R, Celento D. Interdisciplinary by design. Mech Eng. 2008;130(9):30.

Stokols D. Toward a science of transdisciplinary action research. Am J Community Psychol. 2006;38:63–77.

Stokols D. Training the next generation of transdisciplinarians. In: O'Rourke M, Crowley S, Eigenbrode SD, Wulfhorst JD, editors. Enhancing communication & collaboration in interdisciplinary research. Los Angeles, CA: Sage; 2014. p. 56–81.

Stokols D, Misra S, Moser RP, Hall KL, Taylor BK. The ecology of team science: understanding contextual influences on transdisciplinary collaboration. Am J Prev Med. 2008;35(2):S96–S115.

Strober MH. Habits of mind: challenges for multidisciplinary involvement. Soc Epistemol. 2006;20:3–4315-331.

Tebes JK, Thai ND, Matlin SL. Twenty-first century science as a relational process: from Eureka! To team science and a place for community psychology. Am J Community Psychol. 2014;53(3–4):475–90.

Thompson JL. Building collective communication competence in interdisciplinary research teams. J Appl Commun Res. 2009;37:278–97.

Uhlenbrook S, de Jong E. T-shaped competency profile for water professionals of the future. Hydrol Earth Syst Sci. 2012;16:3475–83.

Ulibarri N, Cravens AE, Cornelius M, Royalty A, Nabergoj AS. Research as design: developing creative confidence in doctoral students through design thinking. Int J Dr Stud. 2014;9:249–70.

Vogel AL, Stipelman BA, Hall KL, Nebeling L, Stokols D, Spruijt-Metz D. Pioneering the transdisciplinary team science approach: lessons learned from national cancer institute grantees. J Transl Med Epidemiol. 2014;2(2):1027.

Weber EP, Khademian AM. Wicked problems, knowledge challenges, and collaborative capacity builders in network settings. Public Adm Rev. 2008;68(2):334–49.

Wiek A, Withycombe L, Redman CL. Key competencies in sustainability: a reference framework for academic program development. Sustain Sci. 2011;6:2013–218.

Winowiecki L, Smukler S, Shirley K, Remans R, Peltier G, Lothes E, King E, Comita L, Baptista S, Alkema L. Tools for enhancing interdisciplinary communication. Sustainability. 2011;7(1):74–80.

Woolley AW, Chabris CF, Pentland A, Hashmi N, Malone TW. Evidence for a collective intelligence factor in the performance of human groups. Science. 2010;330(6004):686–8.

Zaccaro SJ, DeChurch LA. Leadership forms and functions in multiteam systems. In: Zaccaro SJ, Marks MA, DeChurch LA, editors. Multiteam systems: an organizational form for dynamic and complex environments. New York: Routledge; 2012. p. 253–88.

The Role of Team Personality in Team Effectiveness and Performance

14

Brooke A. Stipelman, Elise L. Rice, Amanda L. Vogel, and Kara L. Hall

Contents

The original version of this chapter was revised. The correction to this chapter is available at https://doi.org/10.1007/978-3-030-20992-6_46

B. A. Stipelman (✉)
Abrams and Associates, Rockville, MD, USA
e-mail: bstipelman@gmail.com

E. L. Rice
Division of Extramural Research, National Institute of Dental and Craniofacial Research, National Institutes of Health, Bethesda, MD, USA

A. L. Vogel
Clinical Monitoring Research Program Directorate, Frederick National Laboratory for Cancer Research sponsored by the National Cancer Institute, Frederick, MD, USA

K. L. Hall
Division of Cancer Control and Population Sciences, National Cancer Institute, Bethesda, MD, USA

14.1 Introduction

An individual's personality is among the most established predictors of job performance (Barrick and Mount 1991; Hurtz and Donovan 2000; Tett et al. 1999). Given the strength of this finding, it is perhaps not surprising that personality factors in aggregate are predictive of team performance across a range of team types (e.g., Barrick et al. 1998; Bell 2007). However, a recent review of a decade's worth of quantitative and mixed-methods research articles on science teams identified no empirical studies on the impact of personality on science teams (Hall et al. 2018). As such, there is a need to look to the broader teams literature to learn what we can about how personality may impact science teams.

This chapter provides an introduction to the most commonly used framework for understanding personality, the Five Factor Model. It then summarizes what is known from the teams literature about the influence of personality factors on team effectiveness, and considers the potential interactions of personality with team processes and emergent states. Team processes refer to "mechanisms that inhibit or enable the ability of team members to combine their capabilities and behavior," such as communication, cooperation, and coordination (Kozlowski and Bell 2003). Emergent states refer to higher level phenomena that emerge on a team level from the characteristics and interactions of individual team members,

© Springer Nature Switzerland AG 2019
K. L. Hall et al. (eds.), *Strategies for Team Science Success*,
https://doi.org/10.1007/978-3-030-20992-6_14

such as trust and psychological safety (Kozlowski and Bell 2003). The chapter reflects on how personality traits may uniquely impact science teams. Finally, the chapter proposes future directions for research to advance our understanding of the influence of personality factors- as they interact with one another and other critical influencing factors- on the effectiveness of science teams.

14.2   The Five Factor Model of Personality

While many theories of personality exist, the Five Factor Model (McCrae and Costa 1987) is the most commonly used framework for examining personality in the literature on teams. The Big Five personality traits were derived from the Five Factor Model and consist of five broad dimensions that are believed to comprise an individual's personality: extraversion, conscientiousness, agreeableness, emotional stability, and openness to experience (Costa and McCrae 1992). These personality dimensions appear to be biological in origin and relatively stable over time (Costa and McCrae 1992).

Although the Five Factor Model was developed to assess personality at the level of the individual, it has been widely used in the aggregate at the team level in the research on teamwork. Of course, combining personality factors across members of a team introduces an additional level of complexity where measurement is concerned. There is preliminary evidence to suggest that, at the aggregate level, different personality factors are best assessed using different measurement strategies (e.g., mean, variance, or extreme values among team members; Barrick et al. 1998). The mean of a trait indicates the degree to which a personality trait is present (in aggregate) across the team members. This is sometimes referred to as "elevation," as a team is said to "have" a given personality trait if the mean score for that trait is higher than the mean for other traits. Variance in a trait at the team level is typically indicated by the standard deviation of the trait among team members. This is sometimes referred to as heterogeneity, to indicate the degree to which a given trait is or is not consistently "elevated"

among team members. With no current consensus on the best approach to capture and analyze personality traits in team contexts, measurement differences across studies are likely to account for some of the variation in findings. In the current summary, we have chosen to focus primarily on the two most commonly used measures of team personality: mean and variance.

What follows is an introduction to each of the "Big Five" personality traits, and a brief discussion of key findings on how each personality trait impacts team processes, emergent states, and team effectiveness. We then discuss methodological considerations from current research on personality traits and provide recommendations for future research on personality in science teams.

14.2.1   Extraversion

Extraversion refers to the degree to which an individual is sociable and outgoing. It is hypothesized that extraversion plays an important role in the social intra-team processes that influence team functioning (Borman and Motowidlo 1993). For instance, individuals who are extraverted tend to be talkative, outgoing, enthusiastic, and assertive (Costa and McCrae 1992). Such individuals thrive on being around people, and there is evidence that a high mean level of extraversion on a team is associated with greater team viability, cohesion, flexibility, and communication, as well as less conflict (Barrick et al. 1998). Extraverts can help stimulate discussion and foster a climate where team members feel comfortable expressing ideas (Mohammed and Angell 2003; Barry and Stewart 1997). While extraverts provide important contributions, some diversity in the personality traits on a team is useful. Evidence suggests a curvilinear relationship between extraversion and team performance (Barry and Stewart 1997; Neuman et al. 1999), such that too much extraversion on a team can be detrimental to team functioning. It may be that high levels of extraversion on a team may result in a focus on social aspects of the group at the expense of the task at hand (Mohammed and Angell 2003) or greater dissatisfaction in a team (Peeters et al. 2006b). Yet, it appears that the positive social influence of extraversion serves as a protective factor, as evidenced by the relationship between extraversion and greater likelihood a team will continue to function well in the future (team viability) as mediated by social cohesion (Barrick et al. 1998). Overall there is a positive association between variance in team extraversion and team performance, suggesting that a heterogeneous mix of degrees of extraversion within a team is most beneficial (Barry and Stewart 1997; Mohammed and Angell 2003; Peeters et al. 2006a, 2009).

14.2.2 Conscientiousness

Conscientiousness is one of the most consistent predictors of individual performance (Barrick and Mount 1991; Salgado 2003; Hurtz and Donovan 2000). Individuals who score high on this trait are described as hard working, organized, self-disciplined, dependable, and task-oriented (Costa and McCrae 1992). It is believed that team-level conscientiousness exerts its influence on team performance through effort and perseverance in completing tasks and achieving the broader goals of the team (LePine 2003; Molleman et al. 2004; Taggar 2002). Results from numerous studies have shown support for the hypothesis that high overall conscientiousness on a team leads to better decision-making and higher performance (Barrick et al. 1998; Bell 2007; Juhász 2010; Mohammed and Angell 2003; Neuman et al. 1999; O'Neill and Allen 2011; Prewett et al. 2009). With respect to variance, it has been hypothesized that differing levels of conscientiousness among team members may lead to conflict and have a negative impact on team performance, as the more conscientious team members may struggle to interact with the less conscientious team members on shared work (Peeters et al. 2006b). However, findings from studies examining the impact of variability in team conscientiousness have been mixed. Some research has found a significant negative relationship between variability in conscientiousness on a team and team performance (e.g., Barrick et al. 1998), while other research has uncovered no significant relationship between variability in conscientiousness and team performance (e.g.,

Neuman et al. 1999; Peeters et al., 2006b). Indeed, a meta-analysis of 22 studies that assessed variability in conscientiousness and indicators of team performance suggests that the relationship may be null (Prewett et al. 2009).

14.2.3 Agreeableness

Agreeableness can be described, broadly, as a tendency toward compassion and cooperation (Costa and McCrae 1992). Individuals high in this trait are likely to be tolerant, helpful, altruistic, and trustworthy (Costa and McCrae 1992). These characteristics likely promote interpersonal interactions that help to enable team processes such as cooperation, conflict resolution, open communication, and team cohesion (Barrick et al. 1998; Mohammed et al. 2002; Neuman and Wright 1999; Taggar 2002; Van Vianen and De Dreu 2001). Perhaps unsurprisingly, a high level of aggregate agreeableness on a team has been found to be positively associated with team effectiveness (Barrick et al. 1998; Peeters et al. 2006a, b; Van Vianen and De Dreu 2001). In addition, variability in agreeableness among team members appears to be negatively associated with team performance (Barrick et al. 1998; Mohammed and Angell 2003; Peeters et al. 2006a; Prewett et al. 2009). It is important to note that the term agreeableness is not synonymous with agreement. The trait form of agreeableness does not preclude spirited discussion or respectful argumentation. On the contrary, highly agreeable team members may be able to facilitate wide-ranging discussions that engage team members (e.g., junior scientists or those from different backgrounds) who might be less likely to participate under less supportive circumstances.

14.2.4 Emotional Stability

Individuals who score high on emotional stability are considered self-confident, secure, and steady (Costa and McCrae 1992) or well-adjusted (Driskell et al. 1988). It is hypothesized that high levels of this trait among team members foster a climate of cooperation and stability and a relatively relaxed work environment (Mount et al. 1998). Results from a number of studies suggest a positive relationship between emotional stability and team performance (Barrick et al. 1998; Molleman et al. 2004; Neuman et al. 1999). While one might predict that variability in emotional stability would negatively impact team effectiveness by reducing cooperation and team cohesiveness, studies addressing this question have produced inconsistent results. Different studies have found benefits (e.g., Neuman et al. 1999) or detriments of variability in emotional stability depending on the team context (e.g., student vs. professional teams; Peeters et al. 2006a, b), or no relationship at all (e.g., Barrick et al. 1998). This suggests a complicated relationship that may be clarified through future studies that examine this relationship in the context of key moderators (e.g., team leader emotional stability, degree of collaboration needed among team members).

14.2.5 Openness to Experience

Openness to experience involves intellectual curiosity, creativity, imagination, and preference for novelty and variety (Costa and McCrae 1992). As such, substantial representation of individuals with high openness to experience on a team may help to foster a creative and open team climate where members are encouraged to look for alternatives and to be flexible thinkers (Molleman et al. 2004). One would hypothesize that these processes are associated with team effectiveness. Although some studies have produced null or negative results (e.g., O'Neill and Allen 2011; Peeters et al. 2006a), a meta-analysis of 20 studies that evaluated the relationship between mean levels of openness to experience and team performance found a significant positive effect (Bell 2007). Research on the relationship between variability in openness to experience (vs. mean openness to experience) and team performance has not produced evidence of a compelling effect (Bell 2007; Neuman et al. 1999; O'Neill and Allen 2011). The results of one study suggests that there may be value in homogeneous openness to experience (i.e., low variability) on professional teams whereas greater heterogeneity

may be advantageous for student teams (Peeters et al. 2006a). More research is needed to determine how factors such as task type, history of collaboration, task duration, and teamwork experience may influence the salience of variability in openness to experience.

14.3 Methodological Considerations and Recommended Future Directions

In the literature highlighted above, inconsistency in findings across studies is due, in part, to the use of different measurement approaches for both personality factors and team performance. For instance, the effect of team composition on team performance is found to vary depending on the measurement approach (Bell 2007). Despite decades of research, there continues to be a lack of consensus on the best approaches to measure these factors in the team context. Rigorous testing is needed that compares different measurement approaches in the context of teams, in general, and science teams specifically. In addition, testing should consider which measurement approaches are best suited to particular team conditions. For instance, certain measurement approaches for team level personality traits (i.e., minimum and variance) identified relationships in the context of tasks with frequent work exchanges, but not in the context of tasks with few work exchanges, raising questions related to whether the frequency of exchanges is a moderating effect or if the robustness of the measurement approaches is insufficient to detect an effect.

Furthermore, the current state of the science on personality conceptualizes personality traits as co-occurring within individuals, and co-occurring at the aggregate level within teams, but often analyzes their dynamics in isolation (one trait at a time) or without consideration of the particular combination of traits among teams. It will be important, in the future, to carefully and comprehensively consider interactions across multiple factors of personality—both within individuals and in teams—if not more holistic, comprehensive personality profiles altogether.

Modeling the simultaneous influences—whether competing or congruent—of personality factors will yield a more precise understanding of how team composition influences team processes and effectiveness in teams in general, and science teams, specifically.

In addition, the mixed nature of the findings on the relationship between team-level personality factors and team performance suggests the need for research that goes beyond bivariate correlational data and places greater attention on approaches that can illuminate mediators and moderators. Furthermore, there is a need to establish ecological validity and generalizability through less reliance on laboratory studies with student participants and more in vivo studies of science teams. To more richly explore mediators and moderators ranging from team composition to team processes to contextual factors, there is a need for greater use of sophisticated study designs and analytic methods that can account for multi-level, multifactorial influences. Methods such as multi-level analysis, computational modeling, system dynamics modeling, and other system engineering approaches, as well as the development of new methods, are needed. Findings from these approaches will help to generate a more holistic and ultimately more accurate body of evidence that is able to inform recommendations for effective team science, from team assembly to team practices and policies, that aim to maximize scientific advances.

To illustrate the need for more sophisticated treatment of the interacting influences of personality traits on team performance, and more comprehensive studies that take into account moderators and mediators, we can consider the example of a critical team process, such as "back-up" behaviors. Team members who engage in helping or back-up behaviors are found to enhance overall team performance (Stout et al. 2009). Team members high in conscientiousness are more likely to demonstrate back-up behaviors (e.g., Morgeson et al. 2005) whereas team members low on emotional stability are least likely to provide back-up support (Porter et al. 2003). In addition, those high in conscientiousness are more likely to accurately assess when team members "legitimately" need help (Porter et al. 2003).

Furthermore, the ability to support team members when they need it by providing back-up involves communication, as do other types of supportive interactions such as providing feedback, encouragement, and new ideas or solutions to problems. Interestingly, while extroversion is positively associated with certain types of team-process-oriented communication (relation-related and polite utterances), agreeableness is found to be negatively associated with these types of communication. Furthermore, agreeableness is negatively associated with "thinking" or problem-solving-type communications (Juhász 2010). So although overall agreeableness is consistently associated with positive team performance, the mechanisms by which agreeableness enhances team performance are unclear. This example demonstrates how various studies that narrowly examine relationships between particular personality traits, behaviors, team processes, or emergent states in the context of teamwork can be integrated to create rich research questions that can only be explored effectively by more comprehensive, complex future studies.

14.4 Considerations for Future Research on Personality Factors in Science Teams

Key elements of team effectiveness include system context, task interdependence, temporal dynamics, multi-level linkages, organizational structure, workflow design, and virtuality (Kozlowski and Bell 2019 this book). So while "the effects of team personality composition on team effectiveness are stronger for some dimensions of personality (conscientiousness, agreeableness, extraversion) than others (emotional stability, openness to experience)" (Kozlowski and Bell 2019 this book), it is critical to assess the range of key elements when considering the applicability of such findings to science teams. For instance, the results of one meta-analysis were based on professional teams (e.g., flight crews, manufacturing teams) and student teams (e.g., conducting discrete tasks for study purposes) that worked together for durations ranging from one hour to 13 weeks (Peeters et al. 2006a).

The influence of personality on key team effectiveness elements in these teams is likely to be very different than in science teams. Unique conditions in science teams such as the long duration of research projects, the heavy reliance on virtuality, and the interdependent nature of integrative idea generation have the potential to increase the salience of personality traits such as emotional stability and openness to experience.

Contextual factors that influence team effectiveness also are an important source of variability in findings on the influence of personality traits on team effectiveness. Studies have shown differential effects of personality traits on team effectiveness depending on the setting where the study took place (lab vs. field), the type of work (e.g., design vs. service), and the team composition (e.g., professional vs. student; Peeters et al. 2006a). It is likely that science teams in different settings, performing different types of research (e.g., wet lab studies, translational research, community-based participatory research, implementation science), will demonstrate different effects from various team-level personality factors.

The particular scientific goal(s) of a science team may be a critical moderator of the influence of personality on team effectiveness. Given that team goals vary based on the phase of the research (e.g., initial development of the research idea, conceptualization of the research plan, implementation of the research plan, translational applications, development of fruitful spin-offs; Hall et al. 2012), a team may benefit from the inclusion of members with particular personality traits, and in particular roles such as as leaders, consultants, or advisors, at different phases of the research. For example, early in the research process, when there is an emphasis on idea generation, a team will likely benefit from the involvement of team members with openness to experience, whereas once a project is in the implementation phase, the team may benefit more from the involvement of team members high in introversion and conscientiousness (c.f. Stock et al. 2016). With knowledge sharing identified as a mediator of team performance through team learning (Xia and Ya 2012), particularly in cross-disciplinary team science, the finding that conscientiousness hinders diffusion of information among peers (Stock et al. 2016) indicates that careful consideration is needed to facilitate knowledge sharing interactions among team members with high degrees of conscientiousness. Future research will need to explore the interaction of personality traits with key characteristics of the scientific process (e.g., ideation, conceptualization, implementation, etc.) as they influence overall team achievement of scientific goals.

Another example of how the type of scientific work at hand likely mediates the impact of team personality factors on team effectiveness is the degree to which the success of a scientific initiative depends upon creativity. An initiative that aims to achieve high levels of novelty or radical innovation (e.g., integration of theories and approaches from across disciplines, development of new methods, production of an innovative breakthrough), an initiative that aims to advance discovery incrementally, and an initiative that aims to reproduce prior work likely may be influenced very differently by team-level openness to experience and conscientiousness. Future research will benefit from exploring scientific goals as a critical mediator of the relationship between team-level personality factors and scientific outcomes.

In addition, there is a need to disentangle the interaction of personality factors with related variables such as cognitive style in relation to teams' success in achieving their goals. For example, research has found that the presence of team members with high attention to detail reduced team innovation, whereas the inclusion of both creative and conformist members increased innovation, and team potency (efficacy) mediated the effect of cognitive styles on innovation (Bell 2017; Miron-Spektor et al. 2011). Furthermore, team potency and creativity relate to increases in knowledge sharing, and team potency serves as a mediator of the influence of team leadership on creativity (Lam 2012). With self-confidence as a central component to the personality trait of emotional stability, emotional stability is likely to play an influential role in team success, as well.

Finally, a unique contextual factor where team science in academia is concerned is the recognition and reward system (i.e., promotion and tenure policies) by which scientists are recognized for scientific achievement, and the types of achievement (e.g., unidisciplinary, individual contributions vs. cross-disciplinary and/or cross-departmental scientific work) that are rewarded. With traditional promotion and tenure policies continuing to emphasize individual-level contributions over team-level contributions, as well as discipline-specific over cross-disciplinary contributions, future research would benefit from cross-level analyses examining the interrelated influences of team personality traits, team science goals (e.g., innovation vs. replication, unidisciplinary vs. transdisciplinary), team performance, and individual performance in the context of different institutions' promotion and tenure policies (e.g., those that do or do not recognize and reward team-based science and/or cross-disciplinary scholarship). Such research can help to inform policy changes that optimally support the best scientific outcomes given a range of team personality traits and cognitive traits, scientific goals, and other mediators. One approach for advancing this area is to conduct cross-level studies, yet, while "team personality composition can exert meaningful cross-level effects on individual performance, … there is still little empirical research on these effects within organizational team contexts" (Prewett et al. 2009) and none known to date in the context of science teams.

14.5   Conclusions

This chapter briefly highlights what is known about the influence of personality on team performance from the literature on teams, in general. Based on what is known and not known, the chapter provides recommendations for future research directions to advance our understanding of the influence of personality on effectiveness of science teams, specifically. As reflected in this chapter, the study of personality is a large and robust area of research that offers key findings to

inform the practice of team science, and points to needed directions for future inquiry into the influence of team personality in the study of science teams. Our review focused on the Five Factor Model, currently the most widely applied trait-based system in personality research.

Research questions on personality and team effectiveness that have, so far, produced mixed findings point to potential future research directions that may be advanced through utilization of different measurement approaches, introduction of more sophisticated study designs and analytic methods, and the study of both the independent and interacting influences of personality factors as well as a range of mediators of the relationships among team personality factors and team effectiveness in the context of science teams.

Finally, this chapter makes clear that research examining personality, including associated processes, and the effectiveness of science teams is critical to advancing our knowledge due to the unique characteristics of team science, including team composition, research goals, phases of research, and unique influencing factors in the institutional, funding, and policy environments where team science occurs.

Acknowledgments This project has been funded in whole or in part with federal funds from the National Cancer Institute, National Institutes of Health, under Contract No. HHSN261200800001E. The content of this publication does not necessarily reflect the views or policies of the Department of Health and Human Services, nor does mention of trade names, commercial products, or organizations imply endorsement by the U.S. Government.

References

Barrick MR, Mount MK. The big five personality dimensions and job performance: a meta-analysis. Pers Psychol. 1991;44:1–26.

Barrick MR, Stewart GL, Neubert MJ, Mount MK. Relating member ability and personality to work-team processes and team effectiveness. J Appl Psychol. 1998;83(3):377–91.

Barry B, Stewart GL. Composition, process, and performance in self-managed groups: the role of personality. J Appl Psychol. 1997;82:62–78.

Bell S. Deep-level composition variables as predictors of team performance: a meta-analysis. J Appl Psychol. 2007;92:595–615.

Bell S. Tapping into the power of team composition for science teams. Clearwater Beach, FL: Featured presentation at Annual Science of Team Science; 2017.

Borman WC, Motowidlo SJ. Expanding the criterion domain to include elements of contextual performance. In: Schmitt N, Borman WC, editors. Personnel selection in organizations. San Francisco, CA: Jossey Bass; 1993. p. 71–98.

Costa PT, McCrae RR. 4 ways 5 factors are basic. Personal Individ Differ. 1992;13(6):653–65.

Driskell JE, Hogan R, Salas E. Personality and group performance. Rev Pers Soc Psychol. 1988;14:91–112.

Hall KL, Vogel AL, Huang GC, Serrano KJ, Rice EL, Tsakraklides SP, Fiore SM. The science of team science: a review of the empirical evidence and research gaps on collaboration in science. Am Psychol. 2018;73(4):532–48.

Hall KL, Vogel AL, Stipelman B, Stokols D, Morgan G, Gehlert S. A four-phase model of transdisciplinary team-based research: goals, team processes, and strategies. Transl Behav Med. 2012;2(4):415–30.

Hurtz GM, Donovan JJ. Personality and job performance: the big five revisited. J Appl Psychol. 2000;85:869–79.

Juhász M. Influence of personality on teamwork behaviour and communication. Soc Manage Sci. 2010;18(2):63–77. https://doi.org/10.3311/pp.so.2010-2.02.

Kozlowski SWJ, Bell BS. Work groups and teams in organizations. In: Borman WC, Ilgen DR, Klimoski RJ, editors. Handbook of psychology: Industrial and Organizational Psychology, vol. 12. Hoboken, NJ: John Wiley & Sons Inc.; 2003. p. 333–75.

Kozlowski SWJ, Bell BS. Evidence-based principles and strategies for optimizing team functioning and performance in science teams. In: Hall KL, Vogel AL, Croyle RT, editors. Strategies for team science success: handbook of evidence-based principles for cross-disciplinary science and practical lessons learned from health researchers. New York, NY: Springer; 2019.

Lam TK. The influence of team trust, potency and leadership on the intent to share knowledge and team creativity, DBA thesis. Lismore, NSW: Southern Cross University; 2012.

LePine JA. Team adaptation and post change performance: effects of team composition in terms of members' cognitive ability and personality. J Appl Psychol. 2003;88:27–39.

McCrae RR, Costa PT. Validation of the 5-factor model of personality across instruments and observers. J Pers Soc Psychol. 1987;52(1):81–90.

Miron-Spektor E, Erez M, Naveh E. The effect of conformist and attentive-to-detail members on team innovation: reconciling the innovation paradox. Acad Manag J. 2011;54(4):740–60.

Mohammed S, Angell L. Personality heterogeneity in teams: which differences make a difference for team performance? Small Group Res. 2003;34(6):651–77.

Mohammed S, Mathieu JE, Bartlett LB. Technical-administrative task performance, leadership task performance, and contextual performance: considering the influence of team- and task-related composition variables. J Organ Behav. 2002;23:795–814.

Molleman E, Nauta A, Jehn KA. Person-job fit applied to teamwork: a multilevel approach. Small Group Res. 2004;35:515–39.

Mount MK, Barrick MR, Stewart GL. Five-factor model of personality and performance in jobs involving interpersonal interactions. Hum Perform. 1998;11(2–3):145–65.

Morgeson FP, Reider MH, Campion MA. Selecting individuals in team settings: The importance of social skills, personality characteristics, and teamwork knowledge. Personnel Psychology 2005;58(3):583–611.

Neuman GA, Wagner SH, Christiansen ND. The relationship between work team personality composition and the job performance of teams. Group Org Manag. 1999;24(1):28–45.

Neuman GA, Wright J. Team effectiveness: Beyond skills and cognitive ability. Journal of Applied Psychology 1999;84(3):376–389.

O'Neill TA, Allen NJ. Personality and the prediction of team performance. Eur J Personal. 2011;25(1):31–42.

Peeters MA, Rutte CG, van Tuijl HF, Reymen IM. The big five personality traits and individual satisfaction with the team. Small Group Res. 2006b;37(2):187–211.

Peeters MA, Rutte CG, van Tuijl HF, Reymen IM. Designing in teams: does personality matter? Small Group Res. 2008;39(4):438–67.

Peeters MAG, van Tuijl HFJM, Rutte CG, Reymen MJ. Personality and team performance: a meta-analysis. Eur J Personal. 2006a;20:377–96.

Porter CO, Hollenbeck JR, Ilgen DR, Ellis AP, West BJ, Moon H. Backing up behaviors in teams: the role of personality and legitimacy of need. J Appl Psychol. 2003;88(3):391–403.

Prewett MS, Walvoord AAG, Stilson FRB, Rossi ME, Brannick MT. The team personality-team performance relationship revisited: the impact of criterion choice, pattern of workflow, and method of aggregation. Hum Perform. 2009;22(4):273–96.

Salgado JF. Predicting job performance using FFM and non-FFM personality measures. J Occup Organ Psychol. 2003;76:323–46.

Stock RM, von Hippel E, Gillert NL. Impacts of personality traits on consumer innovation success. Res Policy. 2016;45(4):57–769. https://doi.org/10.1016/j.respol.2015.12.002.

Stout RJ, Salas E, Carson R. Individual Task Proficiency and Team Process Behavior: What's Important for Team Functioning? Military Psychology 2009;6(3):177–192.

Taggar S. Individual creativity and group ability to utilize individual creative resources: a multilevel model. Acad Manag J. 2002;45:315–30.

Tett RP, Jackson DN, Rothstein M, Reddon JR. Meta-analysis of bidirectional relations in personality-job performance research. Hum Perform. 1999;12:1–29.

Van Vianen AEM, De Dreu CKW. Personality in teams: its relations to social cohesion, task cohesion, and team performance. Eur J Work Organ Psy. 2001;10:97–120.

Xia L, Ya S. Study on knowledge sharing behavior engineering. Syst Eng Procedia. 2012;4:468–76.

Demographic Diversity in Teams: The Challenges, Benefits, and Management Strategies

15

Kenneth D. Gibbs Jr., Anna Han, and Janetta Lun

Contents

The original version of this chapter was revised. The correction to this chapter is available at https://doi.org/10.1007/978-3-030-20992-6_46

K. D. Gibbs Jr. (✉)
Division of Training, Workforce Development, and Diversity, National Institute of General Medical Sciences, Bethesda, MD, USA

NIGMS Postdoctoral Research Associate Training Program, National Institute of General Medical Sciences, Bethesda, MD, USA
e-mail: kenneth.gibbs@nih.gov

A. Han · J. Lun
Office of Equity, Diversity and Inclusion, National Institutes of Health, Bethesda, MD, USA

15.1 Introduction

Two trends over the past 50 years have inexorably changed the nature of scientific discovery. First is the increasing dominance of interdisciplinary teams in scientific knowledge production. Across all fields of science, research became increasingly conducted in teams (as opposed to by individuals), and team-based research was more impactful than research done by single investigators (Wuchty et al. 2007). Interdisciplinary approaches became increasingly critical to the work of scientific teams due to the increasing complexity of problems that the scientific enterprise sought to address (Sciences TNAo 2005).

Second, and equally significant, are changes in the demographics of the people producing scientific knowledge. Compared to a half-century ago, the demographic diversity of researchers has increased significantly. There are now more women, and scientists from historically underrepresented racial/ethnic groups, with disabilities, or from different countries participating in the research enterprise (National Center for Science and Engineering Statistics 2017). Additionally, technological advances allow for scientific collaborations across continents, significantly reducing the barriers to collaboration once posed by geographic borders, and research collaborations across continents are becoming increasingly common (Adams 2012).

© Springer Nature Switzerland AG 2019
K. L. Hall et al. (eds.), *Strategies for Team Science Success*,
https://doi.org/10.1007/978-3-030-20992-6_15

However, the scientific community continues to have challenges fully leveraging and integrating workforce diversity (Smith-Doerr et al. 2017). Even though the talent pool of scientists from traditionally underrepresented groups has grown significantly in past two decades, the culture and praxis of science still present significant barriers for these scientists to enter and remain in the research workforce, and thus participate in science teams. For example, Ph.D. scientists from historically underrepresented backgrounds (women and underrepresented racial/ethnic minorities) have disproportionately low interest in research-intensive academic careers at the completion of Ph.D. training even when accounting for important objective (e.g., publication record, institutional pedigree) and relational/psychosocial (e.g., advisor relationship, research self-efficacy) factors known to influence career development (Gibbs Jr. et al. 2014). This, in turn, impacts the presence of these scientists in independent research positions where they can influence and contribute to the scientific research agenda. In the life sciences, the percentage of women in entry-level faculty positions lags the percentage in the Ph.D. pool by more than 10% (Valantine et al. 2016). Further, from 1980 to 2013, despite an over ninefold growth in the population of Ph.D. biomedical scientists from URM backgrounds, there was no relationship between the size of the URM talent pool and the number of assistant professors hired in American medical colleges (Gibbs et al. 2016).

This chapter focuses on the role that demographic diversity plays in team science and identifies potential areas of future research. The growth in collaborative research and diversity within the scientific workforce are distinct yet connected trends. The range of twenty-first century health challenges is increasingly complex, and both collaborative efforts and diverse perspectives will be required to meet these challenges. Successful science teams, particularly those involving scientists from different disciplines and backgrounds, hinge upon effective team integration strategies and approaches (e.g.,

O'Rourke et al., this volume; Pohl & Wuesler, this volume, Salazar et al., this volume). The two areas of scholarship overlap and may benefit from a more coordinated approach to integrate both concepts and approaches.

15.2 State of the Science

15.2.1 Defining Demographic Diversity and the Mechanisms Underlying Its Potential Impacts

Within the team science literature, there are distinct ways of categorizing diversity, across dimensions such as social identity, task-relevant knowledge and skills, values and beliefs, personality/cognitive styles, or group status (Mannix and Neale 2005). Traditional demographic factors such as race, ethnicity, country of origin, age, gender, or disability status are varyingly referred to as "surface-level," "visible," "observable," or "bio-demographic" dimensions of diversity. Meanwhile, factors such as education, skills and abilities, values and attitudes, functional background, personality differences, and sexual orientation are often called "deep-level," "non-observable," or "less visible" dimensions of diversity (Mannix and Neale 2005; Horwitz and Horwitz 2007; West et al. 2003). However, these boundaries are not firm, as factors such as organizational or job tenure, level of seniority on a team, and functional background have also been referred to as "demographic" factors (Bell et al. 2011; Lau and Murnighan 1998). In this chapter, we focus our literature review on the traditional demographic factors.

Demographic diversity in teams has enjoyed much theoretical and empirical attention in other fields such as business and psychology (Robinson 2013). Studies on the impact of demographic diversity in science teams are not as rich as in other contexts. Nevertheless, we identified three literature areas to summarize our existing knowledge in demographic diversity in science teams.

15.2.2 Context Mediates the Impact of Demographic Diversity Matters in Science Teams

With mounting evidence that diversity is important in sectors ranging from education to business where solving complex problems is of paramount importance (Galinsky et al. 2015; Gurin et al. 2002; Page 2007a), one line of inquiry is whether demographic diversity matters to science teams. Do demographically diverse science teams perform equally well, better, or worse than demographically homogeneous science teams? The answer, not surprisingly, is context-dependent.

The most extensive studies in this area have focused on examination of gender in science teams. Numerous meta-analyses have shown a contextually dependent impact of gender on science team performance, often measured in terms of publication production (Bear and Woolley 2011). A recent study in ecology, a field where women scientists are still underrepresented, showed that publications with a mix female and male authors (i.e., gender-heterogeneous) received more citations than publications with either all-male or all-female authors (Campbell et al. 2013), while other studies have shown that gender diversity has a null or even negative impact on team productivity (Bowers et al. 2000).

In a study on ethnic diversity, Freeman and Huang (2015) examined ethnic diversity of authorship in 2.57 million scientific papers published between 1985 and 2008 across 11 scientific fields. After controlling for a number of factors (e.g., size of the ethnic groups, number of authors' locations, and number of references), they found that papers published by authors from different ethnic backgrounds received more citations and were more likely to be published in journals with higher impact factors (Freeman and Huang 2015). In a study of the impact of cultural diversity and international collaboration among European life scientists, cultural diversity among junior scientists (i.e., Ph.D. students) showed a curvilinear relationship on team productivity (as measured by number of publications (Barjak and Robinson 2008)). All other factors being equal, teams with moderate levels of diversity among Ph.D. students were more productive than those with very high, or no diversity (there was no impact of postdoctoral cultural diversity). These studies suggest that demographically heterogeneous science teams can result in higher impact research and productivity than demographically homogeneous teams, but that context mediates the effects.

15.2.3 Why and How Demographic Diversity Matters in Science Teams

If demographic diversity can impact science teams, the next questions are why and how. Numerous social and behavioral science research findings shed light on why and how demographic diversity affects teams generally. Many of these studies point to two important conclusions:

- Diversity in teams broadens and increases the range of perspectives, approaches, and information flow to solve a problem (Page 2007a; Reagans and Zuckerman 2001).
- Diversity in teams evokes team and cognitive processing that affords creativity, innovation, and more effective problem-solving (Levine et al. 2014; Phillips 2014; Sommers 2006; Woolley et al. 2010).

These two principles of diversity should be seen as important for teamwork in science as in other sectors. Extant literature on diversity in teams and team processes in industrial and organizational psychology has clearly shown that the impact that diversity has on team-process measures, output quantity or quality, and team cohesion is context-dependent (Horwitz and Horwitz 2007). Diversity is believed to impact team processes and outputs through several psychological processes (Stahl et al. 2010). For example, similarity-attraction theory posits that people desire to work with those they find similar in terms of values, beliefs, and attitudes (Byrne 1971). Social categorization theory asserts that people categorize individuals like themselves as part of the "in" group and those different from themselves as part of the "out" group (Turner et al. 1987). From these viewpoints, diversity may be considered as negative as it can lead to challenging social process that can impair team function.

In contrast, from an information-processing perspective, team members from diverse backgrounds bring new and different perspectives and social networks that can aid in problem solving. In *The Difference*, Scott Page noted that functional diversity in teams is important when dealing with complex, non-routine tasks (e.g., biomedical and behavioral research) where diverse perspectives can lead to enhanced creativity in problem solving (Page 2007b). In many contexts, there is evidence that gender diversity has strong and positive impacts on team process measures, including collective intelligence and communication (Bear and Woolley 2011). Similarly, racial/ethnic and cultural diversity in teams has the potential to promote better decision-making processes. The different perspectives provided by people from different racial/ethnic backgrounds in diverse teams can challenge default cognitive processes and behaviors. That is, racial/ethnic and cultural diversity can enable the consideration of more alternatives and the exploration of different potential consequences of actions (Phillips 2014).

Research shows that people are more likely to think broadly, attribute novelty to dissenting perspectives, and consider alternatives when dissent comes from a group member of a different race rather than the same race (Antonio et al. 2004). Racially and ethnically diverse teams assume less common knowledge, and share more information, which in turn can lead to more effective and careful processing of information (Phillips et al. 2006). Furthermore, teams with more racial/ethnic diversity draw from a larger informational space and engage in greater information elaboration (van Knippenberg et al. 2004).

However, in Scott Page's parlance, there is also a "diversity penalty" in teamwork. As diverse teams invite a wide range of perspectives, they also bring differences in beliefs, attitudes, and preferences that post challenges to team cohesion and coordination (Page 2007a; Reagans and

Zuckerman 2001; Harrison et al. 2002; Reagans et al. 2004). "Diversity facilitates friction that enhances deliberation and upends conformity" (Levine et al. 2014). While friction can increase accuracy and quality of judgment and decision-making in teams, it can also reduce performance due to increased team conflicts and misunderstanding. For example, in a study of hospital-based teamwork, racially diverse teams experienced more conflicts than racially homogenous teams (Sessa et al. 1993). Another study with nursing-care teams showed that black team members were more likely to cite race as a factor in increasing team conflict while white team members cited roles and status (Dreachslin et al. 2000). A large-scale study of 151 teams also showed that racially heterogeneous groups tended to demonstrate lower commitment, less psychological attachment, and increased absenteeism than racially homogenous groups (Tsui et al. 1992). In another evaluation of 122 work teams, Townshend and Scott found attitudinal differences between Black and White team members on perceptions of team commitment, cohesion, and efficacy. These differences correlated with the better performance in all-White teams compared to mixed-race teams (Townsend and Scott 2001). This research suggests that demographic diversity affects the dynamics and productivity of science teams, but the mechanisms by which these effects occur still require further research.

15.2.4 Demographic Patterns in Science Teams

Another central question about demographic diversity in science teams is who participates in science teams. Are scientists from different demographic backgrounds equally likely to engage and participate in science teams? How do scientists of different demographic backgrounds view and value science teams?

Research shows that female and male scientists are equally likely to engage in scientific collaborations (Abramo et al. 2013; Bozeman and Gaughan 2011), but they have different reasons and opportunities to collaborate. A survey study of faculty across scientific disciplines in the U.S. found that after structural factors such as tenure status, professional age, discipline, as well as affiliations to university research centers and industrial institutions were taken into account, female scientists had as many collaborators as male scientists do (Bozeman and Gaughan 2011). The tendency for female and male scientists to collaborate seemed to vary largely by disciplines (Abramo et al. 2013; Prpić 2002) and scientific approaches such as interdisciplinary research (Rhoten and Pfirman 2007).

However, female and male scientists may be motivated to participate in science teams for different reasons. In the aforementioned survey study on collaborations, the number of collaborators was more strongly associated with instrumental (e.g., work with researchers who have strong scientific reputation or complementary skills and knowledge) and experience reasons (e.g., know the collaborator for a long time) among male scientists than female scientists, while both male and female scientists are equally likely to collaborate because of mentoring reasons such as helping graduate students (Bozeman and Gaughan 2011). Therefore, female and male scientists do not seem to differ in their willingness to participate in science teams but they may have different expectations about the functions of science teams.

As mentioned, scientists of different demographic backgrounds may be provided with different levels of opportunities to collaborate scientifically. The source of these differences is complex and could be due to a number of factors such as demographic representation in disciplines and institutions, departmental climates, mentoring opportunities, access to professional networks, and scientific reputation. In the sciences, men publish more papers than women (West et al. 2013), papers published by women as single, first, or last authors received fewer citations than papers published by men in the same authorship positions (Lariviere V et al. 2013). Gender disparities in scientific impact as indicated by bibliometrics have implications for participation in science teams because it suggests

gender imbalance in visibility and perceived productivity. Male scientists could be more likely to be approached as collaborators than female scientists. Gender bias may also play a role in seeking collaborators, as female scientists may not be as readily perceived as providing the leadership and contributions to teamwork, especially in male-dominated scientific fields (Heilman and Haynes 2005).

Another factor that impacts the ability of scientists from different demographic backgrounds to collaborate scientifically is differential access to research networks. A recent study that examined co-authorship networks within an organization found that white male assistant professors have more connections with other faculty members than women and underrepresented minority assistant professors. In addition, those assistant professors who had more connections are also more likely to be promoted (Warner et al. 2016). The growing body of research points to demographic differences in participation of science teams is attributable to the representation and integration of scientists from different demographic backgrounds.

15.3 Future Directions for Research on Demographic Diversity in Science Teams

Although research has made great strides in advancing the understanding of the impacts of demographic diversity in team performance, the research base for understanding diversity in science teams is less extensive. In addition, the knowledge thus far primarily focuses on gender and racial/ethnic diversity; this leaves many questions about the effects of other types of demographic diversity such as age, religion, citizenships, disabilities, and sexual and gender minorities on science teams' dynamics and processes (Smith-Doerr et al. 2017). Beyond this general need for more research, there are also other important research questions that we recommend future research to examine. We highlight and summarize a few of them below.

15.3.1 Knowing the "Where, When, and How" of Demographic Diversity and Science Team Performance

Decades of research have shown mixed findings on the relationship between demographic diversity in teams and team performance (Ely and Thomas 2001; Jackson et al. 2003; Joshi and Roh 2009; Horwitz and Horwitz 2007). That is, context matters for the impact of diversity in science teams. There is an increasing effort to understand the conditions (e.g., contexts, team characteristics, types of diversity) under which demographic diversity in a team would affect team performance, processes, and outcomes (Joshi and Roh 2009; van Dijk et al. 2012). For instance, gender or ethnic diversity was negatively associated with team performance in male- and white-dominated occupations, but has no effect on team performance in gender- or ethnic-balanced occupations (Joshi and Roh 2009). In the same meta-analysis, it was also found that demographic diversity was positively associated with team performance when the team tasks, goals, and outcomes were less reliant on team members to work interdependently. New research has also shown that organizational structure and procedure in promoting diversity can affect team members' attitudes toward diversity (Kaiser et al. 2013; Yogeeswaran and Dasgupta 2014). These studies point to the numerous contingencies in the relationship between demographic diversity and team performance at multiple levels (e.g., organizational, group, interpersonal, individual).

The challenge, moving forward, would be to better understand the contingencies or contexts that are most relevant in moderating the relationship between demographic diversity and outcomes of science teams. For instance, what levels of faculty demographic diversity of an academic department facilitate most scientific collaborations? What kind of institutional structures (e.g., the presence of research centers) and practices (e.g., team teaching) affect demographic composition of science teams? How do scientific methodologies or approaches affect diversity in science teams? In addition to these scientific

contexts, the temporal contexts of scientific process can also moderate how demographic diversity in science teams impacts productivity and outcomes. The effects of demographic diversity at various stages of scientific process such as ideas generation, protocol development, study implementation, analyses, and writing could be different. It is conceivable that demographic diversity may pose more challenges at a certain phase of the process than another.

15.3.2 Translating and Testing Interventions to Enhance Cultural Integration in Diverse Science Teams

The challenges of demographic diversity in teams can be managed. Processes that promote cultural integration and inclusion, and reduce the so-called demographic "faultlines" can be set in place to minimize potential challenges inherent by demographic diversity in teams (Lau and Murnighan 1998). However, these processes are seldom applied to and evaluated in science teams or in institutions with strong scientific cultures and norms. There are well-documented strategies from the intergroup behavior, relations, and communication literature that can be applied and tested to enhance cultural integration in diverse science teams.

For example, research in social psychology has shown that people are more likely to adapt a "we" vs. "them" mindset when competition is high or when people pay more attention to their self-interests than group-interests (Sherif 1966). Kochan and colleagues showed that demographic diversity in teams is especially detrimental when the norm of the organization is highly competitive, but when the organization promotes learning from diversity and cooperative goals, positive effects of diverse team emerged (Kochan et al. 2003). Chatman and Spartaro also demonstrated that team members of demographically diverse backgrounds cooperated more when the norm emphasized the collectivistic vs. individualistic values (Chatman and Spataro 2005). Researchers should explore how to foster cooperation and common goals, and integration in science teams, as well as how academic and research institutions can provide incentive structure that promotes the value of diversity (Harrison and Klein 2007).

Successful cultural integration in diverse science teams also relies on team members' ability to communicate with each other, which are skills that can be learned. A series of studies conducted by Woolley and colleagues have demonstrated that equal contributions during team discussion and the ability of team members to read each other's emotions are key factors that increase a team's collective intelligence (Woolley et al. 2010; Engel et al. 2014). Teams function better when members from minority backgrounds are valued and heard (Ely and Thomas 2001; Eagly 2016) and when misunderstandings due to cultural differences are minimized (Gudykunst 2003). When minority members were seen as an expert, the team is more likely to engage in debate, had more conflict and differing opinions (Sinaceur et al. 2010), exerted more cognitive effort, and thought more creatively (Nemeth and Kwan 1985). This evidence points to the importance of the communication processes that are sensitive to cultural differences in a diverse team. Future work can focus on how these processes can be better integrated and routinized in the practice of science, and the best strategies for wide uptake interventions to facilitate enhanced communication across lines of demography.

15.4 Conclusion

Increasing demographic diversity is a reality that is influencing many aspects of life, and will continue to do so for the foreseeable future. The existing literature focuses on a limited number of "surface-level" demographic differences such as gender, race, and ethnicity and indeed these dimensions of diversity can affect social processes of teamwork. However, there are a number of other diversity dimensions such as age, religion, citizenship, disabilities, and sexual and gender minorities. We know very little about these groups' participation and engagement in science

teams, and their attitudes toward and barriers in working in science teams. As important, future research on demographic diversity in science teams will need to better define and explore the various aspects of demographic diversity and their impacts to further elucidate why diversity matters in science teams. Similar to the large team science literature, there is a strong indication that contexts moderate the effects of diverse teams. This will also be an important future research area. Finally, there should be more opportunity for evidence-based research on translating and testing the best practices of effective management in diverse science teams.

References

Abramo G, D'Angelo CA, Murgia G. Gender differences in research collaboration. J Inf. 2013;7(4):811–22. https://doi.org/10.1016/j.joi.2013.07.002.

Adams J. Collaborations: the rise of research networks. Nature. 2012;490:335–6. https://doi.org/10.1038/490335a.

Antonio AL, Chang MJ, Hakuta K, Kenny DA, Levin S, Milem JF. Effects of racial diversity on complex thinking in college students. Psychol Sci. 2004;15(8):507–10. https://doi.org/10.1111/j.0956-7976.2004.00710.x. PubMed PMID: WOS: 000222822600001

Barjak F, Robinson S. International collaboration, mobility and team diversity in the life sciences: impact on research performance. Soc Geogr. 2008;3(1):23–36. https://doi.org/10.5194/sg-3-23-2008.

Bear JB, Woolley AW. The role of gender in team collaboration and performance. Interdiscip Sci Rev. 2011;36(2):146–53. https://doi.org/10.1179/030801811X13013181961473.

Bell ST, Villado AJ, Lukasik MA, Belau L, Briggs AL. Getting specific about demographic diversity variable and team performance relationships: a meta-analysis. J Manag. 2011;37(3):709–43. https://doi.org/10.1177/0149206310365001. PubMed PMID: WOS: 000289142300003

Bowers CA, Pharmer JA, Salas E. When member homogeneity is needed in work teams. Small Group Res. 2000;31(3):305–27. https://doi.org/10.1177/104649640003100303.

Bozeman B, Gaughan M. How do men and women differ in research collaborations? An analysis of the collaborative motives and strategies of academic researchers. Res Policy. 2011;40(10):1393–402. https://doi.org/10.1016/j.respol.2011.07.002.

Byrne D. The attraction paradigm. New York, NY: Academic Press; 1971.

Campbell LG, Mehtani S, Dozier ME, Rinehart J. Gender-heterogeneous working groups produce higher quality science. PLOS ONE. 2013;8(10):e79147. https://doi.org/10.1371/journal.pone.0079147.

Chatman JA, Spataro SE. Using self-categorization theory to understand relational demography-based variations in people's responsiveness to organizational culture. Acad Manage J. 2005;48(2):321–31. PubMed PMID: WOS: 000229000800008

van Dijk H, van Engen ML, van Knippenberg D. Defying conventional wisdom: a meta-analytical examination of the differences between demographic and job-related diversity relationships with performance. Org Behav Hum Decis Process. 2012;119(1):38–53. https://doi.org/10.1016/j.obhdp.2012.06.003.

Dreachslin JL, Hunt PL, Sprainer E. Workforce diversity: implications for the effectiveness of health care delivery teams. Soc Sci Med. 2000;50(10):1403–14. https://doi.org/10.1016/S0277-9536(99)00396-2. PubMed PMID: WOS: 000085796100005

Eagly AH. When passionate advocates meet research on diversity, does the honest broker stand a chance? J Soc Issues. 2016;72(1):199–222. https://doi.org/10.1111/josi.12163.

Ely RJ, Thomas DA. Cultural diversity at work: the effects of diversity perspectives on work group processes and outcomes. Adm Sci Q. 2001;46(2):229–73.

Engel D, Woolley AW, Jing LX, Chabris CF, Malone TW. Reading the mind in the eyes or reading between the lines? Theory of mind predicts collective intelligence equally well online and face-to-face. PLOS ONE. 2014;9(12):e115212. https://doi.org/10.1371/journal.pone.0115212.

Freeman RB, Huang W. Collaborating with people like me: ethnic co-authorship within the US. J Labor Econ. 2015;33((3)(S1)):S289–318.

Galinsky AD, Todd AR, Homan AC, Phillips KW, Apfelbaum EP, Sasaki SJ, et al. Maximizing the gains and minimizing the pains of diversity. Perspect Psychol Sci. 2015;10(6):742–8. https://doi.org/10.1177/1745691615598513.

Gibbs KD Jr, McGready J, Bennett JC, Griffin K. Biomedical Science Ph.D. career interest patterns by race/ethnicity and gender. PLoS One. 2014;9(12):e114736. https://doi.org/10.1371/journal.pone.0114736. PubMed PMID: 25493425; PubMed Central PMCID: PMCPMC4262437

Gibbs KD, Basson J, Xierali IM, Broniatowski DA. Decoupling of the minority PhD talent pool and assistant professor hiring in medical school basic science departments in the US. Elife. 2016;5 https://doi.org/10.7554/eLife.21393. PubMed PMID: 27852433; PubMed Central PMCID: PMCPMC5153246

Gudykunst WB. Cross-cultural and intercultural communication. Thousand Oaks, CA: Sage Publications; 2003.

Gurin P, Dey E, Hurtado S, Gurin G. Diversity and higher education: theory and impact on educational outcomes. Harv Edu Rev. 2002;72(3):330–66.

Harrison DA, Klein KJ. What's the difference? Diversity constructs as separation, variety, or disparity in organizations. Acad Manage Rev. 2007;32(4):1199–228. PubMed PMID: WOS: 000249754300010

Harrison DA, Price KH, Gavin JH, Florey AT. Time, teams, and task performance: Changing effects of surface- and deep-level diversity on group functioning. Acad Manag J. 2002;45(5):1029–45. https://doi.org/10.2307/3069328. PubMed PMID: WOS: 000178849900012

Heilman ME, Haynes MC. No credit where credit is due: attributional rationalization of women's success in male-female teams. J Appl Psychol. 2005;90(5):905–16. https://doi.org/10.1037/0021-9010.90.5.905.

Horwitz SK, Horwitz IB. The effects of team diversity on team outcomes: a meta-analytic review of team demography. J Manag. 2007;33(6):987–1015. https://doi.org/10.1177/0149206307308587. PubMed PMID: WOS: 000251133200007

Jackson S, Joshi A, Erhardt NL. Recent research on team and organizational diversity: SWOT analysis and implications. J Manag. 2003;29:801–30.

Joshi A, Roh H. The role of context in work team diversity research: a meta-analytic review. Acad Manage J. 2009;52(3):599–627. https://doi.org/10.5465/AMJ.2009.41331491.

Kaiser CR, Major B, Jurcevic I, Dover TL, Brady LM, Shapiro JR. Presumed fair: ironic effects of organizational diversity structures. J Pers Soc Psychol. 2013;104(3):504–19. https://doi.org/10.1037/a0030838.

van Knippenberg D, De Dreu CKW, Homan AC. Work group diversity and group performance: an integrative model and research agenda. J Appl Psychol. 2004;89(6):1008–22. https://doi.org/10.1037/0021-9010.89.6.1008. PubMed PMID: WOS: 000225474100007

Kochan T, Bezrukova K, Ely R, Jackson S, Joshi A, Jehn K, et al. The effects of diversity on business performance: report of the diversity research network. Hum Res Manag. 2003;42(1):3–21. https://doi.org/10.1002/hrm.10061. PubMed PMID: WOS: 000182557700002

Lariviere V, Ni C, Gingras Y, Cronin B, Sugimoto CR. Bibliometrics: global gender disparities in science. Nature. 2013;504(7479):211–3.. (Electronic)

Lau DC, Murnighan JK. Demographic diversity and faultlines: the compositional dynamics of organizational groups. Acad Manage Rev. 1998;23(2):325–40. https://doi.org/10.2307/259377. PubMed PMID: WOS: 000073127100010

Levine SS, Apfelbaum EP, Bernard M, Bartelt VL, Zajac EJ, Stark D. Ethnic diversity deflates price bubbles. Proc Natl Acad Sci U S A. 2014;111(52):18524–9. https://doi.org/10.1073/pnas.1407301111. PubMed PMID: WOS: 000347444400040

Mannix E, Neale MA. What differences make a difference? The promise and reality of diverse teams in organizations. Psychol Sci Public Interest. 2005;6(2):31–55.

National Center for Science and Engineering Statistics. Women, minorities, and persons with disabilites in science and engineering (NSF 17-310). 2017.

Nemeth CJ, Kwan JL. Originality of word-associations as a function of majority vs minority influence. Soc Psychol Quart. 1985;48(3):277–82. https://doi.org/10.2307/3033688. PubMed PMID: WOS:A1985ASM4800009

Page SE. The difference: how the power of diversity creates better groups, firms, schools, and societies. Princeton: New Jersey Princeton University Press; 2007a.

Page SE. Difference: how the power of diversity creates better groups, firms, schools, and societies. Princeton, NJ: Princeton University Press; 2007b. p. 1–424. PubMed PMID: WOS: 000287089400019

Phillips KW. How diversity makes us smarter. Sci Am. 2014;

Phillips KW, Northcraft GB, Neale MA. Surface-level diversity and decision-making in groups: when does deep-level similarity help? Group Process Interg. 2006;9(4):467–82. https://doi.org/10.1177/1368430206067557. PubMed PMID: WOS: 000242158800002

Prpić K. Gender and productivity differentials in science. Scientometrics. 2002;55(1):27–58. https://doi.org/10.1023/A:1016046819457.

Reagans R, Zuckerman EW. Networks, diversity, and productivity: the social capital of corporate R&D teams. Organ Sci. 2001;12(4):502–17. https://doi.org/10.1287/orsc.12.4.502.10637.

Reagans R, Zuckerman E, McEvily B. How to make the team: social networks vs. demography as criteria for designing effective teams. Adm Sci Quart. 2004;49(1):101–33. https://doi.org/10.2307/4131457.

Rhoten D, Pfirman S. Women in interdisciplinary science: exploring preferences and consequences. Res Policy. 2007;36(1):56–75. https://doi.org/10.1016/j.respol.2006.08.001.

Robinson QM, editor. The Oxford handbook of diversity and work. New York, NY: Oxford University Press; 2013.

Sciences TNAo. Facilitating Interdisciplinary Reserach. Washington, DC: National Academic Press; 2005.

Sessa VI, Bennett J, Birdsall C. Conflict with less distress: promoting team effectiveness. Nurs Adm Q. 1993;18:57–65.

Sherif M. In common predicament: social psychology of intergroup conflict and cooperation. Boston, MA: Houghton Mifflin; 1966.

Sinaceur M, Thomas-Hunt MC, Neale MA, O'Neill OA, Haag C. Accuracy and perceived expert status in group decisions: when minority members make majority members more accurate privately. Pers Soc Psychol B. 2010;36(3):423–37. https://doi.org/10.1177/0146167209353349. PubMed PMID: WOS: 000274848000011

Smith-Doerr L, Alegria SN, Sacco T. How diversity matters in the US science and engineering workforce: a critical review considering integration in teams, fields, and organizational contexts. Engag Sci Technol Soc. 2017;3:139–53. https://doi.org/10.17351/ests2017.142.

Sommers SR. On racial diversity and group decision making: Identifying multiple effects of racial composition on jury deliberations. J Pers Soc Psychol. 2006;90(4):597–612. https://doi.org/10.1037/0022-3514.90.4.597.

Stahl GK, Maznevski ML, Voigt A, Jonsen K. Unraveling the effects of cultural diversity in teams: a meta-analysis of research on multicultural work groups. J Int Bus Stud. 2010;41(4):690–709. https://doi.org/10.1057/jibs.2009.85. PubMed PMID: WOS: 000277241800009

Townsend AM, Scott KD. Team racial composition, member attitudes, and performance: a field study. Ind Relat. 2001;40(2):317–37. https://doi.org/10.1111/0019-8676.00210. PubMed PMID: WOS: 000174189900007

Tsui AS, Egan TD, Oreilly CA. Being different—relational demography and organizational attachment. Adm Sci Q. 1992;37(4):549–79. https://doi.org/10.2307/2393472. PubMed PMID: WOS:A1992KG08100002

Turner JC, Hogg MA, Oakes PJ, Reicher SD, Wetherell MS. Rediscovering the social group: a self-categorization theory. Oxford: Blackwell; 1987.

Valantine HA, Lund PK, Gammie AE. From the NIH: a systems approach to increasing the diversity of the biomedical research workforce. CBE Life Sci Educ. 2016;15(3) https://doi.org/10.1187/cbe.16-03-0138. PubMed PMID: 27587850; PubMed Central PMCID: PMCPMC5008902

Warner ET, Carapinha R, Weber GM, Hill EV, Reede JY. Faculty promotion and attrition: the importance of coauthor network reach at an academic medical center. J Gen Intern Med. 2016;31(1):60–7. https://doi.org/10.1007/s11606-015-3463-7.

West MA, Tjosvold D, Smith KG. International handbook of organizational teamwork and cooperative working. Chichester: Wiley; 2003.

West JD, Jacquet J, King MM, Correll SJ, Bergstrom CT. The role of gender in scholarly authorship. PLoS ONE. 2013;8(7):e66212. https://doi.org/10.1371/journal.pone.0066212.

Woolley AW, Chabris CF, Pentland A, Hashmi N, Malone TW. Evidence for a collective intelligence factor in the performance of human groups. Science. 2010;330(6004):686–8. https://doi.org/10.1126/science.1193147.

Wuchty S, Jones BF, Uzzi B. The increasing dominance of teams in production of knowledge. Science. 2007;316(5827):1036–9. https://doi.org/10.1126/science.1136099.

Yogeeswaran K, Dasgupta N. The devil is in the details: abstract versus concrete construals of multiculturalism differentially impact intergroup relations. J Pers Soc Psychol. 2014;106(5):772–89. https://doi.org/10.1037/a0035830.

The Added Value of Team Member Diversity to Research in Underserved Populations

16

William J. Blot, Margaret Hargreaves, and Wei Zheng

Contents

16.1 Overview

In this chapter we describe an example of the added value demographic diversity provides in the conceptualization, design, and conduct of epidemiologic research aimed at clarifying cancer and other chronic disease risks among underserved populations. We report on the Southern Community Cohort Study (SCCS), an ongoing prospective study tracking nearly 86,000 adults seeking to identify and quantify risk factors for cancer and other illnesses and provide information useful toward amelioration of health disparities. Two-thirds of cohort members are African American, and the majority of both black and white participants are generally low-income residents of rural as well as urban areas of the southeastern United States. Herein we outline the goals of the SCCS, describe the diversity of the cohort as well as the scientific research team and collaborating federally qualified community health centers (CHCs), and present summary statistics indicating that several basic measures of health status vary by demographic status. We conclude by presenting lessons learned from conducting research in medically underserved populations

16.2 Disparities in Health Across Diverse Populations

In a recent issue of JAMA, sharp gradients between income and life expectancy were documented, with evidence that differences between the richest and poorest Americans have increased over the past 15 years (Adler and Newman 2002). The income-focused analyses were adjusted for race and ethnicity, but all-cause and disease-specific mortality rates have long been known to be higher among African Americans than other racial/ethnic groups, in part related to lower aver-

W. J. Blot (✉) · W. Zheng
Vanderbilt University Medical Center,
Nashville, TN, USA
e-mail: william.j.blot@vumc.org

M. Hargreaves (Deceased)
Meharry Medical College, Nashville, TN, USA

© Springer Nature Switzerland AG 2019
K. L. Hall et al. (eds.), *Strategies for Team Science Success*,
https://doi.org/10.1007/978-3-030-20992-6_16

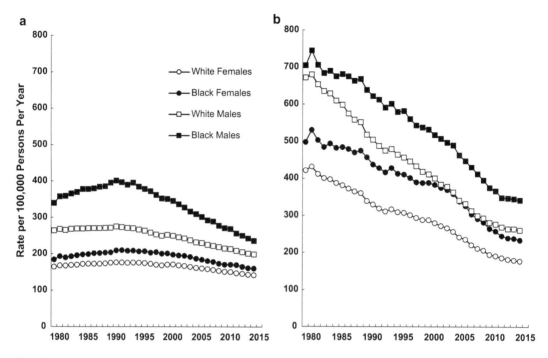

Fig. 16.1 (**a**) Trends in age-adjusted U.S. total cancer mortality rates by sex and race. (**b**) Trends in age-adjusted U.S. major cardiovascular disease (CVD) mortality rates by sex and race

age incomes among blacks than whites (American Psychological Association 2014; Buchowski et al. 2003). Figure 16.1 shows the higher national age-adjusted cancer and cardiovascular disease mortality rates among blacks than whites during 1979–2014. In addition, geographic differences in mortality are apparent (Fig. 16.2), with elevated death rates from both cancer and cardiovascular disease, as well as high obesity prevalences, across broad swaths in the south, overlapping with the SCCS catchment area. Ameliorating such disparities has been a national priority, but the persistence of differences in mortality, as well as in other indices of disease risk and health status, indicates that the task is not easy and suggests a highly complex interplay of medical, social, environmental, lifestyle, biologic, and other causative factors (Chetty et al. 2016). Evaluating determinants of differences in cancer rates and risks among diverse groups, including low socioeconomic populations seldom included in large numbers in prior epidemiologic research, is a major goal of the SCCS (Hargreaves et al. 2006).

16.3 Planning Health Research in Underserved Populations

The SCCS concept arose from discussions in 2000 among staff and leaders of the Vanderbilt University Medical Center (VUMC), Meharry Medical College (MMC), Matthew Walker Comprehensive Health Center (MW), and the International Epidemiology Institute (IEI), all institutions with goals of alleviating the burden of cancer and other illnesses in humans generally and in the populations they serve. Critical to the deliberations were the perspectives brought by the differing backgrounds, experience, and expertise of the investigators. VUMC, MMC, and IEI investigators came from academic research settings accustomed to designing epidemiologic studies to evaluate specific well-defined hypotheses about environmental, behavioral, and host factors in cancer etiology, including the roles of diet and nutrition, smoking and other lifestyle factors, the social and external environment, and how adverse health effects of these factors may vary according

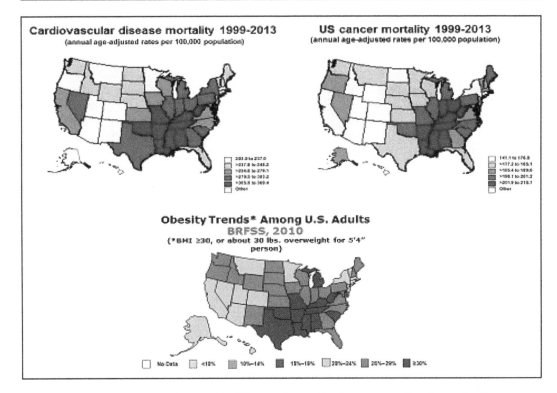

Fig. 16.2 Obesity prevalences and geographic differences in mortality from cancer and cardiovascular disease

to biologic and genetic proclivities. The initial discussions were held at VUMC and MMC and included individuals in leadership positions in both institutions who were interested in expanding VUMC-MMC collaboration. One of the key outcomes was the introduction by MMC staff of the possibility of engaging MW, the largest federally qualified health center in Nashville. The MW director was then contacted and she and her team subsequently became intimately involved in planning the research. The MW director also identified a former colleague with experience in CHC-based research and policy implementation who was then hired by IEI and was later to provide the key role in engagement of additional CHCs. MW investigators were at the front lines of providing basic preventative and healthcare services in medically underserved areas. Representing the "community," they quickly focused on identifying the health and healthcare needs of the populations they served and on practical issues in recruiting and communicating with individuals often with low education levels and

with pressing daily life concerns beyond potential future cancer or other disease risks.

The diversity of the team led to a unique study design for the SCCS. For the first time, a cohort study attempted to recruit large numbers of participants from CHCs like MW which serve populations seldom if ever included in large numbers previously. Because of the study's cancer focus, it was decided to restrict the age range at study entry to 40–79 in order to obtain sufficient statistical power to evaluate risk factors and outcomes in the not too distant future after study initiation. Cancers certainly occurred at younger ages, but at much lower rates so that larger numbers of participants and longer follow-up would have been needed to assess risks among those enrolled in their 20s and 30s. The upper age cutoff was imposed because of practical difficulties in recruiting and the shorter life expectancies among those over age 80. Because of the underrepresentation of African Americans in prior research, it was decided to attempt to have approximately two-thirds of the cohort members be African American, with one-third non-African American to enable direct contrasts between blacks and whites.

The feasibility of an academic–CHC partnership was demonstrated in a pilot study carried out at MW, which showed that the distrust sometimes exhibited toward governmental and academic institutions could be overcome at the local CHC level and that those approached for entry into a health research study were often willing to join (Macinko and Elo 2009). Included in this willingness to participate were African American men, a group greatly underrepresented in prior health studies (Shaya et al. 2007; Signorello et al. 2014).

16.4 Recruiting and Following Hard-to-Reach Populations into Health Studies

The SCCS provides a prime example of partnership with federally qualified health centers, institutions targeting services to the segments of the US population often at highest disease risk and most in need of both healthcare and disease prevention services (Macinko and Elo 2009). In the SCCS pilot study, with the buy-in and encouragement of the MW leadership, staff were hired to approach attendees at the clinic to explain the SCCS rationale and seek their enrollment in this long-term follow-up study assessing cancer risks. Small ($10) monetary incentives were offered, which were highly useful in low-income populations, although many individuals were persuaded that there may be eventual societal benefit from a study attempting to determine the causes of and contributors to cancer. The participants consented to the nearly hour-long computer-assisted personal interview that asked about their medical history, personal habits like smoking, alcohol consumption, diet and exercise, and other characteristics and also requested donation of a biologic sample (preferably blood).

The pilot study showed that CHC-based recruitment was feasible, and thus this approach became the linchpin of the recruitment efforts for the full-scale study (Signorello et al. 2010, 2005; Spence and Oltmanns 2011). Over the period 2002–2009, a total of 71 CHCs partnered in the SCCS, with staff hired in each center to seek enrollment into the SCCS among adults aged 40–79 visiting the CHCs. CHCs in the 12-state (AL, AR, FL, GA, KY, LA, MS, NC, SC, TN, VA, WV) SCCS catchment area were identified in listings of federally qualified health centers maintained by the Health Resources and Services Administration. We then sought interest in joining the SCCS from the CHCs with the largest numbers of adults, particularly African Americans, aged 40–79, with all but a few of the CHCs contacted agreeing to participate. The CHCs themselves were diverse, some covering urban inner city populations, e.g., MW in Nashville TN and Southside Medical Center in Atlanta GA, while others served primarily black, e.g., Delta Health Center in Mound Bayou MS, or white, e.g., Rural Health Services Consortium in Rogersville TN, rural populations.

At the CHCs, the interviewers hired specifically for the SCCS were generally stationed near waiting areas of the clinics and approached persons appearing to be age eligible to ask if they may be interested in joining the SCCS. While the primary qualifications for the interviewers related to experience in health care, social work, survey, or personal services professions, we also considered racial/ethnic and residential concordance between the interviewers and potential SCCS enrollees to be an advantage, especially given the history of recruiting African American participants into health studies. Thus, most interviewers were African American to match the majority black status of the SCCS population. All interviewers received specific training by the study team, itself diverse, in the goals and methods of the SCCS. Among the challenges faced was the integration of the individuals employed specifically for the SCCS into the overall operations of the CHC. The SCCS work could not be disruptive of the patient flow or other CHC tasks, but rather had to fit near seamlessly into routine CHC practices. This was accomplished by close coordination between the interviewers at the CHCs and the VUMC–MMC–IEI study team, with often daily phone and email communication to prevent, and also identify and resolve, any emerging problems. Critical to the smooth operations were the support and encouragement from the CHC directors, which the directors were willing to provide in part because they realized the potential long-term benefits of the research for the populations they served.

Recruitment proceeded by the interviewers providing information about the goals and procedures of the SCCS to potential participants. Those willing to join then reviewed and signed informed consent documents before proceeding to the personal interview about their characteristics and being asked to donate a 20-mL blood specimen. If bloods were to be collected as part of the procedures generating their visit to the CHC, then arrangements were made to draw additional amounts in 10-mL serum and 10-mL EDTA tubes. Those not willing to provide blood specimens were asked to provide mouth rinse or saliva specimen. Beginning in the third year of recruitment, we also began to ask for urine samples. Over 90% of the participants agreed to provide a biologic specimen. This very high biologic specimen donation rate is a distinct advantage for cohort studies attempting to assess molecular or genetic contributors to health risks, since DNA can be extracted for nearly all the participants and molecular biomarkers in blood, urine, and saliva measured for large subsets of the cohort, and is one of the distinct advantages of CHC-based recruitment.

Follow-up of the cohort is ongoing passively and actively, with both activities coordinated centrally for efficiency purposes. Passive follow-up involves linkage with Social Security Administration (SSA) and National Death Index (NDI) registers accessed annually to provide essentially complete ascertainment of vital status and cause of death for the deceased (Spence and Oltmanns 2011), and linkage with cancer registries in each of the 12 states accessed annually to ascertain incident cancers among participants. The cancer registries provide close to complete ascertainment of incident cancers, although efficiencies would be possible if a national cancer registry combining NCI-funded SEER registries and CDC/state-funded registries could be established. Tracking incidence rates for diseases other than cancer has been problematic since there are no standardized national registries monitoring incidence of heart disease, stroke, diabetes, and multiple other chronic illnesses. However, mortality from these diseases is obtainable from the NDI, and, for over two-thirds of the cohort, non-

fatal events can be ascertained from linkage of the SCCS with Medicare or Medicaid claims files. Active follow-up involves attempted contact by mail and then phone with participants themselves approximately every 4 years to update smoking status, weight, and other characteristics and ask about self-reported health events. While passive follow-up is essentially complete, aided by our collection of Social Security Numbers in addition to full names and dates of birth, active follow-up is challenging because of the low incomes and mobility of many cohort members. Nevertheless, over 70% of surviving cohort members have responded to the first or second follow-up surveys conducted up to 12 years after enrollment.

16.5 SCCS Risk Factor Prevalences by Demographic Status

The recruitment strategy resulted in the SCCS population having high percentages of persons with low levels of income and education (Table 16.1). The inclusion of persons resident in cities as well as suburban and rural areas across 12 southern states also resulted in a diverse population of black and white (predominantly non-Hispanic) within the low-end of the socioeconomic status (SES) spectrum, and provides a stark contrast with other longstanding US cohorts comprised mainly of middle and higher income whites, but the recruitment of a portion of the cohort from general population sources expanded the range of demographic characteristics of cohort members. Concomitant with the low SES of CHC-recruited

Table 16.1 Some characteristics of SCCS participants

Indicator	CHC ($n \approx 73,500$)	Gen pop ($n \approx 12,500$)
<12 years education	33%	9%
<$15K household income	61%	20%
Obesity (BMI > 30)	44%	40%
Diabetes	21%	18%
Percent hypertension	55%	49%
Percent current smoker	45%	21%

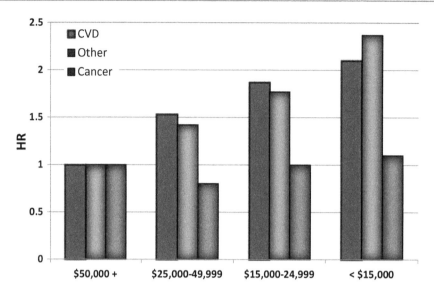

Fig. 16.3 Cause-specific mortality hazard ratios according to household income

Table 16.2 Standardized Mortality Ratios (relative to US age–sex–race-specific general population) among black and white men and women in the SCCS

	Males		Females	
Cause of death	Black	White	Black	White
• All (n = 10,784)	1.46	1.86	1.19	1.70
• All cancer (n = 2663)	1.31	1.43	1.06	1.22
• Lung cancer (n = 896)	1.56	1.70	1.18	1.56
• Diabetes (n = 601)	1.81	2.38	1.51	2.42
• Cardiovascular disease (n = 2533)	1.34	1.88	1.16	1.98
• Stroke (n = 486)	1.36	1.67	1.09	1.12
• Respiratory disease (n = 777)	1.43	2.16	1.11	2.20

Follow up thru 12/31/2013

participants are higher prevalences of smoking, obesity, and other conditions often associated with low SES, with the high obesity and diabetes, but not smoking, prevalences also seen in general population recruits (Table 16.1). The high percentages with obesity in both segments of the cohort correspond to the high southern regional prevalence of obesity shown in Fig. 16.2.

Analyses conducted thus far show that risk of all-cause mortality varies sharply by measures of SES, especially income, with a more than doubled death rate among the poorest (<$15,000) vs. highest (≥$50,000) reported annual household incomes (Fig. 16.3) (Wojcik et al. 2010). The excess is far more prominent for CVD than for cancer. Further, once SES is tightly accounted for, differences associated with race/ethnicity are greatly attenuated. Indeed, within the SCCS,

overall SES-adjusted hazard ratios for all-cause, cancer, and CVD mortality tend to be no higher among blacks than whites (www.southerncommunitystudy.org n.d.).

The combination of low SES, high smoking, and obesity contributes to standardized mortality ratios (SMRs) among black and white men and women each being elevated compared with national race- and sex-specific norms, with the highest SMRs for whites (Table 16.2). The excess death rates and their close ties to SES highlight the importance of improving disease prevention strategies targeting lower income segments of American society. While beyond the scope of this chapter, intense study is underway to explore associations with SES, ancestry, social and local environments, and risks of specific health outcomes all while accounting for lifestyle and biologic factors also associated with disease risks. As the cohort matures, the numbers of cancer and other health events will grow increasingly larger enabling multiple hypotheses about the determinants of risk, outcome, and disparities to be investigated. Further, the SCCS will also provide a population base within which interventions aimed at primary, secondary, or tertiary prevention can be carried out. Already being pilot tested is a randomized trial assessing feasibility of administering a "polypill" to reduce cardiovascular and cancer risk in the community health center setting, which if successful could provide a model for national implementation. The SCCS has established a diverse Intervention Planning Core to bring together study team members and additional experts in behavioral and implementation research with CHC and other community members to develop culturally appropriate strategies to combat smoking, obesity, and other conditions disproportionately affecting underserved populations and to do so in a community-based participatory manner.

16.6   Lessons Learned

Designing, pilot testing, launching, and carrying out the SCCS has provided a series of lessons learned that may be applicable not only for enhancing the continued operation of the SCCS but also useful for other research endeavors aimed at assessing disparities and achieving health equity across diverse populations. The SCCS has demonstrated:

- *The importance and advantages of partnering with CHCs for research studies addressing underserved populations.* A network of CHCs was successfully engaged across 12 southern states, with some of the centers having the effort be its initial contribution to an epidemiologic study and some having the SCCS be one of its largest research projects undertaken. We discovered that CHCs can be willing partners in research, even though their primary mission is health care and even though they often face daily challenges in providing care and preventative services to low-income patients, many without health insurance. Approximately 73,500 adults were enrolled in

the SCCS at CHCs, the largest compilation of mainly low-income adults ever assembled with detailed baseline information and biospecimens undergoing prospective follow-up, providing a clear demonstration that collaboration with CHCs in large-scale research is feasible and highly effective.

- *That conducting health research within communities is not only enabled but also enhanced by working with local representatives of the community and by incorporating diversity in views of what research should be about.* The initial concept of the SCCS to investigate the determinants of elevated cancer rates in socially disadvantaged groups in the south arose in an academic setting, but the key initial discussions about implementation of the research were molded around ideas presented by the community, especially by CHC staff. The academicians among us quickly learned that perceptions persisted in the community about researchers swooping in to seek participants as guinea pigs for their research, with information sought more for the researchers' gain than for actually alleviating the disease burden or suffering of the participants. Being a "researcher" conveyed negative images among some in the community, especially if the researchers were university or government employees. Thus, "giving back" in the sense of providing information that might be beneficial to the participants either directly or indirectly by advancing knowledge of disease risks for the participants, their families, or neighborhoods was essential. Since there were no immediate clinical benefits from participating in the SCCS, we relied in large part on the altruistic values when asking persons to consider enrolling, hoping that the discoveries made would eventually filter back to help improve health status and reduce future chances of developing cancer. Although many of the SCCS participants had more proximal concerns about daily living problems, the message that their participation may in the future help others carried considerable weight.
- *That multiple practical issues arise in conducting epidemiologic field research among a low-income population resident across a broad*

geographic area. Since linkages with national and state health registries may provide nearly complete ascertainment of cancer and other health events, having key identifying information on each participant is crucial. We obtained a social security number (SSN) for over 97% of SCCS participants, a necessity for linkage with SSA, Medicare, or Medicaid rosters and a distinct advantage for linkages with state cancer registries, all of which are based on probabilistic matching of identifying information (SSN plus name, sex, and date of birth). We found that collection of biologic specimens was greatly facilitated by enrolling participants at CHCs, since collecting blood or urine in a clinic setting was routine and we could collect a specimen for research from nearly all persons for whom a biologic sample was requested. This was not the case for those recruited into the SCCS from the general population, although 81% did mail in a mouth rinse sample from which DNA can be extracted. We confirmed that providing even a small monetary compensation for the time and effort to join the study and complete follow-up questionnaires was useful, perhaps particularly so because of the low-income status of many of the participants. We found that direct follow-up via re-contact is challenging, in part because of frequent changes of address and phone numbers among disadvantaged groups, and that multiple modes (direct mail and telephone and indirect linkage with national change of address and other tracing systems) of follow-up are needed to update participant status. We sent repeat mailings to non-responders to mailed follow-up questionnaires. However, we have found that response rates for each subsequent mailing of a particular questionnaire tend to be less than half that of the immediately prior mailing so that the diminishing returns make more than two or three repeat mailings not effective.

• And that a culturally and educationally diverse study team providing multiple points of view can be effective and can coalesce around common goals and approaches to help develop and carry out research in cancer etiology, prevention, and control targeted toward ameliorating

health disparities and reducing the burden of cancer across all groups of Americans.

References

Adler NE, Newman K. Socioeconomic disparities in health: pathways and policies. Health Aff. 2002;21(2):60–6.

American Psychological Association. Committee on Socioeconomic Status. Examining the Complexities between Health Disparities and Poverty; 2014. p. 38. www.apa.org/pi/ses/resources/poverty-bibliography.aspx.

Buchowski MS, Schlundt DG, Hargreaves MK, Hankin JH, Signorello LB, Blot WJ. Development of a culturally sensitive food frequency questionnaire for use in the Southern Community Cohort Study. Cell Mol Biol. 2003;49(8):1295–304.

Chetty R, Stepner M, Abraham S, Lin S, Scuderi B, Turner N, Bergeron A, Cutler D. The association between income and life expectancy in the United States, 2001-2014. JAMA. 2016;315(16):1750–66. PMC4866586

Hargreaves MK, Arnold CW, Blot WJ. Community health centers: their role in the treatment of minorities and in health disparities research. In: Satcher D, Pamies R, editors. Multicultural medicine and health disparities. New York: McGraw-Hill; 2006. p. 485–94.

Macinko J, Elo IT. Black-white differences in avoidable mortality in the USA, 1980-2005. J Epidemiol Community Health. 2009;63(9):715–21.

Shaya FT, Gbarayor CM, Yang HK, Agyerman-Duah M, Saunders E. A perspective on African American participation in clinical trials. Contemp Clin Trials. 2007;28(2):213–7.

Signorello LB, Hargreaves MK, Steinwandel MD, Zheng W, Cai Q, Schlundt DG, Buchowski MS, Arnold CW, McLaughlin JK, Blot WJ. Southern Community Cohort Study: establishing a cohort to investigate health disparities. J Natl Med Assoc. 2005;97(7):972–9. PMC2569308

Signorello LB, Hargreaves MK, Blot WJ. The southern community cohort study: investigating health disparities. J Health Care Poor Underserved. 2010;21(Suppl 1):26–37. PMC2940058

Signorello LB, Cohen SS, Williams DR, Munro HM, Hargreaves MK, Blot WJ. Socioeconomic status, race, and mortality: a prospective cohort study. Am J Public Health. 2014;104(12):e98–e107. PMC4232159

Spence CT, Oltmanns TF. Recruitment of African American men: Overcoming challenges for an epidemiological study of personality and health. Cultur Divers Ethnic Minor Psychol. 2011;1(4):377–80. PMC3192307

Wojcik MC, Huebner WW, Jorgensen G. Strategies for using the National Death Index and the Social Security Administration for death ascertainment in large occupational cohort mortality studies. Am J Epidemiol. 2010;172(4):469–77.

www.southerncommunitystudy.org

Part V
Team Formation

Team Assembly

Marlon Twyman and Noshir Contractor

Contents

17.1 Introduction

The study of team assembly is a crucial area of research for the team science community. Not only are teams an essential component of the scientific enterprise (Falk-Krzesinski et al. 2010; Katz and Martin 1997), but there are now more observational data available to help understand the team assembly process (Pentland 2012). As a result, there is currently a convergence of social science theory, readily available digital data

M. Twyman
University of Southern California, Los Angeles, CA, USA

N. Contractor (✉)
Northwestern University, Evanston, IL, USA
e-mail: nosh@northwestern.edu

traces, and web-based technologies that leverage theories and insights from multiple domains to better understand and enable team assembly (Contractor 2013). The convergence could not have come at a better time. With the uncertainty surrounding scientific research funding, providing researchers with insights into the assembly of effective teams will aid them in maximizing their chances for scientific success and innovation.

Much scientific achievement relies on well-functioning and effective teams (Kozlowski and Bell 2019; Kozlowski and Ilgen 2006; Mathieu et al. 2008; National Research Council 2015; Shneiderman 2016). Science teams are required to effectively combine knowledge to produce novel, high-impact products (Uzzi et al. 2013). Facilitating such high-impact scientific research requires the allocation and coordination of many resources, including people, samples, equipment, and computational facilities (Shrum et al. 2007). Leveraging these scarce and needed resources makes collaboration a necessity, distributed teams more common, and interdisciplinary research essential in the current science environment (Cummings and Kiesler 2014). The prevalence of multi-university science teams who publish high-impact research is indicative of the need to assemble qualified teams despite such constraints (Jones et al. 2008). Additionally, international collaborations have become key for scientific growth (Coccia and Wang 2016). Unfortunately, science teams collaborating in these situations may report less productive out-comes and face higher coordination costs (Cummings and Kiesler 2007).

In addition to the move towards multi-university, geographically distributed teams, science is increasingly turning to interdisciplinary teams. Interdisciplinary research is valuable because taking a problem-based perspective for conducting research focuses on addressing a problem while not being confined within the traditions of a single discipline (Jacobs and Frickel 2009). However, most organizations still maintain disciplinary foci and rely on individuals and teams to span the necessary boundaries to conduct scientific research involving multiple disciplines (Ancona and Caldwell 1992a; Dahlander and McFarland 2013). The organizational structure influences the performance of interdisciplinary teams because locating people with needed knowledge is often the responsibility of people who already have cross-disciplinary and interdepartmental connections (Burt 2004, 2009; Hansen 1999; Reagans and McEvily 2003; Singh et al. 2010). The creation of interdisciplinary research centers is a solution that has been enacted to alleviate some knowledge transfer issues that occur within research organizations (Dahlander and McFarland 2013; Jacobs and Frickel 2009). The presence of such centers is an example of the commitment made to assembling productive interdisciplinary research teams, but coordination challenges still arise due to distance when different center-affiliated departments are not in close physical proximity (Birnholtz et al. 2012; Nomura et al. 2008).

Clearly, assembling interdisciplinary teams is critical for, but not a guarantee of, success. The demand to assemble interdisciplinary teams is stimulated by the increase in interdisciplinary initiatives by funding agencies. Analyses of National Science Foundation (NSF) project proposals for two interdisciplinary initiatives show that researchers who win highly competitive research awards and grants have successful prior collaboration records with team members but cite different bodies of knowledge increasing the odds for offering new insights based on novel combination of ideas (Lungeanu et al.

2014). Collaboration is not the only requirement for success, but assembling a team of people who have demonstrated the ability to work well together and provide different perspectives is essential for winning a research grant. However, even the grant-winning research teams face challenges. One such challenge is the productivity penalty encountered by interdisciplinary researchers. The complexity in navigating across multiple scientific communities results in some researchers having lower productivity (Leahey et al. 2016).

Because specific combinations of people affect performance, developing an understanding of the factors that impact team assembly is crucial. Collaboration in teams has long been an important component of many work tasks in scientific research (Hagstrom 1964; Leahey 2016). Effectively managing relationships within a team plays a key role in team performance, and simply put, assembling the wrong people into a team can derail a project from its beginning (Gewin 2015). To avoid such derailment, developing and openly communicating expectations before beginning a collaborative project is a useful strategy to help increase the chances of having a productive collaboration (Gadlin and Jessar 2002). Considering factors other than expertise when assembling a team is a necessity given the recent empirical evidence showing trends of increasing collaboration (Leahey 2016; Wuchty et al. 2007). As an example, the team size in scientific fields has been increasing over time (Guimerà et al. 2005; Lee et al. 2015; Milojević 2014; Valderas 2007). Additionally, incorporating new team members when assembling teams promotes new ideas and perspectives since performance suffers with repeated collaborations (Guimerà et al. 2005; Reagans et al. 2004; Rink et al. 2013; Skilton and Dooley 2010). We conceptualize team assembly to be broader than the related concept of team composition because we consider not only the individual and team characteristics but also the impact of broader social networks and the organizing processes within which these teams assemble (Humphrey and Aime 2014). Specifically, we delineate the factors influencing team assembly into perspectives operating at

Table 17.1 Key concepts and definitions

Key concept	Concise definition
Team assembly	Factors leading to the formation of teams
Staff-assembled team	A team whose members are staffed by a person either in the team or someone outside the team. The team members have low agency in the selection of the members. In some cases, a manager will staff a team.
Self-assembled team	A team whose members self-select into the team. The team members have high agency in the selection of the members. Research, creative, and consultant teams are more often self-assembled than teams in other industries.
Compositional perspective	Explaining team assembly based on the individual attributes of the members in the nucleating team.
Relational perspective	Explaining team assembly based on prior and current social relationships that exist both among members of the nucleating team as well as with others outside the team.
Ecosystem perspective	Explaining team assembly based on the interlocking structure of teams within which the nucleating team is embedded.
Apprentice-based collaboration	Collaborations that include a senior researcher working with others of lower experience levels, including, –but not limited to –students, technicians, and other researchers
Peer collaboration	Collaborations among researchers at the same career level. For example, student-student collaborations.

three levels: a compositional perspective, relational perspective, and an ecosystem perspective. Our goal for this chapter is to provide a review of the team assembly literature when teams are either staffed or self-assembled. Additionally, we highlight the potential role that technology plays in assembling and studying the team assembly process. The key concepts associated with this chapter are listed and defined in Table 17.1.

17.2 Chapter Roadmap

We begin the chapter by distinguishing between two types of team assembly: *staffed* and *self-assembled*. A staffed team is one that is appointed by a person either outside the team or by a person within the team who mandates participation by others. Self-assembled teams are those where individuals have more agency in self-organizing into teams. It is possible for teams to be a hybrid of both assembly types. As an example, a large research team may form based on the self-assembly into a team by a group of senior researchers. However, they might then staff teams that work on various components of the project. Detailing both *team staffing* and *team self-assembly* provides coverage for how such a hybrid research collaboration is assembled.

Recognizing these differences in the ways in which teams assemble, we next turn to the different perspectives relevant for assembling teams. Clearly, it is important to consider the qualifications, expertise, and abilities of each team member to help ensure the success of projects (Bell 2007; Cooke et al. 2015; Nurius and Kemp 2019; Woolley et al. 2008). The characteristics of team members are then aggregated to give an indication of the entire team's ability to perform (Klein and Kozlowski 2000; Kozlowski and Klein 2000). Using information about individuals' characteristics or attributes as criteria for team assembly reflects what we define as the *compositional* perspective.

However, it is also evident that simply having a collection of individuals with the requisite expertise is a necessary, but not sufficient, condition for success. Research has increasingly considered the relationships, interactions, and the match (similarity or complementarity) of individuals' attributes as important factors influencing team performances. We define the consideration of these criteria for team assembly as the *relational* perspective. There is a growing body of research using the relational perspective. For example, teams whose members have had prior collaborations are more creative and productive across multiple domains (Guimerà et al. 2005; Perretti and Negro 2007; Skilton and Dooley 2010; Uzzi and Spiro 2005), teams composed of friends have more positive work experiences (Jehn and Shah 1997; Ren et al. 2014; Shah and Jehn 1993), and accessing and utilizing diverse knowledge in a team relies on interpersonal networks (Reagans and McEvily 2003; Reagans et al. 2016; Reagans et al. 2004; Reagans and Zuckerman 2001). Quite simply, people's prior relationships influence their assembly into a team and its subsequent performance.

In addition to the compositional and relational perspectives, team assembly is also influenced by the larger networks of prior and current teams where individuals have membership. Working on multiple scientific teams simultaneously is a reality facing most science professionals (González and Mark 2004; Hudson et al. 2002; Scupelli et al. 2005). Individuals on these multiple teams each have members who are in turn on multiple other teams. Some of the membership across these teams overlaps, creating team interlocks. A team interlock exists between two teams that share one or more members (Lungeanu et al. 2018). The collection of teams who are connected by team interlocks to other teams that are in turn connected to even more teams results in an ecosystem of teams. Recent research shows that forces within the ecosystem explain the assembly and performance of teams above and beyond what is explained from a compositional or relational perspective. We refer to this approach as the *ecosystem perspective*. Competing commitments and obligations of the ecosystem often influence a person's ability to collaborate in teams based on the environment (Mortensen 2014). As a result, many professionals have multiteam memberships and competing task dynamics that affect the amount of engagement that one gives to any team at a single point in time (O'Leary et al. 2011; Wageman et al. 2012). On the positive side, information spreading through team interlocks also has the potential to bring new ideas and resources to a team. Therefore, the larger ecosystem in which a team is embedded influences the nature of collaboration and the dynamics of team assembly. To summarize, team assembly must be understood as being influenced by factors operat-

ing at three levels—compositional, relational, and ecosystem perspectives.

Following an elucidation of factors influencing team assembly from these three perspectives, we will consider the potential role of technology in enabling and understanding team assembly. While a much deeper treatment of research networking systems is offered in the following chapter (Weber and Yuan 2019), we focus here on how technology can leverage insights from research on team assembly to facilitate the formation of more effective teams. Many of today's social interactions are mediated through technology, and many teams use online platforms such as communities and forums, social media, shared document editing software, and messaging applications to collaborate and coordinate around their work tasks. Many of these online platforms, such as nanoHUB, GitHub, and other open-source software development networks, require individuals to self-assemble into teams (Dabbish et al. 2012; Hahn et al. 2008; Hertel et al. 2003; Margolin et al. 2012). However, there is a pressing need for these platforms to improve their ability to provide members with evidence-based tools to assemble into effective teams. In other words, there is a need for developing the equivalent of matchmaking tools like match.com, eHarmony, and Tinder to help assemble teams. Lastly and relatedly, the emergence and use of these matchmaking tools to enable team assembly also have the collateral benefit of providing researchers with data to further advance our understanding of team assembly and collaboration at scale.

17.3   Types of Team Assembly

Key Takeaway: An outside authority is responsible for the performance of a staffed team, while self-assembled teams are responsible for their own success.

In scientific research, as in other domains, there are at least two ways in which teams assemble: staff-assembled and self-assembled. People are either assigned to a specific team or self-assemble. In this chapter, staffing a team is analogous to assigning members to a team, and the terms are used interchangeably. There are different considerations to be made by those who need to staff a team in which they may also be a member as compared to those who self-assemble into a team.

17.3.1 Staffed Teams

The staffer of a team may be a principal investigator of a research laboratory, a manager within an organization, or an administrator of scientific research. Additionally, the staffer typically will have responsibility for the team's performance and must attempt to predict a team's potential for achieving the desired goals (Reagans et al. 2004). A staffer, who may or may not be a member of the team, will also seek to ensure that the members of staffed teams meet requirements for skills and diversity, but the team members ultimately have to be willing to utilize the same factors that the staffer and management deem to be necessary requirements for work (Aalbers et al. 2013; Shin et al. 2012). In staff-assembled teams, member understandably feel low agency as compared to self-assembled teams (Contractor 2013; Hackman 1987). Hence, when staffing teams, there is a risk that members will have lower commitment since they did not have much agency to choose the teammates with which they must work (Colquitt et al. 2007; Deci and Ryan 2002). Therefore, a team staffer needs to be cognizant of the planned tasks, requirements for the team members, and expectations for the team processes needed to achieve successful performance outcomes (Stevens and Campion 1999; Thompson 2018).

Staffing a team is a core component of the apprentice-based collaboration model in science where a scientist with some form of authority is making decisions about the students and technicians whose work will be needed to accomplish the scientific goals of the team (Hagstrom 1964). When staffing a team in such a scenario, it is necessary for the staffer to provide well-defined plans and articulate performance expectations because teams vary in their abilities to guide themselves (Hackman et al. 1976). In addition to having a developed task, plans, and expectations, a team staffer will also need to consider the characteristics of the team itself with regard to the abilities of the members, the overall diversity of the team, and imposed constraints from higher levels of management or the organization (Thompson 2018). A team staffer needs to rely upon compositional attributes like the personality, mental ability, and teamwork skills of potential team members when making selections for a team (Stevens and Campion 1999; Zaccaro and Dirosa 2012). Staffing a team places much of the responsibility for the team's performance on a person who the person staffing in the collaboration.

17.3.2 Self-Assembled Teams

Self-assembly generally suggests a bottom-up process where actors self-organize themselves (Pelesko 2007). Some scientific teams are commonly self-assembled and exist in a dynamic environment where people freely work with multiple collaborators (Wang and Hicks 2015). A computational model for team assembly only using team size, the fraction of newcomers, and the tendency to repeat collaborations reproduced the empirical trends of co-authorship in multiple scientific fields (Guimerà et al. 2005). While the self-assembly of these high-impact science teams was explained by simple organizing principles, the teams achieved great impact.

Historically, science has been associated with independence and intellectual freedom for the scientists participating in the enterprise (Fox and Faver 1984). Despite the autonomy of choice, collaboration is necessary for most scientists and self-assembling teams is a manifestation of the agency of people to collaborate with who they choose. People who have such independence are also able to engage in "dating" collaborations where they can learn about new teammates, even strangers, through small projects before agreeing to longer duration, high-commitment projects (Lykourentzou et al. 2017; Lykourentzou et al. 2016). Teams with the autonomy to identify and then select people for the given task requirements have a better understanding of the needed skills and work for a team to be successful, and can adjust to the task requirements through their selection of members (Harrison and Humphrey 2010). The ability to self-assemble is indicative of the peer collaboration model in science where people exercise agency in deciding with whom to collaborate, in contrast with the apprentice-based collaboration model where staffed teams are more prevalent (Hagstrom 1964).

Team members who self-assemble are responsible for making choices based on personal motivations and consider the complementary skills and skill levels of potential team members (Zhu et al. 2013) as well as social norms in a research environment (Kraut et al. 1987). When self-assembled teams are composed of friends and acquaintances, the teams tend to perform better than staff-assembled teams (Jehn and Shah 1997). Self-assembled teams that are successful also tend to collaborate with one another again for knowledge-intensive projects (Hahn et al. 2008). As suggested earlier, the preference of people to self-assemble into teams is related to their self-determination and agency, which positively influences intrinsic motivation (Bandura 1989; Deci and Ryan 2002). Following this logic, people will be more motivated to work on a team if they have agency in assembling it. People who collaborate in autonomous work groups have more positive attitudes and are more socially motivated by their teammates (Cordery et al. 1991; Grant and Berry 2011). Self-assembling teams have responsibility for their own abilities, and they design their own collaborations.

17.4　Perspectives on Team Assembly

Key Takeaway: Team assembly combines compositional, relational, and ecosystem perspectives, resulting in a multilevel, holistic understanding of the process.

Regardless of whether a team is staffed or self-assembled, there are expectations that a given team will be able to perform and achieve a stated goal. For this reason, using all available information when assembling a team will aid the

team in performing well. Designing, or at least understanding, the work context and the tasks being planned for the team is a key consideration in team assembly and requires multiple types of characteristics (Morgeson and Humphrey 2008). There are factors at multiple levels that influence a team, and the science of team science benefits from considering the individual level to the system level (Börner et al. 2010). Using information about the composition of the team (compositional), the collaboration network (relational), and structural features in which the teams are embedded (ecosystem) helps explain productivity and key team processes (Bercovitz and Feldman 2011; Reagans et al. 2004; Stvilia et al. 2011). For many science teams, their work occurs in concert with other teams through the sharing of facilities and resources (Dahlander and McFarland 2013; Jacobs and Frickel 2009; Shrum et al. 2007). Accounting for such interdependencies and contextual factors when assembling teams helps create productive teams for the modern scientific environment.

A helpful example to illustrate the usefulness of using factors at multiple levels is the assembly of teams in the field of cancer research. The demands for diverse skills and perspectives required for cancer research create many opportunities for collaboration and interaction among multiple disciplines (Savage 2018). This results in a large-scale effort of multiple teams to develop solutions to provide better treatment and prevention of cancer (Saporito 2013). There are numerous teams who are composed of highly trained individuals who specialize in some area of inquiry; have interdependencies within the team based on sharing information, results, and research data; and coordinate their research efforts with other science teams researching novel solutions for curing cancer. The fact that science teams are researching in concert with other teams is a manifestation of the notion of "teaming"—the notion that modern, high-impact teams are more dynamic with respect to their membership and individuals are connected to multiple teams based on needs at a given moment (Edmondson 2012a, 2012b). Using the cancer research example to illustrate this point, it is not uncommon for multiple teams to share the same imaging specialist because there may be a finite number of research centers with the resources to perform a specific type of imaging. In such a case, the imaging specialist is a valued team member for multiple teams and focuses her work based on multiple needs of different teams.

There are countless other examples of how reflecting upon a team's composition, relationships, and embeddedness within a larger ecosystem will influence the productivity of a science team. Therefore, a practitioner who is cognizant about factors at each level will be able to apply the different perspectives as needed when assembling a team. The members, team context, and organizational context have long been used as inputs to explain effective teams (Mathieu et al. 2008). Including these types of inputs when reflecting upon team assembly further demonstrates the complexity of teams and how to consider the interactions between members (Arrow et al. 2000; Katz et al. 2004). Recognizing these three perspectives will enable a practitioner to be more knowledgeable about assembling high performance teams.

17.4.1 Compositional Perspective of Team Assembly

Teams are important for scientific research, but how are effective, well-performing teams assembled? There is some risk associated with balancing innovative research approaches with traditional and familiar ones (Foster et al. 2015), and assembling the right team helps mitigate some of this risk. When assembling teams, there are numerous factors to consider, including personality and competence in the team (Cable and Edwards 2004; Humphrey et al. 2007; Moynihan and Peterson 2001; Nurius and Kemp 2019; Rulke and Rau 2000), demography (Duguid 2011; Duguid et al. 2012; Gibbs et al. 2019; Joshi and Roh 2009; Williams and O'Reilly 1998), and the requirements of the project (Thompson 2018).

When assembling teams, the members' individual attributes are important in determining the type of team being assembled and the potential for performance. There are numerous individual attributes that contribute to the assembly of effective teams. Individual cognitive ability is important for the completion of individual work tasks and for consideration when assembling teams. However, in addition to the cognitive ability of team members, there are multiple factors that determine the team-level cognitive ability or intelligence (Devine and Philips 2001; Woolley et al. 2010). For example, the ability to integrate and coordinate expertise within a team (Faraj and Sproull 2000), and the inclusion of teamwork skills, personality, and diversity should all be used when assembling teams because these factors affect team performance (Arrow et al. 2000; Mathieu et al. 2008).

Assembling a team also requires diligence in identifying explicit criteria for composition when selecting the most appropriate members for a given team (Stevens and Campion 1999). Including multiple types of individuals is helpful when predicting the performance of an assembled team. As an example, combining personality traits, such as extraversion and emotional stability, along with the ability of team members, explains positive supervisor ratings for team performance and team viability (Barrick et al. 1998). Decision-making teams with a hierarchy are more accurate in their decisions when the leader and other members have high cognitive ability and conscientiousness (LePine et al. 1997). In addition to cognitive ability, personality, and technical competencies, other knowledge, skills, and abilities (KSA) are needed for productive collaboration in teams. KSA for teamwork are a set of attributes that help account for necessary interactions within a team collaboration environment (Kozlowski and Ilgen 2006; Stevens and Campion 1994). KSA differ from technical competencies because a successful team needs people who are not only capable of accomplishing their tasks, but also performing interpersonal and management functions that help the team collectively accomplish their goals (Klimoski and Jones 1995; Stevens and Campion 1994). Overall, social skills, experience in teams, and personality are important for assembling teams because belonging to a team is a social activity where team members will need to engage beyond the work tasks and the abilities of team members (Lepine and Dyne 2001; LePine et al. 2000; Morgeson et al. 2005).

In addition to surface level composition factors (such as age and gender), combinations of deep-level composition factors explain team performance in a variety of settings (Bell 2007). A meta-analysis of 89 studies showed that the relationship between compositional variables and team performance differed in field and laboratory research settings. Most field settings focused on the performance of physical teams, and the following personality traits emerged as consistent predictors of team performance: team minimum agreeableness and team mean conscientiousness, openness to experience, collectivism, and preference for teamwork. Meanwhile, laboratory settings mostly focused on the performance of intellectual teams, and only negligible effects were observed for the relationships between personality traits and team performance. The important factors related to team performance in laboratory settings were team minimum general mental ability, maximum general mental ability, and team mean emotional intelligence (Bell 2007). The meta-analysis highlights the value of using personality traits and combinations of traits when studying teams in specific types of settings.

In addition, compositional perspectives have also considered the heterogeneity that exists among team members. For science teams, the presence of multiple disciplines within the team is often required or desirable (Jacobs and Frickel 2009; Leahey 2016; Leahey et al. 2016; Lungeanu et al. 2014). The purpose of interdisciplinary teams is to incorporate different perspectives towards a single problem's solution. Appreciating heterogeneity helps to ensure a proper understanding of the team's composition, the roles that members possess within a team, and the expectations for performance of a team (Humphrey et al. 2009; Klein et al. 1994; Stewart 2006; Welbourne et al. 1998). When determining the fit of heterogeneous team members, the fit of members along personality and skills brings deeper understanding to a team's composition

(Cable and Edwards 2004; Hollenbeck et al. 2002; Humphrey et al. 2007).

There are two views of fit that determine whether a team should include a given member: supplementary fit and complementary fit (Kristof 1996; Kristof-Brown et al. 2005; Muchinsky and Monahan 1987). According to Muchinsky and Monahan (1987), supplementary fit suggests that a "person fits into some environmental context because he or she supplements, embellishes, or possesses characteristics which are similar to other individuals in this environment" (p. 269). For a science team, an example of supplementary fit would be assembling a team of researchers who all have demonstrated the ability to independently perform high-impact research in their area of expertise. On the other hand, complementary fit states "the characteristics of an individual serve to 'make whole' or complement the characteristics of an environment. The environment is seen as either being deficient in or requiring a certain type of person in order to be effective" (Muchinsky and Monahan 1987, p. 271). An example of complementary fit in a science team is the inclusion of a team member who has unique technical skills that others do not possess. The presence of the complementary skills in the team expands the types of research that the team can pursue.

Aside from the fit of team members within a team, using diversity along different dimensions when assembling a science team has implications for a team's future performance. Although there is a long tradition of using demography as part of selection criteria in organizations, managers still face challenges when assembling demographically diverse teams (Page 2008; Reagans et al. 2004; Williams and O'Reilly 1998). One such challenge is that demography has ambiguous performance implications since there is a trade-off to consider for a team, a demographically diverse team may not have strong familiarity among team members, but will have access to a broader set of perspectives (Reagans et al. 2004). Sometimes, diversity must be considered after a task has been identified, and a team needs to consciously assemble with qualified members who help achieve some level of diversity. The diversity within a team gives an opportunity to gain exposure to multiple unique perspectives, which results in ideas that may be reflective of different genders, races, or age groups (Harrison and Humphrey 2010). However, diversity within a team has likewise been shown to lead to conflict and diminish team functions, processes, and performance (Harrison and Klein 2007; Williams and O'Reilly 1998). Additionally, the context and industry in which work is being performed is a major determining factor in whether a diverse team will have successful team performance (Joshi and Roh 2009). To further illustrate the importance of context for diverse science teams, increasing the gender diversity of science and engineering teams leads to greater productivity when the teams are in disciplines with more female faculty members (Joshi 2014). In this study, the productivity of gender diverse teams is also influenced by the gender representation of a given discipline, further illustrating the value of considering the work context for assembled teams.

Another key aspect of diversity is functional and skill-based diversity. Returning to the example of the interdisciplinary cancer research team, one member was an imaging specialist creating value for several teams due to the unique skills that the teams gained by including the specialist as a member. The increasing complexity of work tasks makes diverse teams essential because such tasks make crossing functional and disciplinary boundaries a standard part of modern collaboration. There is a trade-off to consider when assembling functionally diverse teams, problem-solving and product development stages may benefit from the unique combinations of functional perspectives, but the speed of implementation is diminished because the team is less equipped for teamwork than homogenous teams (Ancona and Caldwell 1992b). Functional diversity is beneficial to consider in team assembly, but it is also important to specify the different forms of functional diversity. There are at least four different ways to consider functional diversity for team members during team assembly: dominant function diversity, functional background diversity, functional assignment diversity, and intraper-

sonal functional diversity (Bunderson and Sutcliffe 2002). Dominant function diversity is the distribution of functional areas represented by team members. Functional background diversity is the difference between team members with respect to their functional backgrounds. Functional assignment diversity is the extent to which the current assignment covers certain functional areas. Lastly, intrapersonal functional diversity is the diversity within each team member's functional experiences; i.e., is a person a functional specialist or a generalist (Bunderson and Sutcliffe 2002). Science teams, both interdisciplinary and disciplinary, rely upon functional diversity, and using a clear conceptualization of functional diversity when assembling the team will make assembly more consistent with respect to the criteria used to assemble a functionally diverse team.

In summary, the composition of a team with respect to competencies, skills, and traits affects a team's collective properties since diversity, team-level ability, and other features are aggregated from individual-level attributes (Mathieu et al. 2008). However, the aggregation of composition factors results in two different types of team properties: shared and configural (Klein and Kozlowski 2000). Although there are differences, both shared and configural properties are the "experiences, attitudes, perceptions, values, cognitions, or behaviors that are held in common by the members of a team" (Klein and Kozlowski 2000, p. 216). Measuring *shared* team properties requires gathering data from individual team members and aggregating the data to the team level. Examples of shared team properties include team mental models, team cohesion, and team satisfaction. Aggregation indicates the amount of sharedness for a property. On the other hand, measuring configural team properties relies on the "array, pattern, or variability of individual characteristics within a team" (Klein and Kozlowski 2000, p. 217). The key distinction between shared and configural properties is that configural properties capture the differences along individual attributes within the team, but shared properties do not capture the differences. Shared and configural properties help incorporate the compositional perspective into understanding the team at a level beyond the individuals. However, the insights obtained from this compositional perspective can be supplemented by including the relational perspective for a team discussed next.

17.4.2 Relational Perspective of Team Assembly

When assembling teams, the relationships among potential team members inform the performance potential of the team. Therefore, developing an awareness for the impact of relationships when assembling teams is immensely important. A team's ability is not only the aggregation of individual attributes but also results from the combination of members and their interactions (Woolley et al. 2010). For individuals, it is important to recognize the need for creating and maintaining relationships throughout a scientific career. Over the years, a scientist will have countless opportunities to collaborate with colleagues having diverse levels of experience, will need to adjust strategies regarding the pursuit or acceptance of collaborations based on personal experiences, and must make conscious decisions about with whom to re-engage in collaboration when assembling new teams (Petersen 2015). Collaboration relies on the ability and effectiveness of team members when *interacting with one another*.

Teams that generate innovative ideas need to interact with the dissenting and divergent-thinking members to simulate a team's creativity (De Dreu and West 2001), and establishing coordination procedures for various social practices and processes ensure effective communication while in a collaboration (Fussell et al. 1998; Kraut and Streeter 1995). To address the need to have useful collaboration practices, scientific researchers have been shown to commonly work with prior collaborators (Guimerà et al. 2005; Norton et al. 2017; Taramasco et al. 2010). Based on previous experience with certain individuals, the preference to work with prior collaborators can be partially attributed to having a clear understanding of collaborators' behaviors and expecta-

tions for coordination (Cummings and Kiesler 2008; Hahn et al. 2008; Hinds et al. 2000; Lungeanu et al. 2014). Groups where members have strong relationships exhibit different interactions and perform better on decision-making and motor tasks when compared to groups of people with weaker relationships (Shah and Jehn 1993). The importance of strong relationships is present when teams encounter and must work through task conflict because team performance suffers most when there are both task conflict and relationship conflict (De Dreu and Weingart 2003). In another example, the combination of within-team interactions, individual attributes of team members, and the leadership relationships in a team provides a multifaceted and nuanced treatment of how relationships and team processes impact a team's performance (Balkundi et al. 2009; Balkundi et al. 2011; Balkundi and Harrison 2006; Balkundi and Kilduff 2006). These examples demonstrate the benefits of a relational perspective in team assembly and its helpfulness in building firmer expectations for the subsequent interactions that will occur within teams.

Given the importance of relationships to teams and their assembly, we adopt concepts and theory from social network theory to provide a relational perspective. There are numerous theoretical explanations that are used to explain the role of social networks in team assembly: self-interest theories, social exchange or dependency theories, mutual or collective interest theories, cognitive theories, and homophily theories (Contractor 2013; Katz et al. 2004; Monge and Contractor 2003). Each of these theories illustrate different motives that people follow when assembling teams, and all are relevant to the scientist who is assembling or being assembled into a team.

Self-interest theory states that actors will behave to maximize their individual interests, while also accounting for the social structure in which an actor belongs (Coleman 1988). This theory is applicable to team assembly because researchers who are assembling into teams will undeniably have their own personal goals and interests they wish to advance by working within the team. While theories of self-interest explain why one individual would like to assemble into a team with another who maximizes the former's self-interest, it does not take into account the latter's self-interest. In such cases, *theories of social exchange* or dependencies theories provide a frame of reference to think about how individuals assemble into teams where each member contributes resources to, and benefits from, others (Emerson 1976). This frame of reference helps to explain why people with different types of resources will collaborate. If one party has access to technological infrastructure while another person has the specific skills required to efficiently use the technological infrastructure for research, then both parties benefit by exchanging their own resource for another resource that they consider valuable. In contrast, *theories of collective action* suggest that multiple people with a shared interest will assemble not because they need resources from each other (as posited by social exchange theory) but because they believe that acting collectively as a team increases their ability to get resources or other outcomes from a third party (Marwell et al. 1988). Research communities like nanoHUB emerge as a "public good" through the collective efforts of many people who find value in the common resource, and teams assembled within such a community are typically composed of people who share a collective interest around advancing nanotechnology research.

Cognitive theories explain team assembly based at least two motivations: cognitive consistency and transactive memory. The first motivation, *cognitive consistency*, uses balance theory to refer to people's need for consistency and balance in social relationships with respect to the perceptions they share with their close relations. The common example is that two friends should both also be friends with a shared third person to create balance to their relationships (Heider 1958). Based on this perspective, individuals are more likely to assemble into teams with those who have collaborated with their previous collaborators. The second motivation, *transactive memory*, refers to team members' ability to identify who possesses expertise and skills within a team and then develop relevant interaction networks to effectively engage and communicate

with the necessary people (Ren and Argote 2011; Wegner 1987, 1995; Wegner et al. 1991). Based on this perspective, individuals are more likely to assemble into teams with those who they believe (based on their transactive memory system) possess the necessary skills required in the team. *Homophily theories* explain the assembly of teams based on the presence of shared characteristics and belonging to the same social groups (McPherson and Smith-Lovin 1987; McPherson et al. 2001; Ruef et al. 2003). Therefore, people are more likely to build relationships with people who are like them along some dimensions; e.g., have the same gender, race, disciplinary expertise, etc. All five of these theoretical families— self-interest, social exchange, collection action, cognitive theories, and homophily—simultaneous contribute to motivations for team assembly. Therefore, incorporating a relational perspective on team assembly is meaningful since science teams rely on multiple types of relationships and need access to multiple information sources to accomplish their research goals.

The prevalence of interdisciplinary teams underscores the value of being able to access multiple information sources. Interdisciplinary teams are privileged in their social networks because their members are diverse along at least some dimensions that are relevant to the problem. Using a network perspective, a team's performance in generating new ideas results from the structural diversity of a team's members and not a team's demographic diversity (Balkundi et al. 2007). Another benefit of diversity comes not only from the unique contributions of each member but also stems from a diverse team's ability to cross organizational and disciplinary boundaries to access unique, nonredundant information (Cross and Cummings 2004; Podolny and Baron 1997). Teams that effectively communicate outside of the unit gain information that helps them in accomplishing their work. Ancona and Caldwell (1992b) observed that a major benefit of functionally diverse teams was the amount of their communication that occurred outside of the team. The teams that engage in external communication activities organize and schedule their activities in such a way to better support a team's chances of being productive and successful (Ancona and Caldwell 1992a).

Teams that are designed with diversity considerations can be assembled to maximize both a team's internal density and external range with respect to the team's interactions (Reagans et al. 2004). A team's internal density is the amount of connections that exist among team members. A team's effectiveness in coordination is diminished if a team does not have strong relationships among members, has a hierarchy, or there is a lack of communication within the team (Cummings and Cross 2003). Assembling a team that has prior network connections has a positive effect on team performance, most likely due to team members being accessible to one another, able to share information with one another, and having relationships before the start of collaboration. Assembling a team that has diverse networks connections outside the team, or external range, also has a positive effect on performance. External range refers to a team's ability to access different parts of a broader network to utilize nonredundant information. The external range is an essential component for the development of a team's social capital and individual's ability to productively transfer knowledge across boundaries and utilize information from diverse information sources (Cummings and Pletcher 2011; Reagans and McEvily 2003; Reagans and Zuckerman 2001). Assembling interdisciplinary teams that have both internal density and external range are better positioned to have success.

More benefits of the relational perspective are apparent when scientific research is understood to exist within a larger community and network (Shrum et al. 2007). Achieving scientific breakthroughs and innovations depends on both the team itself and the broader network of relationships in which the team is embedded. When selecting collaborators, people have many decision criteria and their choices are dynamic and contingent upon their goals, but also the availability, interest, and expertise of others (Bikard et al. 2015). Inventors with patents are able to generate breakthroughs in part because of extended networks and have higher impact because of team and organization affiliation (Singh and Fleming 2010). The ability of such teams to innovate within a scientific industry is influenced and constrained by the overall structure of the network relations (Ahuja 2000). Teams are valuable products of the social environment in which their members exist before assembling a team, and relationships play an important part in understanding science team assembly as part of a much larger ecosystem discussed next.

17.4.3 Ecosystem Perspective of Team Assembly

The preceding sections have underscored the insights offered by the compositional and relational perspectives on team assembly. In this section, we consider how the assembly of a team and its subsequent performance are shaped by the broader ecosystem in which a team is embedded. The effectiveness of teams is "a function of task, group, and organization design factors, environmental factors, internal processes, external processes, and group psychosocial traits" (Cohen and Bailey 1997). Accounting for all such factors results in increasingly complex conceptualizations of the team and task environments to understand the effectiveness of any team (Crawford and Lepine 2013; Marks et al. 2005; Marks et al. 2001; Mathieu et al. 2008). Therefore, teams must assemble to meet the expectations and goals of the larger ecosystem or organization to which they belong. Assessing the performance or ability of a team is highly dependent upon such factors, and the team will not be considered successful without its goals having a strong alignment with the organization (Hackman 1992; Kozlowski and Ilgen 2006).

The ecosystem encompassing scientific research promotes the assembly of interdisciplinary teams (Cummings and Kiesler 2005). As a result, there is high investment in developing infrastructure and physical spaces to facilitate and support interdisciplinary research (Dahlander and McFarland 2013; Jacobs and Frickel 2009). The interactions that occur between collaborations and their supporting infrastructure affect a team's performance. For example, sharing facility and equipment resources may result in scheduling conflicts and delays, or the reporting requirements of an organization may determine the priority of work tasks for a team (Shrum et al. 2001). Scientific enterprises are organized and managed in ways that promote diverse collaboration styles, e.g., bureaucratic, leaderless, nonspecialized, and participatory (Chompalov et al. 2002). These differences in collaboration styles are useful to reflect upon when assembling teams. *Bureaucratic collaboration* is helpful in multi-university or multi-institution projects to help define goals, determine hierarchy and authority structures, and minimize ambiguity in the collaboration while balancing the interests of all parties. *Leaderless collaboration* delegates tasks to parties deemed competent and responsible, while letting the parties maintain control of their main specialties. *Nonspecialized collaboration* typically has a hierarchy and reporting structure but will not delegate or distribute clear responsibilities. *Participatory collaboration* typically takes place within a single discipline, and the members performing tasks tend to manage themselves and regulate the internal activities needed by a research project. Any of these collaboration styles will be determined by the organizations that host the research teams (Chompalov et al. 2002).

Teams pursuing high-risk interdisciplinary research projects are encouraged and rewarded by the modern science ecosystem (Cummings and Kiesler 2014; Lungeanu et al. 2014; Ma et al. 2015). Lungeanu et al. (2018) characterize the ecosystem in terms of team interlocks. Team interlocks ecosystems comprise teams linked to one another through overlapping membership in teams and/or overlapping knowledge domains. Conceptually, team interlock ecosystems offer novel insights about "how the structural characteristics of embedding ecosystems serve as the primordial soup from which new teams assemble" (Lungeanu et al. 2018, p. 1). Specifically, they found that teams were more likely to assembly if the members of the potential team also belonged to other teams, in the immediate neighborhood, that had minimal overlap. Intuitively, this suggests that the members of the nascent team are able to draw upon the ideas and resources

of diverse nonoverlapping other teams in the local ecosystem in which they are embedded. Concurrently, they also found that teams are more likely to assemble when there is considerable overlap in the overall global ecosystem. That is, a nascent team is more likely to nucleate if the potential members of this team belonged to other teams, who had members belonging to other teams, who have members belonging to yet other teams, and there was considerable overlap in membership in the overall global ecosystem. Taken together, these findings suggests that (i) less overlap in the local ecosystem facilitates the assembly of teams that can engage in innovative ideas drawing upon their diverse nonoverlapping sources in other teams and (ii) more overlap in the global ecosystem facilitates the assembly of teams by providing legitimacy to the broader intellectual enterprise in that scientific domain.

The ecosystem has also lead to the birth of new disciplines that emerge to better integrate multiple areas. Using oncofertility as an example, researchers specializing in fertility preservation and researchers specializing in cancer began assembling into teams to explore questions at the intersection of both topics (Lungeanu and Contractor 2015). The emergence of a new discipline means that a team working in such a space must almost exclusively rely on the information that exists within the originating disciplines, and the assembled team must efficiently synthesize the diverse information with the explicit goal of creating something above and beyond each of the parent disciplines. The teams performing these types of tasks rely on their external connections outside of the team (Ancona and Caldwell 1992a, 1992b; Cummings 2004; Cummings and Pletcher 2011), but the quality of the information is the result of the larger ecosystem.

It is complex to navigate a broader ecosystem when collaborating and interacting. A frequent outcome is the emergence of a "structural fold" that occurs among teams that have overlapping membership; it is important to note that the overlapping teams can potentially have highly different levels of ability and experience different levels of success (de Vaan et al. 2015). The overlapping teams make clear that members must constantly make contributions to multiple teams, which is often typical in scientific research. Making contributions to multiple teams requires nontrivial amount of effort by the members. The interdependence among teams is affected by the individuals' goals and decisions regarding where to put their efforts when balancing the interests from multiple teams (Wageman et al. 2012). The concept of teaming refers to the dynamic and changing membership and team activities in which people in the modern collaboration environment participate (Edmondson 2012a, 2012b). Science team members with specialized skills are often faced with prioritizing tasks for multiple teams and are often participating in different teams on a temporary basis. Belonging to multiple teams requires conscious allocation of time and attention by a person, but productivity and learning of people are influenced by the work contexts of the teams and the connections that exist among the teams (O'Leary et al. 2011). These considerations for individuals mean that all team members are balancing potentially conflicting priorities and maintaining a shared understanding for a given team's progress, status, and membership may be difficult for the members (Mortensen 2014). The ecosystem of science teams is dynamic and requires the people therein to manage their responsibilities and obligations, making team assembly dependent upon the team environment.

In summary, the *compositional* perspective considers the combination of individual's attributes and traits, and with this perspective, a person assembling a team can ensure that the members meet the requisite abilities and personality characteristics needed to successfully accomplish the essential work tasks. The *relational* perspective considers the social relationships and networks in which the team members belong and using relationships among team members means that it is possible to better understand the interactions and the social dynamics that will exist during a collaboration. Both perspectives are augmented by the inclusion of the *ecosystem* perspective, which provides the context in which the assembled team will be working. The

context may include the scientific landscape, large organizations, departments, disciplines of inquiry, or the established work routines that will affect a team. It is important for a practitioner to be cognizant of all three perspectives that contribute to the assembly of effective scientific teams. However, garnering information from all these perspectives and integrating them into the task of team assembly are nontrivial for a single individual. In the following section, we discuss the role of technology and data sources to help make team assembly decisions that use as much available data as possible.

17.5 Technology, Data, and Recommendation Algorithms in Team Assembly

Key Takeaway: Technology is becoming increasingly useful in assembling teams, and there is now a large amount of readily available digital data and growing interest in the development of recommendation algorithms that enable and understand team assembly.

Newly available digital data opens many new opportunities to measure the social interactions encompassing team assembly. The use of digital trace data gathered from our use of technology is a powerful resource for the study of teams and team assembly. People engage in various behaviors when selecting their teammates: searching and screening information about others, extending invitations to others, considering invitations from others, rescinding invitations, and recusing themselves after accepting an invitation. However, much of these "sausage-making" details about the assembly process are well-nigh impossible to glean accurately from retrospective self-reported data, such as surveys and interviews, or in-person observations. Indeed, social networks research has repeatedly shown that respondents are inaccurate in their reporting of network connections (Bernard and Killworth 1977; Bernard et al. 1984; Bernard et al. 1980; Bernard et al. 1982; Humphrey and Aime 2014;

Killworth and Bernard 1976, 1980; Krackhardt 1987; Marsden 1990).

These limitations have the potential of being scaled due to the availability of digital trace data on a large scale, ushering in the era of *computational social science* (Lazer et al. 2009). Computational social science provides new opportunities in the exploration of team assembly through the analysis of web-based platforms that are used for team assembly and collaboration as well as the increased access to digital archives of collaboration records and histories. Team research has historically been at a data deficit when considering preteam communication or interactions, but now digital trace data and accessible longitudinal data in digital archives have the potential to provide rich data about social interactions and individuals engaged in the process of team assembly. These data hold great potential for both studying team assembly and providing an environment for the development of better systems to facilitate team assembly. The two aspects driving this movement are the developments of technology to enable team assembly and the data that fuels their use. These are discussed in the next two subsections.

17.5.1 Technology

Technology is present in many aspects of scientific work, and the presence of social technology has brought many benefits to the modern workplace. Many organizations have implemented web-based social technologies to connect employees to one another and facilitate organization learning, communication, expertise search, and collaboration (Colbert et al. 2016; Leonardi et al. 2013; Lin et al. 2009; Treem and Leonardi 2012). The proliferation of such technology benefits team assembly because people are more able to acquire knowledge and information about their broader organization and the potential collaborators therein (Huang et al. 2013; Leonardi 2015).

Access to such knowledge is invaluable for people who need to assemble teams when performing highly intensive scientific research since

there are many, often competing considerations that must be made (Reagans et al. 2004). The inclusion of technology into team assembly considerations clarifies meaningful selection criteria and effective algorithms to assemble teams that accomplish meaningful outcomes. Technology aids the matching of team members based on their abilities as well as their fit among team members (D'Souza and Colarelli 2010; Spoelstra et al. 2015). To illustrate the value of technology in team assembly, we describe three technologies that improve knowledge availability for people who are assembling teams.

These platforms have applications in businesses, instructor-assigned student teams, and self-assembled research teams. The Pingboard platform allows for organizations to generate and aggregate data on the collaborations that are occurring within the organization instead of having a static reporting chart (Easy, beautiful org chart software | Pingboard n.d.). The application is meaningful because users can recognize the people who collaborate with one another and can use such information to assemble teams based on actual collaborations instead of assumed relationships based on inaccurate information. Another software platform, CATME, is used by instructors who are assigning students to teams and provides value because a single person can use the software to organize information and specify the criteria used to assemble teams (CATME n.d.; Jahanbakhsh et al. 2017; Layton et al. 2010). The MyDreamTeam platform facilitates the self-assembly of project teams for a population of users (Asencio et al. 2014; My Dream Team Assembler n.d.). MyDreamTeam gives agency to those assembling their own teams, provides information about potential collaborators through online profiles and search recommendations, and affords messaging interactions comparable to an online dating application. These three platforms are examples of a growing technology genre focused on team assembly. But there is still much to learn from mature and active online communities where users assemble teams and engage in scientific and technical collaborations to solve real-world problems.

geography

17.5.2 Digital Trace Data

Data generated and tracked on digital platforms, such as messaging applications (e.g., Slack), software repositories (e.g., GitHub), and digital archives such as the Web of Science provide data that fuel the technology to help team assembly. The Internet has simplified access to United States patent records and published academic articles. For example, there are databases available from the US Patent and Trademark Office (USPTO), the Web of Science, Elsevier, US National Institutes of Health (NIH), and the United States National Science Foundation (NSF). These records are especially helpful in the study of teams because they are historical in nature, span the entire careers of some people in the sample, and include clear definitions of teams through authorship lists. The most important fact obtained by analyzing such data is that teams are increasingly becoming more prevalent and impactful. The amount of research done by teams has been increasing over time (Leahey 2016). From analysis of over half a million USPTO patent records, teams are shown to reduce the chance of producing poor outcomes while increasing the chance of having a highly successful invention (Singh and Fleming 2010). Using the Web of Science, researchers have uncovered important facts surrounding teams by leveraging the Web of Science database containing over 20 million records over five decades and 2.1 million patent records over three decades (Jones et al. 2008; Wuchty et al. 2007). Analyzing these research products and learning how the teams were composed and assembled provides a great deal of information about teams that are successful, innovative, and productive.

Another benefit of such data archives is that there is more available data on teams that were not as successful in accomplishing their goals as those who earned patents or publications. To have a comprehensive perspective of science team assembly, it is meaningful to explore teams that were unsuccessful. There are studies using data from the NSF about funded projects and proposals that include both successful and unsuccessful teams in terms of being awarded a research grant. Using data from the NSF, analysis shows geographically distributed teams are becoming more common and have higher impact than co-located teams (Cummings and Kiesler 2007, 2014). However, when accounting for both successful and unsuccessful proposals, it was found that multidisciplinary and geographically distributed teams are less likely to be successful than teams that are less multidisciplinary and geographically co-located (Cummings and Kiesler 2005, 2008). More recent research has been conducted based on 1103 successful and unsuccessful NSF grant proposals submitted to two interdisciplinary initiatives spanning a 3-year period. The results showed that people are more likely to assemble a proposal team with people with whom they already have relationships, but are more likely to be unsuccessful if they cite one another—implying an incestuous intellectual relationship that does not augur well for innovation (Lungeanu et al. 2014). Clearly, without the use of digital data archives, the availability of information regarding less successful or failed teams would not be as readily available.

17.5.3 Recommendation Algorithms

The Internet is a powerful tool for the future of work (Colbert et al. 2016). However, there are countless options and an overwhelming amount of information available online. To help people manage all the options and information, the development of approaches to filter information based on multiple users has been impactful and useful (Resnick et al. 1994). Modern technologies that recommend content are embedded in many web platforms. One would be hard pressed to find an online scenario that does not provide content to a user by making recommendations derived from an algorithm; friend suggestions, future purchases, the next website to visit, and the next content to consume in general are all examples of commonly generated recommendations (Lazer 2015). Using search queries, click-through data, survey responses, prior purchasing behavior, and countless other user data, a person's actions are modeled and compared to other people to generate recommendations that help drive individual choices on the Internet.

Recommendations online are also relevant to social relationships. Major social networking websites, such as LinkedIn, Facebook, Instagram, and Twitter, all recommend people that you may know or people with whom you should connect based on a given individual's interest, demographics, and shared network connections. These same types of algorithmic approaches can be used for the assembly of teams (Contractor 2013; Fazel-Zarandi et al. 2011). Recommendation algorithms use many more data sources and considerations than people can consider, which makes them able to assess numerous team combinations, recommend combinations with some level of confidence, and provide metrics to help assemble the teams with the highest possibility for success (Ghasemian et al. 2016; Lappas et al. 2009). Recent research has also investigated the ability of algorithms to replace members of teams (Li et al. 2015). There is great value in using recommendations to assess different options for a replacement team member that allows people to anticipate how a new addition will influence different team performance measures. The inclusion of technological considerations and recommendations will aid team assembly by making collaborations that may occur within the scientific task environment more responsive to changes.

17.6   Conclusion

There is always been prima facie intuition that team assembly is an important prerequisite to consider in the work of modern science teams. This chapter has sought to marshal the evidence and herald the potential of a more systematic evidence base for this intuition. In this chapter, we have distinguished, and weighed the pros and cons, of two different assembly types—staff-assembly and self-assembly. We have provided the practitioner with evidence for why team assembly must be considered from three perspectives: compositional (individual attributes of potential team members), relational (the prior relations among these members), and ecosystem (the relations of these members with others via their membership in multiple overlapping teams). We also previewed the potential of technology platforms, the proliferation of digital trace data, and the development of recommendation algorithms to dramatically improve our ability to both enable and understand team assembly. Given the ever-increasing need for science to be conducted in teams, the science of team assembly, and the need for practitioners to leverage these insights, will only grow in importance.

Acknowledgment The authors acknowledge the grant award NNX15AM32G from the National Aeronautics and Space Administration (NASA), grant award IIS-1514427 from the National Science Foundation (NSF), and grant award R01GM112938-01 from the National Institutes of Health (NIH).

References

Aalbers R, Dolfsma W, Koppius O. Individual connectedness in innovation networks: on the role of individual motivation. Res Policy. 2013;42(3):624–34.

Ahuja G. Collaboration networks, structural holes, and innovation: a longitudinal study. Adm Sci Q. 2000;45(3):425–55. https://doi.org/10.2307/2667105.

Ancona DG, Caldwell DF. Bridging the boundary: external activity and performance in organizational teams. Adm Sci Q. 1992a:634–65.

Ancona DG, Caldwell DF. Demography and design: predictors of new product team performance. Organ Sci. 1992b;3(3):321–41.

Arrow H, McGrath JE, Berdahl JL. Small groups as complex systems: formation, coordination, development, and adaptation. Thousand Oaks: Sage Publications; 2000.

Asencio R, Huang Y, Murase T, Sawant A, DeChurch L, Contractor N. Enabling teams to self-assemble: the my dream team tool. Presented at the 5th Annual International Science of Team Science (SciTS) Conference;2014.

Balkundi P, Harrison DA. Ties, leaders, and time in teams: strong inference about network structure's effects on team viability and performance. Acad Manag J. 2006;49(1):49–68.

Balkundi P, Kilduff M. The ties that lead: a social network approach to leadership. Leadersh Q. 2006;17(4):419–39. https://doi.org/10.1016/j.leaqua.2006.01.001.

Balkundi P, Kilduff M, Barsness Z, Michael J. Demographic antecedents and performance consequences of structural holes in work teams. J Organ Behav. 2007;28(2):241–60.

Balkundi P, Barsness Z, Michael JH. Unlocking the influence of leadership network structures on team conflict and viability. Small Group Res. 2009;40(3):301–22. https://doi.org/10.1177/1046496409333404.

Balkundi P, Kilduff M, Harrison DA. Centrality and charisma: comparing how leader networks and attributions affect team performance. J Appl Psychol. 2011;96(6):1209.

Bandura A. Human agency in social cognitive theory. Am Psychol. 1989;44(9):1175–84.

Barrick MR, Stewart GL, Neubert MJ, Mount MK. Relating member ability and personality to work-team processes and team effectiveness. J Appl Psychol. 1998;83(3):377–91.

Bell ST. Deep-level composition variables as predictors of team performance: a meta-analysis. J Appl Psychol. 2007;92(3):595.

Bercovitz J, Feldman M. The mechanisms of collaboration in inventive teams: composition, social networks, and geography. Res Policy. 2011;40(1):81–93. https://doi.org/10.1016/j.respol.2010.09.008.

Bernard H, Killworth PD. Informant accuracy in social network data II. Hum Commun Res. 1977;4(1):3–18.

Bernard H, Killworth PD, Sailer L. Informant accuracy in social network data IV: a comparison of clique-level structure in behavioral and cognitive network data. Soc Networks. 1980;2(3):191–218.

Bernard H, Killworth PD, Sailer L. Informant accuracy in social-network data V. An experimental attempt to predict actual communication from recall data. Soc Sci Res. 1982;11(1):30–66.

Bernard H, Killworth PD, Kronenfeld D, Sailer L. The problem of informant accuracy: the validity of retrospective data. Annu Rev Anthropol. 1984;13:495–517.

Bikard M, Murray F, Gans JS. Exploring trade-offs in the organization of scientific work: collaboration and scientific reward. Manag Sci. 2015;61(7):1473–95.

Birnholtz J, Forlano L, Yuan YC, Rizzo J, Liao K, Gay G, Heller C. One university, two campuses: initiating and sustaining research collaborations between two campuses of a single institution. In: Proceedings of the 2012 iConference. ACM; 2012. pp. 33–40.

Börner K, Contractor N, Falk-Krzesinski HJ, Fiore SM, Hall KL, Keyton J, et al. A multi-level systems perspective for the science of team science. Sci Transl Med. 2010;2(49):cm24. https://doi.org/10.1126/scitranslmed.3001399.

Bunderson JS, Sutcliffe KM. Comparing alternative conceptualizations of functional diversity in management teams: process and performance effects. Acad Manag J. 2002;45(5):875–93. https://doi.org/10.2307/3069319.

Burt RS. Structural holes and good ideas. Am J Sociol. 2004;110(2):349–99. https://doi.org/10.1086/421787.

Burt RS. Structural holes: the social structure of competition. Cambridge: Harvard University Press; 2009.

Cable DM, Edwards JR. Complementary and supplementary fit: a theoretical and empirical integration. J Appl Psychol. 2004;89(5):822–34.

CATME. (n.d.). http://info.catme.org. Accessed 19 Oct 2017.

Chompalov I, Genuth J, Shrum W. The organization of scientific collaborations. Res Policy. 2002;31(5):749–67. https://doi.org/10.1016/S0048-7333(01)00145-7.

Coccia M, Wang L. Evolution and convergence of the patterns of international scientific collaboration. Proc Natl Acad Sci. 2016;113(8):2057–61. https://doi.org/10.1073/pnas.1510820113.

Cohen SG, Bailey DE. What makes teams work: group effectiveness research from the shop floor to the executive suite. J Manag. 1997;23(3):239–90.

Colbert A, Yee N, George G. The digital workforce and the workplace of the future. Acad Manag J. 2016;59(3):731–9. https://doi.org/10.5465/amj.2016.4003.

Coleman JS. Social capital in the creation of human capital. Am J Sociol. 1988:S95–S120.

Colquitt JA, Scott BA, LePine JA. Trust, trustworthiness, and trust propensity: a meta-analytic test of their unique relationships with risk taking and job performance. J Appl Psychol. 2007;92(4):909.

Contractor N. Some assembly required: leveraging web science to understand and enable team assembly. Philos Trans R Soc A Math Phys Eng Sci. 2013;371(1987):20120385.

Cooke NJ, Hilton ML, Committee on the Science of Team Science, Board on Behavioral, Cognitive, and Sensory Sciences, Division of Behavioral and Social Sciences and Education, National Research Council. Team composition and assembly. Washington D.C.: National Academies Press; 2015. https://www.ncbi.nlm.nih.gov/books/NBK310388/

Cordery JL, Mueller WS, Smith LM. Attitudinal and behavioral effects of autonomous group working: a longitudinal field study. Acad Manag J. 1991;34(2):464–76. https://doi.org/10.2307/256452.

Crawford ER, Lepine JA. A configural theory of team processes: accounting for the structure of taskwork and teamwork. Acad Manag Rev. 2013;38(1):32–48. https://doi.org/10.5465/amr.2011.0206.

Cross R, Cummings JN. Tie and network correlates of individual performance in knowledge-intensive work. Acad Manag J. 2004;47(6):928–37. https://doi.org/10.2307/20159632.

Cummings JN. Work groups, structural diversity, and knowledge sharing in a global organization. Manag Sci. 2004;50(3):352–64. https://doi.org/10.1287/mnsc.1030.0134.

Cummings JN, Cross R. Structural properties of work groups and their consequences for performance. Soc Networks. 2003;25(3):197–210.

Cummings JN, Kiesler S. Collaborative research across disciplinary and organizational boundaries. Soc Stud Sci. 2005;35(5):703–22.

Cummings JN, Kiesler S. Coordination costs and project outcomes in multi-university collaborations. Res Policy. 2007;36(10):1620–34.

Cummings JN, Kiesler S. Who collaborates successfully?: Prior experience reduces collaboration barriers in distributed interdisciplinary research. In Proceedings of the 2008 ACM Conference on Computer Supported

Cooperative Work. ACM; 2008. pp. 437–446. http://dl.acm.org/citation.cfm?id=1460633.

Cummings JN, Kiesler S. Organization theory and the changing nature of science (SSRN scholarly paper no. ID 2549609). Rochester, NY: Social Science Research Network; 2014. https://papers.ssrn.com/abstract=2549609

Cummings JN, Pletcher C. Why project networks beat project teams. MIT Sloan Manag Rev. 2011;52(3):75.

D'Souza GC, Colarelli SM. Team member selection decisions for virtual versus face-to-face teams. Comput Hum Behav. 2010;26(4):630–5. https://doi.org/10.1016/j.chb.2009.12.016.

Dabbish L, Stuart C, Tsay J, Herbsleb J. Social coding in GitHub: transparency and collaboration in an open software repository. In Proceedings of the ACM 2012 Conference on Computer Supported Cooperative Work. ACM; 2012. pp. 1277–1286. http://dl.acm.org/citation.cfm?id=2145396

Dahlander L, McFarland DA. Ties that last: tie formation and persistence in research collaborations over time. Adm Sci Q. 2013;58(1):69–110. https://doi.org/10.1177/0001839212474272.

De Dreu CK, Weingart LR. Task versus relationship conflict, team performance, and team member satisfaction: a meta-analysis. J Appl Psychol. 2003;88(4):741.

De Dreu CK, West MA. Minority dissent and team innovation: the importance of participation in decision making. J Appl Psychol. 2001;86(6):1191.

Deci EL, Ryan RM. Overview of self-determination theory: an organismic dialectical perspective. In: Handbook of Self-Determination Research; 2002. pp. 3–33.

Devine DJ, Philips JL. Do smarter teams do better: a meta-analysis of cognitive ability and team performance. Small Group Res. 2001;32(5):507–32.

Duguid MM. Female tokens in high-prestige work groups: catalysts or inhibitors of group diversification? Organ Behav Hum Decis Process. 2011;116(1):104–15.

Duguid MM, Loyd DL, Tolbert PS. The impact of categorical status, numeric representation, and work group prestige on preference for demographically similar others: a value threat approach. Organ Sci. 2012;23(2):386–401. https://doi.org/10.1287/orsc.1100.0565.

Easy, beautiful org chart software | Pingboard. (n.d.). https://pingboard.com. Accessed 19 Oct 2017.

Edmondson AC. Teaming: how organizations learn, innovate, and compete in the knowledge economy. Hoboken: John Wiley & Sons; 2012a.

Edmondson AC. Teamwork on the fly. Harv Bus Rev. 2012b;90(4):72–80.

Emerson RM. Social exchange theory. Annu Rev Sociol. 1976:335–62.

Falk-Krzesinski HJ, Börner K, Contractor N, Fiore SM, Hall KL, Keyton J, et al. Advancing the science of team science. Clin Transl Sci. 2010;3(5):263–6. https://doi.org/10.1111/j.1752-8062.2010.00223.x.

Faraj S, Sproull L. Coordinating expertise in software development teams. Manag Sci. 2000;46(12):1554–68. https://doi.org/10.1287/mnsc.46.12.1554.12072.

Fazel-Zarandi M, Devlin HJ, Huang Y, Contractor N. Expert recommendation based on social drivers, social network analysis, and semantic data representation. Presented at the 2nd International Workshop on Information Heterogeneity and Fusion in Recommender Systems. ACM; 2011. pp. 41–48. https://doi.org/10.1145/2039320.2039326.

Foster JG, Rzhetsky A, Evans JA. Tradition and innovation in scientists' research strategies. Am Sociol Rev. 2015;80(5):875–908. https://doi.org/10.1177/0003122415601618.

Fox MF, Faver CA. Independence and cooperation in research. J High Educ. 1984;55(3):347–59. https://doi.org/10.1080/00221546.1984.11777069.

Fussell SR, Kraut RE, Lerch FJ, Scherlis WL, McNally MM, Cadiz JJ. Coordination, overload and team performance: effects of team communication strategies. In: Proceedings of the 1998 ACM Conference on Computer Supported Cooperative Work; 1998. pp. 275–284.

Gadlin H, Jessar K. Preempting discord: prenuptial agreements for scientists. The NIH Catalyst. 2002;10:12.

Gewin V. Collaborations: recipe for a team. Nature. 2015;523(7559):245–7. https://doi.org/10.1038/nj7559-245a.

Ghasemian F, Zamanifar K, Ghasem-Aqaee N, Contractor N. Toward a better scientific collaboration success prediction model through the feature space expansion. Scientometrics. 2016:1–25.

Gibbs K, Han A, Lun J. Demographic diversity in teams: the challenges, benefits, and management strategies. In: Hall KL, Vogel AL, Croyle RT, editors. Strategies for team science success: handbook of evidence- based principles for cross-disciplinary science and practical lessons learned from health researchers. New York, NY: Springer; 2019.

González VM, Mark G. Constant, constant, multi-tasking craziness: managing multiple working spheres. In Proceedings of the SIGCHI Conference on Human Factors in Computing Systems. ACM; 2004. pp. 113–120. http://dl.acm.org/citation.cfm?id=985707

Grant AM, Berry JW. The necessity of others is the mother of invention: intrinsic and prosocial motivations, perspective taking, and creativity. Acad Manag J. 2011;54(1):73–96.

Guimerà R, Uzzi B, Spiro J, Amaral LAN. Team assembly mechanisms determine collaboration network structure and team performance. Science. 2005;308(5722):697–702. https://doi.org/10.1126/science.1106340.

Hackman JR. The design of work teams. In: Lorsch J, editor. Handbook of organizational behavior. Englewood Cliffs, NJ: Prentice-Hall; 1987.

Hackman JR. Group influences on individuals in organizations. In: Dunnette MD, Hough LM, editors. Handbook of industrial and organizational psychology, vol. 3. Palo Alto: Consulting Psychologists Press; 1992.

Hackman JR, Brousseau KR, Weiss JA. The interaction of task design and group performance strategies in determining group effectiveness. Organ Behav

Hum Perform. 1976;16(2):350–65. https://doi.org/10.1016/0030-5073(76)90021-0.

Hagstrom WO. Traditional and modern forms of scientific teamwork. Adm Sci Q. 1964;9(3):241–63. https://doi.org/10.2307/2391440.

Hahn J, Moon JY, Zhang C. Emergence of new project teams from open source software developer networks: impact of prior collaboration ties. Inf Syst Res. 2008;19(3):369–91.

Hansen MT. The search-transfer problem: the role of weak ties in sharing knowledge across organization subunits. Adm Sci Q. 1999:82–111.

Harrison DA, Humphrey SE. Designing for diversity or diversity for design? Tasks, interdependence, and within-unit differences at work. J Organ Behav. 2010;31(2–3):328–37. https://doi.org/10.1002/job.608.

Harrison DA, Klein KJ. What's the difference? Diversity constructs as separation, variety, or disparity in organizations. Acad Manag Rev. 2007;32(4):1199–228. https://doi.org/10.5465/AMR.2007.26586096.

Heider F. The psychology of interpersonal relations. New York: Wiley; 1958.

Hertel G, Niedner S, Herrmann S. Motivation of software developers in open source projects: an internet-based survey of contributors to the Linux kernel. Res Policy. 2003;32(7):1159–77.

Hinds PJ, Carley KM, Krackhardt D, Wholey D. Choosing work group members: balancing similarity, competence, and familiarity. Organ Behav Hum Decis Process. 2000;81(2):226–51.

Hollenbeck JR, Moon H, Ellis AP, West BJ, Ilgen DR, Sheppard L, et al. Structural contingency theory and individual differences: examination of external and internal person-team fit. J Appl Psychol. 2002;87(3):599.

Huang M, Barbour J, Su C, Contractor NS. Why do group members provide information to digital knowledge repositories? A multilevel application of transactive memory theory. J Am Soc Inf Sci Technol. 2013;64(3):540–57. https://doi.org/10.1002/asi.22805.

Hudson JM, Christensen J, Kellogg WA, Erickson T. I'd be overwhelmed, but it's just one more thing to do: Availability and interruption in research management. In Proceedings of the SIGCHI Conference on Human Factors in Computing Systems. ACM; 2002. pp. 97–104. http://dl.acm.org/citation.cfm?id=503394.

Humphrey SE, Aime F. Team microdynamics: toward an organizing approach to teamwork. Acad Manag Ann. 2014;8(1):443–503. https://doi.org/10.1080/19416520.2014.904140.

Humphrey SE, Hollenbeck JR, Meyer CJ, Ilgen DR. Trait configurations in self-managed teams: a conceptual examination of the use of seeding for maximizing and minimizing trait variance in teams. J Appl Psychol. 2007;92(3):885–92.

Humphrey SE, Morgeson FP, Mannor MJ. Developing a theory of the strategic core of teams: a role composition model of team performance. J Appl Psychol. 2009;94(1):48.

Jacobs JA, Frickel S. Interdisciplinarity: a critical assessment. Annu Rev Sociol. 2009;35(1):43–65. https://doi.org/10.1146/annurev-soc-070308-115954.

Jahanbakhsh F, Fu W-T, Karahalios K, Marinov D, Bailey B. You want me to work with who?: stakeholder perceptions of automated team formation in project-based courses. In: Proceedings of the 2017 CHI Conference on Human Factors in Computing Systems. New York, NY: ACM; 2017. p. 3201–12. https://doi.org/10.1145/3025453.3026011.

Jehn KA, Shah PP. Interpersonal relationships and task performance: an examination of mediation processes in friendship and acquaintance groups. J Pers Soc Psychol. 1997;72(4):775–90. https://doi.org/10.1037/0022-3514.72.4.775.

Jones BF, Wuchty S, Uzzi B. Multi-university research teams: shifting impact, geography, and stratification in science. Science. 2008;322(5905):1259–62.

Joshi A. By whom and when is women's expertise recognized? The interactive effects of gender and education in science and engineering teams. Adm Sci Q. 2014;59(2):202–39. https://doi.org/10.1177/0001839214528331.

Joshi A, Roh H. The role of context in work team diversity research: a meta-analytic review. Acad Manag J. 2009;52(3):599–627.

Katz JS, Martin BR. What is research collaboration? Res Policy. 1997;26(1):1–18. https://doi.org/10.1016/S0048-7333(96)00917-1.

Katz N, Lazer D, Arrow H, Contractor N. Network theory and small groups. Small Group Res. 2004;35(3):307–32. https://doi.org/10.1177/1046496404264941.

Killworth PD, Bernard H. Informant accuracy in social network data. Hum Organ. 1976;35(3):269–86.

Killworth PD, Bernard H. Informant accuracy in social network data III: a comparison of triadic structure in behavioral and cognitive data. Soc Networks. 1980;2(1):19–46.

Klein KJ, Kozlowski SW. From micro to meso: critical steps in conceptualizing and conducting multilevel research. Organ Res Methods. 2000;3(3):211–36.

Klein KJ, Dansereau F, Hall RJ. Levels issues in theory development, data collection, and analysis. Acad Manag Rev. 1994;19(2):195–229.

Klimoski R, Jones RG. Staffing for effective group decision making: key issues in matching people and teams. In: Guzzo RA, Salas E, editors. Team effectiveness and decision making in organizations. 1st ed. San Francisco: Jossey-Bass; 1995. p. 291–332.

Kozlowski SWJ, Bell BS. Evidence-based principles and strategies for optimizing team functioning and performance in science teams. In: Hall KL, Vogel AL, Croyle RT, editors. Strategies for team science success: handbook of evidence-based principles for crossdisciplinary science and practical lessons learned from health researchers. New York, NY: Springer; 2019.

Kozlowski SW, Ilgen DR. Enhancing the effectiveness of work groups and teams. Psychol Sci Public Interest. 2006;7(3):77–124.

Kozlowski SW, Klein KJ. A multilevel approach to theory and research in organizations: contextual, temporal, and emergent processes. In: Klein KJ, Kozlowski SW, editors. Multilevel theory, research, and methods in organizations: foundations, extensions, and new directions. San Francisco: Jossey-Bass; 2000. p. 3–90. http://psycnet.apa.org/psycinfo/2000-16936-001.

Krackhardt D. Cognitive social structures. Soc Networks. 1987;9(2):109–34.

Kraut RE, Galegher J, Egido C. Relationships and tasks in scientific research collaboration. Hum. Comput. interact. 1987;3(1):31–58

Kraut RE, Streeter LA. Coordination in software development. Commun. Assoc Comput. Mach. 1995;38(3):69–81.

Kristof AL. Person-organization fit: an integrative review of its conceptualizations, measurement, and implications. Pers Psychol. 1996;49(1):1–49.

Kristof-Brown AL, Zimmerman RD, Johnson EC. Consequences of individuals' fit at work: a meta-analysis of person–job, person–organization, person–group, and person–supervisor fit. Pers Psychol. 2005;58(2):281–342. https://doi.org/10.1111/j.1744-6570.2005.00672.x.

Lappas T, Liu K, Terzi E. Finding a team of experts in social networks. In: Proceedings of the 15th ACM SIGKDD International Conference on Knowledge Discovery and Data Mining. New York: ACM; 2009. p. 467–76. http://dl.acm.org/citation.cfm?id=1557074.

Layton RA, Loughry ML, Ohland MW, Ricco GD. Design and validation of a web-based system for assigning members to teams using instructor-specified criteria. Adv Eng Education. 2010;2(1):n1.

Lazer D. The rise of the social algorithm. Science. 2015;348(6239):1090–1.

Lazer D, Pentland A, Adamic L, Aral S, Barabasi A-L, Brewer D, Van Alstyne M. Computational social science. Science. 2009;323(5915):721–3. https://doi.org/10.1126/science.1167742.

Leahey E. From sole investigator to team scientist: trends in the practice and study of research collaboration. Annu Rev Sociol. 2016;42(1):81–100. https://doi.org/10.1146/annurev-soc-081715-074219.

Leahey E, Beckman CM, Stanko TL. Prominent but less productive the impact of interdisciplinarity on scientists' research. Adm. Sci. Quart. 0001839216665364. 2016. https://doi.org/10.1177/0001839216665364.

Lee Y-N, Walsh JP, Wang J. Creativity in scientific teams: unpacking novelty and impact. Res Policy. 2015;44(3):684–97. https://doi.org/10.1016/j.respol.2014.10.007.

Leonardi PM. Ambient awareness and knowledge acquisition: using social media to learn "who knows what" and "who knows whom". MIS Q. 2015;39(4):747–62.

Leonardi PM, Huysman M, Steinfield C. Enterprise social media: definition, history, and prospects for the study of social technologies in organizations. J Comput-Mediat Commun. 2013;19(1):1–19. https://doi.org/10.1111/jcc4.12029.

Lepine JA, Dyne LV. Peer responses to low performers: an attributional model of helping in the context of groups. Acad Manag Rev. 2001;26(1):67–84. https://doi.org/10.5465/AMR.2001.4011953.

LePine JA, Hollenbeck JR, Ilgen DR, Hedlund J. Effects of individual differences on the performance of hierarchical decision-making teams: much more than g. J Appl Psychol. 1997;82(5):803–11. https://doi.org/10.1037/0021-9010.82.5.803.

LePine JA, Hanson MA, Borman WC, Motowidlo SJ. Contextual performance and teamwork: implications for staffing (Vol. 19). Greenwich, Conn: JAI Press; 2000.

Li L, Tong H, Cao N, Ehrlich K, Lin Y-R, Buchler N. Replacing the irreplaceable: fast algorithms for team member recommendation. In: Proceedings of the 24th International Conference on World Wide Web. Geneva: International World Wide Web Conferences Steering Committee; 2015. p. 636–46. http://dl.acm.org/citation.cfm?id=2741132.

Lin CY, Cao N, Liu SX, Papadimitriou S, Sun J, Yan X. SmallBlue: social network analysis for expertise search and collective intelligence. In: 2009 IEEE 25th International Conference on Data Engineering; 2009. p. 1483–6. https://doi.org/10.1109/ICDE.2009.140.

Lungeanu A, Contractor NS. The effects of diversity and network ties on innovations: the emergence of a new scientific field. Am Behav Sci. 2015; https://doi.org/10.1177/0002764214556804.

Lungeanu A, Huang Y, Contractor N. Understanding the assembly of interdisciplinary teams and its impact on performance. J Informet. 2014;8(1):59–70. https://doi.org/10.1016/j.joi.2013.10.006.

Lungeanu A, Carter DR, DeChurch LA, Contractor NS. How team interlock ecosystems shape the assembly of scientific teams: a hypergraph approach. Commun Methods Meas. 2018;12:1–25.

Lykourentzou I, Wang S, Kraut RE, Dow SP. Team dating: a self-organized team formation strategy for collaborative crowdsourcing. In: Proceedings of the 2016 CHI Conference Extended Abstracts on Human Factors in Computing Systems. New York, NY: ACM; 2016. p. 1243–9. https://doi.org/10.1145/2851581.2892421.

Lykourentzou I, Kraut RE, Dow SP. Team dating leads to better online ad hoc collaborations. In: Proceedings of the 2017 ACM Conference on Computer Supported Cooperative Work and Social Computing. New York, NY: ACM; 2017. p. 2330–43. https://doi.org/10.1145/2998181.2998322.

Ma A, Mondragón RJ, Latora V. Anatomy of funded research in science. Proc Natl Acad Sci. 2015;112(48):14760–5. https://doi.org/10.1073/pnas.1513651112.

Margolin D, Ognyanoya K, Huang M, Huang Y, Contractor N. Team formation and performance on Nanohub: a network selection challenge in scientific communities. In: Vedres B, Scotti M, editors.

Networks in social policy problems. Cambridge, UK: Cambridge University Press; 2012. p. 80–100.

Marks MA, Mathieu JE, Zaccaro SJ. A temporally based framework and taxonomy of team processes. Acad Manag Rev. 2001;26(3):356–76.

Marks MA, Dechurch LA, Mathieu JE, Panzer FJ, Alonso A. Teamwork in multiteam systems. J Appl Psychol. 2005;90(5):964–71.

Marsden P. Network data and measurement. Annu Rev Sociol. 1990:435–63.

Marwell G, Oliver PE, Prahl R. Social networks and collective action: a theory of the critical mass. III. Am J Sociol. 1988;94(3):502–34.

Mathieu J, Maynard MT, Rapp T, Gilson L. Team effectiveness 1997-2007: a review of recent advancements and a glimpse into the future. J Manag. 2008;34(3):410–76. https://doi.org/10.1177/0149206308316061.

McPherson M, Smith-Lovin L. Homophily in voluntary organizations: status distance and the composition of face-to-face groups. Am Sociol Rev. 1987:370–9.

McPherson M, Smith-Lovin L, Cook JM. Birds of a feather: homophily in social networks. Annu Rev Sociol. 2001;27:415–44.

Milojević S. Principles of scientific research team formation and evolution. Proc Natl Acad Sci. 2014;111(11):3984–9. https://doi.org/10.1073/pnas.1309723111.

Monge P, Contractor N. Theories of communication networks. New York, USA: Oxford University Press; 2003.

Morgeson FP, Humphrey SE. Job and team design: toward a more integrative conceptualization of work design. In: Research in personnel and human resources management. Bingley: Emerald Group Publishing Limited; 2008. p. 39–91.

Morgeson FP, Reider MH, Campion MA. Selecting individuals in team settings: the importance of social skills, personality characteristics, and teamwork knowledge. Pers Psychol. 2005;58(3):583–611.

Mortensen M. Constructing the team: the antecedents and effects of membership model divergence. Organ Sci. 2014;25(3):909–31. https://doi.org/10.1287/orsc.2013.0881.

Moynihan LM, Peterson RS. A contingent configuration approach to understanding the role of personality in organizational groups. Res Organ Behav. 2001;23(Supplement C):327–78. https://doi.org/10.1016/S0191-3085(01)23008-1.

Muchinsky PM, Monahan CJ. What is person-environment congruence? Supplementary versus complementary models of fit. J Vocat Behav. 1987;31(3):268–77. https://doi.org/10.1016/0001-8791(87)90043-1.

My Dream Team Assembler. (n.d.). http://sonic.northwestern.edu/software/c-iknow-mydreamteam. Accessed 19 Oct 2017.

National Research Council. Enhancing the Effectiveness of Team Science. Washington, DC: The National Academies Press. 2015. https://doi.org/10.17226/19007.

Nomura S, Birnholtz J, Rieger O, Leshed G, Trumbull D, Gay G. Cutting into collaboration: understanding coordination in distributed and interdisciplinary medical research. In: Presented at the Proceedings of the 2008 ACM Conference on Computer Supported Cooperative Work. New York: ACM; 2008. p. 427–36.

Norton WE, Lungeanu A, Chambers DA, Contractor N. Mapping the growing discipline of dissemination and implementation science in health. Scientometrics. 2017;112(3):1367–90. https://doi.org/10.1007/s11192-017-2455-2.

Nurius PS, Kemp SP. Individual level competencies for team collaboration with cross-disciplinary researchers and stakeholders. In: Hall KL, Vogel AL, Croyle RT, editors. Strategies for team science success: handbook of evidence-based principles for cross-disciplinary science and practical lessons learned from health researchers. New York, NY: Springer; 2019.

O'Leary MB, Mortensen M, Woolley AW. Multiple team membership: a theoretical model of its effects on productivity and learning for individuals and teams. Acad Manag Rev. 2011;36(3):461–78.

Page SE. The difference: how the power of diversity creates better groups, firms, schools, and societies. Princeton: Princeton University Press; 2008.

Pelesko JA. Self assembly: the science of things that put themselves together. Boca Raton: CRC Press; 2007.

Pentland AS. The new science of building great teams. Harv Bus Rev. 2012;(April):60–70.

Perretti F, Negro G. Mixing genres and matching people: a study in innovation and team composition in Hollywood. J Organ Behav. 2007;28(5):563–86.

Petersen AM. Quantifying the impact of weak, strong, and super ties in scientific careers. Proc Natl Acad Sci. 2015;112(34):E4671–80. https://doi.org/10.1073/pnas.1501444112.

Podolny JM, Baron JN. Resources and relationships: social networks and mobility in the workplace. Am Sociol Rev. 1997:673–93.

Reagans R, McEvily B. Network structure and knowledge transfer: the effects of cohesion and range. Adm Sci Q. 2003;48(2):240–67.

Reagans R, Zuckerman EW. Networks, diversity, and productivity: the social capital of corporate R&D teams. Organ Sci. 2001;12(4):502–17.

Reagans R, Zuckerman E, McEvily B. How to make the team: social networks vs. demography as criteria for designing effective teams. Adm Sci Q. 2004;49(1):101–33.

Reagans R, Miron-Spektor E, Argote L. Knowledge utilization, coordination, and team performance. Organ Sci. 2016;27(5):1108–24. https://doi.org/10.1287/orsc.2016.1078.

Ren Y, Argote L. Transactive memory systems 1985–2010: AN integrative framework of key dimensions, antecedents, and consequences. Acad Manag Ann. 2011;5(1):189–229.

Ren H, Gray B, Harrison DA. Triggering faultline effects in teams: the importance of bridging friendship ties and breaching animosity ties. Organ Sci. 2014;26(2):390–404. https://doi.org/10.1287/orsc.2014.0944.

Resnick P, Iacovou N, Suchak M, Bergstrom P, Riedl J. GroupLens: an open architecture for collaborative filtering of netnews. In: Proceedings of the 1994 ACM Conference on Computer Supported Cooperative Work. New York, NY: ACM; 1994. p. 175–86. https://doi.org/10.1145/192844.192905.

Rink F, Kane AA, Ellemers N, Vegt G v d. Team receptivity to newcomers: five decades of evidence and future research themes. Acad Manag Ann. 2013;7(1):247–93. https://doi.org/10.1080/19416520.2013.766405.

Ruef M, Aldrich HE, Carter NM. The structure of founding teams: Homophily, strong ties, and isolation among US entrepreneurs. Am Sociol Rev. 2003;68(2):195–222.

Rulke DL, Rau D. Investigating the encoding process of transactive memory development in group training. Group Org Manag. 2000;25(4):373–96.

Saporito B. The Conspiracy To End Cancer | TIME.com. Time; 2013. http://healthland.time.com/2013/04/01/the-conspiracy-to-end-cancer/.

Savage N. Collaboration is the key to cancer research [News]. 2018. https://doi.org/10.1038/d41586-018-04164-7.

Scupelli P, Kiesler S, Fussell SR, Chen C. Project view IM: a tool for juggling multiple projects and teams. In: CHI'05 extended abstracts on human factors in computing systems. New York: ACM; 2005. p. 1773–6.

Shah PP, Jehn KA. Do friends perform better than acquaintances? The interaction of friendship, conflict, and task. Group Decis Negot. 1993;2(2):149–65. https://doi.org/10.1007/BF01884769.

Shin SJ, Kim T-Y, Lee J-Y, Bian L. Cognitive team diversity and individual team member creativity: a cross-level interaction. Acad Manag J. 2012;55(1):197–212.

Shneiderman B. The new ABCs of research: achieving breakthrough collaborations. Oxford: Oxford University Press; 2016.

Shrum W, Chompalov I, Genuth J. Trust, conflict and performance in scientific collaborations. Soc Stud Sci. 2001;31(5):681–730. https://doi.org/10.1177/030631201031005002.

Shrum W, Genuth J, Chompalov I. Structures of scientific collaboration. Cambridge: MIT Press; 2007.

Singh J, Fleming L. Lone inventors as sources of breakthroughs: myth or reality? Manag Sci. 2010;56(1):41–56.

Singh J, Hansen MT, Podolny JM. The world is not small for everyone: inequity in searching for knowledge in organizations. Manag Sci. 2010;56(9):1415–38. https://doi.org/10.1287/mnsc.1100.1201.

Skilton PF, Dooley KJ. The effects of repeat collaboration on creative abrasion. Acad Manag Rev. 2010;35(1):118–34.

Spoelstra H, van Rosmalen P, Houtmans T, Sloep P. Team formation instruments to enhance learner interactions in open learning environments. Comput Hum Behav. 2015;45(Supplement C):11–20. https://doi.org/10.1016/j.chb.2014.11.038.

Stevens MJ, Campion MA. The knowledge, skill, and ability requirements for teamwork: implications for human resource management. J Manag. 1994;20(2):503–30. https://doi.org/10.1177/014920639402000210.

Stevens MJ, Campion MA. Staffing work teams: development and validation of a selection test for teamwork settings. J Manag. 1999;25(2):207–28.

Stewart GL. A meta-analytic review of relationships between team design features and team performance. J Manag. 2006;32(1):29–55. https://doi.org/10.1177/0149206305277792.

Stvilia B, Hinnant CC, Schindler K, Worrall A, Burnett G, Burnett K, Marty PF. Composition of scientific teams and publication productivity at a national science lab. J Am Soc Inf Sci Technol. 2011;62(2):270–83. https://doi.org/10.1002/asi.21464.

Taramasco C, Cointet J-P, Roth C. Academic team formation as evolving hypergraphs. Scientometrics. 2010;85(3):721–40. https://doi.org/10.1007/s11192-010-0226-4.

Thompson LL. Making the team: a guide for managers. 6th ed. New York: Pearson; 2018.

Treem JW, Leonardi PM. Social media use in organizations: exploring the affordances of visibility, editability, persistence, and association. Communication Yearbook. 2012;36:143–89.

Uzzi B, Spiro J. Collaboration and creativity: the small world problem. Am J Sociol. 2005;111(2):447–504.

Uzzi B, Mukherjee S, Stringer M, Jones B. Atypical combinations and scientific impact. Science. 2013;342(6157):468–72. https://doi.org/10.1126/science.1240474.

de Vaan M, Vedres B, Stark D. Game changer: the topology of creativity. Am J Sociol. 2015;120(4):1144–94. https://doi.org/10.1086/681213.

Valderas JM. Why do team-authored papers get cited more? Science. 2007;317(5844):1496–8. https://doi.org/10.1126/science.317.5844.1496b.

Wageman R, Gardner H, Mortensen M. The changing ecology of teams: new directions for teams research. J Organ Behav. 2012;33(3):301–15. https://doi.org/10.1002/job.1775.

Wang J, Hicks D. Scientific teams: self-assembly, fluidness, and interdependence. J Informet. 2015;9(1):197–207. https://doi.org/10.1016/j.joi.2014.12.006.

Weber G, Yuan L. The power of research networking systems to find experts and facilitate collaboration. In: Hall KL, Vogel AL, Croyle RT, editors. Strategies for team science success: handbook of evidence-based principles for cross-disciplinary science and practical lessons learned from health researchers. New York, NY: Springer; 2019.

Wegner DM. Transactive memory: a contemporary analysis of the group mind. In: Theories of group behavior. New York: Springer; 1987. p. 185–208.

Wegner DM. A computer network model of human transactive memory. Soc Cogn. 1995;13(3):319–39.

Wegner DM, Erber R, Raymond P. Transactive memory in close relationships. J Pers Soc Psychol. 1991;61(6):923–9.

Welbourne TM, Johnson DE, Erez A. The role-based performance scale: validity analysis of a theory-based measure. Acad Manag J. 1998;41(5):540–55. https://doi.org/10.2307/256941.

Williams KY, O'Reilly CA. Demography and diversity in organizations: a review of 40 years of research. Res Organ Behav. 1998;20:77–140.

Woolley AW, Gerbasi ME, Chabris CF, Kosslyn SM, Hackman JR. Bringing in the experts how team composition and collaborative planning jointly shape analytic effectiveness. Small Group Res. 2008;39(3):352–71.

Woolley AW, Chabris CF, Pentland A, Hashmi N, Malone TW. Evidence for a collective intelligence factor in the performance of human groups. Science. 2010;330(6004):686–8.

Wuchty S, Jones BF, Uzzi B. The increasing dominance of teams in production of knowledge. Science. 2007;316(5827):1036–9.

Zaccaro SJ, Dirosa GA. The processes of team staffing: a review of relevant studies. In: Hodgkinson GP, Ford JK, editors. International review of industrial and organizational psychology, vol. 2012. Hoboken: John Wiley & Sons, Ltd; 2012. p. 197–229. https://doi.org/10.1002/9781118311141.ch7.

Zhu M, Huang Y, Contractor N. Motivations for self-assembling into project teams. Soc Networks. 2013;35(2):251–64. https://doi.org/10.1016/j.socnet.2013.03.001.

Innovative Collaboration Formation: The National Academies Keck *Futures Initiative*

Anne Heberger Marino, Kimberly A. Suda-Blake, and Kenneth R. Fulton

Contents

18.1 History and Background

Like most similar programs at other organizations, the National Academies Keck *Futures Initiative* (NAKFI) started with a bold vision: to overcome structural barriers to interdisciplinary research and to enhance opportunities for interdisciplinary collaboration. The original program goals set out for NAKFI included making a positive contribution to the career paths of participants and effecting structural changes throughout the research enterprise. Conferences and seed grants were seen as reasonable tactics to achieve

A. H. Marino (✉) · K. A. Suda-Blake
The National Academies of Sciences, Engineering, and Medicine, Washington, DC, USA
e-mail: ahm@alumni.upenn.edu

K. R. Fulton
National Academy of Sciences, Washington, DC, USA

these goals, and the program design (Fig. 18.1) assumed that increased interactions among people across disciplines and throughout the research establishment would lead to improved communication, connection, and understanding, thereby enhancing opportunities for interdisciplinary researchers.

Known largely as honorific societies and sources of independent, expert advice on topics of national and global significance, the National Academies of Sciences, Engineering, and Medicine also convene programs for scientists, engineers, and medical researchers to explore horizons of knowledge together. While most activities occur independently within each academy, NAKFI's mission focused on topics relevant to all three—recognition that the academies share in the responsibility for providing leadership and vision for the research community. The governing body of the *Futures Initiative* was comprised of the presidents of the National Academy of Sciences, the National Academy of Engineering, and the National Academy of Medicine. Furthermore, the volunteer steering committees involved in planning each NAKFI conference were required to include members of each of the academies.

NAKFI catalyzes inquiry around the interdisciplinary theme of each conference by formulating a series of challenging questions, supporting

© Springer Nature Switzerland AG 2019
K. L. Hall et al. (eds.), *Strategies for Team Science Success*,
https://doi.org/10.1007/978-3-030-20992-6_18

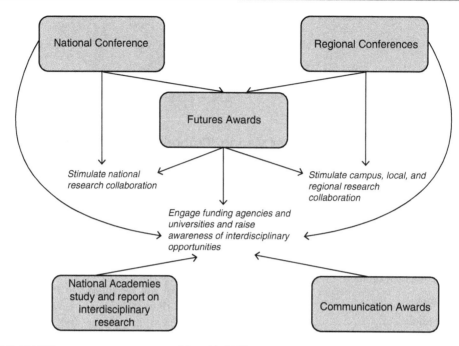

Fig. 18.1 NAKFI program components as envisioned in 2002

the development of a common language, and providing seed funding for high-risk, high-reward projects, which the program referred to as "venture science." This approach drew upon the Academies' capacity to convene experts for workshops, symposia, and consensus studies. Though frequently cited, it is not widely known that the report *Facilitating Interdisciplinary Research* (2005) was one of the first activities supported by the National Academies Keck *Futures Initiative*. Many of the report's recommendations focused on structural changes within universities, funding organizations, and professional societies that were seen as necessary for interdisciplinary research to flourish along with more traditional approaches to academic inquiry. Though support for interdisciplinary research has expanded, many barriers remain, especially in the areas of tenure and promotion (National Research Council 2015).

NAKFI was designed to support interdisciplinary researchers. While others have attempted to classify types of research and researchers (e.g., Aboelela et al. 2007; Choi and Pak 2006; Porter et al. 2006; Rosenfield 1992; Wagner et al. 2011), NAKFI's activities and models can

be applied to other types of integrative, boundary blending research such as "transdisciplinary," "interdisciplinary," "convergence," or "team science" approaches. Since the NAKFI program was intended to serve "interdisciplinary researchers," we have continued to use that term. The definition of "interdisciplinary" used by the program connects to the one set out in *Facilitating Interdisciplinary Research* (2005), which focuses on the various ways teams and individuals bring about integration throughout the research process.

This chapter will describe the key features of the NAKFI conference and seed grants program (Fig. 18.2) and provide specific examples of how evaluation has contributed to the program's development and evolution. Four aspects of the program will be explored: invitation, preparation, convene and seed, and adapt and evolve. Though this presentation does not reflect the iterative, interconnected nature of how the program actually functions, it will provide readers with basic information about the NAKFI approach. Finally, the strengths and limitations of the program will be discussed as well as the strategies that have been used to overcome challenges during its 15-year duration.

TOPIC SELECTION

• Oversight Committee foresight and expertise selecting topics	• Broad audience contributes to topic development	• National Academies' ability to engage esteemed scholars on Steering Committees

CONFERENCE DESIGN & DEVELOPMENT

• National Academies attracts outstanding applicants • Steering Committee expertly vets applicants; identifies key strategic invitees; develops cutting-edge team challenges • Program sponsors attendance; conference size limited to <150 attendees to promote interaction • Applicants already inclined toward interdisciplinary research	• Attendees provide input into preferred team challenge topic • Highly tailored pre-conference communication orients attendees to NAKFI model and expectations • Tutorials provide self-directed learning opportunities to engage with ideas before meeting • Seed grants incentivize collaboration • Beckman Center venue fosters creativity, multiple ways to meet	• Team sessions for focused, small group (8-10 person) idea exchange • Opening reception, poster sessions and breaks for unstructured networking • Full conference sessions for broad perspective; glimpses of other teams • Graduate science writers serve as team rapporteurs • Emergent ideas session incorporated into the agenda

Evaluation includes surveys of applicants and attendees immediately following and 3-months following conference

VENTURE SCIENCE SEED GRANTS

• $ 1 million available; amounts range from $25-$100K; grants are for up to 2 years • Eligibility limited to U.S.-based attendees of each year's conference; collaborators can be from anywhere • Clear online application; responsive staff for questions • Focus on high risk/high reward ideas	• Funding available for workshops and research; quick turnaround on decisions • Flexible terms; investigators can change direction, receive no-cost extension • Mid-cycle grant meeting for course correction and additional networking for grantees, collaborators, graduate students and postdocs • Simple, online final reporting requirements	• Value placed on unexpected and unintended results • Multiple ways of considering and measuring "success" • Recognition that no one source or individual can claim full credit for achievements or "noble failures" • Full scientific and societal impact of projects may not be seen for many years

Evaluation considers multiple outputs and outcomes; examines results as a portfolio of projects and individually.

Fig. 18.2 Current NAKFI conference and seed grant model

18.2   Invitation

The topics (also called "themes") for the first three conferences, held in 2003, 2004, and 2005, were framed and agreed upon by the academies' presidents before the program began. Subsequent topics were selected through a multistage process. Possible topics were submitted by many sources and winnowed down before being presented to the academies presidents for a final decision. Topic descriptions, which may be a brief as a key phrase or as long as a few pages, were sent to a broad group of 30–60 researchers, scholars, and practitioners leaders working in these areas for their input. These themes are sufficiently broad to attract a diversity of applicants, yet focused enough that there is reason to believe that NAKFI's unique conference format can make a contribution to the field. Typically, topic selections were made by the academies presidents a year or more before the intended conference. Figure 18.3 lists the topics of NAKFI

2003: Signals, Decisions and Meaning
2004: Designing Nanostructures at the Interface between Biomedical and Physical Systems
2005: The Genomic Revolution
2006: Smart Prosthetics: Exploring Assistive Devices for the Body and Mind
2007: The Future of Human Healthspan
2008: Complex Systems
2009: Synthetic Biology: Building on Nature's Inspiration
2010: Seeing the Future with Imaging Science
2011: Ecosystem Services: Charting a Path to Sustainability
2012: The Informed Brain in a Digital World
2013: The Future of Advanced Nuclear Technologies: Building a Healthier & Safer Planet
2014: Collective Behavior: From Cells to Societies
2015: Art and Science, Engineering & Medicine Frontier Collaborations
2016: Discovering the Deep Blue Sea: Research, Innovation, Social Engagement

Fig. 18.3 NAKFI conference topics, 2003–2016

conferences from 2003 to 2016. As will be explained in more detail in the section "Adapt and Evolve," shortly after the program's inception, the conference format changed from a standard plenary model to one based on working groups assigned to address real-world problems relevant to the conference theme.

Early topic selection allowed time for the appointment of a steering committee comprised of members—who served without compensation—with relevant expertise in the areas of inquiry covered by the theme and willingness to embrace and contribute to NAKFI's model. They were a working committee, charged with developing key questions to be explored during the conference, selecting attendees, providing input on the conference structure and preconference learning material, and choosing seed grant recipients.

After a steering committee was assembled, NAKFI issued a call for applications that was widely distributed to members of its alumni network, professional societies related to the conference theme, departments and organizations connected to the topic, and through social media. The steering committee worked to develop a series of ambitious challenges that would be explored, though not necessarily solved, during

the course of the 3-day meeting. Assignments to working groups to address these challenges were based on participants' preferences and ensured that a variety of disciplines were represented in each one. This is not "forced togetherness," but rather to provide an opportunity for conversation around a question that allows participants to become familiar with others' ways of approaching the topic.

On average, NAKFI received more than 300 conference applications each year, and 60–100 applicants are invited to attend. Demographically, applicants range in age from their early 20s to their mid-70s, with an average age of about 45. Though they represent many employment sectors, 75–80% of participants were employed in academia. The gender distribution of applicants varied depending on the focus of the meeting. Over time, the application process has become more inclusive, focused on applicants' accomplishments in their respective fields, dedication to the topic, and a demonstrated ability to span boundaries and work collaboratively. In addition to invitations issued to applicants, as many as 20 people were invited to attend the meeting as "strategic invitees," who possessed specialized knowledge or experience or who represented key organizations relevant to the theme.

18.3 Preparation

It is well established that training and experience play an important role in the success of collaborative work (National Research Council 2015; American Academy of Arts and Sciences 2013). Before participants arrived, NAKFI staff provided the information and support for attendees to be fully prepared and able to immerse themselves in the conference experience.

Evaluations provided by attendees of the first few conferences revealed that even the "best and brightest" face difficulties communicating across disciplines. NAKFI tried a number of approaches to help attendees bridge this linguistic divide and develop a common language by the time they arrive for the conference. For the second conference, in 2004, organizers held a 2-day bicoastal preconference tutorial 2 months before the November meeting. Although those who were able to attend the preconference did benefit from the gathering, not everyone was willing or able to travel for an additional meeting. Subsequent steering committees approached the common language problem by inviting key thinkers to create presentations specifically for NAKFI's audience. To remove the burden of additional travel for attendees, some of these presentations were broadcast live online. More recently, presentations were made available for download, allowing participants to watch at times that fit their schedule. In 2009 and 2011, the program commissioned interviews of selected experts as podcasts. In more recent years, NAKFI used a combination of curated content from across the web and commissioned podcasts.

Rather than provide the same content for all attendees, the preconference tutorials for the 2015 conference, which explored the frontiers of art and science, included a series of videos about successful art–science collaboration and content tied to each seed idea challenge. In addition to preconference tutorials, participants in the 2015 conference were asked to seek out an experience related to their assigned seed idea prior to the conference. For example, members of the group tasked to "design a learning, caring healthcare system" might visit a newly constructed hospital and an old clinic, paying attention to patients' experience as they enter the building and check in. Each participant chose his or her own experience, and their time during the meeting was devoted to sharing them. In at least one group, members completed this exercise and used it to find common ground before delving into their topic, using their preconference observations as a collective touchstone to move through challenging moments in their conversations.

18.4 Convene and Seed

When NAKFI convened a meeting, it was impossible to know who would answer the call to apply, how well groups would work together, and where they would be individually and collectively at the end of the meeting. The preparation phase described above is designed to provide fertile ground for rich conversations. The agenda seeks to support a kind of facilitated serendipity, combining focused small group interactions with unstructured time.

The seed idea challenges developed by steering committee members provide a framework upon which working groups build during the conference. Often framed as questions, the challenges describe the importance of the issue, summarize what is known, and address what is unknown. Conferences usually included seven to nine "challenges," some of which may be addressed by more than one group. Prior to the meeting, participants indicated their first, second, and third choice topics; almost all attendees were assigned to their first or second choice group.

The following examples illustrate the breadth and focus of seed idea challenges, as well as the variety that may be covered during a single conference. In 2015, one focused on designing a learning, caring healthcare system, while another explored the medical frontier of machines and the human biome. A challenge from the 2014 conference on Collective Behavior explored a question across scales: "From single cells to tissue: What causes organismality to emerge from individual cells, achieving control of conflict at lower levels so the organism becomes the unit of adaptation?"

Nuclear energy and nuclear medicine were the focus of the 2013 conference for which challenges included: "identify improvements in technology and other approaches that will ensure the future development and supply of radionuclides and radiopharmaceuticals for diagnostic imaging and therapy" and "identify a new and practical application of nuclear phenomena for the benefit of humankind." The 2012 conference on The Informed Brain in a Digital World explored the challenges of determining how the digital age will improve health and wellness, and identifying ways in which the Internet positively and negatively affects social behavior. By design, these are challenges cannot be solved in the time allotted, but solutions are not the goal. Rather, the goal is to bring people with diverse perspectives together around an area of shared interest, provide them with tools and space to explore, and see what they will create.

NAKFI conferences tapped the collective wisdom needed to address complex, intractable issues. If any one person or group had the answers, there would be no need for such gatherings. Insights happen by surprise and often after what feels like stagnation and conflict. Groups were encouraged to go where the conversation takes them, which may be in an entirely unexpected direction. Teams were kept small, consisting of seven or eight people—large enough to provide sufficient diversity of perspectives but intimate enough to encourage full participation. Groups shared their progress midway through the conference and again at the end. One member of each group was a graduate student science writer charged with crafting a narrative of the group's approach to their topic. These collected essays were assembled into a conference summary published by the National Academies Press and made available for free download online.

Though typical scientific and academic conferences frequently take place in hotels or conference centers, the Arnold and Mabel Beckman Center of the National Academies of Sciences and Engineering in Irvine, CA, was an important aspect of the NAKFI experience. The Beckman Center is filled with natural light, modern technology, and provides ample outdoor space for meals and group meetings. Attendees are able to use the meeting and outdoor space to suit their needs. Each seed idea team had an assigned room that functioned as a home base and was stocked with variety of tools to help groups translate amorphous ideas into the physical world (e.g., sticky notes, flip charts, computers and related technology, and other aids to creativity). Teams focused on the same seed idea were located in close proximity to encourage interaction during breaks. It was common to see groups meet outside with flip charts and markers or using break time for a game of croquet on the lawn. The 2015 and 2016 conferences further enhanced the creative environment through carefully curated works of art created by conference attendees.

Connections made at the meeting continued to flourish after attendees return home. Though many organizations conduct postevent surveys, NAKFI contacted attendees at two points: immediately after the conference and again 3 months later. In those 3 months, about 75% of attendees reported interacting with someone they first met at the conference. The type and number of interactions varied and might include one participant inviting another to speak on campus, working on a NAKFI seed grant (see below), sharing unpublished research findings, conducting e-mail conversations, or collaborating on a publication.

In the spring following each conference, NAKFI awarded $1 million in 1- to 2-year grants of up to $100,000. The grant application process was straightforward and reporting requirements were kept to a minimum. Principal investigators must have attended the conference though coinvestigators may or may not have been conference attendees. NAKFI encouraged grantees to learn as they went and to make changes to their research plans as appropriate. Projects that experienced unexpected delays or needed more time could request a no-cost extension with a simple e-mail explanation. NAKFI gathered each cohort of grantees for a midcycle grant meeting 1 year into the grant period. The meeting provided an opportunity for grantees to further connect with each other and gave the program crucial information about how projects progressed. Final reports covered a few key areas of interest to the program and encouraged investigators to reflect on what worked, what did not work, and why. Since 2010, NAKFI appointed grant review committees to evaluate the impact and results of these projects.

NAKFI provided more than $14 million to support innovation along the scientific spectrum—HIV prevention, the evolution of language, forecasting epileptic seizures, the liquidity of financial markets, and tactile sensors for robotic hands. NAKFI seed grants served as an incentive for attendees to collaborate after the conference and provided resources for start-up research projects or workshops that explored a facet of the NAKFI conference in more depth or with a different audience. The approach can be thought of as "venture science," an investment in early stage, high-potential projects that have a substantial element of risk. Instead, the goal is to generate many results across a portfolio of projects within each year's theme.

18.5   Adapt and Evolve

From the outset of NAKFI, the academies made a commitment to an evolving model coupled with ongoing evaluation to track the program's progress and summative evaluations after 5 and 10 years. NAKFI's commitment to an evolving model for interdisciplinary research was paired with an evaluation approach adapted to the ongoing development of the program. This made it possible to continuously monitor the success of the program and to make data-informed decisions for improvements and innovations. NAKFI's evaluation approach was adaptable and responsive to the complex environment in which NAKFI operated; it sought to find new ways to understand and document the program's unique approach to fostering and harnessing innovation.

The format of *Futures* conferences evolved from a traditional program of lectures and panel discussions to a meeting focused on providing a variety of venues for conversation. The first conference, which took place in November 2003, focused on *Signals, Decisions, and Meaning in Biology, Chemistry, Physics, and Engineering*. It followed a format similar to many other scientific conferences, rich with presentations. What made this meeting different from others was that the content and participants came from multiple fields and held differing perspectives. In addition to panels on sensory processing and functional genomics, the meeting included talks on interdisciplinary research, science communication, and the first presentation of the awards for communicating science that are also a component of the NAKFI program.

Input from members of the steering committee and feedback from participants led to changes in the format of the second conference, which took place in 2004 and focused on *Nanoscience and Nanotechnology*. During a planning meeting, the steering committee chair suggested changing the format of the conference from presentations to work in small "task groups" focused on specific challenges. This approach would allow participants time to explore a single issue over several days, learning from one another and working together. To build the common language required for such collaborative work without extending the duration of the conference, NAKFI organized the 2-day bicoastal preconference session described earlier in this chapter. Although that approach has evolved significantly in the intervening years, the task group format was so successful in stimulating new ideas and encouraging participants to think in new ways that it has been the model of every subsequent conference.

Over time NAKFI sought to continually broaden the perspectives brought together at its conferences. This evolution is most apparent in changes to the conference application. The wording on early application forms was targeted toward academic researchers and asked applicants to identify their expertise in one of three broad categories: sciences, engineering, or medicine. The number of categories has increased over time to include more specificity and breadth. In 2015 when the conference topic explored the frontier of collaborations across sciences, engineering, medicine, the arts and design, the conference application included 13 areas of expertise including architecture, design, computer science/math, communications/media, humanities, performing arts, and visual arts. The 2016 conference on *Discovering the Deep Blue Sea: Research, Innovation, and Social Engagement* included a similarly diverse set of participants.

On two separate occasions, NAKFI has used evaluation panels to assess its progress. The first panel reviewed the first 5 years of the program by examining reports and evaluation data, and by conducting interviews with participants and committee members. The review committee affirmed the positive effect of the early changes made to the program and concluded that the program model was valuable, unique, and able to positively influence the careers of participants, who came to the program predisposed to conduct interdisciplinary research. The committee found, however, that structural change, though still necessary, is unlikely to result from the NAKFI program in a clear and measurable way. Rather than initiating dramatic change, the program was advised to focus on maximizing the collaborative opportunities available to participants through its conferences and seed grants, paying special attention to lowering barriers to communication across disciplines and fostering connections between grantees. At the same time, increased attention was devoted to broadening participation in NAKFI conferences and capturing the variety of results produced from seed grant projects.

The shift in the program's focus meant shifting the program's evaluation, which had included development and testing of measures of scholarly integration based on the references in published journal articles (see Porter et al. 2006; Porter et al. 2007; Porter et al. 2008). The strengths and limitations of using bibliometric approaches to measuring research interdisciplinarity have been noted elsewhere (e.g., Wagner, et.al 2011, Rosas et al. 2011) and are beyond the scope of this chapter. The intent behind this work was to develop benchmarks measuring the interdisciplinarity in scientific disciplines and compare the level of integration found in articles by NAKFI conference participants or seed grant recipients to the benchmark disciplines. Importantly for NAKFI, bibliometric analyses focus on only one kind of success: published, peer-reviewed papers. Reviews of grantees' final reports indicated that

they produced a wide variety of outputs and held a much broader view of why the NAKFI grant had been valuable to them and their careers.

Not long after the NAKFI Five-Year Review Panel issued its report in 2008, the *American Journal of Preventive Medicine* published a special supplement focusing on the science of team science. The volume drew from the proceedings of a National Cancer Institute–National Institutes of Health Conference on the Science of Team Science held in 2005. Work of Misra et al. (2009) evaluating the interdisciplinary qualities of undergraduate papers and Hall et al. assessing the collaborative readiness of science teams participating in the National Cancer Institute's Transdisciplinary Research on Energetics and Cancer (TREC) program described an approach that could be adapted to the NAKFI context. In 2009, Stokols became an evaluation consultant to NAKFI and a plan was developed to create a NAKFI Written Products Protocol to be used by expert peer reviewers to appraise the scientific originality, generativity, cross-disciplinary scope, integrative quality, and likely scientific and societal impacts of NAKFI seed grant projects.

In moving the work of Misra et al. and Hall et al. into practice, NAKFI's expert reviewers found value in using the data collected on the WPP instrument to inform their conversations about each project's accomplishments rather than strictly as a tool for gathering measurements. Ratings from reviewers were summarized and used to inform a group conversation about each project's goals, progress, and results. In one instance, reviewers gave a project divergent ratings on potential scientific and societal impact. By exploring why the reviewers gave the scores they did it was learned that the reviewers' scores reflected a debate taking place in the scientific community. The review committee concluded these opposing views indicated NAKFI was following through on its commitment to fund bold, risky research. Subsequent review committees have taken a similar approach, using the quantitative scores to inform a rich, qualitative discussion about each project, often revealing important details that would not have otherwise been revealed. Assessments were completed on grants awarded from 2006 through 2011. Together, these grantees leveraged $6 million in NAKFI seed funding into more than $126 million in additional support, 175 peer-reviewed publications, and 4 patents among other results. In addition to internal reports that have communicated findings to the academies leadership and the program's sponsor, the results from the seed grant reviews have helped to craft video narratives illustrating the program's contributions to participants' careers.

18.6 Strengths and Limitations

The value of expert knowledge and experience available to NAKFI through the National Academies of Sciences, Engineering, and Medicine is impossible to quantify. As with the organization's consensus studies, volunteer committee members work with staff over several years to realize their vision and evaluate the results.

The program attracted diverse attendees from around the nation, and there have been many examples of attendees from the same university meeting for the first time at a NAKFI conference. At the same time, attendees' geographic dispersion and the different rules and policies in force at their institutions can inhibit their ability to collaborate after the conference, especially for attendees from outside the United States who are not eligible to be listed as principle investigators on a grant. They can, and do, however, collaborate as coinvestigators.

NAKFI's ability to tailor aspects of the conference to the topic being addressed helped keep the program relevant. Attendees got to know one another in the seed idea groups and experienced remarkable insights individually and collectively. Though not every group worked well together, the meeting provided time for unstructured conversations outside of the group setting: over meals, during transportation to and from the meeting, and during poster sessions and creative engagements around exhibits.

Since its inception, NAKFI collected, reported, and used data to inform decision-making, inspire programmatic innovations, and document the program's impact. Unlike much of the material generated by the conference, which is distributed freely via the program's website and the National Academies Press, the audience for evaluation findings was internal.

The approach of organizing conferences and providing seed grants fills an important gap in the landscape of scientific discourse and funding. Through NAKFI, scholars, researchers, and practitioners from across sectors had the opportunity to surface new questions and stimulate new modes of inquiry. Though the full value of the program will likely not be fully known for years to come, the NAKFI approach has been used as inspiration for another interdisciplinary research initiative, this time a multiyear effort focused on single health issue: age-related macular degeneration (AMD). Launched in 2009 as the Arnold and Mabel Beckman Initiative for Macular Research (BIMR), the Stephen J. Ryan Initiative for Macular Research (RIMR) at the Doheny Eye Institute focuses on improving AMD diagnostics and expanding the prospect of new treatments for the number one cause of visual impairment and blindness in older Americans. The RIMR experience is one way the NAKFI model can be implemented and adapted.

At the time of this writing, the NAKFI program is entering its final years; NAKFI will concluded as a program of the National Academies in 2018. The NAKFI model could be used by other conveners such as associations, universities, foundations, or multistakeholder initiatives to facilitate new conversations and collaborations on a wide variety of topics. The book *Collaborations of Consequence* published by National Academies Press provides in-depth information on the program's evolution and results, as well as supporting material to implement the approach in other contexts (National Research Council, 2018). It is available as a free download at https://www.nap.edu/catalog/25239/. We are now devoted to sharing and propagating this model and the lessons learned in the hope that others might ask new questions and build new communities of inquiry using NAKFI's approach.

References

Aboelela SW, Larson E, Bakken S, Carrasquillo O, Formicola A, Glied SA, Haas J, Gebbie KM. Defining interdisciplinary research: conclusions from a critical review of the literature. Health Serv Res. 2007;42(1 Pt 1):329–46.

American Academy of Arts and Sciences. ARISE 2: Unleashing America's research & innovation enterprise; 2013. http://www.amacad.org/multimedia/pdfs/publications/researchpapersmonographs/arise2.pdf. Accessed 01 July 2016.

Choi BC, Pak, AW. Multidisciplinarity, interdisciplinarity and transdisciplinarity in health research, services, education and policy. Clin Invest Med. 2006; 29(6): 351–64.

Hall KL, Stokols D, Moser RP, Taylor BK, Thornquist MD, Nebeling LC, Ehret CC, Barnett MJ, McTiernan A, Berger NA, Goran MI, Jeffery RW. The collaboration readiness of transdisciplinary research teams and centers: findings from the National Cancer Institute's TREC Year-One Evaluation Study. Am J Prevent Med. 2008;35(2 Suppl):S161–72.

Misra S, Harvey R, Stokols D, Pinea KH, Fuqua J, Shokairb SM, Whiteley JM. Evaluating an interdisciplinary undergraduate training program in health promotion research. Am J Prev Med. 2009;36(4):358–65.

National Research Council. Enhancing the Effectiveness of Team Science. Washington. DC: The National Academies Press. 2015. https://doi.org/10.17226/19007.

Porter AL, Roessner JD, Cohen AS, Perreault M. Interdisciplinary research—meaning, metrics and nurture. Research Evaluation. 2006;15(3):187–95.

Porter AL, Cohen AS, Roessner JD, Perreault M. Measuring researcher interdisciplinarity. Scientometrics. 2007;72(1):117–47.

Porter AL, Roessner, DJ, Heberger AE. How interdisciplinary is a given body of research? Res. Eval. 2008;17(4):273–82. https://doi.org/10.3152/095820208X364553.

Rosas SR, Kagan JM, Schouten JT, Slack PA, Trochim WMK. Evaluating research and impact: a bibliometric analysis of research by the NIH/NIAID HIV/AIDS clinical trial network. PLoS One. 2011;6(3):e17428. https://doi.org/10.1371/journal.pone.0017428.

Rosenfield PL. The potential of transdisciplinary research for sustaining and extending linkages between the health and social sciences. Soc Sci Med. 1992;35:1343–57.

Wagner CS, Roessner JD, Bobb K, Klein JT, Boyack KW, Keyton J, Rafols I, Börner K. Approaches to understanding and measuring interdisciplinary scientific research (IDR): a literature review. J Infomet. 2011;5(1):14–26.

Facilitating Cross-Disciplinary Interactions to Stimulate Innovation: Stand Up to Cancer's Matchmaking Convergence Ideas Lab

19

Suzanne P. Christen and Arnold J. Levine

Contents

S. P. Christen (✉) · A. J. Levine
Simons Center for Systems Biology, School of
Natural Sciences, Institute for Advanced Study,
Princeton, NJ, USA
e-mail: schrist@ias.edu

19.1 Introduction

In the fall of 2014, the leaders of the high-profile nonprofit program Stand Up To Cancer ("SU2C"), whose mission is to raise awareness and funds to increase the pace of groundbreaking translational research that can get new therapies to patients quickly, and a group at the Institute for Advanced Study in Princeton, New Jersey, a world-famous center for theoretical research in physics and mathematics, teamed up to propose a multidisciplinary meeting to explore novel approaches to cancer research. The participants would include quantitative scientists from various areas of the physical sciences (theoretical physicists, mathematicians, computer scientists, and engineers) and clinical oncologists, two groups whose disparate research fields do not traditionally intersect. They would be invited to a multiday meeting in order to develop research projects integrating quantitative approaches and clinical cancer research—an exercise in convergence science. The success of the meeting that eventually resulted from this partnership, in engaging a very diverse group of researchers in developing creative, quantitative science-based approaches to advance cancer research using clinical data, ultimately led to the formation of four cross-institutional, multidisciplinary teams of researchers pursuing novel translational research projects that are being funded through a combination of private–public grants. The collaborative efforts that resulted in the February 2015 Convergence Ideas Lab meeting and these Convergence Teams are described below, and might provide guidance for others seeking to organize and facilitate cross-disciplinary interactions to stimulate innovation.

19.2 Convergence Science in Translational Cancer Research

Convergence science has emerged as a term to describe the importation of perspectives and approaches from the quantitative sciences and engineering to problems in biological research, and the concurrent influence of understanding of complex evolutionary biological systems on the development of the quantitative sciences. As summarized in a recent report published by the National Academy of Sciences:

> Convergence is an approach to problem solving that cuts across disciplinary boundaries. It integrates knowledge, tools, and ways of thinking from life and health sciences, physical, mathematical, and computational sciences, engineering disciplines, and beyond, to form a comprehensive synthetic framework for tackling scientific and societal challenges that exist at the interfaces of multiple fields. By merging these diverse areas of expertise in a network of partnerships, convergence stimulates innovation from basic science discovery to translational application. It provides fertile ground for new collaborations that engage stakeholders and partners not only from academia, but also from national laboratories, industry, clinical settings, and funding bodies (Alexandrov et al. 2013).

Basic biological and clinical research has been revolutionized by the development of novel high-throughput technologies, methods, and approaches used to identify and characterize DNA, RNA, proteins, and other molecules that permit rapid analysis of large numbers of samples. These technologies result in the generation of large-scale data that challenge the expertise of traditional biologists and clinicians. The need for

quantitative expertise in analyzing the data to understand and identify fundamental principles is particularly evident in oncology. Traditional molecular biology laboratories have not had the capacity to focus on the functional characterization of more than one or a few genes, in a mostly descriptive representation of single pathways, rather than as an integrated part of a more comprehensive picture. The generation of large-scale, high-dimensional, and complex data relating to genetic mutations and many other features of cancers, therefore, presents an opportunity for significant contributions from quantitative research. The Cancer Genome Atlas is an example of such data. Quantitative research has allowed the identification of mutational signatures across cancer types, some of which can be attributed to mutagens in smoke, UV radiation, and defects in DNA maintenance (Tanne et al. 2015). Quantitative science also has contributed to the development of technology and methodology for studying single cells, especially the sequencing and analyzing of DNA and RNA from single cells. This allows the study of heterogeneity of tumors, circulating tumor cells, and cell of origin for a tumor. Single-cell RNA sequencing (RNA seq), which reveals the presence and quantity of RNA in a biological sample at a given moment, has been used to study intratumoral heterogeneity (Balachandran et al. 2017). And, single-cell DNA sequencing has been used to study the circulating tumor cells of lung cancer patients, revealing copy number variation patterns of circulating tumor cells that were very similar to the metastases, and similar patterns of copy number variation among different patients with the same lung adenocarcinoma, but different patterns among patients with small-cell lung cancer (Guryanova et al. 2016).

Ultimately, the successful analysis of the large and complex datasets that are being or could be generated depends on *both* asking the right biological questions and knowing what can be done with these data, thus the need for multidisciplinary teams and thinking. Stand Up To Cancer has established a profile of successfully bringing together the best and the brightest cancer researchers and of mandating collaboration among members of the cancer research community in order to accelerate cancer research to help more people diagnosed with cancer become long-term survivors. Among the various innovative approaches that have been pursued by SU2C to promote progress in cancer research was its embrace, starting in 2014, of Convergence science in the form of the Convergence Ideas Lab.

19.3 Formulating the Convergence Ideas Lab Meeting Proposal

The first step in the realization of this Convergence Ideas Lab was to develop a proposal to the Physics of Living Systems program of the National Science Foundation to bring clinicians and quantitative researchers together, in a residential research setting, for a multiday meeting that would foster the exchange of ideas, methods, and knowledge. The meeting would be held on the campus of the Institute for Advanced Study, under the auspices of SU2C, and would include theoretical physicists, mathematicians, computer scientists, and engineers, with strong backgrounds in biological research, and clinical oncologists with a strong understanding of basic science. Participants representing these two groups would be able to meet and interact in such a way as to promote the generation of novel research ideas and methods in cancer research, through the convergence of clinical and theoretical approaches.

It was hoped that the proposals generated at the Convergence Ideas Lab meeting could eventually be funded, and that they would have a large impact on the direction of future research in clinical cancer. The immediate goal of the meeting was to facilitate the creation of three or four mixed and cross-institutional teams of clinical oncologists and quantitative scientists, focused on addressing a set of important problems or questions that arise from clinical cancer research data. These approaches would be articulated in short preliminary proposals by self-assembled groups of scientists in attendance at the meeting.

Following the meeting, these proposals might then be submitted for review and possible funding from both public and private sources. Also, it was hoped that if the meeting was successful and resulted in funded projects, that those projects could include postdoctoral researchers from quantitative backgrounds, and clinical fellows, in what should become a model for the mentoring and training of the next generation of quantitative and clinical cancer researchers.

The possibility of developing an innovative proposal and actually having it funded within a short time frame was sure to be a carrot to attract potential participants. Therefore, Stand Up To Cancer's President and CEO, Sung Poblete, PhD, worked tirelessly with additional parties to create a collaborative public–private network of additional potential funders for evaluation of innovative research proposals that might emerge from the program, in the event NSF appreciated the ideas and funded the meeting. These additional parties included Bristol-Myers Squibb, the Lustgarten Foundation, the V Foundation, and the Breast Cancer Research Foundation. In the end, the Convergence Ideas Lab held at the Institute for Advanced Study from February 13–18, 2015, was funded by the National Science Foundation's Program on Physics of Living Systems, through a grant to SU2C, with additional support provided by the V Foundation and the Institute for Advanced Study.

19.4 Participants/Meeting Structure

After the Convergence Ideas Lab meeting proposal was selected for funding by NSF, SU2C got to work advertising the opportunity to quantitative scientists and clinicians, through published journal advertisements and word of mouth. As has been the case with other SU2C sponsored opportunities, an advertised call for ideas process was employed (i.e., *Nature, Journal of Clinical Oncology*). Applications were reviewed by a panel of experts in the various disciplines, following NSF guidelines. Of close to 100 applicants, 23 scientists, 9 clinical oncologists, 2 engineers,

1 mathematician, and 11 physicists, were invited to participate. The group, composed of both junior and senior scientists, included two Howard Hughes Medical Institute investigators, several members of the National Academy of Sciences (NAS), and the chief physician of one of the top cancer centers in the United States.

Meanwhile, scientists and administrators at the Institute for Advanced Study took the lead in assembling a panel of advisors and mentors, and designing the structure of the multiday meeting. The general goal of the Convergence Ideas Lab structure was to bring together the clinicians and quantitative scientists who would be chosen to participate in such a way as to foster communication, maximize the natural flow of information back and forth among the participants, and allow for the development of new approaches and testable concepts for the field. Locating the meeting on the relatively secluded residential campus of the Institute for Advanced Study, in Princeton, NJ, an hour outside New York City and within reasonable distance of four major metropolitan airports, served the dual purposes of making it accessible to participants, who could arrive by air, train, or car, and minimizing the distraction of their day-to-day responsibilities, particularly for the very busy clinicians who attended. Having had more than 10 years of experience in successfully introducing young postdoctoral researchers of exceptional ability in the quantitative sciences to important problems in biology, the organizers from the Simons Center for Systems Biology at the institute had a strong sense of the kind of meeting structure that would be successful in bridging the cultural and (specialized) language differences between quantitative scientists and clinicians to achieve these goals.

All of the individuals from the quantitative sciences who were chosen to participate in the February 2015 meeting had worked and published papers in cancer biology or the biological sciences, which provided some common ground with the clinicians who were selected to attend, all of whom had a strong background in basic science as well as clinical oncology. A multidisciplinary group of advisors, made up of physicists, biologists, and oncologists, was asked to facili-

tate the meetings. Among other attendees were representatives from SU2C, including its President, Sung Poblete, and patient advocate, Renee Nicolas, leaders from the National Science Foundation's Physics Division, leaders and program representatives of the V Foundation, and representatives from Bristol-Myers Squibb and the Lustgarten Foundation.

This gathering of researchers, representing complementary but different fields, was composed of several groups who had never met before. The meeting began with a collegial dinner in a private dining room, both to make the arriving participants feel welcome and comfortable and to arrange the seating at tables to mix the diverse groups of scientists, in order to enhance communication between clinicians and quantitative scientists from the outset. The schedule included smaller, more informal, but also assigned, dinners for the participants on the other days. This approach was to ensure that everyone met everyone else, to maximize the exchange of ideas, and to promote "jelling" of the group. Unplanned, and well beyond the organizers' control, a blizzard, accompanied by 4 days of bone chilling temperatures, struck within the first 12 h of the meeting, and did just as much as careful planning to foster camaraderie, as the world outside was blanketed in 2 ft. of snow.

Each of the first 2 days started with a discussion that included the entire group to review the important questions that remain to be solved in clinical oncology: How do co-occurring mutations induce malignant transformation? Are there key nodes that are critical for cancer maintenance? Is it possible to develop good analytics to understand mutational interactions in cancer cells? How do cancer cells access genetic, epigenetic, and transcriptional diversity to evade cancer therapies? First, the oncologists presented talks introducing issues they considered most important to be explored in their areas of research. These talks were interspersed with long discussion sessions of an hour or more, to which the entire group actively contributed. The discussion sessions allowed the quantitative scientists an opportunity to test their understanding of the biological questions that were being presented and to probe the potential clinical significance of particular kinds of data. One participant described the rate and content of these discussions as "a fire hose of information." As questions were described by the oncologists, the group started to explore the many paths to solutions of the questions using approaches suggested by the quantitative scientists, including refining the technological tools to generate robust quantitative biological data, capturing and representing high-dimensional genomic data using rigorous mathematical approaches, identifying markers to stratify patients and to identify potential therapeutic targets, integrating different types of large-scale cancer data, generating tools to identify potential therapeutic targets in large datasets beyond recurrence of single gene alterations; for instance, identifying synergistic activities between different genes using large-scale genomic data, and providing quantitative testable models about the evolution of tumors using genomic data; in particular, reconstructing the evolutionary history of tumors from longitudinal and cross-sectional genomic data.

The days were broken up by working lunches and breaks for tea and coffee, which allowed for additional informal connections to be made among the participants. For dinner each evening, at local restaurants in Princeton, the meeting participants were sorted into small groups of four to six individuals, mixing oncologists and physicists who had never met or spoken to each other before. One of the meeting's designated advisors went along with each group to facilitate the discussions. The participants were housed in apartments on the grounds of the Institute for Advanced Study, so that conversations continued well into the night. By the third day, everyone knew each other and they were struggling to learn, digest, and create an interface among the fields. The meeting then broke into smaller groups, which formed and reformed over a couple of days, with guidance from the meeting advisors to define research questions and sets of experiments that could be analyzed by the physicists and engineers and to produce research project proposals. The only requirements for the projects, following the general outlines of traditional SU2C team struc-

ture, were that each group be composed of at least one clinician and one quantitative scientist, with a mix of senior and junior scientists/clinicians. By the fourth day, teams had self-assembled and were putting together short proposals of two to four pages, to be presented to the entire group on the afternoon of the fourth and morning of the fifth days. Teams that put forward proposals that met the criteria of addressing an important question, reflecting scientifically sound principles, and being innovative and feasible, were to be invited to write and submit more detailed proposals.

19.5 Project Proposals

Over the course of the fourth and fifth days of the meeting, four proposals were presented by the individual teams to the entire group of researchers, as well as the representatives of SU2C, the NSF, and the various other attendees. The first proposal, "Liberating T-cell-mediated immunity to pancreatic cancer," was led by Drs. Jeff Drebin, a world-class pancreatic surgeon/researcher at the University of Pennsylvania, Jedd Wolchok, a leader in the field of immunotherapy at Memorial Sloan Kettering Cancer Center (MSKCC), and David Ting, a young oncologist/researcher at Massachusetts General Hospital (MGH), Harvard, who pioneered circulating tumor cells (CTCs). They teamed up with Drs. Harlan Robins, a physicist at the Hutchinson Cancer Research Center (FHCRC), who first showed how to sequence T-cell receptors in a quantitative fashion; Curt Callan, a senior Princeton University physicist and National Academy of Sciences member, who works on the immune system of humans; and Ben Greenbaum, a young physicist at Mount Sinai Medical School, who demonstrated the mechanisms of innate immunity in cancer cells. The goal of the project is to refine potential immunotherapeutic approaches to pancreatic cancer, to enhance the specificity, generalizability, and maintenance of durable responses, using a combination of mouse models and human clinical trials, and novel immunostimulatory noncoding RNAs, and high-throughput immunomodulation assay development. The collaboration involves characterizing the presence of T cells associated with pancreatic tumors and the T-cell receptor repertoire in untreated pancreas tumors and in pancreas tumors treated prior to removal with vitamin D, which reduces the fibrotic tissue that surrounds the tumor and blocks T-cell entry of the immune system. A subsequent publication by some members of the group in the *Proceedings of the National Academy of Sciences, USA*, demonstrated the role of a small noncoding RNA in stimulating the innate immune response (Hata et al. 2016), using complete exomic sequencing data from pancreas cancers to predict potential tumor neoantigens, and conducting a tri-institutional exploratory Phase 1 clinical trial.

The second team focused their efforts upon "the genetic, epigenetic, and immunological underpinnings of cancer evolution through treatment." The oncologists leading this team were Drs. Jeff Engelman, a physician who headed the lung cancer clinic at MGH, Harvard (now at Novartis, and replaced on the team by Drs. Aaron Hata, and Lecia Sequist MGH, Harvard), and Ross Levine, who heads the leukemia/lymphoma service at MSKCC. They were paired with physicists Harlan Robins; Daniel Fisher, a senior scholar at Stanford University and member of the National Academy of Sciences, who studies evolution of cells; Steven Altschuler, Professor in the Department of Pharmaceutical Chemistry at the University of California, San Francisco (UCSF) School of Pharmacy, who is interested in discovering principles underlying cellular individuality, the emergence of collective cellular behaviors, and the evolution of drug resistance; and Chang Chan, a young assistant professor at Rutgers, Cancer Institute of New Jersey (CINJ), who studies the evolution of cancers in people with inherited diseases. This proposal aims (1) to find the reasons why some patients respond to T-cell therapy and others do not, and to quantitate that response by identifying the signals for selective forces that are in the genomes of patients whose cancer cells survive immunotherapy (lung cancers and blood cancers), and (2) to determine whether mutations leading to resistance of thera-

pies preexist in a few cancer cells or are induced by the therapy (persisters). Two subsequent publications from members of this group, in *Nature Medicine* and *Nature Communications*, demonstrated that mutations preexist in the tumors—at least in most cases (Le et al. 2016; Łuksza et al. 2017). A November 2016 *Nature Medicine* paper from the team reflects findings that identify a crucial role for DNMT3AR882 mutations in driving AML chemoresistance and highlight the importance of chromatin remodeling in response to cytotoxic chemotherapy (Ni et al. 2013).

The third proposal, "Rational design of anti-cancer drug combinations with dynamic multidimensional input" paired Drs. José Baselga, the Physician-in-Chief of the Memorial Sloan Kettering Hospital, Levi Garraway, and Anthony Letai, both from Dana Farber Cancer Institute, with two physicists, Raul Rabadan of Columbia University College of Physicians and Surgeons and Reka Albert of Penn State University. The proposal focuses upon the PI-3 kinase pathway, breast cancers and melanoma, and the use of traditional and experimental therapies that could be combined with immunotherapy, with the goal of developing a general theoretical and experimental framework to analyze how to optimize the order of addition, the duration, the concentrations, and the combinations of drugs to achieve a therapeutic outcome without resistance. This has already led to a publication demonstrating a quantitative model of the PI-3 kinase pathway and reconstruction of the evolution of mutations in a tumor under treatment (NRC [National Research Council] 2014).

The fourth proposal, "The ecology of the tumor microenvironment in breast cancer" is led by Dr. Peter Lee, Chair, Department of Immuno-Oncology and Co-leader, Cancer Immunotherapeutics Program of the City of Hope Cancer Center. The other team members include Herbert Levine, senior physicist at Rice University; physicist Mickey Atwal, Cold Spring Harbor Laboratory; senior physicist Clare Yu, University of California at Irvine; and bioengineer Darrell Irvine, Massachusetts Institute of Technology. The proposal focuses upon understanding the complex interactions among the tumor cells, immune cells, and the surrounding stromal cells in the breast tumor microenvironment. The project combines high-resolution microscopy, single-cell genomics, machine learning, mathematical modeling, and nanotechnology and synthetic biology. The goal is to understand the physical landscape and molecular profiles of breast cancer in primary and metastatic sites, and develop novel nanotechnology therapies targeting the tumor microenvironment. Early findings suggest that the stromal cells in the surrounding breast cancer tissue are not just passive players, but also undergo significant gene expression changes that aid the growth of tumors, suggesting that therapies that also target the stroma would be effective in fighting the cancer cells.

After the conclusion of the Convergence Ideas Lab meeting, all four of these proposals were considered worthy of funding by the Scientific Advisory Board of SU2C, and all four teams were invited to submit written proposals with budgets. Because of Stand Up's President Sung Poblete's efforts before, during, and after the meeting, and because representatives of various potential funding organizations had been welcomed to attend the meeting discussions, and had been impressed with the potential for real progress in the field by the innovative approaches proposed then and in subsequent funder reviews of the final proposals, a total of $12.5 million were found from private sources to provide support for all four proposals (one proposal ended up being supported completely by private funds within a couple of weeks of the conclusion of the meeting). Three of the proposals were submitted to NSF, were favorably reviewed, and received NSF funding in addition to the private support. Together, the private and public funding for these four proposals totaled $17.5 million.

The chief factors that account for the successful dynamics of the meeting are reflected in comments from participants:

"The Ideas Lab meeting was the most interesting cancer conference I have been to ever. The intimate setting encouraged rapid fire learning through lectures, extensive Q & A, and conversations over dinner and late into the night. Dr. Levine's commentaries and questions particularly helped

summarize and frame each talk, though participation in discussions was nearly universal among attendees. Together, this led to a fire-hose style of learning new ideas and techniques in cancer biology that was much appreciated. I was initially uncertain about how teams of clinicians and quantitative researchers would self-organize to put forward proposals, but this also flowed naturally from the talks and dinner discussions. The only suggestion I can think of is of providing follow-up mechanisms so that we can continue to build on the momentum generated at the conference—even across teams, whose boundaries were somewhat artificially imposed by the grant exercise. Bravo!"

"My experience at the Ideas Lab was wonderful and very fruitful. The most important part for me as a computational biologist was to meet the clinical oncologists and learn from them what their most pressing problems were. This exchange occurred over lunches and dinners as well as from their talks. One such exchange has already led to collaboration ... to study how resistance arises in targeted therapy. This was something we had agreed to work on whether or not our proposal got funded. My only suggestion for the Ideas Lab is for group formation. As I saw it, the groups form from a few nucleating centers (defined by clinical oncologists) that aggregated additional members over time. I was not sure which group I could associate with and dropped in on all the groups before finding one where I fit in. It all worked out in the end and perhaps this is the best model. An alternative would be to define some areas of interests and ask people to indicate their interests to help with forming the groups which can then change over time. A question I wonder is if we repeat the Ideas Lab many times (as replicates), how similar would the proposals be or the group members? Overall, I did not know what to expect from the Ideas Lab but the results have exceeded my expectations and I would be more than happy to participate in future iterations."

19.6   Sequelae

The teams quickly got to work, and three related meetings took place at the Institute for Advanced Study (under milder weather conditions). The first follow-up meeting was held in April 2016, bringing the four teams' principal investigators back together for an update on their research. A second meeting in June 2016 and a third in June 2017 were the first two of what are planned as annual summer training meetings for the postdoctoral researchers and clinical fellows who are working on the teams, to introduce them to each other, to the work of all of the teams, and to some of the other latest developments in cancer research. Summer meetings have featured talks from the postdoctoral researchers and clinical fellows to each other on their work for the teams, as well as additional talks from outside senior cancer experts.

One of the positive outcomes of the Convergence Ideas Lab meeting is that team members not only developed strong intrateam relationships, but they have also been finding ways to collaborate across teams. As one individual said "Thank you for hosting this amazing workshop. Our team is very excited about working together on this project, and … interact[ing] with the other teams…." One such cross-team interaction (Ben Greenbaum and Jedd Wolchok) resulted in a Phillip A. Sharp Innovation in Collaboration Award made at the SU2C annual scientific summit in January 2016, in support of a method to develop predictive models of immunotherapy response. Two studies resulting from this collaboration were published in the November 23, 2017 issue of the journal *Nature*.

19.7 Conclusion

The Convergence Ideas Lab meeting generated truly novel hypotheses, concepts, and directions for cancer research. It paired individuals who never would have met each other, never would have worked with each other, and who began the meeting not understanding the questions they will now study over the next 3–4 years. This is all the more impressive, because both the clinical oncologists and the quantitative scientists are among the best in the world at what they do. The project proposals generated by participants in the Convergence Ideas Lab demonstrate the guiding principles of SU2C: bring together the best scientists in the world, from diverse institutions, to solve a problem collaboratively, and provide them with the resources needed to get the job done in a rapid time frame. Innovation comes

from the pairing of great minds in different fields, each contributing a portion of the solution. In the words of one participant "I thought the Convergence Ideas Lab was fantastic. The people and diversity of expertise was amazing. Most importantly, being there for 4–5 days allowed us all to get comfortable with the back and forth, and the physicists really impacted us positively with their willingness to engage in discussions without worrying about time, or egos, or credit. That was a great thing…." As the meeting drew to a close, one of the senior physicists said "independent of anything else, lets meet once or twice a year to continue learning from each other and to continue to push the limits of understanding this disease."

The Convergence Ideas Lab meeting is just the beginning of a new way to do science and to foster cooperation and collaboration among scientists for the benefit of patients with cancer. Novel and good things should happen. Optimally, the Convergence team approach will open up a new field of research that can deepen our understanding of disease origin, progression, diagnosis, prognosis, treatment, and outcome, and also lower the costs to society of developing effective therapeutic treatments, and of enhancing quality of life and outcome for cancer patients. This approach should be replicable with similar effect in other fields of medical research, including infectious diseases. The multidisciplinary approach and research projects developed at the Convergence Ideas Lab meeting and that are now underway have the potential to improve the lives and outcomes of disease in patients, to lower the costs to society of developing effective therapeutic treatments, and to enhance the education and training of the next generation of cancer researchers.

References

Alexandrov LB, Nik-Zainal S, Wedge DC, Campbell PJ, Stratton MR. Deciphering signatures of mutational processes operative in human cancer. Cell Rep. 2013;3(1):246–59. https://doi.org/10.1016/j.celrep.2012.12.008.

Balachandran VP, Łuksza M, et al. Identification of unique neoantigen qualities in long-term survivors of pancreatic cancer. Nature. 2017;551:512–6.

Guryanova OA, Shank K, Spitzer B, Luciani L, Koche RP, Garrett-Bakelman FE, Ganzel C, Durham BH, Mohanty A, Hoermann G, Rivera SA, Chramiec AG, Pronier E, Bastian L, Keller MD, Tovbin D, Loizou E, Weinstein AR, Gonzalez AR, Lieu YK, Rowe JM, Pastore F, McKenney AS, Krivtsov AV, Sperr WR, Cross JR, Mason CE, Tallman MS, Arcila ME, Abdel-Wahab O, Armstrong SA, Kubicek S, Staber PB, Gönen M, Paietta EM, Melnick AM, Nimer SD, Mukherjee S, Levine RL. DNMT3A mutations promote anthracycline resistance in acute myeloid leukemia via impaired nucleosome remodeling. Nat Med. 2016;22(12):1488–95. https://doi.org/10.1038/nm.4210.

Hata AN, Niederst MJ, Archibald HL, et al. Tumor cells can follow distinct evolutionary paths to become resistant to epidermal growth factor receptor inhibition. Nat Med. 2016;22(3):262–9. https://doi.org/10.1038/nm.4040.

Le X, Antony R, Razavi P, Treacy DJ, Luo F, Ghandi M, Castel P, Scaltriti M, Baselga J, Garraway LA. Systematic functional characterization of resistance to PI3K inhibition in breast cancer. Cancer Discov. 2016;6(10):1134–47.

Łuksza M, Riaz N, Makarov V, Balachandran VP, Hellmann MD, Solovyov A, Rizvi NA, Merghoub T, Levine AJ, Chan TA, Wolchok JD, Greenbaum BD. A neoantigen fitness model predicts tumour response to checkpoint blockade immunotherapy. Nature. 2017;551:517–20.

Ni X, Zhuo M, Su Z, et al. Reproducible copy number variation patterns among single circulating tumor cells of lung cancer patients. Proc Natl Acad Sci. 2013;110(52):21083–8. https://doi.org/10.1073/pnas.1320659110.

NRC (National Research Council). Convergence: facilitating transdisciplinary integration of life sciences, physical sciences, engineering, and beyond. Washington, DC: The National Academies Press; 2014.

Tanne A, Muniz LR, Puzio-Kuter A, Leonova KI, Gudkov AV, Ting DT, Monasson R, Cocco S, Levine AJ, Bhardwaj N, Greenbaum BD. Distinguishing the immunostimulatory properties of noncoding RNAs expressed in cancer cells. PNAS. 2015;112(49):15154–9. https://doi.org/10.1073/pnas.1517584112.

Retreats to Stimulate Cross-Disciplinary Translational Research Collaborations: Medical University of South Carolina CTSA Pilot Project Program Initiative

20

Damayanthi Ranwala, Anthony J. Alberg, Kathleen T. Brady, Jihad S. Obeid, Randal Davis, and Perry V. Halushka

Contents

D. Ranwala (✉) · K. T. Brady · J. S. Obeid · P. V. Halushka
South Carolina Clinical and Translational Research Institute, Medical University of South Carolina, Charleston, SC, USA
e-mail: ranwala@musc.edu

A. J. Alberg
Epidemiology and Biostatistics Department, University of South Carolina, Columbia, SC, USA

R. Davis
Strategic Research Initiatives, Medical University of South Carolina, Charleston, SC, USA

20.1 Introduction

To stimulate the formation of new interdisciplinary translational research team collaborations and innovative pilot projects, the Medical University of South Carolina's CTSA—South Carolina Clinical & Translational Research (SCTR) Institute—has initiated biannual scientific retreats often with speed dating style networking sessions. The themes of the retreats are cross-disciplinary, address unmet medical needs in South Carolina (SC) and beyond, stimulate formation of new interdisciplinary teams, and are anticipated to generate pilot project grant applications of novel translational research discoveries, technologies, and methodologies. The retreat format is designed to stimulate new research ideas and exchange in small groups to develop new research projects. The retreats are complemented by the SCTR Institute Pilot Project Program funds to support innovative pilot projects that emanate from the retreats. This chapter describes the design of the retreats, novel scientific collaborations and projects that the retreats have stimulated, scientific impacts, challenges, and strategies for success.

© Springer Nature Switzerland AG 2019
K. L. Hall et al. (eds.), *Strategies for Team Science Success*,
https://doi.org/10.1007/978-3-030-20992-6_20

20.2 Design of the Retreats

SCTR Institute encourages academic investigators and other stakeholders in the state of SC to propose retreat themes that have unmet medical needs requiring development of new interdisciplinary research collaborations to solve. Once a theme is proposed, it is evaluated by the SCTR Institute leadership for appropriateness such as whether the objectives set forth for the retreats—development of new interdisciplinary teams and generation of novel project ideas to move forward—are met, timeliness, and scope. After a theme is selected, experts in that area are asked to participate in a retreat planning committee. The planning committee selects keynote speakers, other presentations, panel/workshop, and networking sessions for the retreat. The keynote speaker is a nationally recognized expert in the thematic area who is actively involved in translational research. The presentations are selected from the abstracts received from the statewide stakeholders during the retreat registration. The SCTR Institute provides announcements about the retreat registration and abstract submissions to the statewide stakeholders. The planning committee reviews the abstracts received based on their importance to the retreat theme, scientific quality, potential for development of new interdisciplinary collaborations, and novel research idea generation to plan the platform presentations. Based on the retreat theme and stakeholders needs, the committee also looks into potential panel and/or workshop ideas to further enhance the generation of novel research ideas. The retreat agenda is developed making sure to include presenters from different disciplines and having a mixture of different talks including 2–3 speed dating style networking sessions throughout the day to promote new team formations and collaborations. Once the agenda is finalized, it is sent to the registered attendees along with the presentations' abstracts and attendees' contact information to facilitate potential networking contacts even before the retreat. This is carried out a few weeks before the retreat. Follow-up reminders are sent several times until the day of the retreat to keep the individuals engaged.

The retreat starts with the keynote address of about 45 min followed by 15 min of Q&A. The keynote speech is followed by 3–4 sessions of local, platform research presentation sessions. Each session includes 3–4 platform presentations, limited to 10 min time followed by 5 min Q&A. The presenters are advised to include 1–2 slides at the end of their presentations to show their research-related needs such as what kind of collaborations they are looking to develop and what kind of expertise is needed to continue their research. This is to help the retreat attendees make the connections with the presenters to develop new collaborations. A 20–30 min of speed dating style networking sessions are included in between the research presentation sessions to facilitate networking and sharing research ideas among the presenters and attendees. A presentation about the SCTR Institute Pilot Project Program Funding Opportunities and a panel composed of the experts in the retreat theme, keynote speaker, and session moderators summarizing key points of the retreat and opportunities for collaborations are included at the end of the day to further promote attendees participation. The attendees are also informed about the other SCTR Institute research support services and free consultation services such as biostatistics, budget and regulatory consultations, as well as mock review services of extramural grant applications to facilitate translational research grant applications that may emanate as a result of the retreat. After the retreat is concluded, a summary of the retreat along with the presentation recordings and SCTR Institute Pilot Project Funding announcements are sent to the attendees. The attendees are encouraged to submit new pilot project applications that may have emanated as a result of the retreat while collaborating with at least one investigator who has attended the retreat. Attendees are instructed to indicate in their potential applications whether the application is a result of the retreat. Once the applications are received, a technical review is done to determine whether they are a result of a SCTR Institute held retreat/s, have a new and interdisciplinary collaboration, and proposed novel research ideas. Then they are peer reviewed, as similar to the NIH peer-review process, by the SCTR Institute Scientific Review Committee and/or ad hoc reviewers to determine the scientific merits.

20.3 Novel Scientific Collaborations and Projects That the Retreats Have Stimulated

The SCTR Institute held total of 10 retreats from 2009 to 2014 (Ranwala et al. 2016). Each retreat theme was different and covered a wide range of topics such as bioengineering, mHealth, obesity, patient-centered outcomes research, and tobacco-related research. Each retreat had an average of 100 attendees. Some attendees have participated more than one retreat. We used the number of pilot project applications received as a direct measure of new and interdisciplinary scientific collaborations formed as a result of the retreats. We received 61 applications (i.e., 61 unique PIs and projects) from the 10 retreats. Based on the peer review, 14 applications were funded. In some cases, retreats and pilot projects led to successful extramural applications. For example, the Telemedicine Retreat facilitated the submission of two successful Duke Endowment grants (the Virtual TeleConsult Clinic and Remote Expert Assessment of Lung Cancer); the Neurological Diseases and Injury Retreat facilitated a successful application for an NIH Center of Biomedical Research Excellence in stroke and a National Center of Neuromodulation for Rehabilitation; and the Bioengineering and Obesity Retreats stimulated multidisciplinary investigators from two institutions (bioengineering from the Clemson University's Human Factors & Ergonomics Research Institute and a clinician from the Medical University of South Carolina Weight Management Center) to

collaborate on a proposal to investigate a new device for weight loss which has resulted in a Small Business Technology Transfer grant and a R01grant. The Obesity Retreat also generated collaborative projects between pediatric researchers and community organizations, including a school-based study focused on pediatric obesity that translated into policy changes regarding daily dietary guidelines in two SC school districts. There were active research programs related to the mHealth and Tobacco Control Program ongoing at the Medical University of South Carolina before the respective two retreats were held. The retreats enhanced the subsequent research of the two programs resulting in a number of new extramural grants and new faculty recruitment to the Tobacco Control Program. The average cost per retreat was approximately $5000. A conservative estimate of the total extramural grant funding received from the five retreats listed above, in which we were able to gather outcome data, was $20,228,047 resulting a return on investment of $809 for each dollar spent on the retreats.

20.4 Scientific Impacts

The attendees were asked to evaluate the retreats for their satisfaction with the retreats and achieving its objective—retreats as stimulators of translational interdisciplinary team building. The evaluation data, as a qualitative measure of the retreats impacts, showed favorable feedback for satisfaction with the retreats in achieving its objective. Attendees indicated that some of the new team building and collaborations would not have happened without the retreats. Some commented frequently that the retreats provided a unique opportunity to gather and exchange research ideas freely with other translational researchers and stakeholders throughout the state. Post-retreat communication with the SCTR Institute Pilot Project Program indicates that the retreats facilitated the formation of new interdisciplinary research teams. A few quotes from those communications are exemplars of attendees experiences: "The project overall has grown and would not be where it is now without SCTR Institute's retreats and early help with the pilot funding support." In some cases, retreats have further enhanced ongoing collaborations and/or the translational research by "watering it and helping it grow."

An analysis of bibliometric data from our research networking system (Science of Team Science Conference, Obeid et al. 2015) provides supporting evidence of increased team science among the SCTR Pilot Project Program-funded investigators. The Research Networking System (RNS) analysis was done among 44 randomly selected investigators, who were funded during the period of 2010–2013 and had 140 publications, to assess the development of team science and translational impact. The RNS analysis showed a significantly higher degree centrality (higher number of unique coauthors) for SCTR-funded investigators as compared to a control group with similar total number of publications but non-SCTR Institute funding. Among these 44 investigators included 5 investigators funded as a result of the retreat/s.

20.5   Challenges and Strategies for Success

Although we continue to improve the retreats and anticipate more positive outcomes of the retreats, we face a challenge in gathering retreat evaluation data and post-retreat outcomes data from the attendees. The average percentage of evaluation forms received by the attendees was about 35%. It has been a challenge to gather evaluation forms from the attendees since some leave the retreat in different times of the day and/or do not return the forms or respond when it is sent via electronically after the retreat is over. We have not collected the demographic data of the attendees in all the retreats. Where it is collected, the data show that there is a tendency that the attendees from academia have retuned more evaluation forms than the rest of the state and community partners. We are

requesting attendees to fill out an annual retreat follow-up survey to collect retreat outcomes such as development of new research teams, successful extramural grant applications, and publications that may have emanated from the retreats. The response rate to these surveys is also only about 35%, so the results are likely skewed by those with more favorable views and outcomes being most likely to respond. In order to increase the response rate to the evaluation form, we are looking into providing incentives such as gift cards for those who return the forms. As an additional mechanism that we have employed to gather outcome measures of the retreats, we contacted the retreat planning committee chairs who are the experts of the retreat theme area. We assumed that they may get to know the outcomes of the retreats even if each individual may not respond to the survey. We plan to continue a more a comprehensive analysis of the RNS data for the investigators that we funded as a result of the retreats. We believe that these measures will be helpful to show the outcome data of the retreats even if the attendees' responses are going to be lower.

In conclusion, the SCTR Pilot Project Program has sponsored 10 Scientific Retreats covering a broad range of topics critical to biomedical research and community needs in the state. About 1000 attendees across the state representing different disciplines have attended. The retreat evaluation data revealed favorable feedback from the attendees for satisfaction with the retreat and achieving its objective as a stimulator of translational interdisciplinary research team building. The SCTR Pilot Project Program-sponsored scientific retreat format appears to be effective in building new interdisciplinary research teams and collaborations to develop innovative research projects to advance translational research. Future retreats will continue to target topics of cross-cutting importance to biomedical and public health research.

Acknowledgments This work was supported in part by the South Carolina Clinical & Translational Research (SCTR) Institute, with an academic home at the Medical University of South Carolina, through a

Clinical and Translational Science Award (CTSA) from the National Center for Advancing Translational Sciences (NCATS), National Institutes of Health (NIH) Grant Numbers UL1 TR000062 and UL1 TR001450. The contents are solely the responsibility of the authors and do not necessarily represent the official views of the NIH or NCATS.

References

Obeid JS et al. Using research networking data to assess the impact of translational research funding on collaborative publications. In: Science of Team Science 2015 Conference, Natcher Conference Center, NIH, Bethesda, MD; 2015.

Ranwala D, et al. Scientific retreats with 'speed dating': networking to stimulate new interdisciplinary translational research collaborations and team science. J Investig Med. 2016;65(2):382–90. https://doi.org/10.1136/jim-2016-000261.

Part VI

Team Functioning and Performance

Evidence-Based Principles and Strategies for Optimizing Team Functioning and Performance in Science Teams

Steve W. J. Kozlowski and Bradford S. Bell

Contents

21.1 State of the Science: Team Functioning and Performance

The functioning and effectiveness of small groups and work teams have been a focus of research in psychology, management, and organizational science for well over 60 years, so there is a wealth of actionable knowledge that can be distilled from this literature. It should be noted that, until relatively recently, most of the research has not been specifically focused on scientific research teams per se. Nonetheless, with the exception of some very specific limitations or boundary conditions that we will address later, this substantial research foundation is a source of numerous conceptual insights and actionable recommendations that are directly applicable to science teams (National Research Council 2015). Our goal in this chapter is to provide a broad, integrative review of theory and research drawn from the science of team effectiveness literature that is particularly relevant and applicable to science teams.

Given the size and scope of this research domain, our strategy for this review was to integrate core concepts and insights drawn from several influential contemporary reviews of the team effectiveness literature in organizational science (Ilgen et al. 2005; Kozlowski and Bell 2003, 2013; Kozlowski and Ilgen 2006; Mathieu et al. 2008), supplemented by promising developments from recent research. We also focused our review on topics highlighted in the National Research Council (NRC) report on *Enhancing the Effectiveness of Team Science* (National Research Council 2015) that are particularly relevant to the functioning of science teams. Several chapters in this handbook address some of these topics in detail, such as team assembly (Twyman and

S. W. J. Kozlowski (✉)
Michigan State University, East Lansing, MI, USA
e-mail: stevekoz@msu.edu

B. S. Bell
Center for Advanced Human Resource Study,
Industrial and Labor Relations School, Cornell
University, Ithaca, NY, USA

© Springer Nature Switzerland AG 2019
K. L. Hall et al. (eds.), *Strategies for Team Science Success*,
https://doi.org/10.1007/978-3-030-20992-6_21

Contractor 2019), diversity (Gibbs et al. 2019), competencies (Nurius and Kemp 2019), team training (Fiore et al. 2019), team leadership (Salazar et al. 2019), and institutional influences (Winter 2019) among other issues. Our primary contribution is to organize and integrate the core concepts relevant to team functioning and effectiveness into a coherent heuristic that makes explicit their respective roles, interconnections, and priorities.

21.1.1 Key Concepts and the Review Structure

Key concepts addressed in the review are highlighted and defined in Table 21.1. The review is structured as follows. We begin the chapter by discussing the nature of work teams in general, describing distinguishing features, and then highlighting some characteristics of science teams that—in the very extreme—serve as boundary conditions that may limit generalization of the knowledge drawn from the science of team effectiveness to specific types of science teams. We emphasize these boundaries for two primary reasons. First, it makes salient that most of the research insights from the science of team effectiveness are generalizable and directly applicable to most science teams. Second, those boundaries that do limit generalization identify clearly where future research for enhancing the effectiveness of science teams needs to be targeted.

We then provide a high-level overview of theoretical frameworks that serve to highlight core conceptual issues, topics, and research areas relevant to team effectiveness. For example, an early framework posed by McGrath (1964) organized the literature on small groups and teams around an Inputs-Processes-Outputs (IPO) heuristic, whereas more contemporary efforts have elaborated the IPO model with feedback loops to account for temporal dynamics (e.g., Ilgen et al. 2005; Kozlowski and Ilgen 2006; Mathieu et al. 2008) and interventions or "levers" that can be used to enhance team processes and effectiveness (Kozlowski and Ilgen 2006). Kozlowski and Bell (2003, 2013) orga-

Table 21.1 Key concepts and definitions

Key concept	Concise definition
Input-process-output	Dominant heuristic used to organize the team effectiveness literature
Boundary conditions	Contingencies that limit or change relationships
Critical conceptual foci	System context, multilevel linkages, task interdependence, and temporal dynamics
Organizational structure	Structure of roles, responsibilities, goals, and authority
Workflow design	Structure by which information and effort flow among team members
Virtuality	Distribution of team members across time and space tempered by media bandwidth
Team composition	The pattern of individual differences (e.g., demographics and ability, experience, values, personality, culture, etc.) across team members
Team climate	Strategic imperatives
Team learning	Psychological safety; learning from errors; supportive feedback; open leadership
Knowledge building	Information sharing mechanisms
Team mental models	Shared knowledge structures
Transactive memory	Team distributed memory
Team cohesion	Task commitment and social attraction
Team efficacy	Shared confidence for goal attainment
Team affect or mood	Group emotions
Team coordination, cooperation, and communication	Combination of member actions; information exchange
Team member competencies	Teamwork knowledge, skills, and abilities
Team regulation	Regulation of attention and effort

nized the literature around a team lifecycle heuristic that considers team formation and composition, socialization and development, processes (cognitive, motivational, affective, and behavioral) and effectiveness, motivation and leadership, and continuance and decline. Although the different reviews provide unique insights, there is substantial conceptual overlap across the approaches. We develop an integrative heuristic to organize the topics that are of particular relevance to science teams.

We also highlight critical conceptual foci (i.e., assumptions, boundary conditions) that are an important aspect of conceptualizing individuals working in teams within a broader organizational system or context as team processes and performance emerge (from individual interaction within teams bounded by the system context) and unfold over time. We use the integrative heuristic, with attention to the critical conceptual foci and boundary conditions, to drive the review which follows. Consistent with our theoretical heuristic, we organize the review of team effectiveness research around *inputs and antecedents*—organizational structure, workflow design, virtuality, and composition—and *team processes and team functioning*—cognitive, motivational and affective, and behavioral. We close the chapter with *recommendations* for how science team processes can be aligned with respect to application and research relevant to advancing the science of team effectiveness to science teams.

21.2 Work Teams and Challenges for Science Teams

21.2.1 The Nature of Work Teams

"Work teams and groups come in a variety of types and sizes, cutting across different contexts, functions, internal processes, and external linkages. However, several features provide a foundation for a basic definition. Work teams and groups: (a) are composed of two or more individuals; (b) who exist to perform organizationally relevant tasks; (c) share one or more common goals; (d) exhibit task interdependencies (i.e., workflow, goals, knowledge, and outcomes); (e) interact socially (face-to-face or, increasingly, virtually); (f) maintain and manage boundaries; and (g) are embedded in an organizational context that sets boundaries, constrains the team, and influences exchanges with other units in the broader entity" (p. 415, Kozlowski and Bell 2013).

The definition above helps to distinguish work teams—which are formed to perform organizationally relevant tasks—from informal social groups which form on the basis of mutual attraction (Levine and Moreland 1990). The primary emphasis on task-relevant processes (versus social processes) for work teams implicates the key features of workflow interdependence, unit boundaries, and linkages to the embedding system context. Moreover, work teams are diverse entities and not a unitary type. This diversity makes teams challenging to study, since the underlying differences implicate different factors or contingencies that are more relevant to some teams and less so to others. As a result, several taxonomies have been proposed in an effort to describe, classify, and distinguish different types of teams (e.g., Cohen and Bailey 1997; Sundstrom et al. 1990, 2000). In other instances, researchers have asserted that a particular team form is distinctly different than other normative types of work teams. For example, some scholars have suggested that crews, top management teams, and virtual teams are distinct team types (see Kozlowski and Bell 2013).

Scholars have argued that, although classification via taxonomy is a useful initial step for describing phenomena and distinguishing similar and different types, a more productive approach is to focus on identifying the dimensions that underlie classification distinctions (Hollenbeck et al. 2012; Kozlowski and Bell 2003, 2013). For example, Hollenbeck et al. (2012) followed the suggestion to take a dimensional approach, identifying three dimensions that encompass a wide range of distinct team types. Their dimensions include: "(1) *skill differentiation*—the degree to which members have specialized knowledge or functional capacities that make it more or less difficult to substitute members; (2) *authority differentiation*—the degree to which decision-making responsibility is vested in individual members, subgroups of the team, or the collective as a whole; and (3) *temporal stability*—the degree to which team members have a history of working together in the past and an expectation of working together in the future" (p. 84).

Integrating their prior work (i.e., Bell and Kozlowski 2002; Kozlowski and Bell 2003, 2013; Kozlowski et al. 1999), Kozlowski and Bell (2013) developed a set of dimensions designed to characterize a continuum to distinguish simple teams from those that are more complex and which capture many of the differences that account for classification in the various taxonomies. Their typology, illustrated in Fig. 21.1, is composed of four primary dimensions, each of which has sub-features. First, the nature of the team's task environment or its organizational context is critical for determining (a) the extent of team process dynamics in terms of tempo, pacing, and rate of change and (b) the degree to which the team is loosely or tightly coupled to the task or context. Low dynamics mean that members operate more or less independently, whereas high dynamics necessitate more intensive and time-bound communication, collaboration, and coordination. Similarly, loose coupling means that the team operates more or less independently of the environment or context,

whereas tight coupling entrains team processes to the broader system. Second, workflow interdependence determines the degree to which and how each team member is linked with their teammates, which has implications for the nature of their role on the team, goal interdependence, and process mechanisms. Third, team members bring characteristics that make the team more homogeneous or more heterogeneous. As a collective, team members can be characterized by their (a) composition (based on the configuration of their abilities, personalities, and values), (b) diversity (based on their demographic, geographic, and associational characteristics; Chao and Moon 2005), (c) proximity (based on their distribution in space and time), and (d) stability (based on the rate of "churn" or the replacement rate of old members with new ones). Fourth, teams range on temporal characteristics that determine (a) the nature of performance episodes (i.e., cycle time), (b) the length of time it takes for the team to develop, and (c) the lifecycle—beginning to end duration—for the team.

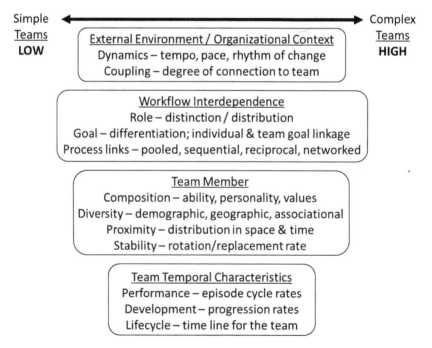

Fig. 21.1 A typology of team complexity. From: Kozlowski, S. W. J., & Bell, B. S. (2013). Work groups and teams in organizations. In N. Schmitt & S. Highhouse (Eds.), Handbook of psychology: Industrial and organiza-

tional psychology (pp. 412-469, Vol. 12, 2nd Ed). London: Wiley. © 2013, 2018 Steve W. J. Kozlowski and Bradford S. Bell. All rights reserved worldwide. Reprinted with permission

21.2.2 The Nature of Science Teams

In the preceding section, we defined work teams and made clear that they are not a unitary form. We highlighted the use of taxonomies to classify different types of work teams, but asserted that there is more conceptual advantage to be had by focusing on dimensions that distinguish different teams rather than on classification, which is merely the first step of scientific understanding. We made these points for a very particular reason. There are instances in which science teams are treated as if they are a distinct type of team. When this view is taken to the extreme, science teams are treated as if they are a fundamentally different entity compared to work teams, such that the established research cannot be generalized to science teams. Such a perspective negates a half century of theory and research. In our view, the goal should be to generalize from the foundational research on work teams and to identify those specific dimensions (i.e., boundary conditions) that are unique or particularly applicable to science teams (Salazar et al. 2012; Stokols et al. 2008).

As we described previously, such thinking harkens back to an earlier point in time when taxonomies were promulgated in an effort to distinguish qualitatively different types of work teams. Those early efforts were supplanted by more contemporary views that emphasized focusing on dimensions that distinguish teams, rather than treating different types as unique foci for study. To be more explicit about the limits of generalization to science teams that can be made from the science of team effectiveness, the NRC report developed a set of dimensions. These dimensions, shown in Table 21.2, represent boundary conditions for generalizing team effectiveness research findings to the functioning of science teams.

In general, the more of the dimensions that are further to the right on the continua, the greater the challenges that a particular science team will face. At the extreme right of the continua, there is a sufficient degree of uniqueness that sets clear boundaries for the application of knowledge from the existing team effectiveness literature. These areas constitute targets for specific research aimed at science teams. However, such instances are more the exception than the rule. Moreover, as we will explicate below, specifying science teams at the far right on some of these dimensions represents a failure to consider the broader set of concepts from organizational science that are relevant to team functioning.

For example, descriptions of a science team composed of 100, 1000, or 10,000 members is a misnomer. Such an entity is not a team; it is an organizational system. A system composed of that many individuals needs a structure to differentiate activities into meaningful clusters (e.g., teams, projects, departments) and to coordinate the goals and activities of smaller work units. Although there is no specific size that distinguishes a team from a larger social entity, many suggested limits for defining a team or small group fall within the "magical seven plus or minus two" heuristic that Miller (1956) identified for the limits of human information processing. Campbell (1958), a sociologist, synthesized a set of concepts that are useful for determining the "entitativity" of meaningful social units that are aggregates of elemental entities, i.e., individuals (Kozlowski and Klein 2000). They include proximity, similarity, common fate, pregnance (i.e., continuance), resistance to intrusion, and greater connectivity and communication within. Wuchty et al. (2007) analyzed authorship teams and concluded that they are becoming increasingly prevalent in science and the size of those teams is growing. Yet, their analysis showed that mean science team size in 2000 ranged from 2 to 3.5 members, depending on the field. Thus, a "team" of 100, 1000, or more individuals is not a team, it is an organization. For such an entity, senior leadership needs to craft an explicit structural design to cluster associated activities into smaller units and to coordinate the units.

Similarly, goal misalignment is most likely to be due to the lack of, or ineffective, structural mechanisms and leadership (March and Simon 1958). Goal misalignment is not an inherent property of teams, but as the diversity of perspectives increase along with size, it would be expected to be an issue in any type of system or

Table 21.2 Dimensions of team science and linkage to relevant team effectiveness topics

Team science dimension	Range		Relevant team effectiveness topic
	Simple	Complex	
Diversity of membership	Homogeneous	Heterogeneous	Team Input—composition
Disciplinary integration	Unidisciplinary	Transdisciplinary	Team Input—composition
Team size	Small (2)	Mega (1000s)	Team Input—system structure
Goal alignment across teams	Aligned	Divergent	Team Input—system structure; Intervention—leadership
Task interdependence	Low	High	Key Consideration—workflow as a constraint; Team Input—task workflow design
Proximity of team members	Co-located	Globally Distributed	Team Input—virtuality
Permeable team and organizational boundaries	Stable	Fluid	This topic has very little research; A clear boundary condition

entity (March and Simon 1958; Salazar et al. 2012). These challenges can and should be rectified with an appropriate system structure. As shown in Table 21.2, these and other team science dimensions map directly to research topics in the science of team effectiveness. Thus, many of the team science dimensions are only boundary conditions for the application of knowledge drawn from the science of team effectiveness *when there are many of them and they are all at the complex end of the continuum*. The one dimension that is a true boundary condition is the issue of fluid and changing membership. There is very little systematic empirical research on that aspect of team collaboration, although there is a substantial case-based literature on project management teams that addresses the phenomenon (Chiocchio et al. 2015).

It is also important to appreciate that a single project team or system incorporating many teams—a multiteam system (MTS)—can cut across the boundaries of a single organizational system (Carter et al. 2019; Luciano et al. in press). Such teams are common in aviation, the military, and medicine where teams form for a short duration event (e.g., emergency medical team) or multiple teams coordinate in real time to accomplish a task (e.g., military operations). This aspect of MTSs—cutting across organizational boundaries—is also relevant to science teams in that a multidisciplinary science team assembled for a specific project will often draw scientists

from different universities or research centers (Jones et al. 2008). In such teams, the connection of the project team (as a collective entity) to the multiple home institutional contexts is likely to be weaker. Moreover, the identification of individual team members with the project team may also be weaker, as each team member likely has multiple strong ties to the home institutional context and to other project teams (Salazar et al. 2012). This has implications for the extent to which science team members identify strongly with the team versus their home institutions.

21.3 An Integrative Theoretical Framework and Critical Conceptual Foci for Team Effectiveness

21.3.1 An Integrative Theoretical Framework

There are many heuristics of team effectiveness and most, in some fashion, have been influenced by the IPO framework posed by McGrath (1964). In this model, *inputs* characterize features of the individual (e.g., demographics; personality; knowledge, skills, and abilities [KSAs]), the team collectively (e.g., composition, workflow design), and the context (e.g., structure, resources, and rewards). *Processes* characterize how team members, given a particular workflow structure,

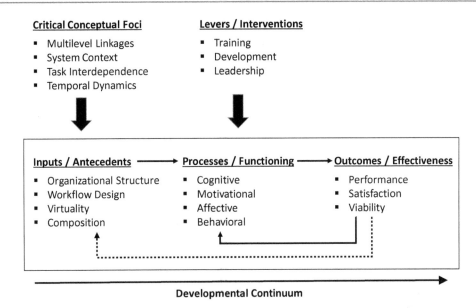

interact to resolve task demands. Although processes have a dynamic flavor, for the most part, researchers have treated processes as retrospective reports of "emergent states" (Marks et al. 2001) or process perceptions (e.g., team mental models, team cohesion, team coordination).[1] *Outputs* characterize cumulative team outcomes that are often organized according to Hackman's (1987) tripartite effectiveness model (e.g., performance [objective or rated by relevant others external to the team], member satisfaction, and viability). Although the IPO heuristic is often regarded as a causal model, that was not intended; McGrath originally developed it to organize research for a literature review (Kozlowski and Ilgen 2006). Nonetheless, the IPO heuristic has been highly influential and is useful for understanding team effectiveness. It forms the core of our integrative heuristic illustrated in Fig. 21.2.

In contemporary treatments, many scholars have noted that the IPO heuristic is static, whereas team effectiveness is much more dynamic in

nature (Ilgen et al. 2005; Kozlowski and Bell 2003, 2013; Kozlowski and Ilgen 2006; Mathieu et al. 2008). For example, Ilgen et al. proposed two key modifications to the IPO heuristic based on the aforementioned limitations. First, they suggested making the mediating role of team processes explicit (i.e., team processes link inputs to outputs). Second, they suggested adding the missing feedback loop between outputs and subsequent inputs to make explicit the iterative and reciprocal relations inherent in the IPO. Thus, they termed their framework as the Input-Mediator-Output-Input (IMOI) heuristic. These modifications have been useful for making explicit what have often been treated as unstated assumptions. The mediating role of processes and the outputs to inputs feedback loop are incorporated in Fig. 21.2.

A key contribution of Kozlowski and Bell (2003, 2013) is that they conceptualized work team functioning from a multilevel theory perspective (Kozlowski and Klein 2000); that is, as a consequence of top-down constraints emanating from the broader organizational system that operate in combination with team processes and outcomes as bottom-up, emergent phenomena. Within this perspective, they emphasized four *critical conceptual foci* (i.e., system context, mul-

---

[1] Most research on team processes uses retrospective perceptions or what Marks et al. (2001) describe as emergent states. We use these terms interchangeably for the purpose of this review.

tilevel linkages, task interdependence, and temporal dynamics [i.e., task episodes and developmental progression]) for understanding factors, both internal and external to the team, that shape team performance cycles and the progressive development of team capabilities. We have incorporated these conceptual foci in Fig. 21.2 as contextual and temporal mechanisms that bound and drive—respectively—IPO linkages. Kozlowski and Bell also used a lifecycle organization that considered team formation and composition, socialization and development, team processes (cognitive, motivational, affective, and behavioral) and effectiveness outcomes, motivation and leadership, and continuance and decline (Kozlowski and Bell 2003, 2013); topics we integrate as appropriate.

Kozlowski and Ilgen (2006) built upon the conceptual features of Kozlowski and Bell (2003) and Ilgen et al. (2005). One notable feature of their approach was the effort to distill the key factors responsible for team effectiveness from the vast literature foundation. They focused specifically on those areas of research with well-established findings based on meta-analytic summaries and on areas with promising progressive lines of inquiry. With that approach, they were able to identify a set of team processes—cognitive, motivational/affective, and behavioral—with well-established, evidence-based contributions to team effectiveness. They then used the same approach to identify evidence-based interventions or "levers" that can be used to shape appropriate team processes. Both features are incorporated in Fig. 21.2.

Finally, to create a framework to organize their review, Mathieu et al. (2008) drew upon many of the features we highlighted previously. For example, they used the IPO as the core of their framework but highlighted the multilevel, nested aspect (i.e., top down and bottom up effects) of teams in organizational settings. In addition, they more explicitly noted the role of time as both a long-term developmental process (Kozlowski et al. 1999) and a shorter term process driven by task episodes or cycles (Kozlowski et al. 1996; Marks et al. 2001; McGrath 1984). Accordingly, we have incorporated these features in our integrative heuristic.

21.3.2 Critical Conceptual Foci for Team Effectiveness

Multilevel linkages. Organizations are multilevel, nested systems composed of lower-level entities (i.e., individuals are the lowest-level meaningful entity) that are hierarchically organized into successively higher-level meaningful social entities (i.e., teams, departments, and larger units). In this conceptualization, a work team or project team is the most proximal social unit for most individuals' interactions. Teams are at the juncture of the higher-level system context and the lower-level behavior of team members. *The higher-level system context influences the team as a collective by exerting top-down effects or constraints that limit the range of likely behavior. Individuals interacting over time within those constraints give rise to phenomena that emerge as collective team characteristics* (i.e., team processes and emergent states; Kozlowski and Klein 2000).

System context. As we highlighted in the previous discussion about team typology dimensions, the higher-level system can exhibit considerable top-down constraint on team behavior when the team is tightly coupled to the context. However, when teams are loosely coupled to the system context, context creation will be much more under the influence of the team itself. Thus, for example, teams that are highly coordinated and embedded in a research center at a single university will experience strong top-down effects from the context. In contrast, a project team composed of investigators drawn from multiple institutions are only loosely coupled to the organizational system features at each home institution. Their interactions as a project team will be much more responsible for context creation in the form of normative expectations and shared perceptions that will operate as contextual constraints. *One needs to consider the nature of the team context, where it originates, and the force it can apply on the team.*

Task interdependence. The structure by which team members combine their expertise, knowledge, skill, and effort to accomplish collective performance is at the core of team processes. Team processes, perceptual states, and performance outcomes emerge from the interactions and exchanges among team members, driven by the interdependence structure, that are required to accomplish the team task. *The nature of task interdependence for the team is the most critical feature for understanding relevant team processes.* We discuss this focus in-depth below as an input.

Temporal dynamics. Finally, the temporal dynamics that shape emergent phenomena in teams is a key consideration. There are two types of temporal dynamics that are of most relevance: (a) developmental and (b) episodic. First, at formation, a group of individuals is a team in name only. They have yet to interact, learn how to coordinate expertise and effort, or to develop shared perceptual states. Processes and coordinated patterns of behavior will emerge, but they will do so over time. "Teams have a developmental lifespan; they form, mature, and evolve over time" (p. 416, Kozlowski and Bell 2013). Second, team tasks can vary with respect to task episodes or cycles. "Episodes are distinguishable periods of time over which performance accrues and feedback is available" (p. 359, Marks et al. 2001). Multiple tasks or problem states that repeatedly confront the team represent episodic task cycles. Such episodes can ebb and flow in their intensity, the load they place on team member resources, and the need for the team to adjust its effort or to radically adapt to the unexpected. *The more episodic the task, the more likely it is that members are tightly coupled together and the team is coupled to the context.*

21.4 A Review of Team Effectiveness Research

21.4.1 Inputs and Antecedents

Organizational structure. As we have previously noted, most work teams are embedded in an organizational system that has structural linkages connecting the teams. That is, they are embedded in a higher-level hierarchical system that integrates, coordinates, and controls activities across teams and across levels of the system. The degree to which the structural mechanisms are formal (i.e., tight, bureaucratic, rule-bound) versus informal (i.e., loose, flexible, negotiated) creates contextual differences that have clear implications for team functioning (Burns and Stalker 1961; Lawrence and Lorsch 1967). Teams that are embedded in formal structures are more highly constrained in terms of work activities and goals, as well as timing of goal accomplishment. Discretion is more limited. In contrast, teams embedded in informal structures have more internal control over work activities, goals, and timelines. As a general rule, formal organizational structures are a better fit and, thus, more likely when the organization's mission environment is stable and predictable, whereas informal structures are a better fit and more likely when the environment is unstable and uncertain.

Science teams are often at the intersection of multiple organizations (e.g., a project "team" that cuts across multiple universities). In this example, there is no single organizational structure and the coupling of the team to any one organization is likely to be loose. How is organizational structure relevant to such science teams? It is relevant because of the size of the entity. Such project teams can be much larger than the magical seven plus or minus two. Whether a structure is rationally designed or simply emerges informally, a structure will develop that is clustered around common activities and goals. We assert that it is better to design the structure intentionally rather than to accept whatever develops on its own.

Thus, if one is focusing on an entity that has more than ten members,[2] it is useful to apply some basic structural design principles. Galbraith (1972) provides a set of robust structural design principles based on task complexity that are useful in this regard. The first and most basic principle is to use standard operating procedures (SOPs)—rules—to coordinate multiple teams. SOPs enable teams to address *predictable* coordination problems that

---

[2] Beyond approximately ten team members, the structural principles are relevant; they become increasingly applicable as the number of personnel comprising the entity increases.

arise without a need for information processing, uncertainty reduction, and problem solving. However, with increasing complexity, more anomalies are likely to arise than can be predicted in advance. Thus, the second principle is to add a formal managerial role to coordinate unanticipated problems that arise beyond SOPs. The role is to monitor for exceptions, collect information from affected teams, and render a decision that resolves the issue across all affected units. With additional complexity, the managerial role gets overloaded and a new mechanism is needed. The third principle is coordination via goals and deadlines. Coordination is then inherent in the interconnections of the goals and their timetable. When one or more teams fail to achieve a goal specification, the entire goal-timeline structure has to be revised and updated. Such revisions are manageable so long as they are reasonably infrequent. However, as complexity increases, more frequent revisions become necessary thereby creating overload. At this point, Galbraith (1972) indicates that organizations need to select one of two very different structural strategies: (1) reduce the need for information processing by reducing complexity demands (e.g., slack resources, self-containment) or (2) increase information processing capacity to better manage complexity demands (e.g., communication protocols and systems, liaison roles). The details of these two strategies are beyond the scope of our review. However, the basic principles provide an understanding of the implications of organizational structure for team functioning and an architecture for structure when needed to rationalize coordination for large project entities.

Workflow design. As a distinguishable unit, a team also has an internal structure of work interdependence. Although there are a variety of interdependence structures by which individual effort, information, and output can be combined to represent a group product (e.g., Steiner 1972; Kozlowski and Klein 2000), a workflow conceptualization—how work flows across team members—is very robust. Extending a typology developed by Thompson (1967), Van de Ven et al. (1976) proposed four workflow interdependence structures—pooled, sequential, reciprocal, and intensive—for group work. As shown in Fig. 21.3,

Bell and Kozlowski (2002) combined that workflow conceptualization with additional features—task dynamics, external coupling, internal coupling—to integrate task complexity and workflow. The least complex end of the continuum is represented by pooled/additive tasks that present the lowest interdependence demands—task activities are essentially performed separately by team members and then pooled together for a team product—and weak internal linkages, loose external coupling, and a largely static task environment. Sequential task structures increase the interdependence demands in that each team member makes a unique contribution and work flows unidirectionally and incrementally from one team member to another. Such structures are feasible when the input–output linkages are relatively well known and predictable. Reciprocal task structures increase interdependence further by adding feedback linkages to represent the mutual adjustments that have to be made across the task sequence. Feedback and adjustments are necessary when the input–output linkages and timing are not well known and well defined. Finally, the most complex end of the continuum is represented by intensive task structures—task activities are performed simultaneously and flexibly by the entire team—in the context of strong internal linkages, tight external coupling, and a dynamic task environment. Team workflows at the more complex end of the continuum place much greater demands on teams to enact appropriate process mechanisms to resolve the workflow demands and achieve team performance.

Virtuality. One important feature to acknowledge is that the nature of teamwork is changing substantially by virtue of technological advances—in particular, advances in communications bandwidth and connectivity—that enable teams to be virtual; far flung across time and space around the globe. This feature of teaming is largely a development that has occurred over the last couple of decades. Early views of virtual teams treated them as a type of team, distinct from face-to-face or co-located teams. However, Bell and Kozlowski (2002) asserted that virtual teams had unique features and consequent challenges, but were otherwise like co-located teams

**Task
Environment:**   • Static   • Dynamic

**External
Coupling:**   • Loosely Coupled   • Tightly Coupled

**Internal   • Asynchronous   • Synchronous
Coupling:**   • Weak Linkages   • Strong Linkages

**Workflow
Interdependence:**

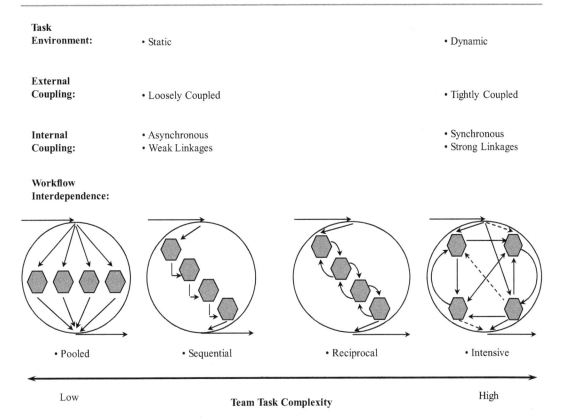

   • Pooled   • Sequential   • Reciprocal   • Intensive

Low   **Team Task Complexity**   High

Fig. 21.3 Characteristics of simple vs. complex team work-flows. From: Bell, B. S., & Kozlowski, S. W. J. (2002). A typology of virtual teams: Implications for effective leader-ship. *Group and Organization Management, 27*, 14-49. © 2002, 2018 Bradford S. Bell and Steve W. J. Kozlowski. All rights reserved worldwide. Reprinted with permission

in many other ways. They argued that the key issue was to focus on the underlying dimensions that distinguish virtual teams from co-located teams and to also address characteristics that distinguish a range of virtual teams from one another.

Bell and Kozlowski (2002) proposed two key dimensions that distinguished virtual and co-located teams: (a) spatial distance and (b) technology-mediated communication and exchange. They also proposed that more and less complex virtual teams, respectively, were distinguished by four characteristics: (a) workflow conducted in real time versus work that was temporally distributed, (b) a team lifecycle that was continuous versus discrete, (c) member roles that were singular versus multiple, and (d) team boundaries that were stable versus permeable. Bell and Kozlowski (2002) argued that the bandwidth and responsiveness of the communication

technologies had to match the workflow demands of the team for virtual teams to be effective. For example, intensive teams with complex work-flows need high bandwidth, real time, synchronous communications, whereas pooled teams with simple workflows could coordinate effort with low bandwidth, asynchronous tools (e.g., email).

In related work, Kirkman and Mathieu (2005) proposed a three-dimensional typology of virtual teams based on: (a) the use of virtual tools to accomplish teamwork, (b) the informational value of the tools, and (c) the degree to which communications were synchronous. Gibson and Gibbs (2006) proposed four dimensions of virtuality: (a) geographic dispersion, (b) electronic dependence, (c) dynamic structures (i.e., changes in members and roles), and (d) national diversity. O'Leary and Cummings (2007) proposed a typology with three dimensions: (a) spatial distance among members,

(b) temporal differences among members, and (c) configuration differences among members (i.e., where the number of members at different locations is different). With the exception of national diversity (which is arguably not unique to virtual teams) and configuration differences (which is), one can see that there is a high degree of convergence across these typologies that traces back to Bell and Kozlowski (2002). In their comprehensive review of the virtual team literature, Kirkman et al. (2012) noted that research on virtuality dimensions was limited. They asserted that team researchers should shift from comparing co-located and virtual teams to decomposing the effects of the different aspects of virtuality on virtual team effectiveness.

Given that many science teams are likely to be virtual to some degree, this is an area that merits further research for team science. Bell and Kozlowski (2002) highlighted that the characteristics of virtuality would make the role of being a team leader more challenging and that the lack of face-to-face contact would necessitate leadership adaptations. For example, they proposed that effective virtual team leaders would create structures, routines, and goals to guide member actions in the absence of face-to-face contact, and that leaders would distribute leadership functions (i.e., shared leadership) and action regulation to team members. Subsequent research has provided support for their assertions (Hoch and Kozlowski 2014). Thus, the research on ways that team leaders can better adapt to the challenges of virtuality are good targets for improving science team effectiveness.

Composition. Teams can differ on a wide variety of individual difference characteristics that—collectively—represent the composition of the team; the overall pattern of differences across team members. When such factors are explicitly considered for team selection, the process can be viewed on one of team assembly (Twyman and Contractor 2019). Among the many characteristics in question, those that have generated the most research attention include cognitive ability, personality, and demographic diversity.

Team members' collective cognitive ability has been shown to consistently predict the effectiveness of teams engaged in many different types of work (Kozlowski and Bell 2013). Cognitive ability exhibits a moderate, positive relationship with team performance and this relationship is relatively stable regardless of whether one focuses on the average level of cognitive ability in the team or the score of the highest or lowest member (Bell 2007; Devine and Phillips 2001). Teams higher in cognitive ability also learn more (Ellis et al. 2003) and are better able to adapt to unexpected changes in the task environment (LePine 2005). Although research is still uncovering the conditions under which team-level cognitive ability has more or less of an impact on team performance, there is reason to expect that it may serve as a particularly potent predictor of the effectiveness of science teams. Research conducted at the individual level has shown that task complexity moderates the cognitive ability-performance relationship, such that cognitive ability has a stronger relationship with performance as task complexity increases (Hunter and Hunter 1984). This suggests that members' cognitive ability may be crucial for science teams engaged in highly complex and unfamiliar work.

The personality composition of a team has also been linked to team effectiveness. However, the effects of aggregate team personality tend to be weaker and less consistent than those for team-level cognitive ability (LePine et al. 2010). In particular, the effects of team personality composition on team effectiveness are stronger for some dimensions of personality (conscientiousness, agreeableness, extraversion) than others (emotional stability, openness to experience) (Bell 2007). Also, the average level of a personality trait across team members is generally a stronger predictor of team effectiveness than other team personality configurations (e.g., lowest/highest member on the attribute, heterogeneity) (Bell 2007; Prewett et al. 2009). The exception is agreeableness, which has equally strong effects when examined as either the team mean or minimum, supporting the idea that one disagreeable member can disturb the social harmony of the team and undermine team performance. Finally, there is some evidence that team personality composition may have stronger effects on team processes than team outcomes and may matter more for performance when tasks require high team interdependence (Prewett et al. 2009).

Substantial research has explored the extent to which team processes and outcomes are shaped by differences in team member *demographic diversity* (see also Gibbs et al. 2019). Although studies in this area have historically yielded conflicting findings, more recent work has begun to untangle the relationship between diversity and team effectiveness. In a comprehensive review of this literature, Mannix and Neale (2005) conclude that differences in surface-level characteristics, such as race and sex, tend to have a negative effect on team effectiveness, whereas differences in deeper-level characteristics, such as functional background and personality, are more often positively related to team performance, but only as long as the group process is carefully managed. As they state, "Unless diverse teams are able to overcome the disruptive effects of their differences or avoid the tendencies to drive out distinctiveness and move toward similarity, they will be unable to engage in effective and creative problem solving" (p. 43). A recent meta-analysis by Bell et al. (2010) provided further support for these patterns, finding that variety in race and sex relate negatively to team performance, whereas variety in functional and educational backgrounds have more positive effects. Research on group faultlines has also advanced a more integrative view of diversity in teams by showing that the configuration of multiple types of diversity can influence the formation and strength of subgroups and ultimately team processes and performance (Lau and Murnighan 1998; Thatcher and Patel 2012).

In order to understand the implications of diversity for team effectiveness, it is also important to consider the nature of both the task and team context. Bell et al. (2010), for example, found that functional and educational background diversity had stronger positive effects in contexts where these differences were likely to be more salient (e.g., cross-functional and design teams) and on creativity and innovation tasks where multiple perspectives and divergent thinking were critical for performance. Another meta-

analysis by Joshi and Roh (2009) found that surface-level diversity was positively related to performance in short-term teams and those with low interdependence but negatively related to performance in long-term teams and those moderate or high in interdependence. In addition, recent research on diversity in team member's temporal orientation suggests that this composition characteristic can negatively influence team cognition and performance (Mohammed et al. 2015; Mohammed and Nadkarni 2014). This factor could be particularly relevant for science teams. These findings suggest that characteristics of both the team and the task serve as boundary conditions that determine whether a particular type of diversity is beneficial or detrimental to team performance.

21.4.2 Team Processes and Team Functioning

Cognitive team processes. Significant attention has been focused on cognitive constructs that reflect the structure of collective perception, cognitive structure or knowledge organization, and knowledge or information acquisition within teams (Kozlowski and Ilgen 2006). In this section, we review five primary cognitive team mechanisms: climate, team learning, knowledge building, team mental models, and transactive memory. *Climate* refers to "cognitively based, descriptive, interpretive perceptions of salient features, events, and processes (James and Jones 1974) that characterize the 'strategic imperatives' (Schneider et al. 1992) of the organizational and team context" (Kozlowski and Ilgen 2006, p. 81). Collective perceptions of strategic imperatives, such as technical updating and innovation, diversity, customer service, and safety, within a team have been shown to play an important role in shaping goal-relevant processes and various facets of team effectiveness. Hofmann and Stetzer (1996), for example, demonstrated that teams in a chemical processing plant that perceived a stronger climate for safety engaged in fewer unsafe behaviors and had fewer actual accidents. The emergence of a strong team climate depends on team members' interactions with leaders and one another. For example, members who have good relationships with their leader develop climate perceptions that are not only more similar to the leader but also more consensual with each other (Kozlowski and Doherty 1989). Also, frequent social interaction among team members tends to create climate perceptions that are more consensual (González-Romá et al. 2002).

Team learning refers to a change in a team's collective knowledge, skills, and performance capabilities that occurs through interaction and shared experience (Ellis and Bell 2005; Wilson et al. 2007). It is a critical mechanism through which teams expand their repertoire of potential behaviors, adapt to changes in their surrounding context, and continually renew their performance over time (Bell et al. 2012). Research has identified a number of behaviors that underlie the team learning process, including sharing information, experimenting, systematically and deliberately processing information, and discussing errors (e.g., De Dreu 2007; Ellis et al. 2003; Wilson et al. 2007). A key determinant of whether a team engages in these activities is psychological safety, which is a shared perception that the team is a safe context for interpersonal risk taking (Edmonson 1999). When team members perceive a supportive interpersonal climate, they are more willing to take risks and confront failures openly, both of which are critical to team learning (Cannon and Edmondson 2001; Edmonson 1999). In this sense, psychological safety is also relevant to a climate for safety. Although a number of factors have been shown to influence perceptions of psychological safety, leader actions appear to play a particularly crucial role. Leaders who actively minimize power differences within the team, encourage others' contributions, and engage in effective coaching are better able to build team psychological safety (Edmondson et al. 2001; Edmondson and Lei 2014; Nembhard and Edmondson 2006).

Another way to view team learning that is particularly relevant to science teams is as a process of information sharing and *knowledge building*. Science teams are often composed of members with differential (i.e., distributed) expertise.

Individual team members apply their expertise to learn about the problem in question, but they also have to convey their understanding to other members of the team if synergy is to be realized. One of the key challenges for teams with distributed expertise is how to facilitate the process of sharing unique information such that all team members develop a common understanding that can be applied to solving the collective problem. There is a substantial literature demonstrating that team members are more likely to focus on discussing commonly held information during deliberations, rather than the unique information that is critical to reaching an optimal decision (Mesmer-Magnus and DeChurch 2009; Stasser and Titus 1985, 1987). Some research has shown that when team members perceive that their outcomes are interdependent, they share more information—but only if they engage in systematic information processing (De Dreu and Carnevale 2003). More recently, Grand et al. (2016) have shown that computational modeling, coupled with agent-based simulation, is an effective methodology for identifying information-sharing bottlenecks in teams. Based on their modeling research, they were then able to design knowledge building interventions that significantly improved team learning and information sharing.

Team mental models and transactive memory both refer to team cognitive structures that are outcomes of team learning (Bell et al. 2012) which reflect how information that is critical to team functioning is organized, represented, and distributed within the team (Kozlowski and Ilgen 2006). Team mental models capture members' shared, organized understanding and mental representation of knowledge or beliefs about key elements of the team's task environment (Klimoski and Mohammed 1994). Research suggests that teams perform better when members possess an appropriate shared understanding of the task, team, equipment, and situation (Mohammed et al. 2010). A variety of interventions, including leader pre-briefs and debriefs as well as training, can be used to enhance the development of shared team mental models (e.g., Blickensderfer et al. 1997; Marks et al. 2000).

Whereas team mental models refer to information that members hold in common, transactive memory deals with knowledge that is distributed among team members. In particular, transactive memory systems consist of two main components: (1) internal memory, or the knowledge held by particular team members; and (2) external memory, or the shared awareness of who knows what (Wegner 1995). Transactive memory systems are thought to benefit teams by enabling a higher degree of specialization and an increase in overall cognitive capacity. Indeed, a recent meta-analysis by De Church and Mesmer-Magnus (2010) suggests that transactive memory may be more important for team performance than shared mental models. However, research has yet to provide much insight into ways to enhance transactive memory, other than increasing interaction and shared experience among members (Kozlowski and Ilgen 2006).

Motivational and affective team processes. Researchers have examined a number of processes in an effort to understand how motivational tendencies, relations among members, and affective reactions influence team effectiveness. In this section, we examine four constructs—team cohesion; team conflict; team efficacy; and team affect or mood—that represent important motivational and affective team mechanisms.

Team cohesion is a multidimensional construct that captures the bond that exists among members of a group. Prior research has tended to distinguish among three types of team cohesion: (1) interpersonal cohesion—shared attraction to or liking for the members of the group; (2) task cohesion—shared commitment or attraction to the group task or goal; and (3) group pride—shared importance of being a member of the group (Kozlowski and Bell 2013). A meta-analysis by Beal et al. (2003) found that all three dimensions of cohesion were significantly and positively related to team performance and the magnitude of these effects was comparable across the different dimensions. In addition, they found that the cohesion-performance relationship became stronger as team workflow interdependencies increased. In other words, having a strong bond among the members of the group becomes increasingly important as one moves along the continuum from pooled/additive tasks to more intensive task structures due to the increased importance of coordination for achieving team performance. There is some evidence to suggest that the composition of a team, particularly in terms of personality, may be an important determinant of interpersonal cohesion (Barrick et al. 1998). Further, setting clear goals and norms may be an effective means of helping teams develop strong task and interpersonal cohesion (Kozlowski and Bell 2013).

Whereas cohesion represents a force that pushes team members together, *team conflict* focuses attention on divergent processes that can threaten to push a team apart. Past research has tended to differentiate among two types of team conflict: (1) task conflict—disagreements about task content; and (2) relationship conflict—interpersonal incompatibilities (Jehn 1995). Although conflict is typically assumed to be detrimental to team performance, some work has suggested that under certain conditions it may prove beneficial. In particular, there is some evidence that conflict focused on task-relevant issues may reveal different perspectives and points of view that helps the team perform nonroutine tasks (Amason 1996; Jehn 1995). A meta-analysis by De Dreu and Weingart (2003), however, found that both task and relationship conflict negatively predicted team member satisfaction and team performance. In addition, they found that conflict had more detrimental effects on the performance of teams working on complex tasks. Overall, these findings suggest that in most situations conflict will undermine team effectiveness and, therefore, attention should be focused on strategies for managing task and interpersonal disagreements. Although much of the work in this area has focused on reactive strategies that can be used to address conflict after it manifests in a team, preemptive conflict management strategies may allow teams to prevent the destructive effects of conflict from emerging in the first place. For example, teams can develop rules or agreements about how team members will handle difficult situations (Marks et al. 2001; Smolek et al. 1999).

Team efficacy refers to a team's shared belief in its ability to organize and execute the actions needed to successfully perform a task (Bandura 1997; Lindsley et al. 1995). Team efficacy shapes the goals that a team sets, how much effort is devoted to achieving those goals, and the extent to which a team persists in the face of failure (Chen et al. 2009; DeShon et al. 2004). Just as self-efficacy has been shown to serve as an important predictor of individual performance (Stajkovic and Luthans 1998), team efficacy has been identified as a robust determinant of team performance (Gully et al. 2002). Team efficacy has a positive effect on team performance and this relationship grows stronger as team interdependence increases. There is also some emerging evidence that team efficacy may facilitate team learning (Bell et al. 2012). Shared perceptions of team efficacy are more likely to emerge when team members are more interdependent and interact more frequently (Paskevich et al. 1999). In addition, research suggests that team efficacy can be developed by team training as well as the actions of leaders in shaping team experiences and interactions (Kozlowski and Ilgen 2006).

Team affect or *mood*, which captures the emotions or affective tone that exist within a group (see Barsade and Knight 2015), may have a more distal impact on team effectiveness through effects on other affective mechanisms, such as cohesion and conflict (Kozlowski and Ilgen 2006). Although it is clear that emotions play a major role in teams, the precise nature of these effects remains somewhat unclear. Whereas some research has found that affective similarity among members positively predicts team outcomes (e.g., Barsade et al. 2000), other studies suggest that affective heterogeneity may be beneficial for certain outcomes (e.g., creativity) or that it may be best for team members to possess complementary affective qualities (e.g., low energy and high energy) (Barsade and Gibson 1998; Jackson 1992). There is also evidence that the emotions of a single person can infect the mood of the entire team (Barsade 2002). Similar to many of the affective processes already discussed, research suggests that mood convergence is more likely when team members are more interdependent

and interact over extended periods of time (Bartel and Saavedra 2000). Also, leaders' mood can shape the affective tone of the team (Sy et al. 2005).

Behavioral team processes. In this final section, we focus attention on the behavioral processes that capture what teams do in order to respond to task demands and achieve their goals. These processes have typically been studied in the context of action teams (e.g., cockpit crews, military units, surgical teams), in which members with highly specialized roles need to synchronize their actions with one another as well as external counterparts to carry out complex and often brief performance events (Sundstrom et al. 1990). Although these processes may be less critical in the context of science teams due to longer work cycles and reduced demands for synchronization, they are important to consider as they represent fundamental elements of team performance (Kozlowski and Ilgen 2006). We also examine individual team member competencies that underlie effective teamwork.

Kozlowski and Bell (2013) identified three key team behavioral processes—*coordination*, *cooperation*, and *communication*. Coordination refers to the activities required to manage interdependencies in the team workflow, whereas cooperation has been defined as "the willful contribution of personal efforts to the completion of interdependent jobs" (Wagner 1995, p. 152). Although both concepts address the combination of team-member actions and efforts to achieve interdependent tasks, coordination is distinguished by a focus on the temporal entrainment (i.e., linked rhythms) and synchronization of these actions (Kozlowski and Ilgen 2006). Interactive processes indicative of coordination, such as making plans, assigning tasks, and backing up other team members, have been found to relate positively to team performance (Stout et al. 1994). Similarly, higher levels of cooperation in teams have been positively linked to various measures of effectiveness (e.g., Seers et al. 1995; Smith et al. 1994). Communication is often viewed as a means of supporting coordination and cooperation in teams. Taskwork communication (e.g., exchange of task-relevant information) underlies the synchronization of team activities, whereas as teamwork communication (e.g., establishing high-quality relationships) can help induce cooperative tendencies in groups.

In recent years, there have been several advances in our understanding of how action and behavioral processes unfold over time. First, Marks et al. (2001) developed a taxonomy that provides a more highly differentiated conceptualization of team behavioral processes. The taxonomy elaborates a temporal structure that distinguishes between behavioral processes that are most relevant during transition (i.e., preparation) phases of task execution, such as goal specification and strategy formulation, and those that are most relevant during action (i.e., engagement) phases of tasks, such as monitoring goal progress and backing up behavior. In addition, they highlight three interpersonal processes—conflict management, motivation and confidence building, and affect management—that support both the transition and action phase processes. The Marks et al. (2001) taxonomy has received meta-analytic support (LePine et al. 2008) and is being used as a tool for conceptualizing and assessing behavioral team processes across many different domains (e.g., military, aviation, medicine). Second, Kozlowski and colleagues (e.g., Kozlowski et al. 1996, 1999) have introduced theoretical frameworks that offer greater insight into how teams allocate cognitive, motivational, and behavioral resources to respond to task demands that vary throughout a task cycle as a result of shifting environmental contingencies. In particular, these frameworks tie processes of individual and team regulation and goal striving to the task performance cycle, thus delineating the processes that are critical at different stages of task performance.

A somewhat different yet complementary perspective on behavioral team processes is offered by research that has focused on identifying the competencies (i.e., knowledge, skills, and abilities) that underlie effective teamwork and collaboration (see Nurius and Kemp 2019). Salas, Cannon-Bowers, and their colleagues (Cannon-Bowers et al. 1995; Salas and Cannon-Bowers 1997), for example, identified eight teamwork skills, including performance monitoring and feedback, communication, and decision-making. Stevens and Campion (1994, 1999) selected 14 competencies that were organized into three categories of interpersonal skills (conflict resolution, collaborative problem-solving, and communication) and two categories of self-management skills (goal setting and performance management). Although efforts to validate these competencies have produced somewhat mixed findings, there is evidence that training designed to develop these competencies can lead to gains in team effectiveness (Ellis et al. 2005).

21.5 Aligning Team Processes: Practical Considerations and Research Recommendations

We have endeavored, in this concise review, to make a strong case that there is a substantial research foundation and evidence base for the science of team effectiveness that is directly applicable to science teams. We have acknowledged that most of the research has not studied science teams per se, but that most of the findings for team processes and their influence on team effectiveness nonetheless apply to most science teams under most normative conditions. As we highlighted in Table 21.2, unless your particular science team is on the far right of the continuum for multiple dimensions, the knowledge summarized in this chapter and other more comprehensive reviews (Ilgen et al. 2005; Kozlowski and Bell 2003, 2013; Kozlowski and Ilgen 2006; Mathieu et al. 2008) is relevant to you. We conclude the chapter by discussing (a) how this knowledge can be used to improve science team effectiveness and, where there are knowledge gaps, (b) what research targets are recommended. Given the limited scope of this chapter, we cannot be comprehensive. In particular, we do not consider the levers/interventions that shape team processes—training, development, and leadership—in a separate section. Rather, these interventions have been discussed throughout where relevant. Using the integrative heuristic

(Fig. 21.2) as a guide, we offer a concise road-map for navigating practical issues and targeting specific research recommendations for advancing science team effectiveness.

21.5.1 Critical Conceptual Foci Issues

From a pragmatic perspective, a good point of departure is to assess the nature of the system, and its key characteristics, within which a science team is embedded. We discussed four key foci: (a) multilevel linkages, (b) system context, (c) task interdependence, and (d) temporal dynamics. These are critical conceptual foci for researchers to consider when they design studies, but they are also useful practical considerations. For example, the first two foci are external and address how tightly bound a team is in a multi-level system—that is, the system context and the extent to which the higher level limits the range of team behavior potential (i.e., rules, regula-tions, monitoring) or leaves it much more open—has a substantial impact on whether a team and its leadership shape processes (open) or whether it is largely a consequence of the higher-level constraints. One expects science teams to thrive under more open systems. The last two foci are internal and address how tightly connected team members are in terms of information exchange and effort in terms of the consequences of action (or non-action) and time. Loose connections pro-vide much more discretion and slack for team members, whereas tight connections are far more demanding and challenging. To the extent possi-ble, these foci are factors that team leaders need to consider.

21.5.2 Inputs/Antecedents Issues

Table 21.3 summarizes practical considerations and research recommendations for inputs to team processes. We considered four primary inputs including organizational structure, workflow design, virtuality, and team composition.

Organizational structure. Basically, designing an organizational structure that aligns with the overall mission and coordination requirements of an entity is relevant whenever the entity is larger than approximately 10 people. Smaller teams (approximately five to seven to nine people) may form informal subgroups as necessary, but in general those relationships are manageable. As teams increase in size, a rational design that applies the principles outlined previously aids communication, cooperation, and coordination of information and action (Galbraith 1972).

Workflow design. For well-defined tasks, workflow designs are often directed by the most efficient and effective means for accomplishing the goal. In contrast, science teams are often embarked on a discovery process where the workflow may not be obvious in advance or even considered when the team was composed. However, once a team is formed, goals, roles, and linkages among team members should be ratio-nally considered rather than simply allowed to emerge. The tighter linkages and timelines asso-ciated with more complex workflows necessitate more active leadership to support communica-tion, cooperation, and coordination (Hackman 1987; Kozlowski et al. 2016; McGrath 1984).

Virtuality. Distributing team members across locations, time, and space makes the team leader-ship role of coordinating and motivating much more challenging. Theory and research suggest that structural supports can substitute for more conventional leadership actions (Bell and Kozlowski 2002; Hoch and Kozlowski 2014; Kirkman et al. 2012). In addition, the concept of shared leadership, which distributes leadership responsibilities to team members, is useful for teams with complex workflows and for virtual teams (Kozlowski et al. 2016).

Team composition. The complex pattern of individual difference characteristics (e.g., demo-graphics, knowledge, skills, abilities, personality, values, experiences, etc.) is a critical input factor; this is one topic for which additional research is needed. People are often added to a science team based solely on their expertise; however, there are many other relevant characteristics they pos-sess that influence how well they interact so it is a critical team process input. It is an all too com-mon experience to be on a team where one or two

Table 21.3 Input application and research recommendations

Input	Concept	Evidence	Recommendations
Organizational structure	Structure of roles, responsibilities, goals, and authority	Substantial research foundation	• Application ready; Apply design principles for larger science "teams"
Workflow design	Structure by which information and effort flow among team members	Substantial research foundation	• Application ready; More complex workflows necessitate more active leadership, coordination, and communication protocols
Virtuality	Distribution of team members across time and space	Substantial research foundation	• Places increased demands on science team leaders to coordinate effort • *Additional research needed*
Team composition	The pattern of individual differences (e.g., demographics and ability, experience, values, personality, culture, etc.) across team members	Meta-analyses	• A critical input for team effectiveness • *Additional research needed*; there are so many important potential differences; difficult to study • *Candidate for computational modeling research*

members impeded progress, promoted conflicts, or otherwise made group work problematic. The challenge for studying composition is that there are so many potentially relevant individual differences to study that it is nearly impossible to conduct systematic, cumulative research. That makes team composition a prime candidate for computational modeling research which can conduct very large-scale virtual experiments to systematically explore the full theoretical space (Kozlowski et al. 2013).

21.5.3 Team Processes/Functioning Issues

Table 21.4 outlines practical applications and research recommendations related to the various cognitive, motivational/affective, and behavioral we reviewed above. Key considerations in each of these three areas are reviewed below.

Cognitive processes. Given the complex, knowledge-based work carried out by science teams, cognitive mechanisms represent an important target for practical interventions. In particular, such efforts should aim to promote shared perceptions of the team's strategic imperatives, encourage members to share their knowledge and information, and develop structures that serve to

organize and distribute critical information within the team. To this end, there are two main levers that can be used to shape and develop the cognition of science teams. First, science team leaders play an integral role in setting and reinforcing the goals and priorities that shape team climate, developing a psychologically safe environment that encourages members to engage in critical learning behaviors, and enacting prebriefs and debriefs that enhance the development of shared mental models (Kozlowski et al. 1996; Zijlstra et al. 2012). Second, team training and development strategies can be used to enhance cognitive team processes. Cross-training, for instance, has been shown to facilitate the development of shared team-interaction models (Marks et al. 2002). Also, team building interventions can be used to engage teams in goal-setting and role clarification, which may help to improve team cognitive processes (Klein et al. 2009).

Although research has provided evidence into levers that can be used to shape certain cognitive processes, such as mental models and team learning, future work is still needed to specify interventions for other mechanisms, such as knowledge building and transactive memory. As described earlier, the computational modeling approach utilized by Grand et al. (2016) holds significant promise for guid-

Table 21.4 Team process/functioning application and research recommendations

	Concept	Evidence	Recommendations
Cognitive processes			
Team climate	Strategic imperatives	Meta-analysis; Substantial research foundation	• Application ready; Train science team leaders to build a strong team mission climate
Team learning	Psychological safety; learning from errors; supportive feedback; open leadership	Substantial systematic research foundation	• Application ready; Train science team leaders to create psychological safety to support team learning
Knowledge building	Information sharing mechanisms	Meta-analysis; Computational modeling	• Develop communication and knowledge sharing protocols; Research needed on interventions
Team mental models	Shared knowledge structures	Meta-analysis	• Application ready; Train science team leaders to conduct pre-briefs and debriefs; Provide team training
Transactive memory	Team distributed memory	Meta-analysis	• Facilitate interaction and shared experience; Research needed on interventions
Motivational/affective processes			
Team cohesion	Task commitment and social attraction	Multiple meta-analyses	• Research needed on cohesion formation and maintenance
Team efficacy	Shared confidence for goal attainment	Meta-analysis	• Application ready; Train science team leaders to build and instill team efficacy; Provide team training
Team affect or mood	Group emotions	Theory and emerging research	• Research needed on factors that influence mood convergence
Behavioral processes			
Team coordination, cooperation, and communication	Combination of member actions; information exchange	Systematic research foundation	• Application ready; Design supporting goal and feedback systems; Train science team leaders to develop team regulatory skills; Provide team training
Team member competencies	Teamwork KSAs	Systematic research foundation	• Application ready; Provide teamwork skills training to science team members
Team regulation	Regulation of attention and effort	Systematic research foundation	• Application ready; Train science team leaders to develop team regulatory skills

ing the design of interventions that can impact these processes. In the meantime, we know that many cognitive processes, including transactive memory, emerge through the interactions and shared experiences of team members. Thus, science team leaders should arrange frequent opportunities for members to interact, particularly face-to-face, and members should be trained together as an intact team whenever possible.

Motivational and affective team processes. Current research and theory provides varying lev-els of guidance on how to influence the various motivational and affective team processes we have examined. For example, there is clear evidence that both team training and leader actions represent potent levers for developing team efficacy (Kozlowski and Ilgen 2006). Science team leaders should create mastery experiences that allow members to develop their self-efficacy and then shift attention toward facilitating more collective experiences in order to build team efficacy (Kozlowski et al. 1996). As noted earlier, research has also identified strategies that can be used to manage conflict in teams, although most of the attention has been focused on reactive efforts to diffuse conflict after it has pervaded the team. Given the evidence that both task and relationship conflict typically have negative implications for team effectiveness (De Dreu and Weingart 2003), science teams would be well served by adopting preemptive conflict management strategies. For instance, when the team is first coming together, time could be spent to create rules or agreements about how members will tackle disagreements when they arise.

Future research is needed to clarify the levers that can be used to build cohesion in teams, although there is some evidence that both team composition and leader actions (e.g., goal setting) may play a role. Barrick et al. (1998), for example, found that teams higher in extraversion and emotional stability exhibited higher levels of interpersonal cohesion. Work on team affect and mood is still in its early stages, so the potential levers in this area are also less clear. Yet, there is evidence that affect will be a more important consideration in science teams that are highly interdependent and have an extended lifespan. Mood convergence becomes more likely as both the intensity and duration of member interactions increases, and these conditions also likely increase the chances of a single member's emotions permeating the rest of the team.

Behavioral team processes. A body of systematic theory and research provides insight into three main levers that can be used to shape behavioral and action team processes within science teams. First, team design factors, such as the structure of the group task, will influence coordination, communication, and other important behavioral processes in science teams. In addition, support structures can be integrated into the team environment to facilitate team regulation. PROMeas, for example, is an application tool that helps teams to understand their work, develop strategies for accomplishing their goals, and monitor performance feedback (Pritchard et al. 2008). Second, science team leaders can initiate task structures that facilitate team performance and can also help develop the capability of the team to regulate its performance. Kozlowski

et al. (1996), for instance, describe how the role of leaders shifts from setting goals at the onset of the task, to monitoring performance discrepancies during task engagement, to ultimately helping the team reflect on their performance after task completion. Finally, both team training and team building can be powerful levers for shaping the behavioral processes that underlie team performance. Team training strategies, such as team adaptation and coordination training (TACT) and crew resource management (CRM), have been specifically designed to enhance coordination, communication, and other behavioral team mechanisms, and meta-analytic studies have demonstrated their positive impact on team effectiveness (Salas et al. 2008, 2007). In addition, transportable teamwork skills training can be used to enhance the teamwork competencies of science team members (Ellis et al. 2005).

21.6 Conclusion

We opened this chapter by noting that there was a wealth of actionable knowledge that can be distilled from some 65 years of research on the science of team effectiveness that is directly relevant to improving the effectiveness of science teams. We developed an integrative framework—critical conceptual foci, inputs, processes, outcomes, and interventions—to organize the relevant literature. We then concisely reviewed research-based evidence based on meta-analytic summaries and promising lines of cumulative findings. We closed with a focused discussion targeting how the knowledge can be applied to improve science team effectiveness and to highlight knowledge gaps that merit research attention. We hope that the chapter provides a useful roadmap for those interested in improving science team effectiveness by both of those pathways.

Acknowledgments We gratefully acknowledge the U.S. Army Research Institute for the Behavioral and Social Sciences (ARI; W911NF-14-1-0026, S.W.J. Kozlowski & G.T. Chao, Principal Investigators), the National Aeronautics and Space Administration (NASA; NNX13AM77G, S.W.J. Kozlowski, Principal Investigator), and the National Science Foundation (NSF,

1533499, S.W.J. Kozlowski & G.T. Chao, Principal Investigators) for support that in part contributed to the composition of this chapter. Any opinions, findings, conclusions, and recommendations expressed are those of the authors and do not necessarily reflect the views of ARI, NASA, or NSF.

References

Amason AC. Distinguishing the effects of functional and dysfunctional conflict on strategic decision making: resolving a paradox for top management teams. Acad Manag J. 1996;39:123–48.

Bandura A. Self-efficacy: the exercise of control. New York: Freeman; 1997.

Barrick MR, Stewart GL, Neubert JM, Mount MK. Relating member ability and personality to work-team processes and team effectiveness. J Appl Psychol. 1998;83:377–91.

Barsade SG. The ripple effect: emotional contagion and its influence on group behavior. Adm Sci Q. 2002;47(4):644–75.

Barsade SG, Gibson DE. Group emotion: a view from top and bottom. In: Gruenfeld DH, et al., editors. Composition. Research on managing groups and teams, vol. 1. Stamford, CT: JAI Press; 1998. p. 81–102.

Barsade SG, Knight AP. Group affect. Annu Rev Organ Psych Organ Behav. 2015;2:21–46.

Barsade SG, Ward AJ, Turner JDF, Sonnenfeld JA. To your heart's content: a model of affective diversity in top management teams. Adm Sci Q. 2000;45(4):802–36.

Bartel CA, Saavedra R. The collective construction of work group moods. Adm Sci Q. 2000;45(2):197–231.

Beal DJ, Cohen RR, Burke MJ, McLendon CL. Cohesion and performance in groups: a meta-analytic clarification of construct relations. J Appl Psychol. 2003;88(6):989–1004.

Bell ST. Deep-level composition variables as predictors of team performance: a meta-analysis. J Appl Psychol. 2007;92(3):595–615.

Bell BS, Kozlowski SWJ. A typology of virtual teams: implications for effective leadership. Group Org Manag. 2002;27:14–49.

Bell ST, Villado AJ, Lukasik MA, Belau L, Briggs AL. Getting specific about demographic diversity variable and team performance relationships: a meta-analysis. J Manag. 2010;37:709–43.

Bell BS, Kozlowski SWJ, Blawath S. Team learning: a review and integration. In: Kozlowski SWJ, editor. The oxford handbook of organizational psychology, vol. 2. Oxford: Oxford University Press; 2012. p. 859–909.

Blickensderfer E, Cannon-Bowers JA, Salas E. Theoretical bases for team self-corrections: fostering shared mental models. In: Beyerlein MM, Johnson DA, editors. Advances in interdisciplinary studies of work teams, vol. 4. Greenwich, CT: JAI Press; 1997. p. 249–79.

Burns T, Stalker GM. The management of innovation. London: Tavistock Publications; 1961.

Campbell DT. Common fate, similarity, and other indices of the status of aggregates of persons as social entities. Behav Sci. 1958;3:14–25.

Cannon MD, Edmondson AC. Confronting failure: antecedents and consequences of shared beliefs about failure in organizational work groups. J Organ Behav. 2001;22(2):161–77.

Cannon-Bowers JA, Tannenbaum SI, Salas E, Volpe CE. Defining team competencies and establishing team training requirements. In: Guzzo R, Salas E, editors. Team effectiveness and decision making in organizations. San Francisco: Jossey-Bass; 1995. p. 333–80.

Carter D, Asencio R, Trainer H, DeChurch L, Zaccaro S, Kanfer R. Best practices for researchers working in multi-team systems. In: Hall KL, Vogel AL, Croyle RT, editors. Strategies for team science success: handbook of evidence-based principles for crossdisciplinary science and practical lessons learned from health researchers. New York, NY: Springer; 2019.

Chao GT, Moon H. The cultural mosaic: a metatheory for understanding the complexity of culture. J Appl Psychol. 2005;90:1128–40.

Chen G, Kanfer R, DeShon RP, Mathieu JE, Kozlowski SWJ. The motivating potential of teams: test and extension of Chen and Kanfer's (2006) cross-level model of motivation in teams. Organ Behav Hum Decis Process. 2009;110:45–55.

Chiocchio F, Kelloway EK, Hobbs B. The psychology and management of project teams. New York: Oxford University Press; 2015.

Cohen SG, Bailey DE. What makes teams work: group effectiveness research from the shop floor to the executive suite. J Manag. 1997;23:239–90.

De Church LA, Mesmer-Magnus JR. The cognitive underpinnings of effective teamwork: a meta-analysis. J Appl Psychol. 2010;95(1):32–53.

De Dreu CKW. Cooperative outcome interdependence, task reflexivity, and team effectiveness: a motivated information processing perspective. J Appl Psychol. 2007;92(3):628–38.

De Dreu CKW, Carnevale PJD. Motivational bases for information processing and strategic choice in conflict and negotiation. In: Zanna MP, editor. Advances in experimental social psychology, vol. 35. New York: Academic Press; 2003. p. 235–91.

De Dreu CKW, Weingart LR. Task versus relationship conflict, team performance, and team member satisfaction: a meta-analysis. J Appl Psychol. 2003;88(4):741–9.

DeShon RP, Kozlowski SWJ, Schmidt AM, Milner KR, Wiechmann D. A multiple goal, multilevel model of feedback effects on the regulation of individual and team performance. J Appl Psychol. 2004;89:1035–56.

Devine DJ, Phillips JL. Do smarter teams do better? A meta-analysis of cognitive ability and team performance. Small Group Res. 2001;32(5):507–32.

Edmondson AC, Lei Z. Psychological safety: the history, renaissance, and future of an interpersonal construct. Annu Rev Organ Psych Organ Behav. 2014;1:23–43.

Edmondson AC, Bohmer RM, Pisano GP. Disrupted routines: team learning and new technology implementation in hospitals. Adm Sci Q. 2001;46:685–716.

Edmonson AC. Psychological safety and learning behavior in work teams. Adm Sci Q. 1999;44:350–83.

Ellis APJ, Bell BS. Capacity, collaboration, and commonality: a framework for understanding team learning. In: Neider LL, Shriesheim CA, editors. Understanding teams: a volume in research in management. Greenwich, CT: Information Age; 2005. p. 1–25.

Ellis APJ, Hollenbeck JR, Ilgen DR, Porter COLH, West BJ, Moon H. Team learning: collectively connecting the dots. J Appl Psychol. 2003;88(5):821–35.

Ellis APJ, Bell BS, Ployhart RE, Hollenbeck JR, Ilgen DR. An evaluation of generic teamwork skills training with action teams: effects on cognitive and skill-based outcomes. Pers Psychol. 2005;58:641–72.

Fiore SM, Gabelica C, Wiltshire T, Stokols D. Training to be a (team) scientist. In:In: Hall KL, Vogel AL, Croyle RT, editors. Strategies for team science success: handbook of evidence-based principles for cross-disciplinary science and practical lessons learned from health researchers. New York, NY: Springer; 2019.

Galbraith J. Organization design: an information processing view. In: Lorsch J, Lawrence P, editors. Organizational planning: cases and concepts. Homewood, IL: Irwin-Dorsey; 1972. p. 530–48.

Gibbs K, Han A, Lun J. Demographic diversity in teams: the challenges, benefits, and management strategies. In: Hall KL, Vogel AL, Croyle RT, editors. Strategies for team science success: handbook of evidence- based principles for cross-disciplinary science and practical lessons learned from health researchers. New York, NY: Springer; 2019.

Gibson CB, Gibbs JL. Unpacking the concept of virtuality: the effects of geographic dispersion, electronic dependence, dynamic structure, and national diversity on team innovation. Adm Sci Q. 2006;51:451–95.

González-Romá V, Peiró JM, Tordera N. An examination of the antecedents and moderator influences of climate strength. J Appl Psychol. 2002;87:465–73.

Grand JA, Braun MT, Kuljanin G, Kozlowski SWJ, Chao GT. The dynamics of team cognition: a process-oriented theory of knowledge emergence in teams [monograph]. J Appl Psychol. 2016;101:1353–85.

Gully SM, Incalcaterra KA, Joshi A, Beaubien JM. A meta-analysis of team-efficacy, potency, and performance: interdependence and level of analysis as moderators of observed relationships. J Appl Psychol. 2002;87(5):819–32.

Hackman JR. The design of work teams. In: Lorsch J, editor. Handbook of organizational behavior. New York: Prentice Hall; 1987. p. 315–42.

Hoch J, Kozlowski SWJ. Leading virtual teams: hierarchical leadership, structural supports, and shared team leadership. J Appl Psychol. 2014;99:390–403.

Hofmann DA, Stetzer A. A cross-level investigation of factors influencing unsafe behaviors and accidents. Pers Psychol. 1996;49:307–39.

Hollenbeck JR, Beersma B, Schouten ME. Beyond team types and taxonomies: a dimensional scaling conceptualization for team description. Acad Manag J. 2012;37:82–106.

Hunter JE, Hunter RF. Validity and utility of alternative predictors of job performance. Psychol Bull. 1984;96(1):72–98.

Ilgen DR, Hollenbeck JR, Johnson M, Jundt D. Teams in organizations: from i-p-o models to imoi models. Annu Rev Psychol. 2005;56:517–43.

Jackson SE. Team composition in organizational settings: issues in managing an increasingly diverse workforce. In: Worchel S, Wood W, Simpson J, editors. Group process and productivity. Newbury Park, CA: Sage; 1992. p. 138–73.

James LR, Jones AP. Organizational climate: a review of theory and research. Psychol Bull. 1974;81(12):1096.

Jehn KA. A multimethod examination of the benefits and detriments of intragroup conflict. Adm Sci Q. 1995;40:256–82.

Jones BF, Wuchty S, Uzzi B. Multi-university research teams: shifting impact, geography, and stratification in science. Science. 2008;322(5905):1259–62.

Joshi A, Roh H. The role of context in work team diversity research: a meta-analytic review. Acad Manag J. 2009;52(3):599–627.

Kirkman BL, Mathieu JE. The dimensions and antecedents of team virtuality. J Manag. 2005;31:700–18.

Kirkman BL, Gibson CB, Kim K. Across borders and technologies: advancements in virtual teams research. In: Kozlowski SWJ, editor. Oxford handbook of industrial and organizational psychology, vol. 1. New York: Oxford University Press; 2012. p. 789–858.

Klein C, DiazGranados D, Salas E, Le H, Burke CS, Lyons R, Goodwin GF. Does team building work? Small Group Res. 2009;40:181–222.

Klimoski R, Mohammed S. Team mental model: construct or metaphor? J Manag. 1994;20:403–37.

Kozlowski SWJ, Bell BS. Work groups and teams in organizations. In: Borman WC, Ilgen DR, Klimoski RJ, editors. Handbook of psychology: industrial and organizational psychology, vol. 12. London: Wiley; 2003. p. 333–75.

Kozlowski SWJ, Bell BS. Work groups and teams in organizations. In: Weiner IB, Schmitt NW, Highhouse S, editors. Handbook of psychology, Industrial and organizational psychology, vol. 12. 2nd ed. Hoboken, NJ: Wiley; 2013. p. 412–69.

Kozlowski SW, Doherty ML. Integration of climate and leadership: examination of a neglected issue. J Appl Psychol. 1989;74(4):546–53.

Kozlowski SWJ, Ilgen DR. Enhancing the effectiveness of work groups and teams (monograph). Psychol Sci Public Interest. 2006;7:77–124.

Kozlowski SWJ, Klein KJ. A multilevel approach to theory and research in organizations: contextual, temporal, and emergent processes. In: Klein KJ, Kozlowski SWJ, editors. Multilevel theory, research, and methods in organizations: foundations, extensions, and new directions. San Francisco, CA: Jossey-Bass; 2000. p. 3–90.

Kozlowski SWJ, Gully SM, McHugh PP, Salas E, Cannon-Bowers JA. A dynamic theory of leadership and team effectiveness: developmental and task contingent leader roles. In: Ferris GR, editor. Research in personnel and human resource management, vol. 14. Greenwich, CT: JAI Press; 1996. p. 253–305.

Kozlowski SWJ, Gully SM, Nason ER, Smith EM. Developing adaptive teams: a theory of compilation and performance across levels and time. In: Ilgen DR, Pulakos ED, editors. The changing nature of work performance: implications for staffing, personnel actions, and development. San Francisco: Jossey-Bass; 1999. p. 240–92.

Kozlowski SWJ, Chao GT, Grand JA, Braun MT, Kuljanin G. Advancing multilevel research design: capturing the dynamics of emergence. Organ Res Methods. 2013;16:581–615.

Kozlowski SW, Mak S, Chao GT. Team-centric leadership: an integrative review. Annu Rev Organ Psych Organ Behav. 2016;3:21–54.

Lau DC, Murnighan JK. Demographic diversity and faultlines: the compositional dynamics of organizational groups. Acad Manag Rev. 1998;23:325–40.

Lawrence PR, Lorsch JW. Differentiation and integration in complex organizations. Adm Sci Q. 1967;12:1–47.

LePine JA. Adaptation of teams in response to unforeseen change: effects of goal difficulty and team composition in terms of cognitive ability and goal orientation. J Appl Psychol. 2005;90:1153–67.

LePine JA, Piccolo RF, Jackson CL, Mathieu JE, Saul JR. A meta-analysis of teamwork processes: tests of a multidimensional model and relationships with team effectiveness criteria. Pers Psychol. 2008;61:273–307.

LePine JA, Buckman BR, Crawford ER, Methot JR. A review of research on personality in teams: accounting for pathways spanning levels of theory and analysis. Hum Resour Manag Rev. 2010;21:311–30.

Levine JM, Moreland RL. Progress in small group research. Annu Rev Psychol. 1990;41:585–634.

Lindsley DH, Brass DJ, Thomas JB. Efficacy-performing spirals: a multilevel perspective. Acad Manag Rev. 1995;20(3):645–78.

Luciano MM, DeChurch LA, Mathieu JE. Multiteam systems: a structural framework and meso-theory of system functioning. J Manag. in press.

Mannix E, Neale MA. What differences make a difference? The promise and reality of diverse teams in organizations. Psychol Sci Public Interest. 2005;6(2):31–55.

March JG, Simon HA. Organizations. New York, NY: John Wiley & Sons; 1958.

Marks MA, Zaccaro SJ, Mathieu JE. Performance implications of leader briefings and team interaction training for team adaptation to novel environments. J Appl Psychol. 2000;85:971–86.

Marks MA, Mathieu JE, Zaccaro SJ. A temporally based framework and taxonomy of team processes. Acad Manag Rev. 2001;26:356–76.

Marks MA, Sabella MJ, Burke CS, Zaccaro SJ. The impact of cross-training on team effectiveness. J Appl Psychol. 2002;87:3–13.

Mathieu JE, Maynard MT, Rapp T, Gilson L. Team effectiveness 1997–2007: a review of recent advancements and a glimpse into the future. J Manag. 2008;34:410–76.

McGrath JE. Social psychology: a brief introduction. New York: Holt, Rinehart, & Winston; 1964.

McGrath JE. Groups: interaction and performance. Englewood Cliffs, NJ: Prentice-Hall; 1984.

Mesmer-Magnus JR, DeChurch LA. Information sharing and team performance: a meta-analysis. J Appl Psychol. 2009;94:535–46.

Miller GA. The magical number seven, plus or minus two: some limits on our capacity for processing information. Psychol Rev. 1956;63:81–97.

Mohammed S, Nadkarni S. Are we all on the same temporal page? The moderating effects of temporal team cognition on the polychronicity diversity-team performance relationship. J Appl Psychol. 2014;99:404–22.

Mohammed S, Ferzandi L, Hamilton K. Metaphor no more: a 15-year review of the team mental model construct. J Manag. 2010;36(4):876–910.

Mohammed S, Hamilton K, Tesler R, Mancuso V, McNeese M. Time for temporal team mental models: expanding beyond "what" and "how" to incorporate "when.". Eur J Work Organ Psy. 2015;24:693–709.

National Research Council. Enhancing the Effectiveness of Team Science. Washington. DC: The National Academies Press. 2015. https://doi.org/10.17226/19007.

Nembhard IM, Edmondson AC. Making it safe: the effects of leader inclusiveness and professional status on psychological safety and improvement efforts in health care teams. J Organ Behav. 2006;27:941–66.

Nurius PS, Kemp SP. Individual level competencies for team collaboration with cross-disciplinary researchers and stakeholders. In: Hall KL, Vogel AL, Croyle RT, editors. Strategies for team science success: handbook of evidence-based principles for cross-disciplinary science and practical lessons learned from health researchers. New York, NY: Springer; 2019.

O'Leary MB, Cummings JN. The spatial, temporal, and configurational characteristics of geographic dispersion in teams. MIS Q. 2007;31:433–52.

Paskevich DM, Brawley LR, Dorsch KD, Widmeyer WN. Relationship between collective efficacy and team cohesion: conceptual and measurement issues. Group Dynamics. 1999;3:210–22.

Prewett MS, Walvoord AA, Stilson FR, Rossi ME, Brannick MT. The team personality–team performance relationship revisited: the impact of criterion choice, pattern of workflow, and method of aggregation. Hum Perform. 2009;22(4):273–96.

Pritchard RD, Harrell MM, DiazGranados D, Guzman MJ. The productivity measurement and enhancement system: a meta-analysis. J Appl Psychol. 2008;93:540–67.

Salas E, Cannon-Bowers JA. Methods, tools, and strategies for team training. In: Quiñones MA, Ehrenstein A, editors. Training for a rapidly changing workplace:

21 Evidence-Based Principles and Strategies for Optimizing Team Functioning...

293

applications of psychological research. Washington, DC: APA; 1997. p. 249–79.

Salas E, Nichols DR, Driskell JE. Testing three team training strategies in intact teams a meta-analysis. Small Group Res. 2007;38(4):471–88.

Salas E, DiazGranados D, Klein C, Burke CS, Stagl KC, Goodwin GF, et al. Does team training improve team performance? A meta-analysis. Hum Factors. 2008;50(6):903–33.

Salazar M, Widmer K, Doiron K, Lant T. Leader integrative capabilities: a catalyst for effective interdisciplinary teams. In: Hall KL, Vogel AL, Croyle RT, editors. Strategies for team science success: handbook of evidence- based principles for cross-disciplinary science and practical lessons learned from health researchers. New York, NY: Springer; 2019.

Salazar MR, Lant TK, Fiore SM, Salas E. Facilitating innovation in diverse science teams through integrative capacity. Small Group Res. 2012;43(5):527–58.

Schneider B, Wheeler JK, Cox JF. A passion for service: using content analysis to explicate service climate themes. J Appl Psychol. 1992;77(5):705–16.

Seers A, Petty MM, Cashman JF. Team-member exchange under team and traditional management: a naturally occurring quasi-experiment. Group Org Manag. 1995;20:18–38.

Smith KG, Smith KA, Olian JD, Smis HP Jr, O'Bannon DP, Scully JA. Top management team demography and process: the role of social integration and communication. Adm Sci Q. 1994;39:412–38.

Smolek J, Hoffman D, Moran L. Organizing teams for success. In: Sundstrom E, editor. Supporting work team effectiveness. San Francisco: Jossey-Bass; 1999. p. 24–62.

Stajkovic AD, Luthans F. Self-efficacy and work-related performance: a meta-analysis. Psychol Bull. 1998;124(2):240–61.

Stasser G, Titus W. Pooling of unshared information in group decision making: biased information sampling during discussion. J Pers Soc Psychol. 1985;48:1467–78.

Stasser G, Titus W. Effects of information load and percentage of shared information on the dissemination of unshared information during group discussion. J Pers Soc Psychol. 1987;53:81–93.

Steiner ID. Group process and productivity. New York: Academic Press; 1972.

Stevens MJ, Campion MA. The knowledge, skill, and ability requirements for teamwork: implications for human resource management. J Manag. 1994;20:503–30.

Stevens MJ, Campion MA. Staffing work teams: development and validation of a selection test for teamwork settings. J Manag. 1999;25:207–28.

Stokols D, Hall KL, Taylor BK, Moser RP. The science of team science: overview of the field and introduction to the supplement. Am J Prevent Med. 2008;35:S77–89.

Stout RJ, Salas E, Carson R. Individual task proficiency and team process behavior: what's important for team functioning. Mil Psychol. 1994;6:177–92.

Sundstrom E, DeMeuse KP, Futrell D. Work teams: applications and effectiveness. Am Psychol. 1990;45:120–33.

Sundstrom E, McIntyre M, Halfhill T, Richards H. Work groups from the Hawthorne studies to work teams of the 1990's and beyond. Group Dyn Theory Res Pract. 2000;4:44–67.

Sy T, Côté S, Saavedra R. The contagious leader: impact of the leader's mood on the mood of group members, group affective tone, and group processes. J Appl Psychol. 2005;90(2):295–305.

Thatcher SM, Patel PC. Group faultlines a review, integration, and guide to future research. J Manag. 2012;38(4):969–1009.

Thompson J. Organizations in action. New York: McGraw-Hill; 1967.

Twyman M, Contractor N. Team assembly. In: Hall KL, Vogel AL, Croyle RT, editors. Strategies for team science success: handbook of evidence-based principles for cross-disciplinary science and practical lessons learned from health researchers. New York, NY: Springer; 2019.

Van de Ven AH, Delbecq AL, Koenig R. Determinants of coordination modes within organizations. Am Sociol Rev. 1976;41:322–38.

Wagner JA. Studies of individualism-collectivism: effects on cooperation in groups. Acad Manag J. 1995;38:152–72.

Wegner DM. A computer network model of human transactive memory. Soc Cogn. 1995;13:319–39.

Wilson JM, Goodman PS, Cronin MA. Group learning. Acad Manag Rev. 2007;32:1041–59.

Winter S. Organizational perspectives on leadership strategies for the success of cross-disciplinary science teams. In: Hall KL, Vogel AL, Croyle RT, editors. Strategies for team science success: handbook of evidence- based principles for cross-disciplinary science and practical lessons learned from health researchers. New York, NY: Springer; 2019.

Wuchty S, Jones BF, Uzzi B. The increasing dominance of teams in production of knowledge. Science. 2007;316(5827):1036–9.

Zijlstra FR, Waller MJ, Phillips SI. Setting the tone: early interaction patterns in swift-starting teams as a predictor of effectiveness. Eur J Work Organ Psy. 2012;21:749–77.

Conflict Prevention and Management in Science Teams

22

L. Michelle Bennett and Howard Gadlin

Contents

Team Science is an exercise in difference, and difference can scatter seeds of discontent. As has been illustrated and argued in the many chapters that precede this one, there are many benefits to bringing individuals from different disciplinary backgrounds together to solve complex multilevel problems. Scientific diversity is one dimension of difference that is necessary for maximizing problem-solving and bringing new perspectives to focus on a challenge (Hong and Page 2004; National Research Council 2015). We can leave it to the imagination to envision the many other facets of diversity possible extending from methodologies, frameworks, and philosophies to personalities, gender, and race/ethnicity (Freeman and Huang 2014). While almost every aspect of diversity presents challenges, when managed well diversity leads to effective functioning, higher achievement, and strong group morale (Campbell et al. 2013).

In this chapter, we will introduce several frameworks, practical strategies, and resources that can be used to prevent, pre-empt, and/or resolve conflict in scientific teams. Because conflict can adversely affect group interactions and undermine the collaboration necessary for effective team functioning, the earlier that tools and approaches are used, the better.

22.1 Stages of Team Development

Bruce Tuckman introduced a framework for understanding the evolution of a team, which included forming (coming together around a shared interest), storming (becoming aware of and managing difference), norming (developing group norms for working together), and performing (achieving the state of successful team functioning) (Tuckman 1965; Tuckman and Jenson

L. M. Bennett (✉)
Center for Research Strategy, National Cancer Institute, Bethesda, MD, USA
e-mail: LMBennett@nih.gov

H. Gadlin
Bethesda, MD, USA

© Springer Nature Switzerland AG 2019
K. L. Hall et al. (eds.), *Strategies for Team Science Success*,
https://doi.org/10.1007/978-3-030-20992-6_22

1977). Introduced in the 1960s, it is still a very useful framework for thinking through the team dynamic at the level of individuals working together. Beyond the team, we have also found it useful for considering the institutional level elements required to support collaborative approaches in the academic setting.

Forming, the initial stage, is often a period of shared excitement as the scientific vision is elaborated and a team is assembled. It is during the storming phase of Tuckman's model that the team begins to realize the honeymoon may be over. Tensions begin to emerge, words can be misinterpreted, and fairness questioned as each person experiences events through their own individual lenses. This particular stage of team development is crucial in at least three ways. First, it is necessary for the team to uncover and bring to light the differences that exist. Second, it is by becoming aware of and working through differences that the team can successfully evolve to the norming stage. And third, successful transition to the norming phase is a sign that there is a foundation of trust that can be further built upon. Without trust, the team cannot engage in the open and honest communication required to move the science to the next level. Team members are not only getting to know their colleagues better but they are also developing some self-awareness around how they function as members of a team.

22.2 Minimizing Affective Conflict and Encouraging Productive Collision

Creating an environment where open and honest discussion about differences of opinion, scientific strategy, and research direction is essential. Conflict in and of itself is not a problem. It is the management of conflict that can become tricky. Its perceived value can get masked as individuals struggle with the affective (personal) and cognitive (intellectual) forms. Scientists are often emotionally invested in their scientific ideas. Consequently, when colleagues disagree, they can easily take that as a personal attack rather than an intellectual difference. Science

thrives on disagreement and therefore cognitive conflict must be embraced in the academic setting. It is the foundation upon which healthy discussions about research approach, methodology, generation of results, and interpretation can be had. The solution is in depersonalizing conflict, focusing on substantive disagreements about methodology, forming data analysis hypothesis, and resisting the inevitable temptation to focus more on winning arguments than getting to the best answer (Fiore et al. 2015). Teams are most at risk of engaging in affective conflict during the Tuckman storming phase, prior to the establishment of trust. During the norming and performing stages with a strong foundation for interpersonal relationships, cognitive conflict that has the potential to propel the team forward can thrive. But there is a lot of work to be done to get to the point where disagreement can be productive. In the early phases, when the team is first being formed, it is important that teams establish modes of communication that help them to understand how their conceptual and methodological differences will strengthen their scientific work and, in so doing, build the sort of trust they will need to work together compatibly.

As we have worked more and more with individuals, teams, and institutions interested in collaboration and team science, we have become increasingly aware of how the Tuckman model can be used at the personal, interpersonal, and institutional levels (see Fig. 22.1).

22.3 Intrapersonal Influences on Conflict in Teams

As described above, Tuckman's model originally addressed the interpersonal dimension of team formation. But there is also an important personal component associated with deciding whether or not to participle in a collaborative effort termed motivators and detractors. Motivators are those elements that encourage or entice an individual to engage whereas detractors could be characterized as those factors that discourage participation, i.e., what one loses when collaborating with others. (Mallinson et al. 2016; Lotrecchiano et al. 2016).

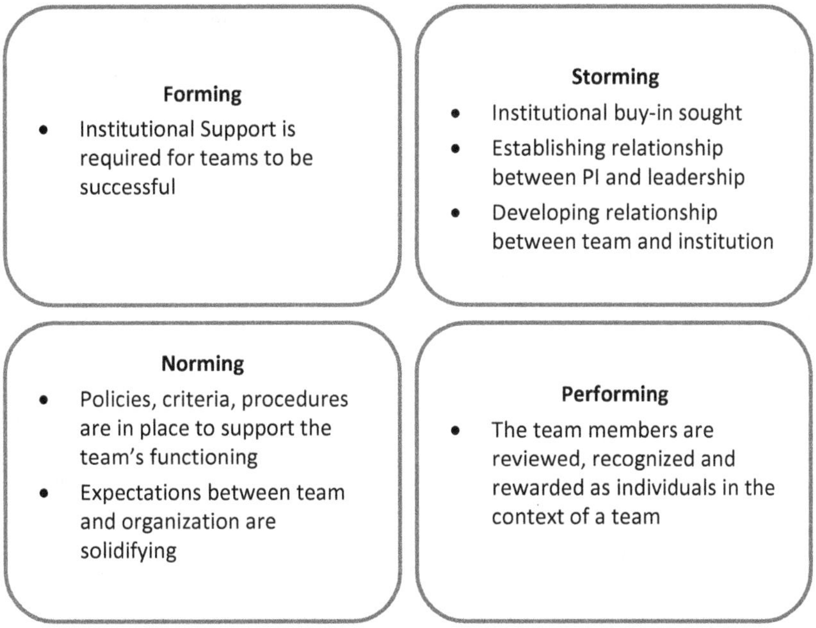

Fig. 22.1 Tuckman model applied to the organizational level

At the personal level, one can compare the forming stage to the courting phase of a romantic relationship. At the start, there seem to be so many reasons to get together and the match seems so perfect. In science, the motivators for participating in a collaborative effort would far outweigh the detractors and could include a shared goal, the promise of achieving greater accomplishments together, benefits of pooling resources, and intellectual stimulation, just to name a few.

As the relationship develops, one becomes aware of what they might have to give up. In team science, anyone participating in a collaborative effort must confront the detractors that emerge. Such detractors include, but are not limited to, a preference to work autonomously, fears of not being appropriately credited for contributions, and threats to power and autonomy. As the collaborators become aware of significant differences with their colleagues, the potential for conflict increases. Identifying and deciding how to manage differences, both conceptual and affective, at the scientific and personal levels become central challenges during the storming phase. As alluded to previously, some degree of self-awareness and emotional intelligence contributes positively to successful participation in collab-

orative ventures. One needs to be aware of one's impact on others as well as of one's own areas of sensitivity and vulnerability.

22.4   Organizational Influences on Conflict in Teams

The team development stages can also be considered in the context of the organization as a whole. Effective team functioning depends on more than managing the personal and interpersonal dynamics of team creation and activity. Institutional support for the formation of and maintenance of collaborative teams is helpful as people come together to work on a joint project. Without top-down support, it is hard for teams to function and receive the status and recognition they require. Individuals recognize quickly when there is no institutional support for such entities, and they turn their attention to efforts for which they will receive backing, especially as it is related to their career growth and advancement.

Some of the elements that come into play during the storming phase include organizational self-awareness (relationship of the team to the organization) buy-in to the activity, trust that the effort will benefit the organization, autonomy for the team, and relationship between the PIs and the leadership. Institutional support at this stage could also be reflected in their support of appointments that help support the team such as lab managers (described in Chap. 49) or creating offices for conflict prevention and resolution. At the NIH, the Center for Cooperative Resolution exists and is staffed with skilled facilitators and mediators (ombudsmen) who serve as a resource to those engaged in conflict. Other institutions take different approaches by providing conflict coaches or other points of contact for people to engage when they need help working through a tricky problem involving other people.

In the norming and performing stages, it is crucially important that the individual team members are confident that policies, criteria, and procedures are in place to support the team's functioning and they will be reviewed, recognized, and rewarded for the collaborative work they are performing.

22.5 Practical Strategies to Prevent or Manage Conflict

In order to prevent or manage conflict, the team must anticipate conflict before it arises. This can be a challenge for scientists and researchers who tend to be conflict adverse (Cohen and Cohen 2012). Even the supposition that conflict could arise can cause unease, and there is discomfort with the notion of having explicit conversations to clearly spell out how the team will deal with conflict when it does emerge. We are not suggesting that scientists working in teams need to have the skills and sensitivity of therapists or social workers. Fortunately, there is a certain predictability to some of the conflicts or possible points of tension in scientific collaborations. For example, the order of authorship and allocation of credit is almost always an issue and needs to be addressed directly and explicitly. And we know from Tuckman's work that there are certain stages that scientific teams must go through to become productive.

Straightforward strategies can be put in place to help individuals, teams, and institutions pre-

vent or at a minimum preempt conflict at its earliest stages. Among the most useful approaches, if people are willing to put them in place, are agreements that clearly set out the goals and objectives as well as roles and responsibilities for all the parties. Collaborative Agreements, affectionately called Prenuptial Agreements for Scientists, can address any topic that the collaborative team thinks useful (Bennett and Gadlin 2012). Often such agreements include goals and objectives, expectations for each of the team members in the form of roles and responsibilities, how data will be generated, shared, and stored, how authorship and media requests will be handled, and how the team will communicate internally as well as with outside groups and manage issues such as conflict of interest or financial matters (Gewin 2015).

We often use a case study (text box) with workshop participants to help them experience how the collaborative agreement can benefit them in their group work. We introduce the case study, have them discuss it in small groups, and then ask them to imagine they are working with the two researchers to develop a Collaborative Agreement. Their assignment is to discuss with their group members how they would approach this and to reflect on what aspects of the interactions presented in the case study require the most immediate attention. This exercise is especially useful prior to helping groups launch their own teams or improve their own team dynamics wherein we encourage them to use the Collaborative Agreement framework.

Dr. Klinik and Dr. Bench

Preface
 Any scientific research collaboration requires open communication and ways of reaching decisions about a wide range of matters. Among the most common are manuscript authorship, abstract and journal submissions, meeting presentations, ways to address disagreements about methodology, data analysis and interpretation, and decisions about further collaboration with other researchers.

Case Study

Two researchers had an idea for a high risk and potentially exciting research project and decided to establish a collaboration. Dr. Tony Bench had performed a preliminary translational experiment in animals with a new agent he developed in his lab that generated some intriguing results. Dr. Irma Klinik was excited about the results of Dr. Bench's study and was eager to move the research into the clinical setting by conducting an early phase clinical trial to test the new agent. The clinical trial would be a "first in man" study. While the agent showed promise in the mouse experiment, the biologic mechanism of action of the agent was still not clear. Although interested in the human studies, Dr. Bench thought it was imperative to fully understand the underlying mechanism of action before moving into human studies.

Drs. Bench and Klinik each had their own staff and it was clear from their discussions that the project would entail both joint and separate research-related activities. Dr. Bench, a PhD, trained in genetics and cell biology and was currently the head of his department. His research was focused primarily in cell lines and animal models. His colleague, Dr. Klinik, an MD, was a gastroenterologist with training in patient-oriented research, and while still a junior investigator, she had earned her colleagues' respect as being thoughtful and thorough.

Although excited about the idea of the joint research project, these potential collaborators were experiencing certain tensions and facing some challenges in putting the team together. To begin with, Drs. Bench and Klinik had very different temperaments. Dr. Bench was direct, even outspoken, and quick to come to judgments and conclusions. Dr. Klinik was much more reserved and accustomed to taking time to mull things over before forming and voicing her opinions. When the two of

them spoke, each found they were frustrated by the other's style and struggled over whose style would dominate their interactions. When there were points of disagreement, even small ones, Dr. Bench had a very competitive approach. He enjoyed engaging in lively discussion and debate and seemed to relish disagreements as an opportunity to win. When it came to conflict or disagreement, Dr. Klinik had a more avoidant or accommodating style. As a result, Dr. Klinik resisted getting pulled into the debates around fine points that Dr. Bench initiated whenever possible, and often avoided raising issues where she feared they might differ. At other times, she often yielded to Dr. Bench's preference when issues were of lesser importance to her so as to minimize overt conflict and disagreement.

There were other differences as well. Dr. Bench wanted a complete fusion of their two teams, as well as the integration of anyone new who joined the collaboration. He insisted that there be one large group meeting with all personnel assembled. Dr. Bench wanted all of the team members, researchers, and clinicians, to have a good grasp of all aspects of the research project. He saw himself as an author on every paper or abstract that was developed as part of this collaboration and was happy to debate the topic when raised. Dr. Klinik preferred separate group meetings and was especially concerned that her team be the one to discuss patient care. With respect to publications, she believed that authorship on papers should be attributed based on intellectual contribution and effort, not based on association with the collaboration. She was especially concerned that she, or other people from her team as appropriate, be the lead and senior authors on any papers discussing clinical trials or patient data.

(continued)

(continued)

Finally, there were questions of autonomy. Both Drs. Bench and Klinik were accustomed to being in charge of their own units and staff and neither had experience in joint decision making. While Dr. Bench wanted a tightly integrated team, Dr. Klinik was accustomed to having her way and enjoyed being a sole decision maker. Finding themselves accountable to each other added to the tensions they were experiencing.

The incident that brought things to a head was one where Dr. Bench, thinking he was saving time and effort for Dr. Klinik, submitted an abstract without running it by her. While the work described in the abstract was largely done prior to the initiation of the formal collaboration, Dr. Klinik had been meeting with Dr. Bench and she had contributed intellectually to the design of some of the experiments included in the submission. Dr. Klinik was irate when she found out and saw this action as an extreme betrayal. She went to discuss this matter with an impartial member of the senior leadership at the institution. The leader chose to call a meeting with Drs. Bench and Klinik.

In addition to the prenuptial agreement, we recently introduced the concept of the Welcome to My Team Letter as another tool to support team functioning (Bennett et al. 2014). This is a document that a team can craft together or can be generated by the leader(s) to share with the rest of the team. It is one additional approach to helping teams function at their fullest by encouraging transparency and explicit discussion at many different levels about the norms of the group. In this way, no one can say they were not aware. They may not agree and if that is the case they can propose a discussion with the group to revisit the matter.

Agreements between individuals and the organization can also provide a sense of safety and security with respect to participating in team science. In the form of offer letters or pretenure agreements, the documents can clarify expectations, list criteria, and provide a framework within which collaborations can be supported in the context of the structure of the organization as a whole. Most importantly, as it relates to individual career growth and development, for early stage investigators these agreements can spell out how the individual will be recognized, reviewed, and rewarded in the context of team efforts (Bennett and Gadlin 2012).

For institutions that want to support team science and collaboration, they can consider the evolution of team development and consider the policies, processes, and procedures they have in place and reflect on whether they support or hinder individual participation in collaborative efforts. Aligning the administrative elements with the overall goals of the organization can go a long way to harmonize institutional messages with the behavior of the leadership and the trust of the research community (Gadlin and Bennett 2013).

Conflict cannot be avoided, and in fact it should be embraced as just one element of the complex human condition. Self-, other-, and organizational awareness provides a foundation for preventing, pre-empting, and if needed, managing conflict when it occurs. Learning to deal with conflict is another matter entirely. Some individuals thrive on conflict while others are avoidant in their stance related to it. As individuals work more in the context of teams, they will have ample opportunities to step into and try on for size different and varied approaches to dealing with disagreements. The more practice one has, the more diverse their repertoire will become for managing it. In the end, they can place their focus on productive collision or encouraging disagreement about the substance of the collaborative work and minimize affective, or personal conflict that gets in the way of progress. For this reason, it is important for each scientist to become conscious of his or her individual ways of handling conflict.

Another activity we will often do in workshops is to assess individual conflict styles using the Thomas-Kilmann Conflict Mode Instrument (Thomas and Kilmann 1974). We work with the group to debrief the results and engage them in conversations about both the pros and cons of each of the five styles: competitive, avoidant, accommodating, compromising, and collaborative. Indeed, each style has strengths and weaknesses for individuals engaged in team science. This assessment helps people become aware of their own conflict style, understand the other styles, and gain an appreciation that when working in teams one must be accepting and tolerant of other group members who have dramatically different approaches.

22.6 Managing Conflict

However, although important, successful management of conflict is just one component of effective teams. Conflict cannot be managed if it cannot be surfaced. The research literature on group performance points to one key factor that appears to underlie effective team functioning—psychological safety. There is a dialectical relationship between managing conflict and creating the conditions for psychological safety (Edmondson and Lei 2014). Expressing views, offering criticisms, challenging other's ideas, and admitting mistakes is risky in groups. But at the same time, it takes skill in conflict management to do these things in a way that does not threaten others or inhibit their ability to do the same.

Members of a team need to feel that they can participate in discussions without creating enemies, risking their reputations or damaging their careers (Edmondson and Lei 2014). Skill at conflict management is an attribute of good team members but psychological safety is quality of effective teams.

22.7 Conclusion

In summary, as a team comes together and begins working toward a common goal there are several predictable stages it will go through before achieving the state of high productivity.

Fortunately, the stages can be anticipated by the leaders of the team which makes working through them a bit easier. We shared in this chapter a few of the tools and approaches we have used with teams as well as individuals interested in establishing their own collaborative science groups. By no means do these represent the full body of approaches that can be used. They do provide a starting point and help individuals develop self- and other-awareness, both critical for working in a team setting.

References

Bennett LM, Gadlin H. Collaboration and team science: from theory to practice. J Investig Med. 2012;60:768–75.

Bennett LM, Maraia R, Gadlin H. The 'Welcome Letter': a useful tool for laboratories and teams. J Trans Med Epidemiol. 2014;2:1035.

Campbell LG, Mehtani S, Dozier ME, Rinehart J. Gender-heterogeneous working groups produce higher quality science. PLoS One. 2013;8(10):e79147. https://doi.org/10.1371/journal.pone.0079147.

Cohen CM, Cohen SL. Lab dynamics: management and leadership skills for scientists. 2nd ed. Cold Spring Harbor: Cold Spring Harbor Laboratory Press; 2012.

Edmondson A, Lei Z. Psychological safety: the history, renaissance, and future of an interpersonal construct. Annu Rev Psychol Organ Behav. 2014;1:23–43.

Fiore SM, Carter DR and Asencio R Conflict, trust and cohesion: examining affective and attitudinal factors in team science. Research on Managing Groups and Teams, Vol. 17, Team Cohesion: Advances in Psychological Theory, Methods and Practice. 2015.

Freeman RB and Huang W. Collaborating with People like Me: Ethnic co-authorship within the US. NBER Working Paper, No. 19995; 2014.

Gadlin H, Bennett LM. Supporting interdisciplinary collaboration: the role of the institution. In: Crowley S, Eigenbrode S, O'Rourke M, Wulfhorst JD, editors. Enhancing communication and collaboration in interdisciplinary research; 2013.

Gewin V. Recipe for a team. Nature. 2015;523:245–7.

Hong L, Page S. Groups of diverse problem solvers can outperform groups of high ability problem solvers. PNAS. 2004;101:16385–9.

Lotrecchiano GR, Mallinson T, LeBlanc-Beaudoin T, Schwartz L, Lazar D, Falk-Krzesinski HJ. Individual motivation and threat indicators of collaboration readiness in scientific knowledge producing teams: a scoping review and domain analysis. Heliyon. 2016;2(7):1–51. https://doi.org/10.1016/j.heliyon.2016.e00105.

Mallinson T, Lotrecchiano GR, Furniss J, Schwartz L, Lazar D, Falk-Krzesinski HJ. Pilot analysis of the motivation assessment for team readiness, integration, and collaboration (MATRICx) using rasch analysis. J Investig Med. 2016;64:1186–93. https://doi.org/10.1136/jim-2016-000173.. Epub 2016 Jul 7

National Research Council. Enhancing the Effectiveness of Team Science. Washington. DC; The National Academies Press. 2015. https://doi.org/10.17226/19007.

Thomas KW, Kilmann RH. Thomas-Kilmann Conflict Mode Instrument Mountain View, CA. Xicom, a subsidiary of CPP, Inc; 1974.

Tuckman B. Developmental stages of small groups. Psychol Bull. 1965;63:384–97.

Tuckman B, Jenson MA. Stages of small group development. Group Org Studies. 1977;2:419–27.

Precollaboration Framework: Academic/Industry Partnerships: Mobile and Wearable Technologies for Behavioral Science

23

Praduman Jain and Dave Klein

Contents

The idea of a "gap" between the cultures of academia and industry is well known. In this chapter, we discuss the value of academic/industry partnerships, including the unique perspectives, challenges, skills, resources, and approaches brought to the table by each partner. The Science of Team Science (SciTS) field has generated evidence-based principles for success in team-based collaboration, which we apply to the partnership framework that we created based on years of participation in these collaborations. The framework aims to support academic and industry partners in initiating, growing, and sustaining collaborations to drive mobile and wearable technologies for behavioral science forward. We highlight a successful case study of this sort of partnership.

Industry and academic partners experience different pressures and have different mindsets, beliefs, motivations, and goals. The open nature of academic science is at times in conflict with companies' need to protect technologies they use. Industrial R&D is driven by time-sensitive product development projects and day-to-day project solving, while academic research focuses on long-term challenges and thus may move more slowly. As a result, companies and universities can sometimes struggle to form strong partnerships. However, we encourage both academic and industry partners to embrace and appreciate these factors that make them different.

The rapid pace of technology development is leveling the playing field, as both industry and academia can achieve more independently. However, industry increasingly recognizes that to successfully innovate they cannot exclusively rely on their internal R&D. Working with external partners, such as academic centers, allows industry to access different pools of talent and knowledge and save R&D costs. Great science and technology only go so far—the right people with the right expertise are critical.

Academic and industry partnerships are especially needed in the behavioral and social sciences.

P. Jain (✉) · D. Klein
Vibrent Health, Fairfax, VA, USA
e-mail: pj@vibrenthealth.com

© Springer Nature Switzerland AG 2019
K. L. Hall et al. (eds.), *Strategies for Team Science Success*,
https://doi.org/10.1007/978-3-030-20992-6_23

Private industry is playing an important role in advancing the field of behavioral health, particularly through mHealth interventions, which focus on the use of mobile phones for improving health outcomes. These mHealth interventions require significant human subjects testing that academic institutions have access to through their affiliations with health care systems, public health research facilities, and clinics. This combination of strengths of academia and industry make these partnerships ideal to advance mobile and wearable technologies for behavioral science.

23.1 The Industry/Academic Partnership Framework

The first step to forming a successful industry/academic partnership is to come equipped with the right frame of mind. As opposed to thinking of the creation of an academic/industry partnership as a one-time event, we recommend considering it an ongoing process. We have found that the best approach to starting and maintaining a healthy partnership is to realize that, like any relationship, it takes work, focus, and continued dedication. Every project will include challenges and hurdles along the way, but these challenges are surmountable when you start with a healthy approach and recognition that both sides of the partnership are needed to be successful.

As discussed earlier, the mindset and goals of industry and academia are different. Consider two people from different parts of the world, speaking different languages, attempting to form a relationship. One could argue that these differences make communication extremely difficult. These challenges are exacerbated when the partnership discussions are conducted remotely rather than spending time face-to-face forming and solidifying the relationship.

Through our experiences of forming and maintaining many industry/academic partnerships and relationships, we realized that a standardized framework that facilitates communication could be very helpful to both partners. To that end, we invented the Industry/Academic Translational Science Partnership Framework © ("Framework") as shown below.

The Framework has been used in over a dozen project of different lengths including R01 projects, SBIR projects, pilot projects, and government projects. A printable version is available online at: www.vibrenthealth.com

The key goal of the framework is keeping each other's interests aligned by promoting and maintaining a healthy industry/academic partnership. This plays out during the collaboration process. The Framework guides each partner to better communicate and understand the goals, motivations, and pressures of the other. It helps the partners transition their individual missions and goals into shared missions and goals (Fig. 23.1).

23.2 How to Use the Industry/Academic Translational Science Partnership Framework

The Framework itself can be presented in PowerPoint form in a single slide. Both partners in a joint meeting complete the Framework during the discussion. We recommend the following steps to complete the framework and determine if there is a good fit between the parties:

1. Explain the value of the Framework exercise to your partner.
2. Set aside at least a dedicated 60-min meeting with your partner for the exercise.
3. Complete the framework during the meeting (we recommend screen-sharing).
4. Share the completed version.

Both partners should have the Framework in front of them during the meeting. One person should volunteer to complete the Framework live during the meeting by overwriting the gray text in the template as you go along. We recommend reading the "mission statement" of the Framework aloud during the meeting to help emphasize the potential value of the partnership and the goals of this conversation, using the Framework as a tool:

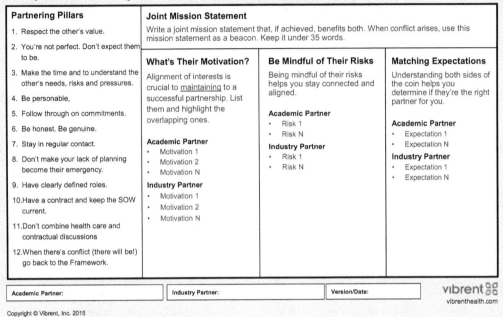

Fig. 23.1 Industry/Academic Translational Science Partnership Framework: The goal of partnering is to create value for both partners. The purpose of the Framework is help both parties become mindful that partnering for better science is a journey. And it's HARD. Setting the right expectations and foundation up front is an investment that will pay dividends throughout the journey, especially when you hit a bump in the road. A well-groomed partnership remains devoid of assumptions

The goal of partnering is to create value for both partners. The purpose of the Framework is help both parties become mindful that partnering for better science is a journey. And it's HARD. Setting the right expectations and foundation up front is an investment that will pay dividends throughout the journey, especially when you hit a bump in the road. A well-groomed partnership remains devoid of assumptions.

The next step is to read each one of the partnering Pillars aloud and briefly discuss each one. We identified each Pillar through years of industry/academic partnering experiences. The list below demonstrates how we explain each Pillar to our partner. Each Pillar is designed to get the partnership in alignment and keep the partners in alignment over time. Understanding what each party values is essential to create a mutually beneficial partnership.

23.3 Partnering Pillars

1. *Respect the other's value.* Understanding the value that the other partner brings to the relationship is the first step toward a foundation of mutual respect. A possible discussion question might be "what value do you believe that we bring to the partnership?"
2. *You're not perfect.* Don't expect your partner to be. Don't set the bar so high that they are destined to fail. Understanding and accepting that there will be mistakes made along

the way will help you to retain alignment. A possible discussion question might be "what limitations can you predict from the get-go?"

3. *Make the time to understand the other's needs, risks, and pressures.* Many academics have never worked in industry and many industry professionals have never worked in academia. These are different worlds that speak different languages. Accept up front that you need a "Rosetta stone" and a healthy attitude to bridge this chasm. Take the time before the Framework meeting to try to understand a bit more about what it's like to be "them." And take the time during the meeting to validate your assumptions and close your knowledge gaps. If you go into the relationship assuming you know exactly what it's like to be in "their" shoes, then you are already risking misalignment from the outset. A possible discussion question might be "what will be our system to make the time?"

4. *Be personable.* Many people would be surprised how many challenges can be overcome by just being friendly and personable. Find things in common to talk about outside of the partnership context. Show your sense of humor. It goes a long way. This may be the most powerful Pillar. A possible discussion question might be "what will be our system to quality check that we're following through on commitments?"

5. *Follow through on commitments.* Trust (or lack of trust) can make or break an industry/academic partnership. Stay vigilant about actively promoting and protecting bonds of trust. One of the easiest and quickest ways to erode trust is to over-commit and under-deliver. Consider each commitment that you make to be an extension of your personal brand. If you cannot meet a stated commitment, then be up-front and communicate with your partner. Conversely, if your partner is up-front about not being able to meet a commitment, then it would be good to remember Pillar #2 to keep you in the right partnership frame of mind. If commitments cannot be met, then the Framework provides a foundation for conducting discussions in a positive, collaborative manner. If irreconcilable differences evolve then there is the ability to part ways amicably. A possible discussion question might be "what is our system to update each other about project delays related to stated commitments?"

6. *Be honest. Be genuine.* This is similar to Pillar #5 in that honesty is an extension of your personal brand. It is tough to regain the trust of your partner once that trust bond is broken. Being genuine is easy when you truly consider the other party as a partner. Because you both come from different "worlds" there is a risk of objectifying the other based on pre-existing assumptions. Being genuine is a way to prevent this from occurring. A possible discussion question might be "do both partners feel that the tone in this meeting is honest and genuine?"

7. *Stay in regular contact.* Everyone is busy. However, keeping in contact, if even with a quick email, will go a long way in promoting and maintaining healthy communication. A reduction in contact should be a red flag in any partnership relationship. A possible discussion question might be "what is our system to do this?"

8. *Don't make your lack of planning become their emergency.* Be mindful that everyone is busy. When you put time pressure on your partner because of lack of planning, you risk fraying the bonds of trust in your relationship because you will be perceived as valuing your time higher than theirs. A possible discussion question might be "what system of project management will be used?"

9. *Have clearly defined roles.* This Pillar cannot be over-emphasized. Be open and realistic about the role of each team member. Aspects of role definition can include responsibilities, work tasks, percent time allocated to the project, and other contributions. State it verbally and, even better, in writing—which leads to the next Pillar. A possible discussion question might be "what are the roles of the key personnel in the project?"

10. *Have a contract and keep the SOW current.* Keeping written agreements current and available to both parties is a fundamental tool that you should use to keep in alignment and resolve conflict—which leads to the final two Pillars. A possible discussion question might be "how will we keep it current?"

11. *Don't combine project and contractual discussions.* Our partners are usually surprised by this Pillar. This advice comes from years of experience. In a contractual discussion, you each have the duty to represent the best interests of your respective organization. You are on opposite sides of the negotiating table by design. This process will go more smoothly if you do not commingle it with working discussions about the project itself. When it comes time to actually do the work together, then you are on the same team and on the same side of the table. A possible discussion question might be "what is our system for doing this?"

12. *When there's conflict (there will be!) go back to the Framework.* If you are experiencing a positive start to the partnership and you assume that it will always be this smooth then you are setting up the partnership for failure. You would not expect this of a marriage and you should not expect this of an industry/academic partnership. There will be bumps in the road. Verbalize this up front, accept it, and plan for it. Better yet, when you experience a challenge, then redo the same Framework exercise to help regain alignment. A possible discussion question might be "what is our system for doing this?"

In just a 60-min exercise, the Framework can be a predictor of future health of the industry/academic partnership. The next step is to discuss the shared mission statement, and record motivations, risks, and expectations of each partner to further the process of understanding one another's goals and pressures and ultimately align interests. This process is described in the case study provided below.

23.4 The Partnership Framework: A Case Study

One of the partnerships where we utilized the Framework, with success, was in a partnership between Vibrent and Laurie Buis, Ph.D., Assistant Professor at the University of Michigan Department of Family Medicine.

Dr. Buis expressed interest in partnering for a NIH R01 grant submission to fund an innovative hypertension intervention using smartphones and wearable devices. The Framework exercise was used to form the foundation of this partnership that continues to broaden and strengthen over time. This case study discusses the mechanics of how the Framework was used in this partnership and how it facilitated the formation of a healthy relationship based on trust, mutual respect, and alignment of interests.

In the absence of the Framework, the initial partnership meeting would have focused on budget discussions and partnering logistics, as is common in introductory industry/academic partnering meetings. The Framework exercise, however, provided a structure that guided the initial discussion in ways that have had lasting effects. Through discussion of the Pillars, the partnering groups realized that there is a shared, common passion for combining the best of what science has to offer with the best of what technology has to offer to truly effect lasting change in populations. The process of sharing our personal stories about how we ended up in our careers led to this insight and created a bond that set the tone for the rest of the Framework exercise, and the partnership.

Joint Mission Statement

The joint mission statement is a 35-word paragraph that both partners create in collaboration. It is meant to be a prototype test of how both partners will collaborate in the partnership.

In this case study, we swapped personal and professional stories while talking through the Pillars, then quickly agreed on the following mission statement: "Fill an immediate need to optimize an R01. But create a long-term stable partnership to effect change in different ways to large populations. No throw-away work. A foundation to broadly build upon." Our confidence around the potential partnership was quickly at a high level. The discussion was grounded and the tone was collaborative, creative, and optimistic. The discussion would have been very different if we started by talking about an R01 budget. This mission statement has become the immutable foundation of the partnership. It has become a kind of "brand" of the partnership itself.

What's Their Motivation?

Alignment of interests is crucial to maintaining a successful partnership. The instruction for the Motivation segment of the Framework exercise is for each partner to list their top two to three motivations. The partners then discuss their overlapping motivations and identify whether any motivations are in opposition. If there are opposing motivations, the partners can either reconcile this dissonance or amicably part ways.

In this case study, the motivations of both partners were strikingly similar but not at all obvious to each other before the Framework exercise. The top motivations of the academic partner revolved around finding a stable partner, letting researchers be researchers instead of getting bogged down with technology, winning an R01 grant, and translating the research into standard of care to have a broad effect on African American hypertensive populations. The top motivations of the industry partner revolved around forming a long-term strategic partnership, conducting high impact research that could translate into a dissemination contract, including the company's name in scientific journals to increase brand awareness, and using technology as an engine for social justice. The amount of overlap was striking to both parties.

Be Mindful of Their Risks

This specific sequence of the segments in the Framework is by design, with discussion of risks following discussion of mission and motivations. The intent is to build a positive tone for the first part of the Framework exercise that carries through as the exercise moves into potentially tougher segments. In this case study, the exercise

worked in exactly this way as the positive tone and collaborative approach carried into the risk segment. The risk segment of the Framework exercise is designed to jump-start empathy for the other party. It forces each party to try to step into the shoes of the other.

In this case study, the academic partner stressed the risks of applying for a highly competitive funding vehicle with a historically low percentage win rate. The industry partner stressed the opportunity cost of partnering for an R01 submission vs. spending the time on a different less risky grant submission or other funded project. Again, it was apparent that there was significant overlap, specifically around both parties being cautious of how they spend their time. We acknowledged this overlap and tied it back to many of the Pillars that stress the importance of being aware that the other partner's time is as valuable as yours. In this case study, this segment worked as designed because it enabled both parties to verbalize a sensitive topic that is frequently not discussed, and to do so in a cordial and respectful way.

Matching Expectations

We have found that this segment frequently becomes a mirror image of the Risk segment. Therefore, if the discussion is positive up until this point, this segment usually is concluded quickly. As with any relationship, it is healthy to state expectations up front and write them down for future reference.

In this case study, the partners discussed their mutual expectations prior to embarking on the program. They agreed to dedicate the requisite amount of time to create a grant submission that they both feel excels in significance, innovation, and approach.

Intellectual Property

This segment is an interesting one because it is a topic that both parties are aware of but naturally gravitate away from discussing initially because it has the potential to be controversial. However, the strategy of ignoring it at the outset is fundamentally flawed; there is no reason to shy away from this topic. In a vast majority of the cases, this is actually the easiest segment to agree upon. A partnership founded on mutual respect will naturally seek to afford proper intellectual property protections. This is a segment about fairness. And if there cannot be an agreement about the fundamental elements of fairness in your partnership, then it is best to end the partnership before it begins, because it is likely to be fatally flawed.

In this case study, both parties agreed they would retain any intellectual property that they each brought to the partnership, and any jointly created intellectual property from the project would be jointly owned.

The case study continues to this day because the R01 was indeed funded and the project will have begun by the time of publication. In fact, we have revisited the partnership Framework a few times in the year that has gone by since the original Framework meeting. The partnership moves forward on solid footing and we have every expectation that this will continue throughout the duration of the R01 grant project.

In summary, we have utilized the Framework successfully in many partnerships and will continue to utilize it to maintain our existing partnerships and form new ones. We believe that the tool will help to keep our industry/academic partnerships in alignment over time and will help to maintain a strong foundation of mutual trust and respect. The more times we conducted the Framework exercise, the better we understood the pressures, challenges, and risks of academia. Additionally, the more times we shared our own pressures, challenges, and risks of industry, the better we have gotten at explaining them to academics. We have become better communicators and better listeners.

A partnership is a relationship. The formal contract is between two organizations, but the day-to-day partnership is between human beings. This is obvious, but subtle at the same time. We have found that approaching a partnership with this relationship management engagement frame of mind helps to foster a creative and energetic atmosphere.

Part VII

Leadership and Management of Teams

Leader Integrative Capabilities: A Catalyst for Effective Interdisciplinary Teams

24

Maritza R. Salazar, Karen Widmer, Kathryn Doiron, and Theresa K. Lant

Contents

24.1 Introduction

Interdisciplinary (ID) medical teams are increasingly used to research and treat complex medical conditions (National Research Council 2015; Wuchty et al. 2007). Interdisciplinary teams in medicine are engaged in a range of endeavors from discovering novel approaches to treating

M. R. Salazar (✉)
Paul Merage School of Business,
University of California, Irvine, CA, USA
e-mail: smaritza@uci.edu

K. Widmer · K. Doiron
Claremont Graduate University, Claremont, CA, USA

T. K. Lant
Lubin School of Business, Pace University,
New York, NY, USA

complex diseases such as cancer,[1] to understanding and finding treatments for rare and neglected diseases,[2] to advancing the use of technology in modeling physical systems, diagnosis, and treatment.[3] The NCATS Chemical Genomics Center,[4] which investigates small molecule chemical probes, provides a vivid illustration. The center is composed of three teams, each specializing on a DNA nucleobase. The teams include specialists in biology, chemistry, and informatics. Each team has three leaders, one from each discipline. The center collaborates with disease-focused research labs around the world. Since their formation in 2008, they have been engaged in collaborations that developed a 3D model of ovarian cancer, made significant progress in understanding Gaucher disease, and have recently received funding from the HHS Innovative Ventures Fund to enhance the web-based Collaborative Use Repurposing Engine (CURE) which supports crowdfunding information on treating tropical diseases. The number and complexity of the network of collaborations that the center must manage begs the question of how to provide effective

[1] Stopping Metastasis in its tracks (Nature Communications, Feb 5, 2015)

[2] Breathing Easier, NCATS feature story 2016

[3] Modeling the Female Reproductive Tract in 3D, NCATS feature story 2015

[4] NCGC Teams, ncats.nih.gov/ncgc

© Springer Nature Switzerland AG 2019
K. L. Hall et al. (eds.), *Strategies for Team Science Success*,
https://doi.org/10.1007/978-3-030-20992-6_24

leadership for the center, its teams, and its collaborative relationships.

The transformation of the medical ecosystem toward the use of large-scale collaborative interdisciplinary teams has been fueled by federal funding agencies (NIH, NCATS) and private foundations (StandUp2Cancer, SolveCFS, CEPI5) that believe the key to scientific breakthroughs to treat complex and intractable diseases depends on a collaborative approach to medical research and practice (Zerhouni 2003; Saporito 2013). The heterogeneous knowledge available in interdisciplinary teams provides the raw material to tackle complex problems that cannot be solved within a single discipline (Kerr and Tindale 2004; van Ginkel and van Knippenberg 2012). This trend is especially true today, an era in which rapid scientific advancement and technological change create increasingly narrow specializations, requiring expertise-diverse collaboration to address a wide range of complex social and scientific problems (Jackson 1992; Jones 2011; Williams and O'Reilly 1998).

Research has demonstrated that knowledge-diverse teams often find the goal of knowledge integration and innovation to be elusive due to cognitive, motivational, and social differences (Balakrishnan et al. 2011; Cronin and Weingart 2007; Okhuysen and Eisenhardt 2002). For instance, collaboration between scientists and physicians, who are accustomed to working in silos on distinct aspects of a disease problem, faces barriers to effectively integrating knowledge because of distinct norms, goals, and approaches (Salazar et al. 2012). Specialized experts find it difficult to share and elaborate upon expertise with teammates from other disciplines because of the limited overlap in shared understanding (Cronin et al. 2011). Coordination of projects can also be difficult. For example, coordination difficulties can arise during efforts to divide responsibilities, share data and specialized equipment, and transfer emerging knowledge through venues such as training, publishing, and conferences (Cummings and Kiesler 2007). These challenges are even more pronounced where geographic dispersion, permeable mem-

bership boundaries, and pluralistic goals of team members from different disciplines exist (National Research Council 2015; see Morgeson et al. 2010, for further discussion of functional challenges). Given the inherent difficulties of generating boundary-spanning ideas and solutions, it is critical to identify the contingency factors that enable some disciplinary diverse teams to collaborate, integrate knowledge, and achieve scientific breakthroughs.

This chapter adds to a growing body of literature that seeks to understand the role of leaders in disciplinary diverse teams (Kearney and Gebert 2009; Nishii and Mayer 2009; Shin and Zhou 2007), and extends research that documents the importance of leaders for enhancing team effectiveness (Börner et al. 2010; National Research Council 2015; Falk-Krzesinski et al. 2010). We propose that leaders with *integrative capabilities* will have greater success in helping disciplinary diverse teams overcome the obstacles of cross-boundary collaboration. We define *leader integrative capability* as a set of skills and behaviors that a team leader can use to bridge intellectual distance and enable knowledge sharing and integration. Throughout this chapter, we detail the integrative capabilities and behaviors that leaders can exhibit to enhance team members' ability to recognize, share, and integrate their knowledge resources more effectively.

Interdisciplinary teams struggle to integrate their diverse knowledge so that their collective knowledge will be greater than the sum of the parts (Balakrishnan et al. 2011; Kozlowski and Chao 2012). By shaping the social context of the team (Hackman 2012), team leaders with integrative capabilities can foster interaction and discussion among team members to generate affective, motivational, and cognitive emergent states (such as trust and shared understanding) that are essential for knowledge integration and creation. We build on input–mechanism–output–input (IMOI) models (Ilgen et al. 2005) that view leader behaviors as key inputs that shape the knowledge elaboration process. We suggest that these behaviors are key to ensuring that team members' uniquely held knowledge can spiral up for use by the entire interdisciplinary team. In the section that follows, we offer tangible and evidence-based recommendations for leaders seeking to help teams of diverse experts reach their fullest potential.

24.2 Background Literature

Interdisciplinary projects promise to enhance the probability of scientific breakthroughs in medicine due to the juxtaposition of ideas, tools, and professionals from different fields of research and areas of practice. To yield these breakthroughs, such as integrating basic science and technological discoveries to find novel approaches to problems (Hargadon 1998; Henderson and Clark 1990) an integrative team leadership approach is needed (NCGCTeams ncats.nih.gov/ncgc). Integrative leadership requires effort to support the synthesis of the team's vision with the heterogeneous inputs of the team leader(s) and members (Mainemelis et al. 2015). *Integrative leadership* is distinct from other types of creative leadership. Under *directive leadership* (e.g., conductors or haute cuisine chefs) leaders drive the creative process. Under *facilitative leadership,* the focus is almost exclusively on the team members' creativity. The concept of integrative leadership builds on a growing body of scholarship that illustrates how collective creativity can occur through a process of combining the experiences, perspectives, and ideas of both team leaders and members via integration (Hargadon and Bechky 2006; Harvey 2014; Taylor and Greve 2006).

Integrative leadership is also distinct from several relationship-based approaches to leadership (e.g., LMX) that focus on the leader–follower relationship (Basu and Green 1997; Clegg et al. 2002; Scott and Bruce 1994; Tierney 2015). Several studies have examined the influence of leader member exchange (LMX) on employee creativity and a recent review suggests that it does have a moderately positive influence on employee creativity and innovative performance (Hammond et al. 2011). Despite the value of this relational approach to creativity of either the follower or the leader, LMX does not explore the creative synthesis that can arise from of the dyad itself. Rather, studies focus on how leaders bring out the creative potential of subordinates through a number of facilitation-oriented behaviors, such as providing creative direction (Mumford et al. 2002) or general support for creativity (Amabile et al. 2004; Basadur 2004; Mumford 2003). Thus, LMX research does not inform us about the collective creativity that can emerge when leaders and followers mutually influence one another through sharing and combining their unique ideas and inputs.

A small set of studies that focused on the role of transformational leadership on the creativity of demographically and educationally diverse teams (Kearney and Gebert 2009; Shin and Zhou 2003) is relevant to leadership in interdisciplinary teams. These studies have demonstrated that leaders who adopt a transformational style are able promote creativity by garnering commitment to a well-articulated vision, and by inspiring followers to develop new ways of thinking about complex problems (Dinh et al. 2014; Piccolo and Colquitt 2006). However, this research neglects to identify causal links between theoretically murky dimensions of transformational leadership and team outcomes (Van Knippenberg and Sitkin 2013). Furthermore, these studies do not consider other leadership dimensions that can be critical for developing scientific discoveries, such as environmental scanning and strategy formulation (Antonakis and House 2014). Thus, the current operationalize of transformational leadership dimensions limit our ability to isolate the capabilities of leaders that are fostering idea integration and innovation.

Perhaps most related to the notion of integrative leaders is a growing body of literature on shared leadership. Studies of shared leadership have several common characteristics: The presence of multiple leaders within a team, a variety of leadership roles, functions and relationships, and a leadership process that exhibits shared or alternating leadership roles, depending on the needs of the team over (Mainemelis et al. 2015). Integrative leadership can involve the synthesis of the creative vision and inputs of a leader with the heterogeneous inputs of not only followers, but other leaders present in a team as well. Despite this possibility, relatively few studies have explored shared leadership in teams working to generate creative outputs through a process of integration of leader and member expertise and insights (Davis and Eisenhardt 2011; Hauschildt and Kirchmann 2001). We tackle this question in the remainder of this chapter, where we elaborate a model of integrative leadership capabilities and *behaviors* that can facilitate knowledge consideration, elaboration, and integration in interdisciplinary teams.

24.3   Theoretical Model

Following existing dynamic models of team inputs, processes, and outputs (Marks et al. 2001; Salazar et al. 2012), we split team emergent states into two categories: social (e.g., trust, cohesion, shared team identity) and cognitive (e.g., knowledge consideration, shared mental models, information elaboration). Cognitive emergent states and social emergent states can independently and jointly help facilitate knowledge exchange and the willingness of members to consider and use the insights of diverse team members. Motivation and capability to elaborate upon diverse knowledge within the team (van Kleef et al. 2004; van Knippenberg et al. 2004), facilitated by a leader with integrative capacity, can help interdisciplinary teams generate new ideas and solutions. Our theoretical model is depicted in Fig. 24.1.

We focus on five potential integrative leadership capabilities that can positively influence interdisciplinary team performance: (a) visioning, (b) reflexivity, (c) perspective-seeking, (d) conflict management, and (e) coordination. For each integrative capability discussed, we provide background from current team's research, as well as ideas for specific behavior that leaders can exhibit to increase the cognitive and social emergent states that facilitate knowledge elaboration and integration. Next, this chapter will briefly cover the performance and team effectiveness in interdisciplinary teams, followed by implications for practice as well as future directions for research on leadership in interdisciplinary teams.

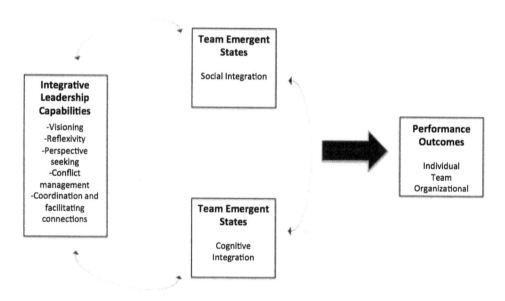

Fig. 24.1 Theoretical model of leader integrative capabilities, team emergent states, and outcomes

24.4   Leader Integrative Capabilities

24.4.1 Visioning

Visioning is one of the integrative behaviors the leader can exhibit to help an interdisciplinary team define its problem parameters, clarify its goals, and identify steps for the effective exchange of member knowledge (Salazar et al. 2012; Zaccaro et al. 2001). Through visioning, leaders help the team conduct "mission analysis" to prevent misalignment among team members regarding their purpose and direction (Marks et al. 2001, p. 363; Morgeson et al. 2010). To ensure alignment, the leader can (re)specify and (re)prioritize sub-goals to ensure that everyone continues to share the same mental model (Zaccaro et al. 2001, p. 461) as they move forward on a team task. The leader might use stories to help develop the shared model, particularly when working with creative projects (Mumford et al. 2002). As the team discusses relevant issues, ambiguous situations will no doubt surface (Morgeson et al. 2010); astute leaders can then remind the team of the purpose and direction of their work. Mumford et al. (2002) suggested that the leader should express the team's vision and direction as tangible products rather than as lofty ideals. Notably, the more unfamiliar or loosely defined the group's task, the more important it may be for the leader to help the team envision the kind of solutions that are appropriate for the team task (Mumford et al. 2002). Given the need to unify and motivate interdisciplinary team members, each of whom has their own specialized knowledge and individual goals, we suggest that visioning is a key integrative behavior that leaders of interdisciplinary teams can utilize.

The interdisciplinary team literature has highlighted three approaches to visioning as a problem conceptualization process that adds traction to team efforts when members hold unique knowledge. The first approach characterizes the team's vision as a task representation, that is, a shared understanding of how the team might use the information resources held by each team member (van Ginkel and van Knippenberg 2012).

Here, the leader's role is to advise the team that high performance will require the elaboration of member contributions during the ensuing discussion. For instance, in van Ginkel and van Knippenberg's (2012) laboratory study, each team member in three-member groups was given unique information regarding a shared market center. Teams who were told that the team task would require the careful exchange, discussion, and integration of each member's information made superior decisions regarding logistical concerns, compared to the decisions of teams who were told that the task required an effort to find common ground. More importantly, however, the leader role was introduced as an experimental condition. When the leader was given the elaboration representation (exchange, discuss, integrate), the team "followed" the leader, regardless of the condition for which they themselves had been instructed. This study underscored the value of the leader's own representation of the task, and how well the leader communicates the importance of that representation.

Goal setting offers a second approach to exceptional team information processing through developing a shared vision of the team task. It is well established that setting goals with challenging performance standards is a strong motivator of both individual and group performance (Weingart and Weldon 1991), ostensibly through directing the attention of the team, increasing their effort, and encouraging their persistence. Indeed, in a meta-analysis, it was determined that when team goals were specific and set at a level difficult enough that current goal attainment was at least one standard deviation lower than the new goal, team performance was higher than when less challenging goals were set (Kleingeld et al. 2011). Similarly, in a field study of nurse surveyors, the accuracy level of health inspection reports was higher when the nurses set a combination of long- and short-term goals (Weldon and Yun 2000). However, there is limited empirical evidence regarding the role of leadership in facilitating goal setting. For instance, Kleingeld et al.'s (2011) meta-analysis showed no significant difference in team performance when the leader unilaterally, partially, or fully delegated the decision regarding achievement standards to the team. However, an early laboratory study showed that when the leader played a coordinator role (rather than a commander role) in a tank battle simulation, members participated more in the goal-setting decisions, reported better use of recommended team tactics, and demonstrated superior performance (Durham et al. 1997). This suggests that the leader's role is to facilitate the team's active selection of their shared goals.

A third approach to visioning draws on a relational perspective. Members tend to *categorize* themselves into subgroups based on differences in observable surface traits (Harrison et al. 2002). This reaction can hinder collaboration, as members tend to favor like-member input, and oppose, feel threatened by, or retreat from the viewpoints of other subgroups (Hogg et al. 2012). Leadership behavior can play a promising role in helping teams manage this kind of relationship, which can often be divisive (Klein and Ziegert 2014). According to Hogg et al. (2012), visioning can include rhetoric that unifies groups containing two or more subgroups, by motivating action toward a unified vision and sense of purpose. For example, the leader might frame the task, while simultaneously crafting a new relational identity that helps team members to view the collaboration as an intertwined partnership connecting each member to a shared outcome, while preserving their unique contributions and making the joint effort greater than the sum of its parts.

24.4.2 Reflexivity

A team process that has been linked to team effectiveness is reflexivity (Carter and West 1998). Team reflexivity is the explicit and purposeful reflection on the team's knowledge, strategy, and progress toward goals; as well as the adaptation of current working methods in response to negative aspects of this reflection (Schippers et al. 2015; West 1996).

Although the role of reflexivity in interdisciplinary teams has not been investigated, studies point to the importance of reflexivity in teams with diverse knowledge. For example, reflexivity

can increase the propensity to redistribute knowledge in teams to meet task demands (West 1996). In addition, it can facilitate the formation of transactive memory systems, or team members' understanding of who knows what, in knowledge-diverse teams with permeable membership (Lewis et al. 2007). However, much of the research on team reflexivity has focused on reflexivity as a team process, without the acknowledgment of leader influence.

Some research, however, suggests that leadership styles can increase team reflexivity (e.g., transformational leadership: Carmeli et al. 2014; Schippers et al. 2008; and authentic leadership: Lyubovnika et al. in press). The overall project management skills of the team leader have also been found to be related to reflexivity (Hoegl and Parboteeah 2006). In addition, some theory and empirical research has pointed to specific behaviors that leaders can practice to increase team reflexivity. Widmer et al. (2009) listed several concrete communication behaviors that leaders should use to increase the quality of reflexivity in teams. These behaviors include discussing errors, creating an environment for exploration and experimentation, and promoting respect among team members.

Reflexivity has been linked to several cognitive emergent states, which are more distally linked to performance outcomes such as knowledge integration and innovation. For example, Salazar et al. (2012) proposed that reflexivity in teams increases the knowledge assimilation and accommodation of team members with diverse knowledge and disciplinary backgrounds. Several studies have also linked reflexivity to shared mental models among team members (Gurtner et al. 2007; Konradt et al. 2015) and shared understanding of the information elaboration requirements of the team's task (Konradt et al. 2016; van Ginkel et al. 2009). A few social emergent states (e.g., trust) and other integrative leadership behaviors (e.g., visioning) have also predicted increased reflexivity (Schippers et al. 2008); these findings show the relationship between the integrative leadership behaviors and the cognitive and social emergent states in the theoretical model proposed in this chapter.

24.4.3 Perspective-Seeking

Literature on creative processes in teams (Mannix et al. 2009; Paulus and Coskun 2012; Paulus and Nijstad 2003) has provided evidence to demonstrate how leaders can foster innovative outcomes by facilitating information sharing and by helping team members to pool their diverse sources of knowledge. For instance, leader interventions have been shown to effectively elicit dissenting views (Schulz-Hardt et al. 2006), facilitate access to team members' knowledge by prompting reflection on group tasks (van Ginkel and van Knippenberg 2008), and enhance the use of varied cognitive capabilities of team members through collaborative planning (Woolley et al. 2008). We propose that perspective-seeking is an additional and underexplored team leader behavior that can foster information elaboration in interdisciplinary teams.

Perspective-seeking is defined as actively seeking out the viewpoints of the other members of the team. This action, in turn, can help a team leader and other members to gain a general understanding of the diverse viewpoints of other members (Davis 1996; Grant and Berry 2011). In their study examining predictors of knowledge sharing and integration, Okhuysen and Eisenhardt (2002) compared the effectiveness of several microinterventions consisting of instructions for members to either share their own uniquely held information, inquire about the knowledge of fellow teammates, or manage their time efficiently. Of these microinterventions, asking others to share information, along with managing time, were found to facilitate information integration. This experimental study illuminates the key role that perspective-seeking can play in fostering knowledge sharing and integration, which are necessary processes for team creativity. Similarly, other scholars have shown an increase in team perspective-seeking when the team is instructed to seek the other team members' perspectives (Hoever et al. 2012), and that knowledge sharing and the development of new ideas may naturally increase in teams with diverse perspectives, through the intense discussion that emerges (Miller et al. 1998; Smith et al. 2005).

Perspective-seeking on the part of the leader can also function to increase the willingness of disciplinary diverse team members to consider the ideas and perspectives contributed by their teammates. As is well documented, perceived dissimilarity tends to decrease the desire to favorably evaluate the contribution of other members of the team (Williams et al. 2007). Heterogeneity of professions leads to less knowledge sharing due to power and status differences, lack of shared language, and less knowledge of who is an appropriate recipient of shared expertise (Wu et al. 2015). To combat these tendencies in interdisciplinary teams, leaders' efforts to engage in perspective-seeking can demonstrate interest in the ideas of others and can set an example regarding the value of diverse perspectives. This role modeling in public settings such as meetings (Gross and Kluge 2014) can positively influence the propensity of team members' willingness to inquire about other team members' perspectives, and to be open to alternative approaches and ideas.

Perspective-seeking has been linked to several cognitive emergent states included in the theoretical model for this chapter, including information elaboration (Hoever et al. 2012), transactive memory (Gockel and Brauner 2013), and shared mental models (Gross and Kluge 2014). Again, showing the dynamic nature of the leader behaviors and team emergent states, transactive memory can also increase the effectiveness of suggesting ideas, as knowing who has the expertise that is needed at a particular point in time is important to the effective use of expertise (Faraj and Sproull 2000).

24.4.4 Conflict Management

In interdisciplinary teams, there is a tendency for conflict to arise as differences in language and methodology between disciplines are uncovered (Cronin and Weingart 2007). Differences in the language, knowledge, and methodology of the team members' disciplines can lead to high-stakes conflict regarding the power and legitimacy that any one discipline has in the group

(Salazar et al. 2012). A discipline may be seen as the "winner" of such a conflict, and team members from that discipline could gain more legitimacy within the team, which in turn could influence the knowledge integration and the overall performance of the team. However, as suggested by Lovelace et al. (2001) findings regarding functional diversity, a team's disciplinary diversity will most likely determine the type of conflict the team will have, but the critical factor in the final outcome of the team's work (e.g., innovation) is how the team leader and team members manage this conflict.

Deciding how to manage conflict effectively can be a complicated challenge for leaders. Different kinds of conflict (e.g., relationship and task conflict; Jehn 1995) lead to positive and negative outcomes for teams. Relationship conflict, which stems from individual differences and disaffection among team members, appears to have only negative consequences in how a team functions, as it can undermine team viability and satisfaction (Amason and Sapienza 1997; Jehn 1995). On the other hand, task-oriented conflict that stems from disagreement about how to complete team tasks has been shown to be more nuanced (Amason and Sapienza 1997). While task conflict has also been shown to lead to lower team satisfaction and willingness to stay on the team (Jehn 1995), it has also been shown to lead to better strategic thinking and team performance in nonroutine tasks (Amason and Sapienza 1997; Jehn 1995). While task conflict can be a tool to increase constructive conversation and innovation in teams, conflict management techniques must approach the introduction of task conflict carefully, as task conflict can also lead to relationship conflict over time (Amason and Sapienza 1997).

In addition to the different kinds of conflict in teams, there are also effective and ineffective ways of dealing with conflict. Tjosvold et al. (2003) found that cooperative (as opposed to competitive or avoiding) conflict management leads to an increase in-role and extra-role team performance. Cooperative conflict management involves framing the goals of the team members who are in conflict as mutually beneficial, where all parties to the conflict "win" if the goals are reached. This leads to the team working together to solve the conflict in a mutual and shared manner. Competitive conflict management (i.e., framing conflict as having a winner and a loser) and avoiding conflict (i.e., attempting to ignore conflict) tend to have worse outcomes (Tjosvold et al. 2003). With all the nuances involved in conflict situations, leaders must have a good view not only of the nature of the conflict, but also of the possible outcomes of stopping the conflict versus attempting to guide the conflict to a healthy debate that has the potential to increase knowledge integration and innovation (Salazar et al. 2012).

Several studies have focused on the types of behaviors leaders should use when attempting to manage conflict in teams, such as encouraging collaborative rather than contentious communication of problems, remaining focused on the task rather than the people, and using visual communication to stimulate discussion if a team has a difficult time finding common language to discuss problems (Klein et al. 2011; Lovelace et al. 2001; Von Glinow et al. 2004). Another potential method of conflict management that can be effective in reducing conflict is emotion management and regulation (Ayoko and Konrad 2012; Meng et al. 2015; van den Berg et al. 2014). Ayoko and Konrad (2012) found that leaders engaging in emotion management interventions with a team decreased both task and relationship conflict, and van den Berg et al. (2014) found that managers using emotion regulation techniques can stop task and process conflict from transforming into a more destructive form of conflict (i.e., relationship conflict). Leaders can also influence how team members manage conflict with one another, without intervention by the leader. For example, Zhang et al. (2011) found that leaders with a transformational leadership style helped teams manage conflict cooperatively.

Several studies have linked cooperative, rather than competitive, conflict management approaches to team reflexivity and team coordination (Tjosvold et al. 2004; Zhang et al. 2011). Effective conflict management experiences could also lead to (a) cognitive emergent states, such as team information seeking (Meng et al. 2015); as well as (b) social emergent states, including lower conflict as well as higher cohesion, collaboration, and even positive feelings toward one another (Lovelace et al. 2001; Salazar et al. 2012; Tekleab et al. 2009). High conflict in a team has been associated with reduced intra-team trust (Langfred 2007) and high levels of trust have been found to both mitigate the negative effects of relationship conflict and amplify the positive effects of task conflict (Simons and Peterson 2000). This interdependence of trust and conflict (Curşeu and Schruijer 2010) means that the development of trust in a team has an impact on and is impacted by the amount of conflict the team has. Team leaders, when approaching conflict and conflict management, should keep this relationship in mind as trust can positively influence willingness to disclose information and knowledge sharing (Lee et al. 2010).

24.4.5 Coordination and Facilitating Connections

Coordination is defined as orchestrating interdependent actions (Marks et al. 2001). For most coordination activities, timing is everything, and more so in a multilevel system where individual members and work teams are situated within a larger organizational context (Kozlowski and Ilgen 2006). Marks et al. (2001) develop a temporally based framework of complex team processes. Rather than viewing teamwork as a simple input–process–output (I-P-O) model, Marks and colleagues demonstrate that many teams have multiple tasks, long-term and short-term goals, and deadlines that they are working toward at the same time. The more dynamic and interdependent the tasks, the more frequent the need to adjust interaction plans to avoid unnecessary process loss. Team leaders must be aware of the temporal nature of teamwork, and help with coordination where it is needed throughout the task planning, task execution, and evaluation of progress toward task completion.

Mumford et al. (2002) have examined the coordination behaviors of leaders of creative ventures. Here too, the leader's social skills (i.e., persuasion, an intuitive sense of others' thoughts, encouraging appropriate peer pressure) and the ability to create cognitive structures (i.e., concrete production missions: planning the structure and timing of a task, but not the conduct of the work) are key. Coordination behaviors suited for creative thinking ranged from providing idea support during the idea generation process, to increasing structures and formalization as projects move from generation to development and implementation, to employing decision rules and norms suited for the creative climate, using intrinsic as well as extrinsic reward, and seeking persons of influence to champion a shared interest.

Interdisciplinary teams working on generating scientific knowledge across disciplinary boundaries pose a particular challenge for coordination, because knowledge and expertise are distributed among team members (Cannon-Bowers et al. 1993; Faraj and Sproull 2000; Moreland 1999). The intellectual distance among team members, coupled with team members' limited experience of working together, can make coordination difficult, because disciplinary diverse team members tend to be unaware of the available knowledge resources at their disposal. Thus, team functioning depends on a team leader's awareness of members' expertise, as well as the ability of the team members to recognize each others' expertise (Moreland and Thompson 2006). In teams where members are made aware at the onset of the expertise possessed by team members, access to knowledge is much easier and uncovers information that enhances team performance (Stasser 1992; Stasser et al. 1995). Enhancing team members' awareness of how they can uniquely contribute to the team's goal, and how their knowledge complements that of their fellow team members, can have a positive impact on team performance. Such awareness can help them not only to recognize that they have different insights that they can apply to the task, but also to accumulate a greater pool of diverse knowledge that can be brought to bear on the team's task (van Ginkel and van Knippenberg 2008).

Although planning and coordinating interactions can require considerable time and resources (Cummings and Kiesler 2007; Morgeson et al. 2010), the integrative capability of leaders who do so can greatly enhance the potential of a team to meaningfully exchange and integrate knowledge. For example, a leader can facilitate the awareness of who knows what by forming and fostering connections between members who may be unfamiliar with one another. This assists the team in open communication across boundaries while buffering them from competing time demands (Morgeson et al. 2010; see also Ancona and Caldwell 1992). As a leadership behavior, this form of networking has been shown to foster more weak ties within the team, which can facilitate creativity (Perry-Smith 2006).

Coordination and facilitating connections between team members can also lead to a crucial affective emergent state: psychological safety. Psychological safety is a shared belief among team members that the team is a safe context for taking risks and sharing ideas without the risk of negative response (Edmondson 1999). Psychological safety has been shown to increase the intention of continually sharing information in a team over time (Zhang et al. 2010), which is an important outcome for most interdisciplinary teams. Several studies have found that inclusive leadership that encourages team members to make contributions and appreciate other team member's contributions increases psychological safety (Carmeli et al. 2010; Nembhard and Edmondson 2006). Relational coordination, which encompasses the establishment of shared goals, shared knowledge, and mutual respect among team members, can also increase psychological safety in teams (Carmeli and Gittell 2009). Coordinating behaviors that leaders undertake can have a huge effect on developing the shared sense of psychological safety.

In summary, integrative capabilities are critical to diverse science teams, such as interdisciplinary medical research teams. Setting a common direction is necessary for coordinated team action (Salas et al. 1992). Given the pluralistic goals of team members working on health-related problems that are translational in nature

(Winter and Berente 2012), visioning can help construct a shared understanding of the problem among clinical care providers, outcome and population researchers and basic scientists, who may all have different agendas. . Perspective-seeking, a form of respectful inquiry, from a team leader can make members feel that their inputs are valued, appreciated, and listened to. This sense of inclusion and acceptance can help team members become more open and attentive to the diverse contributions of fellow teammates. Without this engagement in one another's ideas, creative synthesis cannot occur (Harvey 2014; Homan et al. 2007). While working on a joint problem, heterogeneous perspectives and approaches could potentially reduce team cohesion (Antonakis and House 2014). Reconciling these differences through conflict management can help to support creative synthesis (Tjosvold and Ziyou 2007) by keeping members engaged in the integration process. Finally, enabling access to a variety of diverse associates or colleagues through introductions and referrals both within and outside the boundary of the team can help to provide the team with the relevant skills and knowledge they need to be creative (Perry-Smith and Shalley 2003).

24.5 Performance Outcomes

The last part of the theoretical model included in this chapter (see Fig. 24.1) is how integrative leadership behaviors—as well as the cognitive and social emergent states that stem from these behaviors—lead to performance. Performance in interdisciplinary teams can be difficult to gauge, for many reasons. First, many conventional models of team performance rely on input–process–output models of team functioning, which are less useful in knowledge work environments where the work is nonsequential and the products are less tangible (Slyngstad et al. 2017). Second, interdisciplinary teams may have a variety of purposes and tasks, and these teams may experience difficulties in creating a general understanding of what constitutes "good performance" (Slyngstad et al. 2017). Third, while all interdisciplinary teams have certain aspects of task performance in common (e.g., reciprocal task interdependence, shared mental models, and knowledge integration; Balakrishnan et al. 2011), these aspects of performance are difficult to measure. Fourth, when a diversity of disciplines and expertise is involved in creating the final team product, it is difficult to know who is qualified to judge performance.

Several approaches have attempted to create a way to measure team effectiveness in interdisciplinary teams. Given the difficulty of creating a performance metric that fits all teams of this type, Slyngstad et al. (2017) argued for an evaluation of how useful the team is in terms of creating value for the organization (e.g., fiscal return); the intended user of the team's knowledge product (e.g., client, customer, patient); the team itself (e.g., team viability); and the individuals within the team (e.g., gaining new knowledge or skill). Thus, we encourage scholars to use a variety of measurement techniques (e.g., objective, subjective, self-report, other-report) to examine the impact of a leader's integrative capabilities on team processes and outcomes. We also encourage scholars and practitioners to uncover causation by considering each behavior separately, and examining the influence of each behavior on emergent states and knowledge.

24.6   Discussion

This chapter defines distinct leader capabilities that can be developed and enacted by leader(s) in an interdisciplinary team who wish to facilitate the emergent cognitive and social states that have been shown to enhance team knowledge integration and innovative performance. A clear view of what leaders can do to improve team performance in various kinds of interdisciplinary teams has taken shape throughout this chapter, incorporating the complex elements of contemporary knowledge work in teams. Future theory and research can extend this work in developing theory and practice based around what leaders can actively do to improve team performance in interdisciplinary teams.

As has been shown, integrative leadership capabilities (i.e., the extent to which a team leader has the skills to bridge intellectual distance and enable knowledge sharing and integration) lead to desired team emergent states and team effectiveness. The relationship between integrative leadership capabilities and emergent states is dynamic, evolving over time to ultimately improve a team's integrative capacity. We argue that the development and enactment of integrative leadership capabilities are crucial to the performance of interdisciplinary teams, in terms of individual, team, organizational, and other stakeholder outcomes. Any leader can perform the behaviors detailed in this chapter; however, the specific facets of the interdisciplinary team context, such as team composition, the distribution of members, leadership structure, and team size, can be complicated and must be attended to when choosing how and when to try these behaviors. These contextual conditions must be further explored in future theoretical development and empirical research. The effectiveness of leader integrative capabilities may vary depending on the nature of interdisciplinary collaboration. In the following paragraphs, we offer examples of different contextual elements of teams and what behaviors may be more important in different circumstances.

Interdisciplinary teams vary in the configurations in how their work is accomplished (e.g., distributed or partially distributed teams, multiteam systems, multiple institution collaborations). Such configurations can incur increased coordination costs and result in poor team performance if not managed effectively (Cummings and Kiesler 2007; Stokols et al. 2005). One way to enhance coordination is to adopt a shared team-centric leadership structure (Zaccaro et al. 2009). In the team-centric perspective, two or more team members share responsibility for coordination and action. While this often leads to one individual emerging as a leader, it is still regarded as shared leadership, because leadership is not seen as something that is an input, but as something that emerges from the team experiences and processes. In the team-centric perspective, the development of integrative capabilities would be the responsibility of all team members to foster the cognitive and social emergent states that bolster knowledge integration and innovation. This form of leadership is common in virtual teams and multi-team systems, because they often perform better with this type of leadership structure (Millikin et al. 2010; Ocker et al. 2011). In such teams, we believe that all team members, including team leaders will need to possess integrative capabilities to reach high levels of team integrative capacity.

Similarly, the size of the interdisciplinary team determines which of these leader integrative behaviors will be more critical to the team. It is well documented that interdisciplinary teams can range in size from small teams within one location to large teams that work from different sites all over the world (National Research Council 2015). In small, collocated teams, leaders should focus on team building and process improvement; while in large, dispersed teams, leaders are brokers who should focus on coordination and conflict management (Gray 2008). It could be argued in corollary that leaders in small, collocated teams need to perform behaviors such as reflexivity and perspective-seeking to enhance team performance more often than in larger, more dispersed teams; while leaders in large, dispersed teams should attend more to the coordination and conflict management aspects of team work. We conclude with thoughts for future research. First, leadership scholars should expand their conceptualization of leadership to include behaviors of leaders that foster not only knowledge sharing and transfer, but integration as well. In doing so, scholars should not only identify which capabilities are most critical at various phases of a team's life cycle, but also work to uncover additional capabilities that are important across several domains including the military, for-profit sectors, and in academic settings. Additionally, researchers should consider task, team, and organizational influences that could moderate the effect of a leader's integrative capabilities on team performance, such as the degree to which knowledge integration is essential for team performance, the cognitive distance among members in an inter-

disciplinary team, the degree of (im)permanence or extent to which members expect to work with one another, and rewards for collaborating across boundaries. Additionally, we encourage the exploration of leader integrative capabilities using a variety of methodological approaches to capture when and how they are enacted.

References

Amabile TM, Schatzel EA, Moneta GB, Kramer SJ. Leader behaviors and the work environment for creativity: perceived leader support. Leadersh Q. 2004;15(1):5–32. https://doi.org/10.1016/j.leaqua.2003.12.003.

Amason AC, Sapienza HJ. The effects of top management team size and interaction norms on cognitive and affective conflict. J Manag. 1997;1997:495516.

Ancona DG, Caldwell DF. Bridging the boundary: external activity and performance in organizational teams. Adm Sci Q. 1992;37:634–65.

Antonakis J, House RJ. Instrumental leadership: measurement and extension of transformational–transactional leadership theory. Leadersh Q. 2014;25(4):746771.

Ayoko OB, Konrad AM. Leaders' transformational, conflict, and emotion management behaviors in culturally diverse workgroups. Equality Diversity Inclusion. 2012;31:694–724.

Balakrishnan AD, Kiesler S, Cummings J, Zadeh R. Research team integration: what it is and why it matters. In: Proceedings of the ACM Conference on Computer Supported Cooperative Work (CSCW '11). New York, NY: ACM Press; 2011.

Basadur M. Leading others to think innovatively together: creative leadership. Leadersh Q. 2004;15(1):103–21.

Basu R, Green SG. Leader-member exchange and transformational leadership: an empirical examination of innovative behaviors in leader-member dyads. J Appl Soc Psychol. 1997;27(6):477–99.

Börner K, Contractor N, Falk-Krzesinski HJ, Fiore SM, Hall KL, Keyton J, Uzzi B. A multi-level systems perspective for the science of team science. Sci Transl Med. 2010;2(49):49cm24-49cm24.

Cannon-Bowers J, Salas E, Converse S. Shared mental models in expert team decision making. In: Castellan Jr NJ, editor. Individual and group decision making: current issues. Hillsdale, NJ: Erlbaum; 1993. p. 221–46.

Carmeli A, Gittell JH. High-quality relationships, psychological safety, and learning from failures in work organizations. Journal of Organizational Behavior: The International Journal of Industrial, Occupational and Organizational Psychology and Behavior. 2009;30(6):709–29.

Carmeli A, Reiter-Palmon R, Ziv E. Inclusive leadership and employee involvement in creative tasks in the workplace: the mediating role of psychological safety. Creat Res J. 2010;22:250–60.

Carmeli A, Sheaffer Z, Binyamin G, Reiter-Palmon R, Shimoni T. Transformational leadership and creative problem-solving: the mediating role of psychological safety and reflexivity. J Creat Behav. 2014;48:115–35.

Carter SM, West MA. Reflexivity, effectiveness, and mental health in BBC-TV production teams. Small Group Res. 1998;29:583–601.

Clegg C, Unsworth K, Epitropaki O, Parker G. Implicating trust in the innovation process†. J Occup Organ Psychol. 2002;75(4):409–22.

Cronin MA, Weingart LR. Representational gaps, information processing, and conflict in functionally diverse teams. Acad Manag Rev. 2007;32:761–73.

Cronin MA, Bezrukova K, Weingart LR, Tinsley CH. Subgroups within a team: the role of cognitive and affective integration. J Organ Behav. 2011;32:831–49.

Cummings JN, Kiesler S. Coordination costs and project outcomes in multiuniversity collaborations. Res Policy. 2007;36:1620–34.

Curşeu PL, Schruijer SG. Does conflict shatter trust or does trust obliterate conflict? Revisiting the relationships between team diversity, conflict, and trust. Group Dyn Theory Res Pract. 2010;14(1):66.

Davis MH. Empathy: a social psychological approach. Madison, WI: Westview Press; 1996.

Davis JP, Eisenhardt KM. Rotating leadership and collaborative innovation recombination processes in symbiotic relationships. Adm Sci Q. 2011;56(2):159–201.

Dinh JE, Lord RG, Gardner WL, Meuser JD, Liden RC, Hu J. Leadership theory and research in the new millennium: current theoretical trends and changing perspectives. Leadersh Q. 2014;25(1):36–62.

van den Berg W, Curseu PL, Meeus MTH. Emotion regulation and conflict transformation in multi-team systems. Int J Confl Manag. 2014;25:171–88.

Durham CC, Knight D, Locke EA. Effects of leader role, team-set goal difficulty, efficacy, and tactics on team effectiveness. Organ Behav Hum Decis Process. 1997;72:203–31.

Edmondson A. Psychological safety and learning behavior in work teams. Adm Sci Q. 1999;44:350–83.

Falk-Krzesinski HJ, Börner K, Contractor N, Fiore SM, Hall KL, Keyton J, Uzzi B. Advancing the science of team science. Clin Transl Sci. 2010;3(5):263–6.

Faraj S, Sproull L. Coordinating expertise in software development teams. Manag Sci. 2000;46:1554–68.

van Ginkel WP, van Knippenberg D. Group information elaboration and group decision making: the role of shared task representations. Organ Behav Hum Decis Process. 2008;105:82–97.

van Ginkel WP, van Knippenberg D. Group leadership and shared task representations in decision making groups. Leadership Quarterly. 2012;23:94–106.

van Ginkel W, Tindale RS, van Knippenberg D. Team reflexivity, development of shared task representations, and the use of distributed information in group decision making. Group Dyn Theory Res Pract. 2009;13:265–80.

Gockel C, Brauner E. The benefits of stepping into others' shoes: perspective taking strengthens transactive memory. Basic Appl Soc Psychol. 2013;35:222–30.

Grant AM, Berry J. The necessity of others is the mother of invention: intrinsic and prosocial motivations, perspective-taking, and creativity. Acad Manag J. 2011;54:73–96.

Gray B. Enhancing transdisciplinary research through collaborative leadership. Am J Prev Med. 2008;35:S124–32.

Gross N, Kluge A. Predictors of knowledge-sharing behavior for teams in extreme environments: an example from the steel industry. J Cog Eng Decision Making. 2014;8:352–73.

Gurtner A, Tschan F, Semmer NK, Nagele C. Getting groups to develop good strategies: effects of reflexivity interventions on team process, team performance, and shared mental models. Organ Behav Hum Decis Process. 2007;102:127–42.

Hackman JR. From causes to conditions in group research. J Organ Behav. 2012;33:428–44.

Hammond MM, Neff NL, Farr JL, Schwall AR, Zhao X. Predictors of individual-level innovation at work: a meta-analysis. Psychol Aesthet Creat Arts. 2011;5(1):90.

Hargadon AB. Firms as knowledge brokers: lessons in pursuing continuous innovation. Calif Manag Rev. 1998;40(3):209–27.

Hargadon AB, Bechky BA. When collections of creatives become creative collectives: a field study of problem solving at work. Organ Sci. 2006;17(4):484500.

Harrison DA, Price KH, Gavin JH, Florey AT. Time, teams, and task performance: changing effects of surface- and deep-level diversity on group functioning. Acad Manag J. 2002;45:1029–45.

Harvey S. Creative synthesis: exploring the process of extraordinary group creativity. Acad Manag Rev. 2014;39(3):324–43.

Hauschildt J, Kirchmann E. Teamwork for innovation–the 'troika' of promotors. R&D Manag. 2001;31(1):41–9.

Henderson RM, Clark KB. Architectural innovation: the reconfiguration of existing product technologies and the failure of established firms. Adm Sci Q. 1990:9–30.

Hoegl M, Parboteeah KP. Team reflexivity in innovative projects. R&D Manag. 2006;36:113–25.

Hoever IJ, van Knippenberg D, van Ginkel WP, Barkema HG. Fostering team creativity: perspective taking as key to unlocking diversity's potential. J Appl Psychol. 2012;97:982–96.

Hogg MA, van Knippenberg D, Rast DE. Intergroup leadership in organizations: leading across group and organizational boundaries. Acad Manag Rev. 2012;37:232–55.

Homan AC, Van Knippenberg D, Van Kleef GA, De Dreu CK. Bridging faultlines by valuing diversity: diversity beliefs, information elaboration, and performance in diverse work groups. J Appl Psychol. 2007;92(5):1189.

Ilgen DR, Hollenbeck JR, Johnson M, Jundt D. Teams in organizations: from input-process-output models to IMOI models. Annu Rev Psychol. 2005;56:517–43.

Jackson SE. Diversity in the workplace: human resources initiatives. Guilford Press; 1992.

Jehn KA. A multimethod examination of the benefits and detriments of intragroup conflict. Adm Sci Q. 1995;40:256–82.

Jones BF. As science evolves, how can science policy? Innov Policy Econ. 2011;11:103–31.

Kearney E, Gebert D. Managing diversity and enhancing team outcomes: the promise of transformational leadership. J Appl Psychol. 2009;94:77–89.

van Kleef GA, de Dreu CK, Manstead AS. The interpersonal effects of anger and happiness in negotiations. J Pers Soc Psychol. 2004;86:57–76.

Kerr NL, Tindale RS. Group performance and decision making. Annu Rev Psychol. 2004;55(1):623–655.

Klein KJ, Ziegert JC. Toward a science of leader development. In: Day DV, Zaccaro SJ, Halpin SM, editors. Leader development for transforming organizations: growing leaders for tomorrow. New York, NY: Routledge; 2014. p. 359–82.

Klein KJ, Knight AP, Ziegert JC, Lim B, Saltz JL. When team members' values differ: the moderating role of team leadership. Organ Behav Hum Decis Process. 2011;114:25–36.

Kleingeld A, van Mierlo H, Arends L. The effect of goal setting on group performance: a meta-analysis. J Appl Psychol. 2011;9:1289–304.

van Knippenberg D, de Dreu CKW, Homan AC. Work group diversity and group performance: an integrative model and research agenda. J Appl Psychol. 2004;89:1008–22.

Konradt U, Schippers MC, Garbers Y, Steenfatt C. Effects of guided reflexivity and team feedback on team performance improvement: the role of team regulatory processes and cognitive emergent states. Eur J Work Organ Psy. 2015;24:777–95.

Konradt U, Otte K, Schippers MC, Steenfatt C. Reflexivity in teams: a review and new perspectives. J Psychol. 2016;150:153–74.

Kozlowski SWJ, Chao GT. Macrocognition, team learning, and team knowledge: origins, emergence, and measurement. In: Salas E, Fiore SM, Letsky MP, editors. Theories of team cognition: cross-disciplinary perspectives. New York, NY: Routledge; 2012. p. 19–48.

Kozlowski SW, Ilgen DR. Enhancing the effectiveness of work groups and teams [monograph]. Psychol Sci Public Interest. 2006;7:77–124.

Langfred CW. The downside of self-management: a longitudinal study of the effects of conflict on trust, autonomy, and task interdependence in self-managing teams. Acad Manag J. 2007;50:885–900.

Lee P, Gillespie N, Mann L, Wearing A. Leadership and trust: their effect on knowledge sharing and team performance. Manag Learn. 2010;41:473–91.

Lewis K, Belliveau M, Herndon B, Keller J. Group cognition, membership change, and performance: investigating the benefits and detriments of collective knowledge. Organ Behav Hum Decis Process. 2007;103:159–78.

Lovelace K, Shapiro DL, Weingart LR. Maximizing cross-functional new product teams' innovativeness and constraint adherence: a conflict communications perspective. Acad Manag J. 2001;44:779–93.

Lyubovnika J, Legood A, Turner N, Mamakouka A. How authentic leadership influences team performance: the mediating role of team reflexivity. J Bus Ethics. in press.

Mainemelis C, Kark R, Epitropaki O. Creative leadership: a multi-context conceptualization. Acad Manag Ann. 2015;9(1):393–482.

Mannix EA, Neale MA, Goncalo JA, editors. Creativity in groups. Bingley, England: Emerald Group; 2009.

Marks MA, Mathieu JE, Zaccaro SJ. A temporally based framework and taxonomy of team processes. Acad Manag Rev. 2001;26:356–76.

Meng J, Fulk J, Yuan YC. The roles and interplay of intragroup conflict and team emotion management on information seeking behaviors in team contexts. Commun Res. 2015;42:675–700.

Miller CC, Burke LM, Glick WH. Cognitive diversity among upper-echelon executives: implications for strategic decision processes. Strateg Manag J. 1998;19:39–58.

Millikin JP, Hom PW, Manz CC. Self-management competencies in selfmanaging teams: their impact on multi-team system productivity. Leadership Quarterly. 2010;21:687–702.

Moreland R. Transactive memory and job performance: helping workers learn who knows what. In: Thompson LL, Levine JM, Messick DM, editors. Shared cognition in organizations: the management of knowledge. New York, NY: Psychology Press; 1999. p. 3–32.

Moreland RL, Thompson L. Transactive memory: learning who knows what in work groups and organizations. In: Levine JM, Moreland RL, editors. Small groups: key readings. New York, NY: Psychology Press; 2006. p. 327–46.

Morgeson FP, DeRue DS, Karam EP. Leadership in teams: a functional approach to understanding leadership structures and processes. J Manag. 2010;36:5–39.

Mumford MD. Where have we been, where are we going? Taking stock in creativity research. Creat Res J. 2003;15(2–3):107–20.

Mumford MD, Scott GM, Gaddis B, Strange JM. Leading creative people: orchestrating expertise and relationships. Leadersh Q. 2002;13(6):705–50.

National Research Council. Enhancing the Effectiveness of Team Science. Washington. DC; The National Academies Press. 2015. https://doi.org/10.17226/19007.

Nembhard IM, Edmondson AC. Making it safe: the effects of leader inclusiveness and professional status on psychological safety and improvement efforts in health care teams. J Organ Behav. 2006;27:941–66.

Nishii LH, Mayer DM. Do inclusive leaders help to reduce turnover in diverse groups? The moderating role of leader–member exchange in the diversity to turnover relationship. J Appl Psychol. 2009;94(6):1412.

Ocker RJ, Huang H, Benbunan-Fich R, Hiltz SR. Leadership dynamics in partially distributed teams: an exploratory study of the effects of configuration and distance. Group Decis Negot. 2011;20:273–92.

Okhuysen GA, Eisenhardt KM. Integrating knowledge in groups: how formal interventions enable flexibility. Organ Sci. 2002;13:370–86.

Paulus PB, Coskun H. Creative collaboration, group creativity, and team innovation. In: Levine J, editor. Group processes. Amsterdam: Elsevier; 2012. p. 215–39.

Paulus PB, Nijstad BA. Group creativity: an introduction. In: Paulus PB, Nijstad BA, editors. Group creativity: innovation through collaboration. New York, NY: Oxford University Press; 2003. p. 3–11.

Perry-Smith JE, Shalley CE. The social side of creativity: a static and dynamic social network perspective. Acad Manag Rev. 2003;28(1):89–106.

Perry-Smith JE. Social yet creative: the role of social relationships in facilitating individual creativity. Acad Manag J. 2006;49:85–101.

Piccolo RF, Colquitt JA. Transformational leadership and job behaviors: the mediating role of core job characteristics. Acad Manag J. 2006;49(2):327340.

Saporito B. The conspiracy to end cancer: a team-based, cross-disciplinary approach to cancer research is upending tradition and delivering results faster. Time Magazine. 2013, April;1.

Salas, E., Dickinson, T. L., Converse, S. A., & Tannenbaum, S. I. (1992). Toward an understanding of team performance and training.

Salazar MR, Lant TK, Fiore SM, Salas E. Facilitating innovation in diverse science teams through integrative capacity. Small Group Res. 2012;43:527–58.

Schippers MC, den Hartog DN, Koopman PL, van Knippenberg D. The role of transformational leadership in enhancing team reflexivity. Hum Relat. 2008;61:1593–616.

Schippers MC, West MA, Dawson JF. Team reflexivity and innovation: the moderating role of team context. J Manag. 2015;41:769–88.

Schulz-Hardt S, Brodbeck FC, Mojzisch A, Kerschreiter R, Frey D. Group decision making in hidden profile situations: dissent as a facilitator for decision quality. J Pers Soc Psychol. 2006;91:1080–93.

Scott SG, Bruce RA. Determinants of innovative behavior: a path model of individual innovation in the workplace. Acad Manag J. 1994;37(3):580607.

Shin SJ, Zhou J. Transformational leadership, conservation, and creativity: evidence from Korea. Acad Manag J. 2003;46(6):703–14.

Shin SJ, Zhou J. When is educational specialization heterogeneity related to creativity in research and development teams? Transformational leadership as a moderator. J Appl Psychol. 2007;92(6):1709.

Simons TL, Peterson RS. Task conflict and relationship conflict in top management teams: the pivotal role of intragroup trust. J Appl Psychol. 2000;85:102–11.

Slyngstad DJ, DeMichele G, Salazar MR. Team performance in knowledge work. The Wiley Blackwell handbook of the psychology of team working and collaborative processes; 2017. p. 43–71.Smith KG,

Collins CJ, Clark KD. Existing knowledge, knowledge creation capability, and the rate of new product introduction in high-technology firms. Acad Manag J. 2005;48:346–57.

Stasser G. Information salience and the discovery of hidden profiles by decision-making groups: a "thought experiment.". Organ Behav Hum Decis Process. 1992;52:156–81.

Stasser G, Stewart DD, Wittenbaum GM. Expert roles and information exchange during discussion: the importance of knowing who knows what. J Exp Soc Psychol. 1995;31:244–65.

Stokols D, Harvey R, Gress J, Fuqua J, Phillips K. In vivo studies of transdisciplinary scientific collaboration: lessons learned and implications for active living research. Am J Prev Med. 2005;28:202–13.

Taylor A, Greve HR. Superman or the fantastic four? Knowledge combination and experience in innovative teams. Acad Manag J. 2006;49(4):723–40.

Tekleab AG, Quigley NR, Tesluk PE. A longitudinal study of team conflict, conflict management, cohesion, and team effectiveness. Group Org Manag. 2009;34:170–205.

Tierney P. LMX and creativity. The Oxford Handbook of Leader-Member Exchange 2015 175.

Tjosvold D, Hui C, Yu Z. Conflict management and task reflexivity for team in role and extra-role performance in China. Int J Confl Manag. 2003;14:141–63.

Tjosvold D, Tang MML, West M. Reflexivity for team innovation in China: the contribution of goal interdependence. Group Org Manag. 2004;29:540–59.

Tjosvold D, Yu Z. Group risk taking: the constructive role of controversy in China. Group Org Manag. 2007;32(6):653–74.

Van Knippenberg D, Sitkin SB. A critical assessment of charismatic— transformational leadership research: Back to the drawing board? Acad Manag Ann. 2013;7(1):1–60.

Von Glinow M, Shapiro DL, Brett JM. Can we talk, and should we? Managing emotional conflict in multicultural teams. Acad Manag Rev. 2004;29:578–92.

Weingart LR, Weldon E. Processes that mediate the relationship between a group goal and group member performance. Hum Perform. 1991;4(10):33–54.

Weldon E, Yun S. The effects of proximal and distal goals on goal level, strategy development, and group performance. J Appl Behav Sci. 2000;36:336–44.

West MA. Reflexivity and work group effectiveness: a conceptual integration. In: West MA, editor. Handbook of work group psychology. New York, NY: Wiley; 1996. p. 555–79.

Widmer PS, Schippers MC, West MA. Recent developments in reflexivity research: a review. Psychol Everyday Activity. 2009;2:2–11.

Williams HM, Parker SK, Turner NIH. Perceived dissimilarity and perspective taking within work teams. Group Org Manag. 2007;32:569–97.

Williams KY, O'Reilly CA III. Demography and diversity in organizations. Res Organ Behav. 1998;20:77–140.

Winter SJ, Berente N. A commentary on the pluralistic goals, logics of action, and institutional contexts of translational team science. Transl Behav Med. 2012;2(4):441–5.

Woolley AW, Gerbasi ME, Chabris CF, Kosslyn SM, Hackman JR. Bringing in the experts: how team composition and collaborative planning jointly shape analytic effectiveness. Small Group Res. 2008;39:352–71.

Wu D, Liao Z, Dai J. Knowledge heterogeneity and team knowledge sharing as moderated by internal social capital. Soc Behav Pers. 2015;43:423–36.

Wuchty S, Jones BF, Uzzi B. The increasing dominance of teams in production of knowledge. Science. 2007;316(5827):1036–8.

Zaccaro SJ, Rittman AL, Marks MA. Team leadership. Leadership Quarterly. 2001;12:451–83.

Zaccaro SJ, Heinen B, Shuffler M. Team leadership and team effectiveness. In: Salas E, Goodwin GF, Burke CS, editors. Team effectiveness in complex organizations: cross-disciplinary perspectives and approaches. New York, NY: Taylor & Francis; 2009. p. 83–111.

Zerhouni E. Medicine: the NIH roadmap. Science. 2003;302(5642):63–72.

Zhang Y, Fang Y, Wei K, Chen H. Exploring the role of psychological safety in promoting the intention to continue sharing knowledge in virtual communities. Int J Manag. 2010;30:325–436.

Zhang X, Cao Q, Tjosvold D. Linking transformational leadership and team performance: a conflict management approach. J Manag Stud. 2011;48:1586–611.

Organizational Perspective on Leadership Strategies for the Success of Cross-Disciplinary Science Teams

25

Susan Winter

Contents

25.1 Introduction

Traditional views hold that research is performed by individual scientists; recent work has raised awareness of the importance of science performed in teams of up to nine members (National Research Council 2015). Both solitary researchers and science teams can be found in universities, corporate settings, and federal agencies and labs. Increasingly team members are drawn from across organizational boundaries and may be organized as larger formal and enduring organizations such as centers, institutes, or consortia with designated directors, specified membership and roles, and written policies and procedures

S. Winter (✉)
College of Information Studies,
University of Maryland, College Park, MD, USA
e-mail: sjwinter@umd.edu

(Bolukbasi et al. 2013; Winter et al. 2014). This trend reflects the growing focus on addressing complex intellectual challenges and solving significant societal problems—pursuits that are difficult for individual scientists or short-lived informal science teams to engage.

Teams, centers, institutes, or consortia are science organizations that are subject to many (though not all) of the same dynamics as other organizations, suggesting that insights drawn from extensive research in organizational studies can be beneficial to the field of Team Science. Many date the formal study of organizations to the work of Frederick Taylor on scientific management (Taylor 1910), which inspired generations of researchers to identify principles and techniques to optimize internal efficiency and effectiveness through components such as leadership, job design, incentives, and communication. Later theorists were inspired by developments in the open systems movement that focused on organisms embedded in and open to the influences of their environments. Organizational theorists adapted this view to emphasize the interdependence of organizational units and their environment (Thompson 1967) and developed methods and techniques to assist in the analysis and management of these complex relationships (Pfeffer and Salancik 1978). This chapter follows in the tradition of these open system organizational theorists to highlight the importance of the context within which research is carried out, be it by individuals, science teams, centers, institutes, or consortia.

The open systems view considers the relationship between an organization and its context or environment to be of paramount importance because the environment provides the resources that are needed for organizational survival including both tangible resources such as funding, space, personnel, and equipment and intangible resources such as good will and legitimacy (Pfeffer and Salancik 1978). In return, organizations provide valuable outputs. In science organizations, these are often publications, patents, and trained graduates. Although the traditional view of research has focused on the individual researcher, the role of their environment is widely acknowledged: scientists are successful partly because of the support provided by the organizations that they are embedded in. In the United States, the typical university was created to advance knowledge and provide instruction in a variety of academic disciplines. It is divided into colleges, and subdivided into departments reflecting academic disciplines, because this structure allows individual researchers to be successful. Universities have developed complex policies, practices, structures, and cultures that reflect and support their research mission (Cutcher-Gershenfeld et al. 2016; Winter 2012), but this institutional context can be a hindrance to large-scale, coordinated, and cross-disciplinary research.

Cross-disciplinary research is becoming increasingly important as science is asked to address complex intellectual challenges and significant societal problems that seldom fall neatly into a single academic discipline or department and may require sustained efforts with little immediate economic payoff. Corporations find it difficult to address these challenges and societal problems due to the market forces that keep them focused on short-term profits, not basic research or breakthroughs that cannot be easily monetized. Federal agencies and labs were designed with particular missions in mind so have difficulty quickly addressing emerging issues that may not fit squarely within their mission. Engaging complex intellectual challenges and solving significant societal problems requires building a body of cross-disciplinary scholarship, developing innovative products, processes, or services, delivering these innovations, and changing user behavior (Winter and Butler 2011). Cross-disciplinary teams and institutions such as centers, institutes, and consortia are often created to coordinate efforts and share resources across disciplinary, organizational, state, national, and sector boundaries, but they can be facilitated or hindered by the system of rules, policies, regulations, and practices of their environments—their "institutional context." Some of these cross-disciplinary science teams and organizations survive for decades and are very successful (e.g., CERN), but many last only a few short years and never meet their full potential (Bolukbasi et al. 2014).

In many ways, this is not surprising. Cross-disciplinary teams and organizations share many characteristics with other new ventures that have been studied extensively. Research has found that 50% of new businesses fail within 5 years (Bureau of Labor Statistics 2017)—a phenomenon that has been termed the liability of newness and smallness. We see similarly daunting odds for new ventures that are not specifically focused on profits and are more reliant on volunteer efforts such as online communities like Wikipedia, and citizen science collaborations like NanoHub (Freeman et al. 1983; Gaglio et al. 1998; Olson et al. 2008). Like science teams, new ventures have little control over their institutional contexts, which can be supportive or extremely challenging. We know a lot about what new ventures can do to succeed; this knowledge can be applied to cross-disciplinary science teams and organizations. This chapter presents three robust strategic planning frameworks from the organizational science domain that research leaders can use proactively to improve the success of their boundary-spanning and cross-disciplinary science teams.

25.2 Cross-Disciplinary Science Teams as New and Small Organizations

New organizations face significant challenges including attracting resources, initiating operations, and becoming sustainable. Many universities have created incubators to provide help in meeting these challenges for new businesses, but do not provide equivalent support for interdisciplinary scientific teams and organizations. New business incubators provide a variety of tangible and intangible resources such as seed funding, space, and the legitimacy of being associated with an incubator. Legitimacy—the perception that an organization is pursuing acceptable goals through appropriate means (Suchman 1995)— plays a central role in attracting resources (Starr and MacMillan 1990). More importantly, new venture incubators provide access to managerial and entrepreneurial expertise that helps teach new venture founders how to succeed. This expertise spans topics such as strategic planning, accounting, budgets and finance, operations management, human resource management, and marketing.

Similar to new venture incubators, many cross-disciplinary science teams and organizations at universities are also provided space, seed funding, and legitimacy, all of which can help them in attracting additional resources (Starr and MacMillan 1990). Associating with a respected university may enable cross-disciplinary science teams to gain legitimacy by emphasizing consistency with university goals (advancing knowledge or providing instruction) and means (scientific research, classroom, or online instruction). However, unlike typical new venture incubators, science team leaders are seldom provided access to expertise or training in how to create and manage a successful organization.

Like other organizations, cross-disciplinary science teams also need to attract or gain control over resources in their environments such as space, facilities, equipment, raw materials, and data or financial capital that can be used to purchase these resources (Zimmerman and Zeitz 2002). Space and financial resources for scien-

tific teams, centers, institutes, and consortia are often highly constrained in university settings. Most new businesses are funded through personal debt (founders' credit cards and loans from family and friends), avenues not often available to leaders of cross-disciplinary science teams. Successful leaders may be able to secure additional sources of capital (e.g., research grants, contracts, donations of cash or in kind), but the timing of these resource infusions is critical. Delays in funding can result in the loss of valued personnel when funding runs out followed by a hiring scramble when new funding is secured.

Attracting human capital can also be more complex for science organizations than it is for most new ventures due to the unique mix of paid staff, soft money positions, and volunteers. The success of many university-based cross-disciplinary science teams relies upon volatile soft money positions together with voluntary participation of faculty members and graduate students. Voluntary participation can be particularly difficult to achieve and maintain with over-committed faculty and students whose primary obligations and incentives are only loosely related to their engagement with the science organization. Many universities do not provide incentives to work across boundaries, and cross-disciplinary work, science organization administration, and collaborative science may not be recognized in hiring, promotion, and tenure policies.

In addition to attracting resources, new organizations face challenges in initiating their operations. Processes must be created, job descriptions written, personnel hired, facilities leased, equipment purchased, and products or services created and delivered. Although it sounds obvious, successful organizations need to proactively identify and then manage the products or services that they provide. For many new ventures, the nature of their products and services are relatively straightforward: restaurants serve food. For other new ventures, there is considerable ambiguity: whether Uber provides transportation services or just information exchange is still being contested. For science teams, the products and services are often less obvious but can include disseminating knowledge through white papers, social media posts, publication, patents, and educational programs, importing knowledge through guest speakers, journal clubs, and organized symposia or seminars, or maintaining collaborative writing groups, supplying mentoring, or providing data analytic services or data products, etc. Successful science organizations proactively manage the set of products and services that they provide.

Once the suite of products and services has been identified, processes and structures must be put in place to create and deliver them. Many of the processes that must be created are constrained by, often very complex and conflicting, laws or policies. For example, an urgent hire may be delayed for months because of centralized approval of all job descriptions, minimum job posting times, rules against jobs being split across organizational units, or the negotiation of complex financial agreements between colleges. Similarly, a promising line of research may be impossible to pursue because the institution does not have the ability to handle HIPPA-compliant data. The team may not be able to purchase necessary equipment because procurement has not qualified the vendor, it is not an allowable expense, or a member of the team has a financial conflict of interest with the vendor. Cross-disciplinary science teams need to determine which rules apply and how best to get things done. Science teams that cross organizational boundaries (multi-departmental, multi-college, multi-university, multi-national) will often have to reconcile incompatible rules and processes, which may require complex memos of understanding (MOUs) and legally binding agreements about issues such as division of intellectual property rights, data sharing, export restrictions, joint human subjects reviews, restricted research, and conflicts of interest or commitment (Lutters and Winter 2011).

In addition to these more tactical challenges faced by science teams and organizations, their long-term success and sustainability can be enhanced through robust strategic planning, a topic of long-standing interest in business and entrepreneurship. A number of strategic planning frameworks have been developed to understand why some organizations succeed while others fail and to guide leaders in their strategic planning efforts and enhance the likelihood of their success.

25.3 Strategic Planning Frameworks for Science Leaders

Three frameworks are widely used to help organizations become sustainable: (1) assessing and influencing the environment they are operating in; (2) managing their stakeholders and developing their communication strategy; and (3) fulfilling their value propositions. All three of these frameworks can help leaders of cross-disciplinary science teams achieve sustained success.

25.3.1 Strategy 1: Assessing the Environment for Cross-Disciplinary Science Teams

Organizational science has long recognized that success and longevity is easier in some environments than in others and that effective leaders take actions to improve their environment (Porter 2008; Thompson 1967). Building on Porter's work, we can develop a framework for assessing a science team or organization's environment and identifying components that leaders can influence to make it more likely that the team or organization will survive and thrive. In this framework, it is important to consider all of the relevant stakeholders—the individuals, groups, organizations, or institutions that care about your team's activities and whether or not you succeed. Porter identified the importance of existing competitors, potential customers, potential suppliers, possible substitutes for your product or service, and potential new entrants (Porter 2008). Science leaders should identify analogous stakeholders in their environment and also consider funders and regulators.

Competitors: Initially, it might seem easy to identify existing competitors and determine how fierce the competition is among them, but this is often a very difficult task because it requires an organization to determine what its product or service really is (a topic that we will return to when we talk about building a value proposition). At a minimum, leaders of cross-disciplinary science teams should be aware of other similar teams and how their efforts compare. Are they complementary, competing, or irrelevant? If they are complementary, can you form a partnership that strengthens both of your efforts? If they are competing, how will you differentiate your efforts (more focused on basic research, tailored for a particular use like education or economic development, more policy-oriented, more focused on transition to practice or commercializable products, etc.)? If they are irrelevant, how will you monitor their efforts and influence them to make sure that they do not become competitors? If there are lots of existing competitors in a space and the competition among them is intense, it is less likely that a new science team in this area will be successful.

Customers: Porter (2008) considered the environment to be positive, and, consequently, a new science team is more likely to succeed if there are lots of potential customers who want the things that the team can provide and these customers act independently so they cannot organize to make demands that would be difficult to meet. This means that successful cross-disciplinary science teams must determine who would want the things that they can provide (their potential customers) and whether there are multiple kinds of customers.

Tangible products or services of interest to potential customers could include a center's research publications, colloquium or speaker series, white papers, patents or other intellectual property, contract research services, or educational offerings such as seminars, workshops, and certificates. Intangible benefits of interest to participating members of the research team or center could include mentoring, a sense of community, visibility, intellectual engagement, insights, and motivation. Customers can be funding agencies, graduate students, other researchers, policymakers, companies hoping to buy or license

intellectual property for commercial development, or students hoping to learn specialized skills and their potential employers.

Customers themselves are often not sure what their needs are so a team must first figure out their potential customers' needs (which may be an iterative process) and how to meet them. Many entrepreneurship programs are embracing a "lean start-up" form of new venture creation that rapidly moves between identifying unmet needs, developing products or services that meet those needs, and then seeking feedback on how well the products or services have met those needs (Wilson 2011). Although this iterative process of prototyping and testing various products and services with potential customers may get a new science team started, sustained success often depends upon the team building on what it offers that is unique and difficult to duplicate (Barney et al. 2001). For example, many competitors can produce white papers or publications, but a successful science team will have valued insights that others do not have and cannot easily develop. If these insights are fairly straightforward and are drawn from publicly available data, other teams may be able to provide them faster or more easily. If these insights are unique to the members of the team or to the resources available at a particular university, or stem from a trusted relationship with a funding source or exclusive support from an industry partner, it will be difficult for other teams to duplicate them. Successful sustainable science teams may need to attract and retain key people, affiliate with a particularly prestigious university, build strong ties to funding sources, or develop exclusive industry partnerships.

Resource Suppliers: Just like for customers, Porter (2008) considered the environment to be positive and a new science team is more likely to succeed if there are lots of potential suppliers for each of the needed resources and they act independently so they cannot organize to raise prices or make demands that would be difficult to meet. Potential suppliers for cross-disciplinary science teams can include a variety of providers for resources. For most teams, skilled personnel will be the most important resource. However, some teams may rely on access to scarce or expensive equipment such as the Large Hadron Collider or on computational resources such as valuable datasets and high performance computing services. Even suppliers of more mundane services such as payroll processing are important, but, since many of these services are supplied within the employing institution such as the university, they are not of direct concern to science team leaders. If there is a single source for a critical resource, leaders of cross-disciplinary science institutions should consider taking steps to ensure a continuous supply of that resource by, for example, entering into long-term contracts or including the provider as part of the institution through an MOU, consortium agreement, or some other form of contract.

Substitutes: Porter (2008) also suggests that cross-disciplinary science teams should consider possible substitutes for their products or services. Just as Uber is a viable substitute for car ownership in many large U.S. cities, a science team's potential customers could get their needs met through other means. Readers can easily learn about a topic from Wikipedia instead of from your white papers or publications, so it is important to think about what you can provide that does not duplicate what is in Wikipedia. Maybe a YouTube presentation can present material in a better format or make more complex material more easily understood. Of course, this may not be consistent with the tenure requirements in place at the university and may require advanced marketing skills that would have to be acquired, so science team leaders need to balance these conflicting needs and develop policies that enable the success of both the team and its individual members. Science teams should think about questions like why companies would license intellectual property from you when they can develop their own. Can students gain valuable skills through online videos or a massively open online course (MOOC) instead of relying on your courses, seminars, workshops, or similar offerings?

New cross-disciplinary science teams should also be aware of whether they are a substitute for an existing organization's products or services. New substitutes often disrupt markets and may drive existing organizations out of business or firms that produce the substitute may be acquired to remove the threat. For example, Wikipedia has disrupted the market for printed encyclopedias; flexible, extensible cloud-based data storage and open source statistical software such as R are disrupting university data centers and the market for traditional statistical software such as IBM's SPSS. A science team that creates a new method for handling clinical samples may be a threat to existing services. If a team does pose a threat to a powerful existing group, it should develop strategies to manage this concern.

New Entrants: New cross-disciplinary science teams may not provide a substitute for an existing product or service, but simply be a new entrant into an existing research environment. Porter (2008) suggests that they should consider the likelihood that other new entrants may be emerging who can become competitors for both customers and resources. Although potential new entrants are always a concern, they may be particularly likely when a cross-disciplinary science team focuses on a trendy topic such as big data, personalized medicine, or cybersecurity. New entrants can benefit from the knowledge gained by existing teams and capitalize on that knowledge to avoid the mistakes that were made by first movers, called the second mover advantage (Birger 2006; Epstein 2006). In many fields there are considerable barriers to entry such as expensive facilities or scarce resources such as proprietary data. Teams that can overcome the high barriers that dissuade potential new entrants are more likely to be successful.

Funders: Cross-disciplinary science teams must also consider funding streams. These may be sources of start-up capital such as internal seed grants, competitive research grants, and donations. Some of the sources of start-up capital that are available in the economy but are often not available to new science teams within universities are crowdfunding (the equivalent of angel investors in the entrepreneurship world), banks, and venture capital. These sources can be tapped if the science team pursues commercialization of their innovations, but they require the creation of a legal entity that is separate from the university and considerable entrepreneurial and managerial activity that is not directly linked to supporting the research team itself.

Successful science teams must also develop sustainable funding streams that provide a recurring infusion of funds. Many cross-disciplinary teams rely on a single funding stream leaving them vulnerable to disruptions. A team that has been very successful in receiving funding from a single federal agency program may find its future jeopardized if that program is discontinued. Diversifying across funding sources helps buffer the effects of changes in any single source. Teams could pursue additional revenue-generating arrangements such as technology licensing agreements, industry partnerships, successful grant proposals to a broader array of funders, or user fees.

Although science team leaders seldom think about the legal form of their team, each team is bound by a set of legal constraints. Team leaders should be aware of the different legal forms that are available since they have implications for how their funds can be held, distributed, and taxed. For example, many teams are legally located within a university, which allows the university to handle the funds, create accounts, and designate signing authority. The university handles tax issues, payroll, benefits, and so on, and recoups some of these expenses through overhead. Many funders such as the National Science Foundation (NSF) do not make awards to individual researchers but to their employing organization so a scientist at a university may have no actual legal claim to the funds. The university has designated the scientist as the investigator responsible for carrying out the work, but is well within its legal rights to designate a different investigator (with NSF's approval). Some funders hold the entire PI and co-PI team responsible for late or missing reports. If a science team member changes employment, he or she will have changed their legal status and may become ineligible to receive funds from the grant, access the data that have already been collected, or use research equipment purchased through the grant.

In addition, the relative permeability of work units such as departments and centers may vary, so crossing a university's boundaries may be more difficult in some situations than others. Large, international collaborations may require complex interorganizational contracts, nondisclosure agreements, MOUs, and export control measures. Instead of relying on the university as the home institution, long-lived cross-disciplinary science teams may also use the 501(c)3 organizational form that is available for not-for-profit scientific and educational organizations and formally designate their own officers with authority to receive and disburse funds and to store, curate, and archive research data.

Regulators are more of a concern for some cross-disciplinary science teams than others, but none is entirely unregulated. Those housed within universities take advantage of existing systems to comply with, for example, IRS regulations through proper accounting practices, Institutional Review Board (IRB) policies for proper treatment of human subjects, and Occupational Safety and Health Administration (OSHA) requirements for workplace and lab safety. Funding agencies, accreditors, and licensing organizations may also act as regulators. Cross-disciplinary science teams that are aware of regulators' concerns and work proactively to address them are more likely to be successful.

In sum, there are many ways in which a cross-disciplinary science team's institutional environment can help or hinder its development and survival. Some of these are difficult for a team to influence, but other aspects of the team's situation can be engaged to improve the probability of success. Organization science provides a robust strategic planning framework that can be used by team leaders to better understand and manage their team's situation (Porter 2008).

As this section has shown, Porter's framework considers the organization an open system and can be used to assess the environment for cross-disciplinary science teams. Science leaders can consider the relevant stakeholders in the environment: existing competitors such as similar science teams, potential customers including individuals or organizations that would want the insights, products (e.g., papers, patents, presentations), services (e.g., analysis, recommendations, training) that the science team provides, potential suppliers of needed resources such as skilled personnel or valuable datasets, possible substitutes for a team's products or services, potential new entrants, diverse funding streams (investors), and regulators. Each of these will affect the team's situation within its institutional context and can affect its success. Analyzing the team's environment is the first step toward enabling science leaders to take positive action to improve their likelihood of success and longevity.

25.3.2 Strategy 2: Stakeholder Management

Stakeholder management is a second organizational science framework that provides additional detailed guidance to science team leaders so that they can improve their environment (Donaldson and Preston 1995; Freeman 1984). As with Porter's Environmental Forces framework (2008), stakeholder management grew out of the realization that organizations are open systems so are dependent upon their environment, and that one of the most important functions of a leader is to manage the various stakeholder entities (individuals, organizations, and interest groups) in their environment that control the organization through the exchange of resources (Pfeffer and Salancik 1978). As open systems that are dependent on their environment and are influenced by various stakeholder groups, science team leaders need to identify and manage their stakeholders.

Springman (2011) summarizes best practices in stakeholder management and lays out a set of steps to be taken. First, identify stakeholder groups, and for each identified stakeholder group, develop a value proposition and determine what you want from them in return. Then identify any capabilities that will need to be developed to provide what stakeholder groups want and prioritize them based on the importance of the stakeholder groups whose demands they address. Finally, organizations should track how well they are providing value for their stakeholders.

These steps apply equally well to science teams. Stakeholders should be identified and

their levels of power and interest should be determined. The science team should develop value propositions for each of their stakeholders and what they want from these stakeholders in return. Finally, science teams should create a strategy for stakeholder communications and relationship management. Science teams need to decide how much attention to pay to each of their stakeholder groups and create communication plans that assign communication responsibilities to team members and specifies communication frequency, media, and goals. This plan should include metrics that track how well the team is providing value for its stakeholders.

25.3.2.1 Identifying Stakeholders
Porter's 2008 framework provides categories science team leaders should consider when identifying any relevant stakeholders (including competitors, customers, suppliers, substitutes, potential new entrants, funders, and regulators. Of course, the detailed list of specific stakeholders will be closely tied to the nature of the science team and its activities. Stakeholders that play multiple roles should be considered stakeholders in multiple categories. For example, a faculty member may both disseminate information by writing papers and consume information by reading papers written by other team members. Science teams doing similar or complementary work are significant stakeholders and can be competitors, customers, or partners depending on the details. Customers can also include companies that collaborate with the science team on research projects and those same companies may be potential employers of students who have been trained by the science team.

Other customers may be faculty and student participants, journal publishers, and university administration that benefit from publication and intellectual property (IP) streams. State and federal governments can be important stakeholders when research teams are located in state universities and for intramural researchers in federal or state agencies.

Resource suppliers can include faculty and student participants who provide the knowledge, skills, abilities, and time that make a team successful. Data resources, equipment, and technical support may be provided by IT services or by partners at other institutions. Department chairs, deans, and provosts may provide valuable space and access to crucial administrative expertise for tasks such as preparing grant proposals, processing expenses, handling payroll, and personnel issues.

Science team leaders should also identify new teams that may emerge and could compete for customers and resources. The likelihood of such new entrants will vary. It is easier to assemble a small team of researchers to complete a single project than it is to create a large sustainable center, institute, or consortium. Teams working on currently popular topics will more likely see many more new entrants than those working on areas that are not receiving as much attention. Some activities will require expensive and scarce resources making new entrants less likely, but this can change if costs fall and access increases. Team leaders should consider these factors in identifying potential new entrants. Funders and regulators will also vary depending on the particulars of the research collaboration.

25.3.2.2 Stakeholder Analysis

Mendelow (1991) developed the stakeholder power grid to help leaders visualize the importance of various stakeholder groups. Stakeholders differ in how much they are interested in the science collaboration and in how much power or influence they have with the team (Mitchell et al. 1997). Figure 25.1 provides an overview of the stakeholder power grid. Once research team leaders have identified the relevant stakeholders, each should be assigned to a quadrant of the stakeholder power grid. It is worth revisiting this categorization periodically since a stakeholder group's interests may change.

Stakeholders with low levels of power can be divided into "apathetics" and "defenders" or fans. Apathetic stakeholders with low levels of interest and power such as students unaffiliated with the science team or its topic require (and often prefer) minimal effort. The majority of stu-

dents at a university (those not interested in the topic or involved in the science team's work) will likely fall into this category. They do not need to be actively managed, but should be monitored to make sure that they do not move into one or another category (e.g., developing concerns about the team's ethics or excitement about a new breakthrough).

Defenders or Fans have a high level of interest, but very little power or influence over the science team. They are likely to act as champions and tout the value of the science team and its work. Alumni who worked with the team before graduation may be defenders.

Stakeholders with moderate power and influence will vary in their level of interest. If they are interested, they could make things more or less difficult for the science team. For example, department faculty who are not part of the science team could devalue collaborative research at tenure time, argue to the Department Chair that their space needs outweigh yours, and refuse to serve on your students' dissertation committees or serve and require unnecessary changes that delay your students' time to completion. Because they can affect the collaboration's success and even its survival, stakeholders with moderate levels of power and interest should be actively monitored and steps should be taken to maintain their support.

Stakeholders with high levels of power can be divided into "latents" and "promoters" or key players. Latents are stakeholders who have considerable power and influence over the science collaboration, but relatively little interest. For example, university space allocation and facilities administrators are unlikely to be particularly interested in the science team's success (insights, papers, patents), but may have the power to take away lab and work space. Similarly, often at state universities the state owns the equipment being used by a science team and the land where the lab space is located. Regents and State Legislators can wield enormous power. This means that state officials could make these essential resources unavailable. They usually have relatively little interest in the team and are unlikely to exercise this power. However, these latents should be kept

Fig. 25.1 Stakeholder
power grid

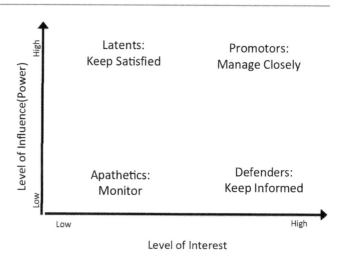

satisfied and it is worth monitoring these stakeholders' levels of interest so that additional steps
can be taken if necessary.

Promoters are key players with considerable
power and influence over the science team and
high interest in it. A major funder may have a
high level of interest and a high level of influence, so is a key player who should be managed
closely.

Promoters and Defenders should be actively
and frequently engaged. Finding roles for them
among the team's leadership, for example, in an
advisory capacity, is an excellent way to ensure
that they are properly included.

25.3.2.3 Developing a Communication Strategy

Successful stakeholder management requires a
communication strategy (Mendelow 1991).
However, many science teams do not systematically consider stakeholder management or
develop a communication strategy. They are
more likely to decide that they need to have a
website than to systematically consider the audience for that website and the messages that they
want to convey (Lutters and Winter 2011). This
focus on the communication medium rather than
the audience or the message can represent a
missed opportunity to influence the institutional
environment and may jeopardize the success of
the team.

Science teams should determine what information each stakeholder or audience would be
interested in hearing. Audiences can be external
or internal and can include the public, politicians,
university administration, customers, staff,
funders, and regulators. For example, a team's
customers would want to hear about the products
or services that are available and the value that
they provide (the value proposition). A major
donor is more likely to want to hear success stories highlighting the team's impact and to be
informed about financial accounts and how their
donation is being used. Board members may
want to hear about all of these and about internal
policies and practices.

Understanding what a stakeholder group
wants to hear will require understanding what
motivates them. Building this understanding can
be done in many different ways, some of which
depend on the specifics of the science team's situation. Informal conversations with faculty and
students can provide a wealth of information.
Conferences and workshops provide valuable
opportunities to collect information from a
broader sample. More formalized data collection
methods such as focus groups and surveys can be
used for current students and alumni. A careful
exploration of websites can help clarify the goals
of funders, regulators, and other science teams.
University development officers can clarify the
goals of alumni, and research development
offices can often provide insight into the con-

cerns of major foundations. Most universities also have offices of legislative affairs that can provide information about the interests and concerns of local, state, and federal governments and may have outreach plans that science leaders can participate in. Some communications offices will provide training in effective communication of research activities and results. Advisory boards can also provide valued insight.

Once the stakeholders have been identified and analyzed, the team can set communication goals for each stakeholder group. Do you want to raise a potential new team member's awareness of what the team has to offer or are you hoping to motivate the University Provost to provide the team with lab space in a central location? An effective message can then be developed that shows how meeting the team's needs will also meet the stakeholder's needs. For example, communicating to a potential new member that if they join the team they will have access to research data that will lead to high quality publications and tenure. Similarly, communicating to the Provost that the new lab in a central location will be a more efficient use of a currently underutilized space.

Finally, research teams should prioritize stakeholders and set appropriate goals for communication frequency. Figure 25.2 shows communication guidelines for stakeholder types.

Apathetic stakeholders require (and often prefer) minimal effort. Receiving an annual newsletter or website update may be sufficient to manage this relationship.

Defenders and Promoters should be the focus of most of the science team's communications efforts. *They* should be communicated with frequently so that they feel informed and it is important to make sure they are provided reasons for any significant changes. Posting breaking news on the team's website or via twitter can help this group stay informed. Likes, comments, and re-tweets can help the team gauge the overall mood of the defenders (the "fans"). This kind of brief, instant communication can be supplemented with more in-depth information provided through an outlet such as a monthly newsletter or annual report. Placing promoters in key leadership or advisory roles enables even more in-depth communication.

Stakeholders with moderate power and high levels of interest should receive communications more frequently than those who have a low level of interest. This could include inviting them to events such as public talks given or hosted by science team members, or "friends of" receptions or lunches at major conferences. They may also appreciate receiving science collaboration products such as annual reports or papers.

Fig. 25.2 Overview of stakeholder communication strategies

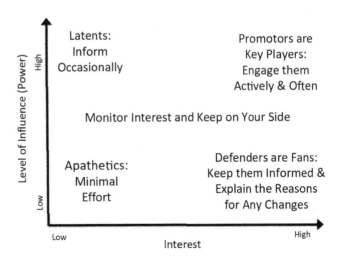

Latents can often be satisfied with targeted, but relatively infrequen communications. For example, providing information to the university that it can incorporate into its annual report to the Regents and to the State may be sufficient.

25.3.2.4 Developing a Communications Plan

The last, and perhaps most important step in developing an effective communication strategy is to create a concrete plan for developing appropriate messages, delivering them via preferred media and in a timely fashion. The team should determine who is responsible for key communications activities and develop a budget, resources, and timeline for implementation. Finally, the team should identify how it will measure success and determine if its communication goals are being met. Are the number of hits on the website sufficient or is the team's goal to get their key messages mentioned in media coverage? Appropriate milestones to measure progress toward these goals should also be developed.

Understanding your team's environment and communicating the team's "value proposition" to stakeholders is extremely important to the success of science teams. Organization science has also found that leaders need to pay attention to their internal operations so that their team can actually make good on their promises and deliver what their stakeholders value. Being able to communicate this value proposition and provide good value will enhance a team's ability to navigate even a difficult institutional environment and achieve success.

25.3.3 Strategy 3: Fulfilling the Team's Value Proposition

Teamwork takes considerable time and effort and may not always result in success. Given these facts, working in a team only makes sense if it results in valuable outcomes that are not otherwise possible. Identifying the benefits that a team will provide and the costs that a stakeholder will incur in garnering those benefits is the value proposition. Although traditionally, value propositions are developed for customer segments (Barnes et al. 2009; Rackham and DeVincentis 1998), science teams should consider both a general value proposition and a set of tailored value propositions for each of their major stakeholder groups—identifying the benefits for team members, funders, and others.

The value chain is one well-known and robust way of thinking about what the collaboration provides and how the value is created and can be enhanced for various stakeholders. It focuses on the activities that a team or organization performs and how value is added at each stage in the chain of activities that links the provision of raw materials to postdelivery maintenance of a finished product (Porter 1985). In manufacturing, the value chain starts with a supplier who provides raw materials. The collaboration then transforms these raw materials into some sort of product or service that is valued by a customer. The guiding question is "Why would a customer buy from your organization instead of buying the raw materials directly from your supplier?" Figure 25.3 shows a typical value chain including direct activities that transform raw materials into a product or service for delivery to a customer and the indirect or support activities that enable the direct activities to take place such as financing the direct activities and accounting for income and expenditures.

Translating the guiding question into a science team context, team leaders should consider questions such as, "In a world of open data, why would a customer/stakeholder read my team's scientific publication instead of analyzing the data for herself?" These are not meant to be rhetorical questions. The answers should be concrete and point the way toward fulfillment of a clear and compelling value proposition. For example, the cross-disciplinary team could add value over and above an open data source by providing multiple perspectives, exercising rare data analytic skills, creating compelling graphics, and/or applying analytic software that is expensive or difficult to master. Any of these would add value for the reader at a lower cost

Fig. 25.3 The direct and indirect value chain

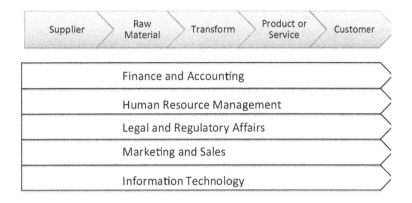

than he or she would have to spend to duplicate these capabilities, so the reader should value the publication.

To take this a step further, leaders should consider whether researchers in the area of study could get more value from other kinds of information products. Leaders should consider whether it would add significant value if your science team also made the results available as presentation slides, as a YouTube video presentation, as an open access publication, or with the option to chat with the authors. Would it add value if your science team made the cleaned and annotated data and analytic codes available? Should these be posted to Github or would another repository add more value for stakeholders?

The team should also consider the needs of other customers/stakeholders such as researchers in other areas, students, alumni, funders, university administrators, and legislators. Could the team expand the kinds of customers/stakeholders it provides value for if the results were translated into a press release or otherwise made more media-friendly? How will the results be integrated into the team's communications strategy? How will they be featured on the website, in the annual report, and in social media postings? Could the materials be made available for use in teaching at the graduate, undergraduate, or K-12 levels? If there are multiple science teams that are addressing similar issues, those that find more ways to add value and reach a wide variety of stakeholders may find that they attract more resources (collaborators, students, funding,

industry partners, space) and are more sustainable.

The science team also has to consider the costs of each of these additional information products and whether they could result in a revenue stream. If these additional information products are provided for free, then the added value would accrue to the customer/stakeholder. If the science team charged for them then at least a portion of the added value could accrue to the team. Of course, team leaders should consider community norms and local regulations. Charging for information products may conflict with the terms and conditions set out by the funders or with university policies. On the other hand, if these information products are intellectual property that is owned by the university, then it may be the university that determines whether they can be made available for free.

25.3.3.1 Value Chain Analysis

Once important stakeholders have been identified and value propositions have been created for each, science teams can systematically look for opportunities to add value. Although scientific output is important, teams that focus solely on scientific publications may miss opportunities to add value in ways that will attract strong collaborators, good students, improved lab space, helpful industry partners, supportive university administrators, and additional funding. To help science leaders consider a wider range of opportunities, the value chain focuses on activities and systems, is divided into stages, and encompasses both primary activities that have an immediate effect on the production of products and services and activities that support and enable these activities. Value chain analysis consists of four steps: activity analysis, value analysis, evaluation, and planning for action (Van Vliet 2010).

Activity analysis involves identifying what the science team does including sub-activities. The focus here is on a step-by-step description of the team's workflow. For example, science teams create knowledge by engaging in research. They also disseminate knowledge by preparing publications and presentations, filing patents, delivering educational programs, authoring research proposals and white papers, and writing social media posts. They could import knowledge through arranging guest speakers, running a journal club, and organizing symposia or seminars. They could provide research support by maintaining collaborative writing groups, supplying mentoring, and providing data analytic services or data products. Each of these activities will involve sub-activities that should be enumerated, identifying the steps that are involved from the beginning of the process to its successful completion. To take a relatively simple example, bringing in guest speakers could start with identifying interesting potential speakers, determining a preferred schedule, contacting speakers, reserving rooms, asking for the talk title and abstract and speaker bio, advertising the event, making travel arrangements, providing appropriate swag, arranging additional meetings as desired, and ensuring that expenses are reimbursed.

A value analysis considers each of the sub-activities and identifies what each customer/stakeholder values in the way that this activity is conducted. For example, the early activity of choosing a speaker has implications for multiple stakeholder groups. Faculty team members likely value innovative speakers in areas that are relevant to their research. Student team members may value established speakers who can help build their professional network and provide mentoring. Development officers may value

speakers that would appeal to wealthy alumni or other potential donors. Administrative staff likely value getting complete and accurate information in a timely fashion so that they can schedule rooms and make travel arrangements.

Science teams should then identify potential changes in primary or support activities that would add the greatest value for their customers/stakeholders and look for links among these to identify those changes that can have the largest impact. For example, setting a regular time and place for guest speakers can help faculty and student team members plan ahead and enable administrative staff to schedule rooms. Posting this on the team's website and tweeting details as they emerge can assist in communicating the event to alumni and potential donors. Science teams may want to develop a process for selecting speakers that results in a mix of innovation, experience, and areas of application. They could also create bundle of activities that maximize the value of each speaker by adding tutorial sessions for enhancing the understanding of new innovations, networking and mentoring opportunities with students, and alumni or donor activities such as lunch with the department chair.

This value analysis would be repeated for each step in each of the team's activities resulting in a large number of potential changes that could add value and fulfill the team's value proposition for its customers/stakeholders. Teams often overlook important activities that are not directly related to producing scientific results so should be sure to consider issues like what they do to recruit and retain the best people, how they motivate team members, how they keep up to date on new innovations, how they decide what new technologies and techniques to adopt, and how they collect feedback from customers/stakeholders. If these are neglected, then the team may have difficulty fulfilling their value proposition as they lose valued team members, decline in motivation, fall behind technically, and fall out of touch with important stakeholders in their environment.

Completing an activity analysis and a value analysis will result in a very large number of possible changes, not all of which can or should be made. The science team should identify those that would add a lot of value for important stakeholders and are relatively quick and easy. These should begin to be put into place immediately. There will also be a set of changes that are impractical or that are very difficult and would yield only marginal added value. These should not be pursued. The team can then prioritize the remaining changes in terms of their degree of difficulty and potential payoff. This list should then be used to create a concrete implementation plan. The plan should be achievable, provide step-by-step guidance, and show continual improvement so that the team remains engaged and enthusiastic.

Large teams and those that wish to grow can follow the same value chain process in planning their growth, but face additional challenges in fulfilling their value propositions. They must consider the impact of this growth on their current activities and identify new activities that may need to be added. In general, the larger and more complex the collaboration, the more elaborate and formalized the management structure and processes need to be to enable fulfillment of the team's value proposition. Many science teams find that their underdeveloped management structures, processes, and capabilities severely limit their scale and impact. Without adequate management, a team can seldom grow larger than a dozen members so cannot fulfill a value proposition that promises to address the most complex and difficult societal problems. Science teams that wish to scale up and increase their impact must develop management capabilities that are adequate to the task and many find that they need to embrace a division of labor with management responsibilities explicitly assigned to team members or provided by the team's university.

Regardless of how large or elaborate a science team is, to successfully fulfill their value propositions, a team must have in place robust management and collaboration plans that assign responsibilities to team members and specify management activities, processes, and reporting. These plans should identify who oversees the team's finances and accounting, what reports are created, how often they are created, and who receives them. Similarly, responsibilities and

Table 25.1 Steps in science team strategic management

Framework
Assessing the environment for the science team
Amount of existing competition
Number of customers
Number of suppliers
Substitutes
New entrants
Funders
Regulators
Managing stakeholders
Identify stakeholders
Analyze stakeholders
Level of interest
Level of power
Motivation
Developing a communication plan
Identify communication goal
Plan message based on motivation and value proposition
Determine communication timing based on interest and power and choose media
Fulfilling the value proposition
Perform a value chain analysis
Activity analysis
Value analysis
Evaluate options and plan implementation

processes for human resource management must be determined. It should be clear who is responsible for hiring, supervising, evaluating, and firing personnel and what processes should be followed. Responsibility for compliance with legal and regulatory constraints must be assigned and it must be clear what these constraints are and how they are addressed. Teams must clarify who provides and maintains the information technology and at what service levels. Responsible for communications, marketing, and any revenue-generating activities must also be specified (Table 25.1).

25.4 Conclusion

Collaboration lies at the heart of the ongoing transformation of science. From small teams to teams of teams, to enduring centers, institutes, and consortia, scientific success increasingly depends upon good leadership. Few team leaders have easy access to appropriate management expertise, but some of the robust frameworks common to organizational studies can be adapted to provide guidance and help leaders of cross-disciplinary science teams achieve sustained success. This chapter has presented three such frameworks that can help team leaders: (1) assess and influence the environment they are operating in; (2) develop their value propositions and communication strategy; and (3) improve their ability to fulfill their value propositions.

Team leaders can think broadly and systematically about their stakeholders and take action to improve their situations. They can identify competitors, customers, suppliers, substitutes, new entrants, funders, and regulators. Each of these can create an environment for the team that is supportive or potentially dangerous. By exploring this space, team leaders can think creatively about their products and services identifying new opportunities and partnerships.

Developing a specific set of stakeholders, determining their levels of power and interest, and understanding their motivations allows leaders to improve their value proposition for those that are most important and, therefore, make their environment more supportive. These value propositions can be combined with communication goals to craft effective messages that can be delivered in a timely fashion via appropriate media. Of course, it is also important that the science team be able to fulfill their value proposition. Teams can analyze their value chain identifying sequences of activities and processes, determining what important stakeholders value about each, thinking creatively about ways to add value at each step in the sequence, and taking action to implement appropriate value-adding changes, thus fulfilling the value proposition.

Using these robust managerial techniques increases a cross-disciplinary science team leader's ability to improve their situational awareness, manage stakeholder relations, and deliver clear value to those that the team depends upon. Organizational science has a long history of studying new ventures and providing tools to help them overcome the liabilities of newness and smallness. Armed with these tools, science team leaders can make better strategic decisions to proactively create supportive institutional contexts and the conditions for success.

References

Barnes C, Blake H, Pinder D. Creating & delivering your value proposition: managing customer experience for profit. London: Kogan Page Limited; 2009. p. 40–1.

Barney JB, Wright M, Ketchen DJ Jr. The resource-based view of the firm: ten years after 1991. J Manag. 2001;27(6):625–41. https://doi.org/10.1177/014920630102700601.

Birger J. Second-Mover Advantage. CNN; 2006. Accessed 23 Nov 2011.

Bolukbasi B, Berente N, Cutcher-Gershenfeld J, Dechurch L, Flint C, Haberman M, King JL, Knight E, Lawrence B, Masella E, McElroy C, Mittleman B, Nolan M, Radik M, Shin N, Thompson CA, Winter S, Zaslavsky I, Allison ML, Arctur D, Arrigo J, Aufdenkampe AK, Bass J, Crowell J, Daniels M, Diggs S, Duffy C, Gil Y, Gomez B, Graves S, Hazen R, Hsu L, Kinkade D, Lehnert K, Marone C, Middleton D, Noren A, Pearthree G, Ramamurthy M, Robinson E, Percivall G, Richard S, Suarez C, Walker D. Open data: crediting a culture of cooperation (29 November). Sci Lett. 2013;342(6162):1041–2.

Bolukbasi B, DeChurch L, Winter SJ. Team Science In Cutcher-Gershenfeld J & King JL, Transformation of the Science Enterprise: Workable and Sustainable? Symposium Presented at the Joint Meeting of the Industry Studies Association and the Labor and Employment Relations Association, 5/29/14, Portland OR; 2014.

Bureau of Labor Statistics. Business employment dynamics, National Industry Level Data, Survival of Private Sector Establishments by Opening Year; 2017. https://www.bls.gov/bdm/us_age_naics_00_table7.txt. Accessed 06 Jan 2018.

Cutcher-Gershenfeld J, et al. Build it, but will they come? A geoscience cyberinfrastructure baseline analysis. Data Sci J. 2016;15:8.

Donaldson T, Preston L. The stakeholder theory of the corporation: concepts, evidence, and implications. Acad Manag Rev. 1995;20:65–91.

Epstein K. Marketing made easy. Epstein; 2006. pp. 116–117. ISBN 978-1-59918-017-5.

Freeman RH. Strategic management: a stakeholder approach. Englewood Cliffs, NJ: Prentice-Hall; 1984.

Freeman J, Carroll GC, Hannan MT. The liability of newness: age dependence in organizational death rates. Am Sociol Rev. 1983;48(5):692–710.

Gaglio CM, Cechini M, Winter SJ. Gaining legitimacy: the symbolic use of technology by new ventures. Front Entrepren Res. 1998:203–15.

Lutters W, Winter SJ. Virtual organizations. In: Bainbridge W, editor. Leadership in science and technology: a reference handbook. Thousand Oaks, CA: Sage; 2011.

Mendelow A. Stakeholder Mapping, Proceedings of the 2nd International Conference on Information Systems, Cambridge, MA (Cited in Scholes,1998); 1991.

Mitchell RK, Agle BR, Wood DJ. Toward a theory of stakeholder identification and salience: defining the principle of who and what really counts. Acad Manag Rev. 1997;22(4):853–88.

National Research Council. Enhancing the effectiveness of team science. Washington, DC: The National Academies Press; 2015. https://doi.org/10.17226/19007.

Olson GM, Zimmerman A, Bos N. Scientific collaboration on the internet. Cambridge, MA: MIT Press; 2008.

Pfeffer J, Salancik G. The external control of organizations. Manhattan: Harper & Row; 1978.

Porter ME. Competitive advantage: creating and sustaining superior performance. New York: Simon and Schuster; 1985.

Porter ME. The Five Competitive Forces that Shape Strategy. In: Harvard Business Review; 2008, pp. 86–104.

Rackham N, DeVincentis J. Rethinking the sales force: refining selling to create and capture customer value. New York, NY: McGraw-Hill; 1998.

Springman J. Implementing a Stakeholder Strategy, Harvard Business Review, July 28; 2011.

Starr JA, MacMillan IC. Resource co-optation via social contracting: resource acquisition strategies for new ventures. Strateg Manag J. 1990;11:79–92.

Suchman MC. Managing legitimacy: strategic and institutional approaches. Acad Manag Rev. 1995;20(3):571–610.

Taylor FW. Scientific management. New York: Harper & Row; 1910.

Thompson JD. Organizations in action: social science bases of administrative theory. New York: McGraw Hill; 1967.

Van Vliet V. Porter's Value Chain Analysis; 2010. ToolsHero: https://www.toolshero.com/management/value-chain-analysis-porter/. Accessed 31 12 2017.

Wilson N. How Eric Ries changed the framework for startup success; 2011. Financial Post. Accessed 4 June 2015.

Winter SJ. The rise of cyberinfrastructure and grand challenges for eCommerce. IseB. 2012;10(3):279–93. https://doi.org/10.1007/s10257-011-0165-5.

Winter SJ, Butler B. Creating bigger problems: grand challenges as boundary objects and the legitimacy of the information systems field. J Inf Technol. 2011;26(2):99–108.

Winter S, Berente N, Butler B, Howison J. Beyond the organizational 'container': conceptualizing 21st century sociotechnical work. Inf Organ. 2014;24(4):250–69.

Zimmerman MA, Zeitz GJ. Beyond survival: achieving new venture growth by building legitimacy. Acad Manag Rev. 2002;27(3):414–31.

How Leadership Can Support Attainment of Cross-Disciplinary Scientific Goals

26

Nathan A. Berger

Contents

N. A. Berger (✉)
Center for Science, Health and Society, Case Western
Reserve University School of Medicine,
Cleveland, OH, USA
e-mail: nab@case.edu

26.1 Introduction

In 2004, at Case Western Reserve University (CWRU) School of Medicine, we started a program to conduct Transdisciplinary Research on Energy Balance and Cancer (TREC). The specific impetus for developing this program was the funding opportunity, RFA CA-05-010, issued by the National Cancer Institute (NCI) in 2004 for establishment of U54 Transdisciplinary Research on Energetics and Cancer (TREC) Centers to integrate diverse disciplines spanning the full range of cancer research, to foster collaboration among transdisciplinary teams, to accelerate progress, and to create new opportunities for interdisciplinary training of scientists at all stages of their careers. During a 5-year NCI funding period, and extending thereafter, this program resulted in development of multiple successful, original research activities including highly productive research initiatives that contributed significantly to understanding the problem, several paradigm shifting concepts, over 300 publications with many articles in high-profile journals, a book series on Energy Balance and Cancer, and a formal course on obesity in the CWRU Epidemiology and Biostatistics curriculum. The CWRU TREC Center likewise launched and promoted multiple scientific research careers, fostered new local, national, and international collaborations, and helped establish an enduring

© Springer Nature Switzerland AG 2019
K. L. Hall et al. (eds.), *Strategies for Team Science Success*,
https://doi.org/10.1007/978-3-030-20992-6_26

culture of team science that focuses on energy balance and related problems and continues to operate and interact through multiple successors, to this date.

26.2 Identifying Challenges

In this chapter, we initially provide Table 26.1 to outline, what in retrospect, were the key challenges to initiate development of our Transdisciplinary Center. This table is somewhat, but not entirely, similar to a recent analysis of pioneering efforts in transdisciplinary science (Vogel et al. 2014), which represented a synthesis of viewpoints provide by the original TREC leaders and participants. Programmatic development will be discussed in terms of identifying the research focus, establishing leadership, defining their roles, engaging the research team, and identifying and securing the resources required for programmatic success. This chapter will focus on how leadership contributed to programmatic success by building an organizational environment

Table 26.1 Initial challenges to development of transdisciplinary research

1. Lack of clarity about what TD is, how to get there and how to know when you are there
2. TD Science stretches intellectual capacity and is time consuming
3. How to integrate different disciplinary cultures-values, language, traditions, rewards and how to foster common language development and collaboration
4. Complexity of project planning
5. How to provide academic incentives, expectations and rewards
6. How to garner resources to support TD initiative
7. What are most effective TD training approaches and how to provide training opportunities and recognition
8. How to identify and recognize strong productive colleagues with mutual trust and respect, willing to establish strong interactive relations. Remember, you can't soar with eagles if you hang out with turkeys
9. How to guide both early and ongoing successes
10. Resistance by Silos (Departments)

that facilitated and nurtured innovation and highly productive cross-disciplinary team-based science, strategies for success and lessons learned.

First, it should be noted that the team of investigators who developed the original CWRU TREC Center did not get together one day and seek a problem to apply a transdisciplinary (TD) approach. Rather, at the time of its initiation, obesity and physical activity had been prominently identified as respectively increasing and decreasing the risk of multiple malignancies with significant impact on cancer incidence and prognosis (Calle et al. 1999, 2003; Friedenreich 2001). Obesity and lack of physical activity were noted to be rapidly growing problems of worldwide proportion, and there were no clear approaches to defining the mechanisms by which either of these factors related to cancer or how to disrupt their cancer linkage. Thus, there was a clear presentation of a problem of pandemic proportions (Balard-Barbash et al. 2010), with no apparent solution residing within any single scientific discipline and the real promise that transdisciplinary teams might make significant contributions.

26.3 Initial Strategies

Based on my background as a translational and multidisciplinary cancer researcher with significant experience in intermediary metabolism, DNA damage and repair research, this RFA appeared to be an interesting and exciting challenge. Moreover, since I had been the founding director of what is now the Case Comprehensive Cancer Center, and had recently completed a term as Dean of the CWRU School of Medicine and CWRU Vice President for Medical Affairs, positions through which I became highly familiar with diverse faculty expertise and talent and knowledgeable about institutional opportunities, it seemed reasonable to attempt to organize this Center initiative. In addition, I was at that time PI on an institutional P20 grant to build a multidisciplinary program in Aging-Cancer Research (Berger et al. 2006).

26.4 Building and Motivating a Team

As Center director, my first responsibility was to assemble a leadership team of investigators with previous multidisciplinary research experience, who were ready and able to interact and saw the potential benefit of collaboration to impact the problem. The initial leadership team consisted of Susan Redline, MD, MPH, Professor of Pediatrics, Epidemiology, and Biostatistics with expertise in childhood obesity, its interaction with sleep disturbances and its impact on multiple systemic health problems (Punjabi et al. 2004); Li Li, MD, PhD, Associate Professor, Family Medicine, Epidemiology, and Biostatistics with expertise in metabolic syndrome, and insulin-like growth factor as cancer risk factors (Li et al. 2003); Joe Nadeau, PhD, Professor and Chair, Genetics, with a highly productive program developing and studying consomic chromosome mouse models to interrogate gene–environment interactions affecting obesity and their consequences including diabetes and cancer (Singer et al. 2004); and Sandy Markowitz, MD, PhD, Professor of Medicine and Genetics who was conducting ground-breaking molecular genetic research in oncogene drivers of colorectal cancer (Grady and Markowitz 2002). This group brought together individuals with different clinical approaches and patient access including medical oncology, family medicine, and pediatrics which together with expertise in genetics (mouse modeling) provided the basis for developing translational studies between mouse and man and across the age span from infancy to adulthood. Moreover, this group brought together a group of investigators with complementary research disciplines of metabolism, genetics, and molecular biology in association with an established pediatric cohort of low birth weight infants with follow-up through their teens, as well as developing cohorts of adults undergoing breast and colon cancer screening, thereby providing a strong basis for transdisciplinary development. Of this group of investigators, Susan Redline was the only one who had not previously pursued the relation between obesity and cancer, having focused her attention on association of low birth weight, development of obesity, cardiovascular risk factors, and sleep disturbances. She was however knowledgeable about the association of sleep disturbances with cancer and, as described below, she was the individual who focused attention of both the CWRU and the national TREC communities on the association of sleep disturbances with obesity and cancer (Redline and Pack 2006). Although in retrospect, initial inclusion of behavioral scientists would have been useful, no member of the original group had a behavioral focus; however, multiple investigators with this orientation became involved once the NCI funding was awarded and significantly contributed to the overall development and productivity.

While these scientists formed the initial group of investigators, they also provided the leadership for development of the TREC effort at CWRU. In addition to an interest and commitment to contribute to better understanding and intervening in the energy balance and cancer challenge, each of the initial group of investigators was attracted and motivated by the opportunities to enhance their own research interest and the potential resources and collaboration that could be developed by a successful response to the NCI RFA. Thus, the second responsibility was to coordinate preparation and submission of the U54 grant application. In this regard, it is important to note that while the ultimate goal was to develop a TD program to effectively study the relation of energy balance and cancer, in this unique situation, the more immediate goal was to secure NIH TREC funding as a necessary prerequisite to enable development and pursuit of the TD studies. Accordingly, an important consideration in assembling the initial leadership team was to engage investigators with strong research experience and successful track records in preparing and securing NIH grant funding. Thus, each member of the initial group had significant grant funding and had served on multiple NIH study sections.

Our initial grant application was approved and funded by NCI in 2005. In addition to the TREC Center at CWRU, NCI funded three other U54 TREC Centers, one each at the Fred Hutchinson

Cancer Research Center (FHCRC), University of Southern California (USC) and University of Wisconsin along with a coordination center at the FHCRC. In addition to sponsoring several major research projects at each institution, the U54 TREC award provided funding for annual granting of pilot projects to develop new transdisciplinary efforts. Moreover, in preparing the grant proposal, leadership was successful in obtaining institutional commitments to provide annual financial resources for TREC initiatives from both the CWRU School of Medicine and the Case Comprehensive Cancer Center. Leadership was subsequently instrumental in helping garner additional support in the form of startup and early phase grants awarded to junior investigators from disease-specific agencies such as American Cancer Society, Susan Komen Foundation, and community-based philanthropy, as well as in kind support from The Gathering Place, a community support program for patients touched by cancer. Although many of these organizations provide grants to support new investigators and/or new initiatives, these proposals fare best when they are supported by preliminary data, which means that it takes upfront investment to even gain agency-based startup grant support. In this regard, in addition to providing junior investigators with guidance and overview for preparation of startup proposals, TREC leadership was able to help secure initial resources, sometimes funding and other times access to techniques or equipment sufficient to generate preliminary data to strengthen applications for startup grants. The NIH-funded CWRU Clinical Translation and Science Award was helpful in this regard by providing core resource services to help support pilot projects. Importantly, funds from the Comprehensive Cancer Center were able to be used for a broad range of academic activities including support for these startup efforts by junior investigators.

26.5   Stimulating Transdisciplinary Interaction

During the early period of grant preparation and before funding was secured, the initial strategy of leadership to encourage interest and interaction among this already successful group of independent scientists was to hold regular, weekly, face-to-face meetings to review areas of expertise, to discuss potential areas of scientific collaboration, to identify areas where integration of disciplines could overcome scientific obstacles, and to define resources and personnel likely to be interested in participating and contributing to this effort. These meetings usually started with a presentation of each investigator's current relevant research focus, expertise, resources and barriers to progress, followed by an interactive discussion how collaborators could interact and/or complement each other's programs. Important aspects of these initial meetings were to understand each other's capacities, languages, and potential contributions to the ultimate goal of defining and disrupting the linkage between obesity and cancer. A most important aspect of these initial meetings was to identify young, undifferentiated investigators (graduate students, post-doctoral fellows, junior faculty) that could be engaged and supported to conduct research at the interface between investigators in the initial group and/or to link members of the initial group with other investigators either within or outside of our institution. Another important aspect of these meetings was to establish a culture where because of our differing disciplines and unfamiliarity with approaches and techniques, everyone felt comfortable asking even the most fundamental questions or posing what seemed to be the most far out concept. Overall, these meetings served to broaden understanding of each other's expertise and discipline, to cross-fertilize ideas across disciplines, to stimulate new collaborations and to engage both senior and junior investigators in these efforts.

As successful independent investigators, each member of the leadership team already had a group of colleagues, junior faculty, and trainees with whom they interacted, many of whom were interested in participating in the TREC program. Once the NCI U54 grant was secured, an important early goal was to expand the group for multiple reasons. First, our approach to develop transdisciplinarity was not focused on getting a small group of investigators to develop shared language, but rather, because of the enormity and multifaceted nature of the challenge, the goal was to engage and incorporate multiple investigators with complementary disciplines to interrogate multiple aspects of the problem. Second, engaging other investigators provided opportunities for expanding into other areas of the issues, such as behavioral interventions, community issues, food availability, exercise, physical activity, and geriatric populations. Third, involving new investigators further challenged evolving concepts so as to reorient our approaches. A critically important fourth aspect of expanding the group was to establish a recognizable and robust institutional presence, the latter helping to further attract collaborators and, more importantly, to provide a platform to influence development of institutional policy such as promotion and tenure standards, to lobby department heads to commit their trainees to work within our program and/or to convince department heads to recruit some of these trainees to junior faculty positions within their departments. This latter ability was clearly enhanced when the TREC Program could contribute to development of recruitment packages and more importantly, to provide mentoring capacity.

To better engage the expanding group and further establish an institutional presence, we initiated a regular, monthly, CWRU TREC Retreat. The meeting was held the first Monday of each month, from 4:00 to 6:00 p.m., a schedule specifically selected to provide an easily rememberable calendar date which did not conflict with any department meetings, was compatible with clinical service demands and teaching obligations and, since it was restricted to only once a month, was acceptable to those with family responsibilities. Participants were provided with a gastronomically appealing dinner buffet, so as to provide an end-of-the-day nutritious pickup and to eliminate the need to rush home to prepare dinner that night. Since dinner was always provided and the conference was scheduled at day's end, there were no obligations to rush and/or to release the room to the next group. Presentations were accompanied and followed by extensive question, answer, and discussion periods. Discussions occasionally extended for one and sometimes two hours.

26.6 Stimulating Idea Exchange Across Disciplines

The agenda for the CWRU TREC Retreat Series was carefully constructed to have at least one main speaker to review areas of relevant expertise at a level that would be understandable and engaging to an audience of significantly different disciplines and different levels of accomplishment. Speakers were selected both from among our own faculty and invited experts from other institutions. In addition to major speakers, sometimes as many as four, opportunities were provided for junior faculty and trainees to present research in progress, ideas for grant proposals, practice for meeting presentations and suggestions—invitations for collaborative efforts.

Regularly incorporating visiting speakers into the retreat programs was designed to introduce concepts from outside CWRU and also to stimulate collaboration across institutions. Opportunities were created for faculty and especially junior faculty to meet individually or in small groups with visiting speakers both before and after the presentations. In addition to providing our faculty with exposure to external expertise, an important goal of the visiting speaker program was to acquaint visitors with the expertise, endeavors, and accomplishments of our faculty. Moreover, the high profile of many of these guest speakers and the audience they attracted to our TREC Retreats, significantly added to the institutional awareness and stature of the TREC program. A partial list of these visiting speakers is included in Table 26.2. As visiting scientists became aware of the quality of the CWRU TREC Retreats and their TD nature, some began to send some of their own trainees to present early concepts and results for discussion. These visiting speakers, sometimes stimulated new research approaches and/or became collaborators on projects and NIH grant applications.

The monthly CWRU TREC Retreats were soon identified as an exciting, educational conference and began to attract both senior and junior investigators and trainees, thereby enhancing our capacity to conduct relevant research. Among the senior investigators who became

Table 26.2 CWRU TREC retreat visiting speakers

Mimi C. Yu, PhD, University of Minnesota
Topic: Epidemiologic Approaches to Cancer
Anne McTiernan, MD, PhD, Fred Hutchinson Cancer Research Center
Topic: Obesity, Energy Balance and Breast Cancer
Henry J. Thompson, PhD, Colorado State University
Topic: Emerging opportunities: From animal models to human populations
W. Todd Penberthy, PhD, University of Cincinnati
Topic: NAD Pharmacotherapeutics: Zebrafish-based small molecule studies of lipid metabolism with implications for cancer and multiple sclerosis
Stephen Hursting, PhD, University of Texas at Austin
Topic: Obesity, Metabolism and Cancer: Trends, Targets and Transgenics
Daniel Medina, PhD, Baylor College of Medicine
Topic: The p53 null model of mouse mammary tumorigenesis
Robert Hegele, MD, Robarts Research Institute
Topic: Phenomics: The role of deep phenotyping in medical research
Robert Hardy, PhD, University of Alabama at Birmingham
Topic: Fatty Acids and Breast Cancer
Lee M. Kaplan, PhD, Harvard Medical School
Topic: Gastrointestinal regulation of metabolic function
Nancy H. Colburn, PhD, National Cancer Institute at Frederick
Topic: Biomarkers for dietary intervention and protection against colon cancer in mice and humans
Andrew J. Dannenberg, MD, Weil Cornell Medical College
Topic: The prostaglandin aromatase connection: implications for breast carcinogenesis
Steven E. Shoelson, MD, PhD, Harvard Medical School
Topic: Obesity-induced inflammation: pathogenesis and target for reversal in T2D and CVD
Giovanni Cizza, MD, PhD, National Institute of Diabetes and Digestive and Kidney Diseases
Topic: Neuropeptide: mediating obesity and sleep disorders
Debra Haire-Joshu, PhD, Washington University, St. Louis
Topic: Policy initiatives to control obesity through change in food and activity environment
Pamela Goodwin, MD, Samuel Lunenfeld Research Institute
Topic: Metformin in breast cancer therapy
Gerald V. Denis, PhD, Boston University School of Medicine
Topic: Bromodomain coactivators in obesity, cancer and inflammation
James Carson, PhD, University of South Carolina
Topic: The regulation of skeletal muscle protein turnover during cancer cachexia: a role for muscle contraction and exercise
Dipali Sharma, PhD, Johns Hopkins University School of Medicine
Topic: Obesity, leptin and breast cancer
Chao-Pin Hsiao, PhD, RN, National Institute of Nursing Research
Topic: Using mitochondria PCR array in determining correlates of cancer-related fatigue
Katherine Schmitz, PhD, University of Pennsylvania
Topic: The impact of exercise on breast cancer prognosis
Francine H. Einstein, Montefiore Medical Center
Topic: Epigenetic effects of abnormal fetal growth
Peixin Yang, PhD, University of Maryland School of Medicine
Topic: Towards understand the molecular mechanism of diabetic embryopathy
Melinda Irwin, PhD, MPH, Yale School of Public Health
Topic: exercise trials in cancer survivors
Carey Lumeng, MD, University of Michigan
Topic: Adipocyte macrophage interaction
Colleen Novak, PhD, Kent State University
Topic: How brain melanocortins enhance physical activity and energy expenditure
Ellen Heber-Katz, PhD, The Wistar Institute
Topic: The impact of regenerative genes on obesity associated cancers

(continued)

Table 26.2 (continued)

Darlene Berryman, PhD, RD, LD, Ohio University
Topic: Fat yet fit: the huge impact of growth hormone on adipose tissue
Satchin Panda, PhD, The Salk Institute
Topic: Circadian Rhythm effects on cancer
Kelle H. Moley, MD, Washington University School of Medicine in St. Louis
Topic: Epigenetic effects of prenatal energy balance on prostate cancer and other diseases in the offspring
Pamela Salsberry, RN, PhD, The Ohio State University
Topic: Poverty, low birth weight and obesity across the life course
Derek LeRoith, PhD, Mt Sinai School of Medicine
Topic: Mouse models for studies of diabetes, insulin and IGF on cancer
Judith Storch, PhD, Rutgers University
Topic: Fatty acid binding protein
David Tuveson, MD, PhD, Cold Springs Harbor Laboratory
Topic: Model systems to study pancreatic cancer
Lei Cao, PhD, The Ohio State University
Topic: Environmental manipulation and neuropeptide effects on cancer
Lorraine T. Dean, ScD, University of Pennsylvania Perelman School of Medicine
Topic: Resources or race? Social determinants of cancer screening and survivorship
Kathleen Sturgeon, PhD, MTR, University of Pennsylvania
Topic: Physical activity to reduce breast cancer risk associated with delayed parity
Leorey Nagac Saligan, PhD, RN, CRNP, NINR/NIH
Topic: Radiation fatigue prevention, pathogenesis and therapy
Melinda Stolley, PhD, Medical College of Wisconsin
Topic: Health promotion in African American breast cancer survivors
William S. Blaner, PhD, Columbia University
Topic: Metabolic disease in transgenic mouse models

regular participants and speakers were Dick Hanson, emeritus Chair of Biochemistry and developer of the Phosphoenolpyruvate Carboxykinase C (PEPCK) Enhanced Exercise Mouse (Hakimi et al. 2007); Chuck Hoppel, Professor of Pharmacology and expert in mitochondrial metabolism (Distler et al. 2006); Hung-Ying Kao, Associate Professor Biochemistry and expert in tumor suppressors and cancer signaling (Reineke et al. 2007); Amitabh Chak, Professor of Medicine in Gastroenterology with expertise in Barrett's esophagus and esophageal adenocarcinoma (Chak et al. 2006); and Shirley Moore, Associate Dean for Research at the CWRU School of Nursing and expert in self-management and system CHANGE (Change Habits by Applying New Goals and Experiences) as an approach to weight management (Moore et al. 2016). Regular participants also included Henri Brunengraber, Professor and Chair Department of Nutrition, PI Mouse Metabolic Phenotyping Center and Expert in Metabolomic Studies;

Satish Kalhan, Staff Member Cleveland Clinic whose research focused on protein and amino acid metabolism (Kalhan and Bier 2008); Ofer Reizes, Associate Member Cleveland Clinic, with expertise in leptin and obesity (Shi et al. 2009); and Noa Noy, Professor of Pharmacology, with expertise in Retinol Binding Protein 4 and its relation to breast cancer (Donato et al. 2007). The program was further broadened by engagement of John Kirwan who coordinated most of the metabolic studies and exercise programs associated with the renowned Bariatric Surgery Program at the Cleveland Clinic (Brethauer et al. 2013), and Pat Catalano, PI of the eminent high risk pregnancy program at the MetroHealth Medical Center that mainly focused on diabetes and obesity during pregnancy and their epigenetic effects (Catalano et al. 1999).

Collaborations with these newly engaged investigators led to pursuit of many new TD initiatives. For example, Dick Hanson with his PEPCK-C transgenic mice provided opportunities to study metabolic mechanisms of exercise on development of aging and colon carcinogenesis (Fiuza-Luces et al. 2016). Collaboration with Hung-Ying Kao led to research on mouse metabolic changes associated with obesity and hepatocellular cancer (Cheng et al. 2013). Collaboration between Li Li, Noa Noy and Berger focused attention on Retinol Binding Protein 4 as a potentially important adipokine contributing to obesity, promotion of breast and colorectal cancer (Abola et al. 2015; Noy et al. 2015). Amitabh Chak, Li Li, Nate Berger developed a study to demonstrate the potential contribution of obesity to the rising rates of Barrett's esophagus and esophageal adenocarcinoma and then Chak went on to lead a study with Navtej Butar, Mayo Clinic, to evaluate insulin resistance and metformin as therapy for Barrett's esophagus (Thompson et al. 2008; Chak et al. 2015). Through the guest speaker program, Ofer Reizes established a relation with Stephen Hursting, University of Texas, Austin, leading to collaborative studies to demonstrate and define mechanisms of leptin promotion of MMTV-Wnt1, Mouse Mammary Carcinoma (Zheng et al. 2011, 2013). A strong example of development of a transdisciplinary focus is provided by Susan Redline, who as noted above, was the only member of the original group of investigators that had little or no research involving cancer. However, Redline, together with Nora Nock, who applied her skills in mathematical modeling, along with Li Li's epidemiological expertise, were able to demonstrate sleep disturbance as an essential and contributing component of the metabolic syndrome, contributing to its redesignation from Syndrome X to Syndrome Z (Nock et al. 2009). In subsequent studies, Cheryl Thompson, Redline and Li, examining a cohort undergoing screening colonoscopy, identified an association of short sleep as a risk factor for colon adenoma (Thompson et al. 2011) following which Thompson and Li were able to demonstrate lack of sleep as a risk factor for aggressive breast cancer as well (Thompson and Li 2012). And, as noted above, Susan Redline was responsible for raising awareness to the TREC community of the important contribution of sleep disturbances to metabolic and neoplastic processes. Redline also went on to coedit the Energy Balance book volume on *Impact of Sleep and Sleep Disturbances on Obesity and Cancer* thus further raising awareness of this important TD relationship to the international community (Redline and Berger 2014).

Another example where TD interaction resulted in a robust program is demonstrated by a study of a breast cancer screening cohort developed by Thompson and Li involving Owusu, Nock and Berger, to show differential levels of physical activity based on ethnic and body habitus characteristics (Thompson et al. 2014). In subsequent studies, Cynthia Owusu, a geriatric oncologist who together with Nora Nock, with personal interest in exercise and physical activity and Nate Berger, developed programs to implement and study Physical Activity in Older Breast Cancer Survivors, particularly those of lower socioeconomic status (Nock et al. 2013, 2015). And after meeting Katherine Schmitz, University of Pennsylvania, as a TREC Retreat visiting speaker, Owusu and Nock with input from Schmitz collaborated on a productive research program and successfully funded NIH RO1 grant. Interactions between Markowitz and Berger and Chak and Berger contributed to successful pursuits in colon cancer, Barrett's esophagus, and esophageal adenocarcinoma. Another example of development of TD interaction is provided by collaboration of John Kirwan, Pat Catalano and Berger which provided the basis for an NIH Nutrition Obesity Research Center grant application with further possibilities for supporting an even broader TD effort relating obesity to metabolic disease, maternal and epigenetic effects as well as cancer. Thus, many of the retreat based interactions led to direct collaborations to provide further insight into the obesity–cancer relationship.

Interestingly, the multiplicity of projects stimulated by the TREC program identified the complexity and multiple issues involved in the energy balance–cancer spectrum. The conduct of multiple initiatives and regular communications among investigators led to development of interactions in which the sum of the projects created an overall transdisciplinary program.

With engagement of many well-established and productive investigators, the network quickly broadened. The monthly retreats soon attracted junior faculty, postdocs and graduate students to the program. Since these participants were just beginning their research efforts, they were somewhat more adventurous and willing to engage in TD projects, especially since the TREC Center had resources to invest in pilot projects. It is noteworthy that Department leaders, who were somewhat skeptical about the TD approach, became quite willing to have their junior faculty members engage in TD research since the TREC Center was able, in many cases, to provide both financial and intellectual support. As the program matured, more senior members provided mentorship and guidance for junior members including manuscript and grant reviewing and career advice. Some of the junior faculty members attracted to the program included Stephanie Doerner, genetics graduate student with Joe Nadeau who conducted her thesis research on inflammatory mechanisms of dietary fat stimulation of colon cancer (Doerner et al. 2016), and Jason Heaney, a Genetics postdoctoral fellow with Nadeau who developed a program to study inflammatory processes in colorectal cancer (Maywald et al. 2015). Nora Nock, along with Anastasia Dimitropoulos, a psychologist who focused on food related behavior in Prader–Willi Syndrome (Dimitropoulos and Schultz 2008), developed a program using functional MRI (fMRI) to analyze neuroregulation of exercise in obese women with gynecologic malignancies (Nock et al. 2014). Other junior faculty members who made important contributions to the program included Carolyn Ievers Landis and Leslie Heinberg, who led the institutional Healthy Kids, Healthy Weight Initiative to prevent childhood obesity (Ievers-Landis and Jelalian 2013), Perrie O'Tierney-Ginn, whose research focused on placental fatty acid metabolism (Yang et al. 2016), and David Buchner, who pursued epigenetic control of diabetes and obesity (Stegemann and Buchner 2015).

26.7 Playmaking and Nurturing for TD Collaboration

Overall, the monthly CWRU TREC retreats became a major focus of interaction for a broad cross-disciplinary sampling of participants, for educating each other about unique disciplinary concepts, approaches, and barriers, and for conception of novel TD initiatives. When new initiatives were sparked spontaneously at retreats or elsewhere, leadership frequently played an important follow up "playmaker" role, which in team sport parlance, like basketball, soccer or hockey, refers to the on-field player who understands each players' skills, capacities, and positions, perceives opportunities and coordinates interactions to successfully score points. The role of playmaker in the TREC program was to ensure contact between key investigators, maintain the interaction, promote the project, identify resources and facilities to support their efforts and either provide or identify mentoring to help guide the initiative to successful completion, including initial preparation and revision of scientific presentations, manuscripts and grant proposals. For example, while the project noted above with Owusu, Nock and Schmitz was clearly developed by these investigators, leadership contributed to bringing them together, advising on preliminary studies to establish a track record of both scientific as well as successful and collaborative interactions, coordinating relations with community-based exercise facilities for support of cancer patients and guiding and critiquing a series of successful grant applications to American Cancer Society, Susan Komen Foundation, ultimately leading to NIH RO1 funding.

The ability of leadership to foster the TD experience was further enhanced, in many ways, by the overall national TREC program. First and foremost were semiannual meetings of all four TREC Centers, along with the Coordination Center and NCI members. These meeting which usually included guest speakers, presentations of major research projects from each of the centers, a poster session for pilot projects, strategy and business sessions were valuable opportunities to learn from each other, to develop cross-institutional collaborations, and to provide opportunities for junior members to meet and receive advice from senior leaders in the field and to communicate directly with NCI leadership.

These national meetings always stimulated novel ideas among both new and established investigators. For example, presentations by investigators from CWRU TREC put consideration of sleep disturbances and their relation to obesity and cancer on the TREC investigators radar, whereas CWRU investigators were alerted to the importance of the built environment on obesity by presentation from USC investigators. Moreover, as a result of these meetings, Markowitz developed a collaborative interaction with both John Potter, Joanna Lampe and Neli Ulrich of the FHCRC to investigate genetic variants and 15-hydroxyprostaglandin dehydrogenase (15-PGDH) levels related to colorectal cancer (Gray-McGuire et al. 2010; Fink et al. 2013).

A very important role of leadership in engaging and nurturing development of junior investigators was by using NCI, institutional and philanthropic resources to support travel, attendance, and presentations by junior investigators at the semiannual national TREC meetings and other important cancer-related meetings. In addition to support of the major research projects supported by TREC, the U54 also provided critically important support, at each institution, for annual pilot projects, specifying that at least one project per year was required to be cross-institutional. Although pilot project proposals were evaluated and awarded by an internal study section, an important function of leadership was to ensure that major portions of these grants were targeted to junior investigators engaged in TD research.

Another national TREC initiative was the establishment of cross-institutional working groups focused on topics such as nutrition assessment, physical activity assessment, biomarkers, animal models, and molecular pathways. These groups usually met by conference call, once per month, and face to face at the semi-annual TREC meetings. Membership in these committees was mostly by self-selection but also strongly supported and stimulated by leadership, who further ensured importance and recognition of these roles by having representatives report on committee activities at the monthly TREC retreats. These working groups provided the basis, with variable degrees of success in different groups, to stimulate cross-center communication, interaction, and collaboration, identify new research opportunities and needs, and establish common language and comparable measurement techniques.

26.8 Stimulating Productivity

In addition to stimulating interaction and encouraging development of a TD approach, an important responsibility for leadership was to foster productivity, recognition, and reward. Since academic productivity is generally measured in terms of publications and grants, we emphasized performance of research that would provide publication data and/or preliminary data for grant applications. We mentored faculty, especially junior members in manuscript and grant preparation, submission, revision and resubmission. While classes for developing these skills are already in existence in association with multiple training programs at our institution, the service provided by TREC leadership was individualized mentoring based on needs and faculty expertise and experience. In almost all cases, junior faculty were encouraged to emphasize the TD aspect as a unique advantage of new proposals.

In addition to reports of their own research, we encouraged faculty to identify "low hanging fruit" where investigators could analyze existing data in a TD fashion to make important publishable contributions and guarantee some early successes. We encouraged working group members to identify publishable topics based on their cross-center interactions. By starting a book series on Energy Balance and Cancer, we were able to provide a transdisciplinary resource and educational tool to the scientific research community as well as opportunities for many junior investigators, throughout the TREC network, to author pertinent review articles which not only helped sharpen their own focus, but also afforded them widespread international exposure. The book series on Energy Balance and Cancer, recently having published Volume 14, Energy Balance and Cancer: Focus on Gynecologic Malignancies, with over 47,000 copies downloaded, has not only had an international impact, but has acted locally, as well, to enhance the status of the TREC Center.

26.9 Recognition and Rewards

Academic recognition, frequently accompanied by salary increments, primarily centers on promotion and tenure (P&T). Factors considered in the evaluation of candidates for P&T usually include individual scholarship and productivity, grant funding, teaching, service and national and international reputation. Realizing the challenge to P&T for individuals engaged in team science, leadership engaged, from the beginning, in developing the CVs of participants. Increasing bibliometric productivity, as noted above, was one of the most important strategies to prepare candidates for P&T. Arranging and encouraging young investigators to present at national meetings and introducing them to the national investigator community was another. When junior investigators were ready, we suggested their names to be journal reviewers and whenever possible we nominated them to serve as study section ad hoc reviewers, ultimately leading to study section appointments. To help faculty learn the skills associated with grant reviews and learn how study sections function, we had junior investigators serve as reviewers for our pilot project series. With the overall TREC program, we established an annual recognition system for Best Trainees, where appropriately selected individuals were recognized and provided with a plaque at national meetings. At CWRU, we made sure that these awards were duly recognized and published in the school electronic newspaper. By establishing an Epidemiology and Biostatistics course on Obesity, we provided opportunities for faculty to engage in formal TD teaching exercises and further broadened the attraction for student engagement in TREC activities.

At CWRU, promotion and tenure was traditionally awarded to independent scientists for a body of work for which they had been the major intellectual driver. With the NIH promotion of translational and transdisciplinary science and the funding of multi-investigator grants, institutions began to recognize the value of Team Science. At the same time, many other programs involving Team Science were developing at CWRU. An important role for leadership of all these programs was to advocate for recognition and reward of team scientists in the P&T process. At CWRU, P&T guidelines were ultimately changed such that in addition to recognizing independent scientists, P&T could be granted to team scientists whose original, creative and unique, independent research accomplishments were made with a group of other scientists. A critically important role for leadership then became to write P&T support letters, clearly explaining each candidate's unique and integral contributions to the team effort. At this point, I am happy to say that all of our candidates have successfully passed through the P&T processes at multiple levels and no one has been refused P&T because of their efforts as a Team Scientist. Judged by the numbers of requests we get to write letters of support for TD investigators at other institutions, it is clear these testimonials provide an important mechanism by which leadership contributes to success of individual investigators and the overall TD effort as well.

26.10 Sustainability and Expansion Post Funding

Ongoing funding for research initiated with TREC financial and intellectual support has utilized a variety of mechanisms. As a result of national and international meetings, sponsored both by us and by other investigators, on a worldwide basis, as well as by our book series on Energy Balance and Cancer (see Table 26.3 for list), a number of collaborations have been established including highly productive and funded research projects with investigators both in the US and in places ranging from Spain to Shanghai

Table 26.3 Energy balance and cancer book series

Vol. 1: Cancer and Energy Balance, Epidemiology and Overview
Ed. Nathan A. Berger; 2010

Vol. 2: Insulin Resistance and Cancer
Ed. I. George Fantus; 2011

Vol.3: Physical Activity, Dietary Calorie Restriction, and Cancer
Ed. Anne McTiernan; 2011

Vol. 4: Energy Balance and Gastrointestinal Cancer
Ed. Sanford D. Markowitz, Nathan A. Berger; 2012

Vol. 5: Energy Balance and Hematologic Malignancies
Ed. Steven D. Mittelman, Nathan A. Berger; 2012**

Vol. 6: Exercise, Energy Balance, and Cancer
Ed. Cornelia M. Ulrich, Karen Steindorf, Nathan A. Berger; 2013

Vol. 7: Obesity, Inflammation, and Cancer
Ed. Andrew J. Dannenberg, Nathan A. Berger; 2013

Vol. 8: Impact of Sleep and Sleep Disturbances on Obesity and Cancer
Ed. Susan Redline, Nathan A. Berger; 2014

Vol. 9: Impact of Energy Balance on Cancer Disparities
Ed. Deborah Bowen, Gerald V. Denis, Nathan A. Berger; 2014

Vol. 10: Murine Models, Energy Balance, and Cancer
Ed. Nathan A. Berger; 2015

Vol. 11: Epigenetic Mechanisms, Energy Balance, and Cancer
Ed. Nathan A. Berger; 2016

Vol. 12: Adipocytokines, Energy Balance, and Cancer
Ed. Ofer Reizes, Nathan A. Berger; 2017

Vol. 13: Energy Balance and Prostate Cancer
Ed. Elizabeth Platz, Nathan A. Berger, 2017

Vol. 14: Energy Balance and Gynecologic Malignancy
Ed. Karen H. Lu, Ann H. Klopp, Nathan A. Berger; 2017

(Fiuza-Luces et al. 2013, 2015; Sanchis-Gomar et al. 2015; Wang et al. 2013). Interestingly, the Shanghai research project, with Li Li as CWRU PI has been supported by funding from the government of Zhabei District, Shanghai (Wang et al. 2013). Moreover, at CWRU where TREC activities continue without specifically designated NCI funds, there are, nonetheless, several NIH-funded multi-investigator team science spin offs, and successors and funding applications in various stages of development and review. These include the Specialized Program on Research Excellence in GI Malignancies, PI Sandy Markowitz; Barrett's Esophagus Translational Research Network, PI Amitabh Chak; Prevention Research Center for Healthy Neighborhoods, PI Elaine Borowski; Prevention of Functional Decline in Older Breast Cancer Survivors, PI Cynthia Owusu. In addition to those multiple successor programs at CWRU, Susan Redline moved to Harvard where she continued research with the Harvard TREC Center and now continues to focus on genetic epidemiology of sleep disorders and their relation to systemic diseases; Joe Nadeau is now at Pacific Northwest Diabetes Research Institute, where he studies the genetic, epigenetic and systems control of complex traits in mouse models of common human diseases and Leslie Heinberg moved to Cleveland Clinic (CWRU) where she is a CoPI with Phil Schauer and investigators at University of North Carolina, Kent State and Brown University to investigate importance of macrobiome, and behavioral variables on weight loss trajectory in patients undergoing bariatric surgery.

26.11 Conclusions

The following summary highlights some of the principles noted above and lessons learned in retrospect.

Leadership including PI and lead investigators should include scientists with successful academic, research and organizational track records, with broad knowledge base, preferably with commitment to translational and transdisciplinary research, who are willing to push beyond their personal boundaries, willing to share credit with a team, willing to let others conceive ideas and set goals, willing to take and invest the time to educate and develop TD investigators, and willing to serve as spokespersons and advocates for local, institutional and national goals. A bit of charisma and a "can do" inspirational attitude are helpful as well.

As in the case of TREC, leadership was not responsible for selecting the problem, since it was predetermined by NCI. However, in general, when deciding to implement a TD approach, it is important for leadership to ensure that it is not easily solvable by a traditional approach, for providing initial vision, guidance, and strategies, for engaging and involving all participants in developing the TD approach, for identifying opportunities for support, and to promote an environment of trust and openness, where all participants are comfortable that they will be heard, appropriately considered, and credited for their contribution. An important challenge for leadership is to provide opportunities for different institutions and different disciplines to understand and integrate their values, languages, cultures, approaches, and traditions.

Leadership should likewise help to recruit junior faculty and trainees, provide opportunities, and encourage their participation and contribution to TD research and build collaborations using face-to-face meetings and foster participation in national meetings.

Leadership is also responsible for establishing and maintaining an interactive environment, for identifying opportunities for support, to encourage both top down and bottom up approaches, for identifying and fostering early and sustained successes and to assure recognition, both for the group and individuals and to promote individual rewards and advancement.

While leadership played a critical role in conceptualizing, guiding, and establishing the CWRU TREC Center and faculty, trainees and students provided the building blocks, NCI clearly provided the resources to fuel programmatic development, accelerate the research, and overcome the obstacles to TD research. Thus, we thank all the participants who contributed to the success of the CWRU TREC and the overall TREC program. We sincerely appreciate the funding and guidance provided by NCI and we hope that NCI sees the wisdom of sustained support for this type of initiative, especially, since despite significant gains, obesity and lack of physical activity remain major problems with profound impact on cancer morbidity and mortality. Much more remains to be done to even better understand the multiple pathways by which energy balance is linked to cancer, to disrupt the obesity cancer linkage and to promote physical activity as a cancer prevention strategy.

Acknowledgment Supported in part by NCI TREC Grant #U54 CA116867.

References

Abola MV, Thompson CL, Chen Z, Chak A, Berger NA, Kirwan JP, Li L. Serum levels of retinol-binding protein 4 and risk of colon adenoma. Endocr Relat Cancer. 2015;22(2):L1–4. https://doi.org/10.1530/ERC-14-0429.

Balard-Barbash R, Berrigan D, Potischman N, Dowling E. Obesity and cancer epidemiology. In: Berger NA, editor. Cancer and energy balance, epidemiology and overview. 1st ed. New York: Springer; 2010. p. 1–44.

Berger NA, Savvides P, Koroukian SM, Kahana EF, Deimling GT, Rose JH, Bowman KF, Miller RH. Cancer in the elderly. Trans Am Clin Climatol Assoc. 2006;117:147–55; discussion 155–6

Brethauer SA, Aminian A, Romero-Talamás H, Batayyah E, Mackey J, Kennedy L, Kashyap SR, Kirwan JP, Rogula T, Kroh M, Chand B, Schauer PR. Can diabetes be surgically cured? Long-term metabolic effects of bariatric surgery in obese patients with type 2 diabetes mellitus. Ann Surg. 2013;258(4):628–36; discussion 636–7. https://doi.org/10.1097/SLA.0b013e3182a5034b.

Calle EE, Thun MJ, Petrelli JM, Rodriguez C, Heath CW Jr. Body-mass index and mortality in a prospective cohort of U.S. adults. N Engl J Med. 1999;341(15):1097–105.

Calle EE, Rodriguez C, Walker-Thurmond K, Thun MJ. Overweight, obesity, and mortality from cancer in a prospectively studied cohort of U.S. adults. N Engl J Med. 2003;348(17):1625–38.

Catalano PM, Huston L, Amini SB, Kalhan SC. Longitudinal changes in glucose metabolism during pregnancy in obese women with normal glucose tolerance and gestational diabetes mellitus. Am J Obstet Gynecol. 1999;180(4):903–16. 26.

Chak A, Ochs-Balcom H, Falk G, Grady WM, Kinnard M, Willis JE, Elston R, Eng C. Familiality in Barrett's esophagus, adenocarcinoma of the esophagus, and adenocarcinoma of the gastroesophageal junction. Cancer Epidemiol Biomarkers Prev. 2006;15(9):1668–73.

Chak A, Buttar NS, Foster NR, Seisler DK, Marcon NE, Schoen R, Cruz-Correa MR, Falk GW, Sharma P, Hur C, Katzka DA, Rodriguez LM, Richmond E, Sharma AN, Smyrk TC, Mandrekar SJ, Limburg PJ, Cancer Prevention Network. Metformin does not reduce markers of cell proliferation in esophageal tissues of patients with Barrett's esophagus. Clin Gastroenterol Hepatol. 2015;13(4):665–72.e1–4. https://doi.org/10.1016/j.cgh.2014.08.040.

Cheng X, Guo S, Liu Y, Chu H, Hakimi P, Berger NA, Hanson RW, Kao HY. Ablation of promyelocytic leukemia protein (PML) re-patterns energy balance and protects mice from obesity induced by a Western diet. J Biol Chem. 2013;288(41):29746–59. https://doi.org/10.1074/jbc.M113.487595.

Dimitropoulos A, Schultz RT. Food-related neural circuitry in Prader-Willi syndrome: response to high- versus low-calorie foods. J Autism Dev Disord. 2008;38(9):1642–53. https://doi.org/10.1007/s10803-008-0546-x.

Distler AM, Kerner J, Peterman SM, Hoppel CL. A targeted proteomic approach for the analysis of rat liver mitochondrial outer membrane proteins with extensive sequence coverage. Anal Biochem. 2006;356(1):18–29.

Doerner SK, Reis ES, Leung ES, Ko JS, Heaney JD, Berger NA, Lambris JD, Nadeau JH. High-fat diet-induced complement activation mediates intestinal inflammation and neoplasia, independent of obesity. Mol Cancer Res. 2016;14(10):953–65.

Donato LJ, Suh JH, Noy N. Suppression of mammary carcinoma cell growth by retinoic acid: the cell cycle control gene Btg2 is a direct target for retinoic acid receptor signaling. Cancer Res. 2007;67(2):609–15.

Fink SP, Yang DH, Barnholtz-Sloan JS, Ryu YM, Mikkola D, Potter JD, Lampe JW, Markowitz SD, Myung SJ. Colonic 15-PGDH levels are stable across distance and time and are not perturbed by aspirin intervention. Dig Dis Sci. 2013;58(9):2615–22. https://doi.org/10.1007/s10620-013-2670-5.

Fiuza-Luces C, Garatachea N, Berger NA, Lucia A. Exercise is the real polypill. Physiology (Bethesda). 2013;28(5):330–58. https://doi.org/10.1152/physiol.00019.2013.

Fiuza-Luces C, Garatachea N, Simpson RJ, Berger NA, Ramírez M, Lucia A. Understanding graft-versus-host disease. Preliminary findings regarding the effects of exercise in affected patients. Exerc Immunol Rev. 2015;21:80–112.

Fiuza-Luces C, Simpson RJ, Ramírez M, Lucia A, Berger NA. Physical function and quality of life in patients with chronic GvHD: a summary of preclinical and clinical studies and a call for exercise intervention trials in patients. Bone Marrow Transplant. 2016;51(1):13–26. https://doi.org/10.1038/bmt.2015.195.

Friedenreich CM. Physical activity and cancer prevention: from observational to intervention research. Cancer Epidemiol Biomarkers Prev. 2001;10(4):287–301.

Grady WM, Markowitz SD. Genetic and epigenetic alterations in colon cancer. Annu Rev Genomics Hum Genet. 2002;3:101–28.

Gray-McGuire C, Guda K, Adrianto I, Lin CP, Natale L, Potter JD, Newcomb P, Poole EM, Ulrich CM, Lindor N, Goode EL, Fridley BL, Jenkins R, Le Marchand L, Casey G, Haile R, Hopper J, Jenkins M, Young J, Buchanan D, Gallinger S, Adams M, Lewis S, Willis J, Elston R, Markowitz SD, Wiesner GL. Confirmation of linkage to and localization of familial colon cancer risk haplotype on chromosome 9q22. Cancer Res. 2010;70(13):5409–18. https://doi.org/10.1158/0008-5472.CAN-10-0188.

Hakimi P, Yang J, Casadesus G, Massillon D, Tolentino-Silva F, Nye CK, Cabrera ME, Hagen DR, Utter CB, Baghdy Y, Johnson DH, Wilson DL, Kirwan JP, Kalhan SC, Hanson RW. Overexpression of the cytosolic form of phosphoenolpyruvate carboxykinase (GTP) in skeletal muscle repatterns energy metabolism in the mouse. J Biol Chem. 2007;282(45):32844–55.

Ievers-Landis CE, Jelalian E. Novel frameworks for understanding pediatric obesity. J Dev Behav Pediatr. 2013;34(8):539–40. https://doi.org/10.1097/01.DBP.0000436477.92552.86.28.

Kalhan SC, Bier DM. Protein and amino acid metabolism in the human newborn. Annu Rev Nutr. 2008;28:389–410. https://doi.org/10.1146/annurev.nutr.28.061807.155333.

Li L, Yu H, Schumacher F, Casey G, Witte JS. Relation of serum insulin-like growth factor-I (IGF-I) and IGF binding protein-3 to risk of prostate cancer (United States). Cancer Causes Control. 2003;14(8):721–6.

Maywald RL, Doerner SK, Pastorelli L, De Salvo C, Benton SM, Dawson EP, Lanza DG, Berger NA, Markowitz SD, Lenz HJ, Nadeau JH, Pizarro TT, Heaney JD. IL-33 activates tumor stroma to promote intestinal polyposis. Proc Natl Acad Sci U S A. 2015;112(19):E2487–96. https://doi.org/10.1073/pnas.1422445112.

Moore SM, Jones L, Alemi F. Family self-tailoring: applying a systems approach to improving family healthy living behaviors. Nurs Outlook. 2016;64(4):306–11. https://doi.org/10.1016/j.outlook.2016.05.006.

Nock NL, Li L, Larkin EK, Patel SR, Redline S. Empirical evidence for "syndrome Z": a hierarchical 5-factor model of the metabolic syndrome incorporating sleep disturbance measures. Sleep. 2009;32(5):615–22.

Nock NL, Owusu C, Kullman EL, Austin K, Roth B, Cerne S, Harmon C, Moore H, Vargo M, Hergenroeder P, Malone H, Rocco M, Tracy R, Lazarus HM, Kirwan JP, Heyman E, Berger NA. A community-based exercise and support group program in African-American breast cancer survivors (ABCs). J Phys Ther Health Promot. 2013;1(1):15–24.

Nock NL, Dimitropoulos A, Rao SM, Flask CA, Schluchter M, Zanotti KM, Rose PG, Kirwan JP, Alberts J. Rationale and design of REWARD (revving-up exercise for sustained weight loss by altering neurological reward and drive): a randomized trial in obese endometrial cancer survivors. Contemp Clin Trials. 2014;39(2):236–45. https://doi.org/10.1016/j.cct.2014.08.008.

Nock NL, Owusu C, Flocke S, Krejci SA, Kullman EL, Austin K, Bennett B, Cerne S, Harmon C, Moore H, Vargo M, Hergenroeder P, Malone H, Rocco M, Tracy R, Lazarus HM, Kirwan JP, Heyman E, Berger NA. A community-based exercise and support group program improves quality of life in African-American breast cancer survivors: a quantitative and qualitative analysis. Int J Sports Exerc Med. 2015;1(3):020.

Noy N, Li L, Abola MV, Berger NA. Is retinol binding protein 4 a link between adiposity and cancer? Horm Mol Biol Clin Invest. 2015;23(2):39–46. https://doi.org/10.1515/hmbci-2015-0019.

Punjabi NM, Shahar E, Redline S, Gottlieb DJ, Givelber R, Resnick HE, Sleep Heart Health Study Investigators.

Sleep-disordered breathing, glucose intolerance, and insulin resistance: the Sleep Heart Health Study. Am J Epidemiol. 2004;160(6):521–30.

Redline S, Berger NA. Impact of sleep disturbances on obesity and cancer. New York: Springer; 2014.

Redline S, Pack AI. Rising to meet an unmet public health need: sleep medicine and the pulmonary community. Am J Respir Crit Care Med. 2006;174(5):487–8. 25.

Reineke EL, Liu H, Lam M, Liu Y, Kao HY. Aberrant association of promyelocytic leukemia protein-retinoic acid receptor-alpha with coactivators contributes to its ability to regulate gene expression. J Biol Chem. 2007;282(25):18584–96.

Sanchis-Gomar F, Lucia A, Yvert T, Ruiz-Casado A, Pareja-Galeano H, Santos-Lozano A, Fiuza-Luces C, Garatachea N, Lippi G, Bouchard C, Berger NA. Physical inactivity and low fitness deserve more attention to alter cancer risk and prognosis. Cancer Prev Res (Phila). 2015;8(2):105–10. https://doi.org/10.1158/1940-6207.CAPR-14-0320.

Shi H, Akunuru S, Bierman JC, Hodge KM, Mitchell MC, Foster MT, Seeley RJ, Reizes O. Diet-induced obese mice are leptin insufficient after weight reduction. Obesity (Silver Spring). 2009;17(9):1702–9. https://doi.org/10.1038/oby.2009.106.

Singer JB, Hill AE, Burrage LC, Olszens KR, Song J, Justice M, O'Brien WE, Conti DV, Witte JS, Lander ES, Nadeau JH. Genetic dissection of complex traits with chromosome substitution strains of mice. Science. 2004;304(5669):445–8.

Stegemann R, Buchner DA. Transgenerational inheritance of metabolic disease. Semin Cell Dev Biol. 2015;43:131–40. https://doi.org/10.1016/j.semcdb.2015.04.007.

Thompson CL, Li L. Association of sleep duration and breast cancer OncotypeDX recurrence score. Breast Cancer Res Treat. 2012;134(3):1291–5. https://doi.org/10.1007/s10549-012-2144-z.

Thompson CL, Khiani V, Chak A, Berger NA, Li L. Carbohydrate consumption and esophageal cancer:an ecological assessment. Am J Gastroenterol. 2008;103(3):555–61.

Thompson CL, Larkin EK, Patel S, Berger NA, Redline S, Li L. Short duration of sleep increases risk of colorectal adenoma. Cancer. 2011;117(4):841–7. https://doi.org/10.1002/cncr.25507.

Thompson CL, Owusu C, Nock NL, Li L, Berger NA. Race, age, and obesity disparities in adult physical activity levels in breast cancer patients and controls. Front Public Health. 2014;2:150. eCollection 2014. https://doi.org/10.3389/fpubh.2014.00150.

Vogel AL, Stipelman BA, Hall KL, Nebeling L, Stokols D, Spruijt-Metz D. Pioneering the transdisciplinary team science approach: lessons learned from national cancer institute grantees. J Transl Med Epidemiol. 2014;2(2):1027.

Wang GR, Li L, Pan YH, Tian GD, Lin WL, Li Z, Chen ZY, Gong YL, Kikano GE, Stange KC, Ni KL, Berger NA. Prevalence of metabolic syndrome among urban community residents in China. BMC Public Health. 2013;13:599. https://doi.org/10.1186/1471-2458-13-5.

Yang X, Li M, Haghiac M, Catalano PM, O'Tierney-Ginn P, Hauguel-de Mouzon S. Causal relationship between obesity-related traits and TLR4-driven responses at the maternal-fetal interface. Diabetologia. 2016;59(11):2459–66. https://doi.org/10.1007/s00125-016-4073-6.

Zheng Q, Dunlap SM, Zhu J, Downs-Kelly E, Rich J, Hursting SD, Berger NA, Reizes O. Leptin deficiency suppresses MMTV-Wnt-1 mammary tumor growth in obese mice and abrogates tumor initiating cell survival. Endocr Relat Cancer. 2011;18(4):491–503. https://doi.org/10.1530/ERC-11-0102.

Zheng Q, Banaszak L, Fracci S, Basali D, Dunlap SM, Hursting SD, Rich JN, Hjlemeland AB, Vasanji A, Berger NA, Lathia JD, Reizes O. Leptin receptor maintains cancer stem-like properties in triple negative breast cancer cells. Endocr Relat Cancer. 2013;20(6):797–808. https://doi.org/10.1530/ERC-13-0329.

The Interdisciplinary Executive Scientist: Connecting Scientific Ideas, Resources and People

27

Christine Ogilvie Hendren
and Sharon Tsai-hsuan Ku

Contents

27.1 Introduction

We invest in research as a society in order to generate knowledge—often, knowledge that will be useful for solving complex challenges, improving the human condition, and navigating competing constraints. Marked increases in cluster funding and interdisciplinary organizational designs reflect a growing recognition that many of our most critical research needs require us to assimilate complex information and harness expertise that spans boundaries in multiple directions, including disciplines and sectors.

This growing focus on interdisciplinary science is evidenced in a multitude of new centers for grand scientific challenges including sustainable energy generation, sustainable agriculture, water treatment and availability, translational medical efforts, and risk forecasting of emerging technologies. These organizations and projects have been funded with the specific aim of bringing together interdisciplinary and inter-sectoral teams to apply their collective expertise to research on these complex topics, often serving multiple goals of advancing basic science as well as policy guidance.

Within these efforts lies an explicit recognition of critical connections between the moving parts of the team, but often also an implicit assumption that these connections will be successfully made by the individuals residing within those moving parts. In other words, in the typical box and arrow diagram depicting teams, the boxes represent the disciplines and the arrows signify the knowledge flow between disciplines. The experts assigned to the team reside within the boxes, whereas nobody is explicitly assigned to the arrows. This chapter is about a class of professional we call an Interdisciplinary Executive Scientist (IES), whose expertise and career path is defined by being those connective arrows.

The set of responsibilities that must be navigated by an IES can range widely and often overlap with other established roles. Several key aspects of practicing interdisciplinarity in a role

C. O. Hendren (✉)
Department of Civil & Environmental Engineering, Duke University, Durham, NC, USA
e-mail: christine.hendren@duke.edu

S. T. Ku
Department of Engineering, University of Virginia, Charlottesville, VA, USA

© Springer Nature Switzerland AG 2019
K. L. Hall et al. (eds.), *Strategies for Team Science Success*,
https://doi.org/10.1007/978-3-030-20992-6_27

that operates at the interstices of organizations include constant cross-boundary communication, project leadership and management, research, administration, and outreach to a variety of constituents. These requirements result in an integrated workload that includes management of both scientific and interpersonal issues, and importantly, spans tasks that would fall across multiple levels of hierarchy within a typical research organization. A key goal of this chapter is to better articulate the particular mix of expertise necessary to act at the boundaries of many different disciplines and institutional placements, which entails balancing work for a diverse array of people with different roles and institutions, and is essential to maximizing the output from scientific endeavors at the boundaries of disciplines.

It is particularly important to articulate value contributions from the work of an IES because it is challenging to demonstrate counter-examples or quantify the productivity that may be left on the table in the absence of such a role. This is true in part because research teams in need of IES roles are tackling complex problems that may in some cases not be addressed by any other teams, anywhere. In those cases, there simply aren't possible comparisons, so there will not be opportunities to look back and see how teams performed with or without an individual assigned to make connections and facilitate knowledge flow across boundaries. And in part, articulating the value of IES work is difficult because so much of the contribution arises by nature within interactions rather than standing alone as explicit tasks. These include listening to and diagnosing disconnects between team members that lie at the root of frustrations; developing a strategy to bring both parties to a better mutual understanding; and brokering discussions and changes needed to bridge the disconnect. Tools and best practices are being developed to intentionally navigate such conversations, but realistically these moments often occur during the course of meetings and communications with other goals. Without intervention, there is a very real risk that the original disconnect could result in a continued misunderstanding resulting in lost time before the issue is addressed, or even the possibility that it is never addressed to the detriment of the greater research effort.

The researchers within individual fields of complex science teams may be preeminent experts in their areas of knowledge. In such a team endeavor, they typically also display a willingness to collaborate with experts across other fields.

Figure 27.1 illustrates an idealized knowledge flow within a generic interdisciplinary team. The boxes represent the disciplines and the arrows signify the knowledge produced within and flowing between disciplines. The researchers involved in each box are considered domain experts in their disciplines; they are undoubtedly named as individuals, whether PIs or project collaborators. In such a team endeavor, domain experts are encouraged to collaborate with experts across other fields, moving their knowledge out of their own box to engage with experts in other boxes. Within this type of framework that we see so commonly in teams lies an explicit recognition of critical connections between each discipline involved in the team. However, notice that there are no names or roles written into the connecting arrows. The idea that demonstrated competence and willingness to collaborate will be sufficient to ensure the type of rich information exchange and knowledge synthesis necessary to fully capitalize on collective expertise belies a naiveté toward the time requirements and specific boundary spanning expertise[1] needed to make such translation and synthesis happen. The implicit assumption in such a diagram is often that these connections will be spontaneously made by the individuals residing within those segments; whereas experts assigned to the team reside within the boxes, typically nobody is explicitly assigned

---

[1] "Boundary spanning expertise" is a term originating from social science and organizational management literature beginning with Tushman (1977). The expression began within theories of innovation, referring to the skill-sets necessary for translation and conveyance of knowledge across departments and companies, but the use has since expanded in scope. For our purposes, we use the notion of boundary spanning, and related expertise, to refer to all of the skills inherent in the successful movement of knowledge from one silo to another. These "silos" could include any boundary with the potential to impose an artefactual barrier to seamless knowledge transfer, including boundaries across: disciplinary domains, sector cultures (government, academia, advocacy, commerce), stages of career hierarchy, or institutional sub-units.

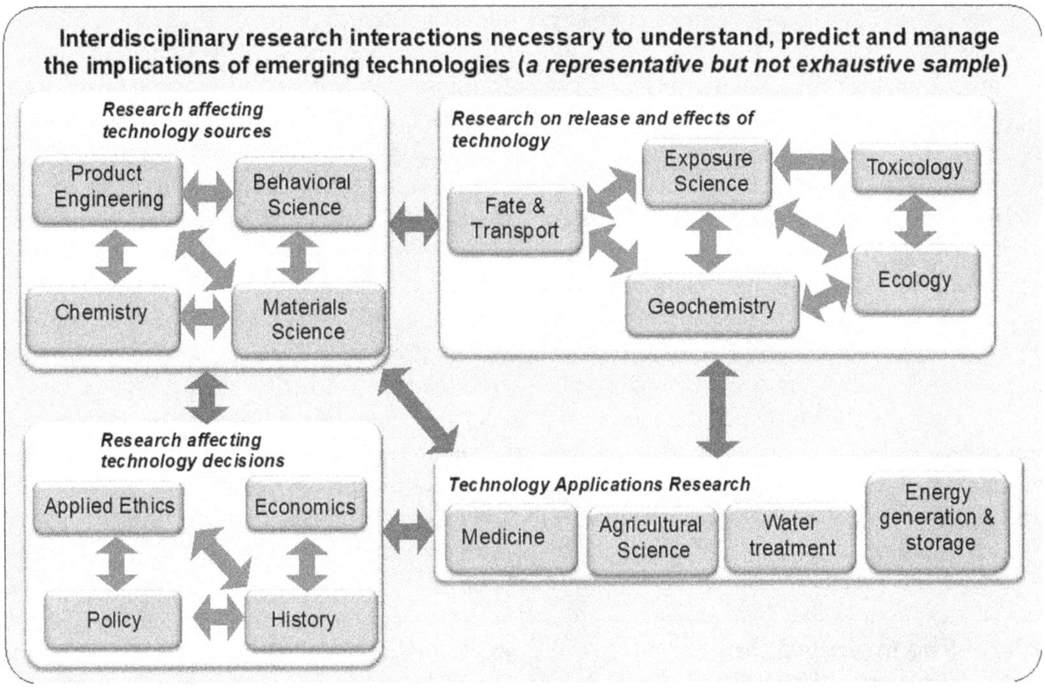

Fig. 27.1 Generic interdisciplinary team schematic illustrating the anonymity and implicit assumptions of boundary-spanning knowledge transfer in teams

to the arrows. Indeed, the tagline for Intereach (Interdisciplinary Integration Research Careers Hub), the community of practice and research for roles dedicated to spanning the boundaries in complex teams, is simply: Be The Arrow.

In the absence of an acknowledged and dedicated professional assigned to integration, synthesis, translation, and cross-boundary coordination, how do these activities currently happen? Sometimes, they simply don't. In smaller groups, perhaps these boundary activities may be taken on by one or more project leaders with the skills and disposition to address these needs as they become apparent. Sometimes the boundary spanning needs may align well with the individual's disciplinary expertise, or fall within standard project management activities inherent to directing a multi-person effort. In more complex organizations, basic coordination activities may be carried out suboptimally by participating researchers at the expense of their "real" responsibilities, with a series of diffusely distributed or ad hoc tasks.

Should we only acknowledge and invest funding in building domain expertise with the idea of training domain experts to translate and interpret research across boundaries, or is there equal value in acknowledging and supporting boundary work defined by those connective arrows, and cultivating professionals to supply boundary expertise? How do we conceptualize such boundary work and boundary expertise such that they appear alongside other domain experts as named roles in our mental models of successful interdisciplinary collaboration teams?

We assert that a need exists to acknowledge and consider boundary-spanning roles and possible career paths from multiple different vantage points, including:

- Interdisciplinary practice from the organization perspective—how do we structure and plan collaborations in relation to boundary-spanning activities?
- Interdisciplinary practice from the human resource perspective—how do we staff our teams so that these boundary-spanning tasks are explicitly owned?
- Funding policy around interdisciplinary efforts—how does a funding body request,

evaluate, and extract value from boundary-spanning roles and tasks?

- Funding policy from the human resource perspective—who pays "the arrows"?

This chapter focuses on articulating the work and the value of spanning such boundaries. Here we discuss a hybrid set of responsibilities within a class of professionals we call Interdisciplinary Executive Scientists (IES), whose expertise and career path are defined by operating to manifest those cross-boundary arrows, enabling synthesis of better collective science outcomes. The functions, skillset, and challenges of IES deserve a full articulation to inform infrastructure building and human resource management in team science.

27.2 The Interdisciplinary Executive Scientist Role

27.2.1 Defining IES

An Interdisciplinary Executive Scientist (IES) requires a mixture of specialized project management skills, deep fluency in the type of scientific problem being addressed, and skills and training in interdisciplinary science approaches. Like the chapter in this volume by Carter, Carlson, Crockett, et al. on Research Development Professionals (RDP), and like previous discussions of the traditional academic career role of Integration and Implementation Specialist (I2S) (Bammer 2012), this chapter asserts that the definition and support of a career path is critically important to successful team science outcomes. However, while the I2S and RDP roles have been defined and discussed in a number of prior publications(Bammer 2012; Bammer 2016; Bass and Stogdill 1990), and there are developing communities of individuals who identify with these roles (Bennett et al. 2010; National Research Council 2015), this chapter focuses on a closely related role that is only very recently being defined—a set of leadership, administrative, and research tasks focused on the *boundary work* at the interface of

different research units.[2] IES practitioners apply and expand integrative methodologies to create an epistemic and social space where cross-boundary intellectual exchange and communication can be planned, executed, and managed. In other words, IES practitioners do not take the existing disciplinary or institutional boundaries as a *given*; instead, they actively participate in boundary negotiation, spanning, and stabilization among the involved disciplines, and between the research centers and the external stakeholders, creating an inreach–outreach balance to execute the intellectual commitment made by the center directors or PIs. They share many of these dynamic integration responsibilities with I2S and RDP practitioners, but the role also carries a lasting organizational tie to the interdisciplinary team and its specific collective mission that spans the duration of the team science research initiative and includes leadership and management. The expression of these integrative methodologies, the driving success metrics of the position, and the scope of the managerial functions differ widely across those who have thus far self-identified as the IES role, but some broad categories are shared. Though the IES role was recently named, there are multiple extant rich sources of literature to be drawn upon as this class of professionals coalesces and seeks to better define and optimize the role, including organizational psychology, management, sociology, and social ecology. Some of these resources are tapped throughout this chapter, and many further opportunities exist to draw together existing knowledge with the community of IES practitioners who need its insight (Box 27.1).

Currently, efforts are underway to explore and further define the IES role on its own and in relation to its "cousin" roles mentioned above. A

----

[2]Here we borrow the concept "boundary work" from the Science Studies literature, which defines boundary work as boundary work as the "attribution of selected characteristics to an institution of science (i.e., to its practitioners, methods, stock of knowledge, values and work organization) for purposes of constructing a social boundary that distinguishes some intellectual activities as outside that boundary." (Farr-Wharton and Brunetto 2009; Gieryn 1983)

Box 27.1 IES Competencies

The IES career path can be linked to a stand-alone body of knowledge to develop boundary-spanning experts with competency around:

- Translation skills between a diverse group of scientists
- Effective knowledge synthesis between disciplines
- Balancing intellectual leadership with key administrative responsibilities between disciplines

workshop devoted to the formation of a community of practice for IES, I2S, and RDP roles, held at the 2016 Science of Team Science (SciTS) conference, kicked off the foundation of a community of practice with an associated listserv called the Interdisciplinary Integration Research Careers Hub (Intereach),[3] which will be discussed further later in the chapter. In addition to drawing upon relevant literature and accumulated experiences across multiple exploratory research panels and workshops(Gieryn 1999; Goleman 1998), ideas put forth in this chapter will include insight from interactions and early surveys of the approximately 50 attendees of the 2016 workshop, the approximately 60 attendees of the 2017 workshop, and the approximately 350 subscribers (at the time of this chapter publication) to the Intereach listserv (Hendren 2015). Future efforts will continue to crystallize similarities, distinctions, and shared needs across the three roles.

---

[3] The Interdisciplinary Integration Research Careers Hub (Intereach) listserv provides a mechanism for communication for those interested in a community of practice around the interdisciplinary and integrative functions critical to team research, steeped in the valuable knowledge offered from team science research, and informed by administrative and institutional insights. It is maintained at Duke University, and is open to all interested stakeholders globally.

27.2.2 IES Functions and Skills

Broadly speaking, an Interdisciplinary Executive Scientist role is characterized by three classes of key functions: epistemic, managerial, and interpersonal. It is the combination of these three aspects that defines the IES role in a meaningful way as distinct from the cousin roles of I2S or RDP.

27.2.2.1 Epistemic Functions

Individuals acting in an IES role are often viewed as research administrators, or may be confused with RDP (less frequently with I2S). We argue this confusion can be clarified in part by examining the epistemic functions IES offers to team science in the context of the hybrid research and managerial task set. We leverage the SciTS literature as an explanatory tool to justify the epistemic functions and values IES bring into the team.

The job of an IES is to carry out the "boundary work" assigned to the connecting arrows seen in Fig. 27.1, by creating social and technical infrastructures that make domain knowledge and information travelable, shareable, and communicable, and then navigating these infrastructures to lead the process of synthesizing this knowledge. A key point of this chapter is to express that although coordination is a key role of the IES, so is knowledge making. Sharing and synthesizing knowledge across boundaries depends on more than simply a transfer of facts. The backdrop of what information is necessary, how we know that we have this information, and the language and disciplinary cultures employed to communicate these aspects are just as critical as high quality information within the participating disciplinary knowledge domains. In other words, IES practitioners do not just move ready-made knowledge from A to B, or simply act as a facilitator or cheerleader advocating collaboration but remaining peripheral to the knowledge production process. Rather, they carry administrative and managerial duties but also participate actively as knowledge makers, negotiating and navigating epistemic boundaries to shape the process and products of interdisciplinary collaboration.

Performing epistemic boundary work demands specific skills, as well as time and resource investment. The concept of "epistemic cultures" proposed by Knorr-Cetina (1999) offers a theoretical foundation to explain the practice of interdisciplinarity and justify the epistemic functions performed by the IES. She argues that different scientific fields exhibit different epistemic cultures constituted by their preferred theories, experiments, peer review systems, or other technical and social standards. This further suggests that what an IES faces is not just communication issues among individual scientists; rather, they are dealing with the issue of "incommensurability (Hughes and Terrell 2009)" among different epistemic cultures. Their epistemic functions are demonstrated through identifying and inventing shared research questions, terminology, methods, or guiding visions across different domains of expertise or disciplines, utilizing them as "bridges" to connect various "cultures of knowing," making them coexist harmoniously and complementarily.

Beyond discipline-based boundary work, an IES may be called upon to translate between researchers and external stakeholders to the individual or combined scientific outcomes. Such "macro-epistemics" (Knorr-Cetina 2007) underscores another critical aspect of an IES' epistemic function: the importance of orienting the synthesized knowledge and its communication outwardly from the research body to broader networks of stakeholders, including government, industry, advocacy groups, and various publics. The administrative functions of an IES in an ongoing capacity throughout the duration of the organization means that they play the role of a dynamic boundary spanner who constantly redraws, renegotiates, and tests the boundary between the research center and external societal knowledge stakeholders.

27.2.2.2 Managerial Functions

In the current way of thinking about the IES role, the administrative project and team management functions of an IES make up a primary distinc-

tion between this and other integrative roles. The kind of management and leadership associated with an IES often differs from the primary Project Director or lead Principal Investigator (PI) position as recognized by the funding body within large team science projects. These primary Project Director or PI roles are often performed by senior scientists with internationally recognized expertise and significant leadership experiences, but who typically are not directly involved in performing the research or the administration.[4] An IES may be brought into the team, reporting to the project director, with a title such as Executive Director or Managing Director. For an IES, the epistemic functions keep them and their work closer to the detailed execution of project activities, by directly engaging with the research strategy, design, and execution. However, in addition they also perform high-level managerial work codirecting teams with the primary directors, coordinating intellectual and sometimes social activities within the organization, and exploring new partnerships with external stakeholders.

Some of these managerial functions, such as convening meetings, identifying mutually interesting research questions and conversations that need to happen in a timely manner to advance research goals, are not vastly different from those of an RDP. The primary difference lies in the fact that IES support begins post-award and includes embedded, active participation in the generation of the resulting scientific work products, whereas the RDP often participates more heavily (or exclusively) in assembling teams and pre-award team science support.

The level of intellectual leadership and authority conferred on an IES is a matter of wide variability thus far. Typically IES practitioners identify as the only individual within their organization that holds this type of position, often reporting that they have "created their own job", organically growing the job description and responsibilities to fit the otherwise unmet needs

---

[4]For example, Oppenheimer who led the Manhattan Project (Knorr-Cetina 2007); James Watson who led NIH Human Genome Project.

of facilitating the operations of the organization. A wide variety of managerial responsibilities may be included in these positions. Some IESs carry budgetary, event planning, and/or laboratory management. Many seem to shoulder administrative reporting responsibilities. Some also take responsibility for leading research groups within their organization or acting as a chair in national or international research fora. Drawing on input from the Intereach workshops held at the 2016 and 2017 SciTS Conferences, self-identified IESs have indicated that communication between different parts of a broader organization falls within their role. In some cases, the person is also responsible for defining tasks and milestones and holding team members accountable (or at least informed of the status) for their particular project areas.

The organic origin story of many of these roles means that an IES often provides complementary leadership and managerial functions to execute the authority of a more highly ranked director position, but does so from a service standpoint rather than an understood position of authority. Because the project director is often a person with very high scientific status, and may have multiple leadership positions as well as a heavy travel schedule, he or she typically is not involved in the center's daily routine practice. Many people acting in an IES role sit in staff or research administration roles, rather than principal investigator roles.

The dynamics of this leadership model can sometimes put an IES in a position of uncertainty in terms of role, responsibility, and status, which in turn can affect one's ability to clearly target and evaluate success. This administrative functions included in the scope of IES activities can create a status-based cultural boundary within academia, aligning the IES more closely with what faculty researchers recognize as a staff role than that of a peer contributor to the intellectual leadership of the team as a whole. A common report from people in the IES role is that with regard to the managerial functions, they often hold responsibility without authority. Their administrative and coordinating responsibilities consume a significant enough portion of their

time that they have diminished time to publish in the peer-reviewed literature. For some in an IES role, staying "academically viable" by maintaining a publication record is not a concern and thus diminished publications do not present an issue. For others, the dual responsibilities of carrying out managerial functions and associated organizational activities as well as conducting research and writing publications, whether as a success metric or as a hedge against the impermanence of these roles, presents a tension. Navigating this perceived status boundary and competing priorities is a nontrivial aspect of succeeding in the IES role, and effective approaches to doing so can be heavily dependent on individual personalities and organizational cultures. This represents a rich area for future research and practical exploration within communities of practice.

27.2.2.3 Emotional/Interpersonal Functions

Communication across boundaries requires more than epistemic understanding and adept management. As with all communication between humans, navigating these channels requires emotional and interpersonal navigation. In terms of team science success, emotional intelligence, and skills have been proven to play an equally important role as technical expertise (Knorr-Cetina 1999). Scholars of public organizations have begun to examine the role of broad interpersonal skills, such as empathy, social skills, and tact, in team building and evaluating leadership effectiveness (Levin 2011; Mørk et al. 2008). Possessing emotional and social skills was also associated with higher quality social relationships and more supportive social support systems (National Organization of Research Development Professionals n.d.; Newell 2001; Riggio and Zimmerman 1991). These aspects are particularly important for large-scale interdisciplinary collaborations, where disciplinary hierarchies and tensions are hard to avoid. In the National Institutes of Health (NIH) published field guide on Collaboration & Team Science, emotional preparedness is recognized as an important quality of team building (Riggio and Reichard 2008). However, in most science-focused centers, researchers are not formally encouraged to examine their emotional reactions and the role emotions and dispositions can play in navigating communication and scientific outcomes. As a result, these issues can become like the proverbial elephant in the room: obviously influential to the way a research team functions, but seldom discussed or explicitly appreciated. With the distribution of responsibilities between PIs and the groups they lead, it is often students and postdoctoral fellows who serve as the frontline researchers executing collaborative projects, and staff who carry out daily coordination and infrastructural support for loosely organized research teams.

IESs with their hybrid professional identity of faculty/staff/researcher witness these interpersonal and emotional dimensions of interdisciplinary collaboration. During the discussion at the SciTS 2016 Conference workshop on the roles of the IES, I2S, and RDP, many participants expressed that interdisciplinarity ultimately is an issue about people. The extent to which team members are willing to open the disciplinary boundaries and be accommodating and integrative to other epistemic cultures very much depends on the level of personal trust between them. Facilitating trust-building is a part of the IES role that could be optimized with the development and training of best practices, allowing for a shift from what is currently a more ad-hoc application of tacit knowledge toward more intentional emotional navigation.

Psychologist Daniel Goleman (1998) suggested that emotional intelligence among leaders might be more important than how smart they are otherwise (Riggio et al. 1993). For the IES role, though indeed the emotional/interpersonal functions are key aspects of effective performance as an intellectual leader, it is important to note that in this case the emotional skillset must be fully integrated with the epistemic functions for success. This means that an IES must function as more than an emotionally intelligent facilitator; deep domain knowledge and organizational familiarity are required as well. The translational tasks necessary to span boundaries require that in addition to excellent communication skills and the ability to listen and receive feedback, the IES brings a specific transdisciplinary knowledge base to understand to recognize potential disconnects that may be barring effective translation. This knowledge can include insights into the nuances beneath different knowledge claims, how different fields use the same language differently, or when to elevate useful opinions across hierarchical diversity which might otherwise be obfuscated by power dynamics (such as technicians' experience). Some IESs also work with social scientists connecting the emotional aspects to broader societal issues and scientists' social responsibilities within the research team, gleaning insight from ethnographic methodologies and the broader comparative understanding these methods can provide.

The interpersonal/emotional management an IES offers a team can build both personal and scientific trust among the team members, and provide a conduit for effective communication across disciplines and across the hierarchical spectrum in the organization.

27.3   Challenges and Inefficiencies

The critical role of the IES brings up a series of challenges to current knowledge infrastructures and human resource processes implemented in interdisciplinary research centers. Often, if such integrative work is being done, it is carried out by people who are providing invisible leadership from a supporting or administrative role within the organizational hierarchy, commonly characterized by having responsibility without authority. In many cases, these roles will be unique to the organization, and will grow organically to fill in the unmet needs of the particular team science endeavor. While the person in such a role may be a critical part of the organizational functions and be personally appreciated, their career path may be unclear.

Based on our interviews with many research scientists with IES positions in academia, long-term job insecurity is a primary issue. These people often hold a PhD in sciences or engineering, and must often perform academic duties such as publishing and supervising students or postdoctoral fellows to remain academically viable within an established field, while at the same time devoting most of their efforts to their jobs in the IES role. Currently, this represents a tension common within this class of jobs.

One solution to this conundrum is articulated in the establishment of the previously mentioned discipline of Integration and Implementation Sciences (I2S), where publications and grants are undertaken specifically on the integrative work and knowledge synthesis contributed by the I2S specialist. For the IES though, with additional managerial and administrative duties that are often tied to a temporary funding scenario, the experience, skills, and technical and social networks they pour a large portion of their time and energy into building will not be preserved once their contracts end with the termination of project funding.

In addition, their success metrics are often tied solely to the satisfaction of their direct supervisor, and they may lack the broader support and the training and best practice resources of a defined specialization. Left unnamed, the work of this class of boundary spanning professional can be diminished to a list of the outwardly visible tasks, without an understanding of the value added by the tacit knowledge and the intellectual scaffolding provided by their contributions. And diminished to a list of tasks, while the individual domain experts reap the benefits of the synthesized knowledge, the work of the IES may be viewed only as a coordinator or facilitator, so that only the administrative functionality is recognized. The development of objective, measurable evaluation metrics represents another rich opportunity for research and for exploration within communities of practice. Leveraged funding, while diffuse in its potential for direct attribution to IES interventions, provides one opportunity. Documentation of individual testimonials from researchers who experience increased efficiency and newly sparked ideas upon working with an IES may represent an opportunity to provide an interim qualitative dataset, as well as a source of ideas for potential impact metrics.

While those functions are crucial for managing a team, they do not capture the intellectual leadership or the specifically critical boundary-spanning expertise necessary to guide and optimize science

outcomes. We must define this skill set and recognize its added value and training needs on a pragmatic level before we can hope to optimize contributions to science outcomes. Further, this career path definition and acceptance is equally important in order to appropriately value and support the individuals in these roles in terms of training, organizational placement, and compensation.

Existing at a boundary, free of definition and beholden to disparate epistemic cultures and power dynamics, creates difficulties and inefficiencies for many who currently hold IES roles. Without an established career path, the support they provide is often invisible support and their intellectual contributions, which may fundamentally shape and build the content of the science outcomes, are often implicitly classified as "service" rather than "science." Further compounding these challenges has been the lack of intentional training or a peer group to draw upon in navigating these tensions.

27.4 Next Steps

This discussion illustrates that there is work to be done establishing definitions, resources, and thriving communities of practice for IESs, and that a first step toward this will be drawing on a rich body of existing expertise as the roles and the career pathways of the IES are developed.

Theoretical constructs born outside of natural science and engineering can be applied to provide concrete, practical utility in defining and training an IES. By channeling concepts from the SciTS literature, applied philosophy, and interdisciplinary studies, we can appreciate the critical role that epistemic environment and cultures play in interdisciplinary scientific endeavors. As boundary spanning experts better understand the epistemic forces at play, we can more artfully and intentionally navigate those boundaries in multiple directions including between disciplines or sectors, within an organization or externally.

Examining team science from the angle of epistemic cultures therefore enables us to address both theoretical and practical questions about team science operation in broad socio-political contexts. It extends the current team science analysis from interdisciplinary activities in academics to "public epistemology" at the interface of science and public policy, and recognizes the common translational skill sets required to successfully span multiple classes of boundaries. Through this lens, the role of the IES is appropriately cast as a powerful actor who brings in multiple societal actors into the process of knowledge generation, creating orders, and cultivating bridges across diverse epistemic cultures.

Among other bodies of insight to draw upon in working across epistemic cultures and knowledge domains is the Association for Interdisciplinary Studies (https://oakland.edu/ais/). Founded in 1979, its core values include exploration of theory and best practices for integrating knowledge across disciplines (Thorpe and Shapin 2000). Useful institutional as well as individual best practices can also be mined from the 2015 National Research Council report, Enhancing the Effectiveness of Team Science (Tushman 1977). The I2S specialist role, more advanced in their process of self-defining but adjacent to the knowledge, skills, and disposition of an IES, can bring a great deal of useful theoretical and practical understanding that can be further developed and applied by IES practitioners (Bammer 2012).

It was with the intention to draw collectively from the expertise of more established boundary-spanning roles of I2S and RDPs, while advancing the understanding of IES career paths, that the Intereach community was founded to pursue the dual missions of:

1. Developing the profession—making the case these roles add value and warrant institutional investment.
2. Professional development—gathering resources and sharing experiences to train and educate those who currently serve in or aspire to hold boundary-spanning roles.

The Intereach community hosts a website (www.intereach.org) and a webinar series focused on advancing both goals. The group has begun with this simple method of open communication between interested members, and it is hoped that this forum provides a path toward coalescing people interested in the IES, I2S, and RDP roles. These three career paths share a great deal in terms of the tacit and explicit knowledge, the skills, and the dispositions of those who are successful in boundary spanning roles. Combining discussion of all three roles in context of a focus on intentional career paths is useful during the current exercise of coalescing and defining particularly the IES role; similarities between the roles provide direct opportunity to leverage knowledge, and differences can help crystalize the identity and needs of IESs.

Future efforts within this group could help address some of the challenges introduced in this chapter, aiding the community in efforts such as:

- Understanding what distinguishes this role from others, and what constitutes a healthy responsibility map.
- Developing metrics for success that transcend stand-alone staff performance reviews.
- Exploring how the value added from this work can be made visible.
- Developing best practices for leveraging the IES role to maximally contribute to the success of the team.
- Collecting and developing training materials to support and grow a future cadre of professionals dedicated to this important integrative work.

References

Association for Interdisciplinary Studies. http://wwwp.oakland.edu/ais.

Bammer G. Disciplining interdisciplinarity: integration and implementation sciences for researching complex real-world problems. Canberra: ANU Press; 2012.

Bammer G. Negotiating boundaries, leadership, and integration and implementation sciences (I2S). J Environ Stud Sci. 2016;6(2):432–6.

Bass BM, Stogdill RM. Bass & Stogdill's handbook of leadership: theory, research, and managerial applications. New York: Simon and Schuster; 1990.

Bennett LM, Gadlin H, Levine-Finley S, Collaboration & team science: a field guide. NIH Office of the Ombudsman, Center for Cooperative Resolution; 2010.

National Research Council. Enhancing the Effectiveness of Team Science. Washington. DC; The National Academies Press. 2015. https://doi.org/10.17226/19007.

Farr-Wharton R, Brunetto Y. Female entrepreneurs as managers: the role of social capital in facilitating a learning culture. Gender in Management: an international journal. 2009;24(1):14–31.

Gieryn TF. Boundary-work and the demarcation of science from non-science: strains and interests in professional ideologies of scientists. Am Sociol Rev. 1983:781–95.

Gieryn TF. Cultural boundaries of science: credibility on the line. Chicago: University of Chicago Press; 1999.

Goleman D. Working with emotional intelligence. New York: Bantam; 1998.

Hendren CO, How an Interdisciplinary Executive Scientist Can Help Enable Effective Team Science. In 6th Annual Science of Team Science Meeting. Bethesda, MD; 2015.

Hughes M Terrell JB, Coaching with emotional and social effectiveness. Handbook for developing emotional and social intelligence: Best practices, case studies, and strategies; 2009: p. 3–20.

Knorr-Cetina K. Epistemic cultures: how the sciences make knowledge. Cambridge: Harvard University Press; 1999.

Knorr-Cetina K. Culture in global knowledge societies: knowledge cultures and epistemic cultures. Interdiscip Sci Rev. 2007;32(4):361–75.

Levin J. The emergence of the research-development professional. In The Chronicle of Higher Education. Washington, D.C.; 2011.

Mørk BE, et al. Conflicting epistemic cultures and obstacles for learning across communities of practice. Knowl Process Manag. 2008;15(1):12–23.

National Organization of Research Development Professionals. http://www.nordp.org/. Accessed 05 June 2018.

Newell WH. A theory of interdisciplinary studies. Issues Integrative Studies. 2001;19(1):1–25.

Riggio RE, Reichard RJ. The emotional and social intelligences of effective leadership: an emotional and social skill approach. J Manag Psychol. 2008;23(2):169–85.

Riggio RE, Zimmerman J. Social skills and interpersonal relationships: influences on social support and support seeking. Adv Personal Relationships. 1991;2:133–55.

Riggio RE, Watring KP, Throckmorton B. Social skills, social support, and psychosocial adjustment. Personal Individ Differ. 1993;15(3):275–80.

The Interdisciplinary Integration Research Careers Hub (Intereach) listserv Established 2016.; https://lists.duke.edu/sympa/subscribe/intereach.

Thorpe C, Shapin S. Who was J. Robert Oppenheimer? Charisma and complex organization. Soc Stud Sci. 2000;30(4):545–90.

Tushman ML. Special boundary roles in the innovation process. Administrative science quarterly; 1977: p. 587–605.

The Role of Research Development Professionals in Supporting Team Science

28

Susan Carter, Susan Carlson, John Crockett,
Holly J. Falk-Krzesinski, Kyle Lewis,
and Barbara Endemaño Walker

Contents

S. Carter (✉)
Santa Fe Institute, Santa Fe, NM, USA
e-mail: scarter@santafe.edu

S. Carlson
Office of the President, University of California, Oakland, CA, USA

J. Crockett
San Diego State University, San Diego, CA, USA

H. J. Falk-Krzesinski
Global Strategic Networks, Elsevier Inc., New York, NY, USA

Philanthropy and Nonprofit Fundraising Program, School of Professional Studies, Northwestern University, Chicago, IL, USA

K. Lewis · B. E. Walker
Technology Management Program, College of Engineering, University of California Santa Barbara, Santa Barbara, CA, USA

During the past decade, partially in response to the increasingly competitive funding climate for extramural scientific research (Levin 2011; AAAS 2013), there has been a significant increase in the number of research and academic institutions that have invested in providing support to faculty in developing research collaborations through the establishment of research development offices (NORDP 2016).

Research development is defined as a set of strategic, proactive, and capacity-building activities designed to facilitate individual faculty members, teams of researchers, and central research administrations in attracting extramural research funding, creating relationships, and developing and implementing strategies that increase institutional competitiveness and facilitate research excellence (Mason and Learned 2006). The professional workforce in research development offices—research development professionals—works directly with faculty to support their efforts to secure extramural research funding and initiate and nurture scientific collaborations within their institutions, among institutions, and with external stakeholders (NORDP website n.d.; Leeming 2016) The basic strategies and roles of research development professionals in advancing research through cross-disciplinary team science are essentially the same across the disciplines, including social and behavioral health research.

Research development as a professional field in its own right is relatively new; however, the scientific literature has long recognized the role of research administration in building and supporting successful collaborations; and there is a small but growing body of literature that focuses specifically on the role played by research development professionals (Mason and Learned 2006; Laughlin and Sigerstad 1990). Facilitation of the expansion of research development strategies, programs, and services can help institutions thrive in an increasingly competitive environment (Mason and Learned 2006). The research development enterprise could also help address the growing importance of teamed scientific collaboration that includes representation from the broader community and external nonacademic institutions in order to address increasingly complex scientific questions (Mason and Learned 2006; Hall et al. 2008).

Several journal articles give detailed descriptions of the service process and outcomes of research development activities (Havermahl et al. 2015); and numerous articles describe and quantify the benefits to the discipline, cross-disciplinary teams, institution, and individual faculty members from the types of activities that are promoted and facilitated by research development professionals, both in the United States and globally (Walker and Pandya-Wood 2015; Dorling et al. 2014; Chung and Shauver 2008; Porter 2009; Porter 2005; Campbell et al. 2013). Research development efforts have existed in the United States for many years, with some institutions providing strategic support for writing extramural research grant proposals and coordinating research teams as early as the 1970s (Levin

2011; NORDP website n.d.). However, there has been rapid growth in the research development profession in recent years, as reflected in the fact that the research development professional association, the National Organization of Research Development Professionals (NORDP) was established as a small grass-roots organization in 2010 with a core group of individuals representing 37 participating institutions, and has since grown to include almost 1000 national and global members (Levin 2011; NORDP website n.d.). Not surprisingly, a large number of the NORDP membership is composed of research development professionals at doctoral granting research institutions; however, an increasing portion of the membership represent predominantly undergraduate institutions, master's granting institutions, hospitals and other nonteaching research institutes, community colleges, and the National Laboratories (NORDP Member database). This diversity among the NORDP membership reflects a growing understanding of the important role of research development at facilitating collaborations across a broad spectrum of research institutions. These research development professionals are sometimes housed in central administrative offices focused only on research development, but a significant number may be affiliated with colleges, departments, or research centers within the institution (NORDP Member database). Twenty-two percent of the NORDP membership indicated that the staff in their affiliated research development office totaled at least five persons, indicating institutional investment in research development efforts, even in times of generalized university budget tightening.

28.1   Credibility and Reputation of the Research Development Professional

The role of the research development professional includes at its core establishing and building relationships to facilitate the development and growth of research collaborations. Research development professionals cultivate influence and effectiveness by maintaining trust and credibility in their academic community. Depending on the type of institution and scope of the research development office, credibility may be obtained in different ways. At some institutions, having knowledge of grant administration activities such as budgeting, online submission portals, and research compliance issues, can enhance the reputation of the research development professional. At other institutions, proven writing and copy-editing skills are considered necessary. At the majority of research intensive, doctoral-granting institutions, disciplinary expertise as demonstrated by a Ph.D. or comparable doctoral degree, research experience, and publications are required to maintain credibility. According to 2010, 2012, and 2015 surveys of members of the National Organization of Research Development Professionals (NORDP), members with a Ph.D. were more likely to have leadership titles in the profession (Director of Research Development or Associate Vice President for Research, for example) than members with a Masters or Bachelor degree respectively (42% of members with a Ph.D. compared to 38% and 15% for members with a Masters or Bachelors respectively). Similarly, members with a doctoral degree garnered approximately 25% higher salaries and were more likely to work at institutions with over $300,000,000 in annual sponsored projects (NORDP website/resources). Moreover, many research development professionals maintain concurrent faculty appointments and may also contribute to the literature of their field and/or serve as key personnel or PIs on relevant externally funded programs. These are indicators that particularly at R-1 institutions, research development professionals are required to have comparable academic experience as the faculty members and teams with whom they work and are expected to provide a high level of scholarly advice along with strategic guidance.

28.2   Role of the Research Development Professional in Creating and Supporting Science Teams

Research Development Professionals (RDPs) play an integral role in identifying, developing, and managing Team Science collaborations both within their own institutions, and between and among institutions. They perform this responsibility through four priority duties:

- Helping institutional scientists build collaborations with other institutional scientists
- Building cross-disciplinary and cross-institutional bridges
- Helping to create cross-disciplinary and cross-field research concepts
- Building relationships with external stakeholders and funders

RDPs can be situated in departments, centers, schools/colleges, or at the campus-wide level. It is part of their job to understand research strengths and clusters, as well as more specific areas of research undertaken by individual faculty members. With such knowledge, they are in a position to understand and conceptualize potential collaborations among and between disciplines in response to new cross-disciplinary calls for funding, or in emerging areas of research.

In addition to such campus roles, research development professionals are often involved in regional consortia or statewide systems, and also communicate with research development professionals from other institutions when multi-campus collaborations are called for. Research development professionals then act as key intermediaries at the crossroads of a variety of research actors, from faculty members, to Deans and Vice Presidents/Chancellors for Research, and even with other research development professionals.

Research development professionals secure, maintain, and deploy a number of tools to support the needs and desires of faculty and other researchers to build collaborations both within and among colleges and departments. These tools are listed below in rough order of ease of management, and, not coincidentally, in reverse order of potential impact.

28.2.1 Knowing Who Is Doing What

It may seem obvious, but of critical importance is to know consistently what research is active or in development on campus. This can be equally challenging for campus-wide (discipline agnostic) as well as disciplinary-situated research development professionals. In some cases, keeping up-to-date on institutional research can be more difficult for discipline-specific research development professionals because they are more focused on their disciplinary responsibilities, but that is not always the case. The most successful research development professionals are able to communicate, network, and build credibility, whether in a single research center or in an Office of Research with campus-wide scope.

Effective communications are essential, and research development professionals use a number of digital and in-person tools to improve their ability to support faculty in identifying new collaborative opportunities. Close coordination with the institutional Marketing and Communications (MarCom) function is critical, including participation in key social media campaigns, such as those on Facebook or Twitter. MarCom divisions often highlight developing research, collaborations, or recent publications, and may publish commentary from disciplinary experts on current events, even in the absence of funded research or recent publication, giving research development professionals both real-time and anticipatory insight into the research capabilities of their institutions.

RDPs participation in campus intellectual networks is also a basic tool and may include participating in conferences hosted on their campuses, informal or formal faculty presentations, tracking institutional areas of excellence and "cluster" faculty hiring, and being present at campus settings where informal research opportunities are developed such as Faculty/Staff clubs or luncheons.

Such networking also includes staying appraised of ongoing Technology Transfer activity on campus, including tracking presentations at institutional patenting committees and coordinating with tech transfer professionals to track provisional patent applications. Because of publication and patenting rules, these milestones can often point to new research programs before any public publication or research funding request.

28.2.2 Hiring in Areas of Excellence

RD Professionals can often contribute to more generalized hiring strategies developed at the institutional, college, or departmental level. These efforts are variously characterized as "Areas of Excellence," "Cluster Hires," or "Interdisciplinary Faculty;" terms that highlight the strategy of identifying faculty that, through their research programs, can bridge multiple disciplines to create synergy. While it is beyond the scope of most research development professionals to direct a cluster hire, they are deliberate about investing time, training, and resources in quickly integrating the new hires into the research culture and strategic directions of the larger organization.

28.2.3 Building Cross-Disciplinary or Cross-Institutional Bridges

RDPs can influence institutional research teams in a number of ways but are most effective when facilitating teams on which members are willing partners. Fundamentally, collaborations have to be enthusiastically entered by the relevant faculty. That being said, research development professionals do have important roles in stimulating cross-disciplinary and cross-institutional bridges.

Due to their position responsibilities, research development professionals are in a better position to track multidisciplinary research opportunities than discipline-focused faculty. And they often build teams through open-invitation campus-wide sessions which facilitate brainstorming or mental-mapping to identify specific high-value opportunities. One potentially useful tool for this function is Coggle.it—an easy and straightforward mental-mapping tool that can create program maps like the one below (Fig. 28.1).

Electronic brainstorming can lead to more ideas through the process of comparing, rearranging, combining, reducing, and evaluating concepts (Kerr and Murthy 2004). Cross-disciplinary research is a good example of "ill-structured" problems that abound in knowledge-based organizations for which Group

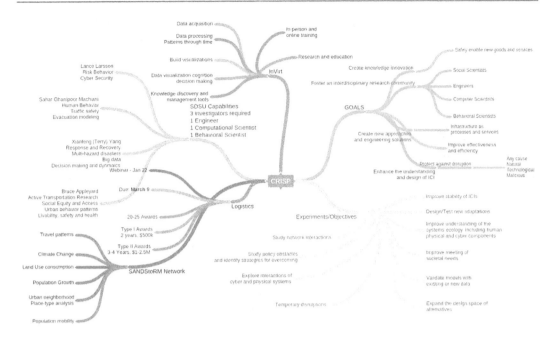

Fig. 28.1 Example of mental map generated using Coggle.it

Support Systems (GSS) or Electronic Brainstorming (GBS) can facilitate vertical and lateral thinking (DeBono 1967), or knowledge expansion or knowledge restriction (Nov and Jones 2005). The research development professional can serve as a facilitator for the deployment of the GSS in a "decision room" setting at a specially arranged meeting (George 2003). The process involves idea generation, consolidation, and voting. The space of information visualization includes Concept Maps (Cañas et al. 2005), Information Visualization (Card et al. 1999), and Knowledge Visualization (Burkhard 2005). While it is not our intention to give a comprehensive review of these technical tools and disciplines, visualization tools have documented effectiveness in fostering collaboration (Fischer et al. 2002) and are an important tool in the research development arsenal.

RDPs also lay the groundwork for interdisciplinary team-based funding opportunities before a Solicitation or Request for Proposals (RFP) is released. The research development professional stays abreast of funding agency priorities and strategic plans and gleans advance information from agency contacts. Research development professionals typically form relationships with key agency program directors/officers and stay apprised of agency reports and meetings that might shed light on future funding directions (Levin 2011; Mason and Learned 2006) (Laughlin and Sigerstad 1990; Porter 2009). Armed with this information, a research development professional might start building relationships among potential collaborators in a variety of ways. This could range from a semi-social event (lunch or cocktail hour) with a short, facilitated ice-breaker to get scholars talking about their overlapping research interests, to a day-long symposium where many scholars across a given transdisciplinary topic give short "lightning talks" on their current research, and describe their specific collaboration goals. These tools to facilitate team formation include the following:

28.2.4 Discovery Slams

RD offices facilitate the building of cross-disciplinary and inter-departmental relationships by supporting institution-wide updates regarding past successes and sharing information on current and future research trends and activities. Successful past efforts often lend credibility and institutional capital to the research development office that can be used to stimulate future participation in large research program efforts. These faculty-led and future-focused experiences are often named "Discovery Slams," "Lighting Talks," "Fast Pitch," or "Elevator Speeches," to emphasize the general audience targeted in the talks, along with the short-form of the presentation. Usually, three to five rapid faculty presentations with Q&A can be managed within an hour. When the presentations are organized around a broad topic, for example neuroscience, faculty may present from a variety of disciplines and perspectives (psychology, neurology, imaging, public health, music).

28.2.5 Regional Networking Events

Beyond the campus, universities can play an important "convening" role as a neutral party bringing together business and industry leaders with municipal stakeholders (e.g., city, county, or state governments), and even engaging additional academic regional partners in networking events that can build the foundation for future functional collaborations. The dividends of hosting such events can be substantial in having appropriate partners identified for future multidisciplinary, multisectoral, and/or multilocation collaborative projects.

One of the most substantial roles that universities can play is as "Convener." With some creativity, research development professionals can play a pivotal role in designing, hosting, or supporting regional conferences centered around innovation—either from an economic development perspective, which can be discipline agnostic, or from a specific disciplinary perspective targeting core capabilities of the institution or region. These conferences can be magnets for regional academic partners, industry collaborators, and federal agency program officers that can help guide future research initiatives.

28.3 Role of the Research Development Professional in Building and Supporting the Team Proposal Development Process

While key activity is in developing new institutional capacity for team science, as detailed in the previous section, much of the research development professional's work is in the proposal development process. Sometimes the research development professional builds an entirely new team for the work, but the most functional and productive teams are those that have been around for a while, and that have developed group trust, instincts, and roles (Huckman et al. 2009). Therefore, a research development professional may be involved in galvanizing an existing team around a new funding opportunity, re-building or healing a broken team, introducing new actors to an existing team, or building a team from scratch.

In working with both old and new teams, research development professionals use various forms of communication depending on the geographic locations of research team members. Some studies show that geographically co-located and thus more frequently face-to-face teams are more robust, as more frequent personal encounters build the trust and familiarity that is critical to successful teams (Pan et al. 2012; Onal Vural et al. 2013; Perry 2014). On the other hand, with increasingly sophisticated technology available to connect team members, such as electronic voice and video platforms, in-person encounters are potentially less important now than they have been in the past (Olson and Olson 2000; Finholt 2003). Within these varying spaces of communication, the research development professional works in various ways to foster smooth collaborations in crafting funding applications. The intensity of the research development professional's involvement often depends on the research team leader (or lack thereof), his/her style of leadership, and his/her ability to provide effective project management.

Thus, depending on the team composition and the research and/or funding opportunity at stake, a research development professional's job may consist of a range of the following project management responsibilities:

- Understanding the time constraints, strengths, and weaknesses of individual team members in relation to the work at hand.
- Translating and synthesizing a long RFP into a short, digestible outline for proposal conceptualization and writing.
- Assigning team members writing sections and other work tasks.
- Developing a work schedule and timeline, scheduling meetings, and motivating team members to meet deadlines.
- Writing or providing "boilerplate" sections of the proposal narrative.
- Liaising with Office of Research and Sponsored Projects personnel regarding budgets, compliance, institutional permissions and signatures, cost-share requirements, etc.
- Communicating with funding program directors/officers about questions that come up in the course of developing the proposal.
- Arranging for an internal "red team" or internal peer review of a draft proposal, coordinating the necessary expert reviewers, and helping investigators synthesize and incorporate the mock panel feedback into their final proposal. In a red team review, key members of the local research community evaluate the research proposal and offer critical developmental feedback for improving it.
- Arranging logistics for an agency site visit.
- Problem solving and trouble-shooting when challenges arise.
- Working behind the scenes to understand potential team tensions or bottlenecks, and judiciously and diplomatically resolving them.

In the case where a research development professional is attempting to start a new team from scratch, especially around an emerging transdisciplinary area, it is necessary to invest time in getting all parties "on the same page." Building new teams can be particularly difficult and precarious, especially if the research development professional (or Vice President for Research or Dean) has the strongest interest in developing the team. Therefore, strategic leadership is critical to align interests, motivations, and languages, around a central and shared vision. Making collaboration worthwhile to a group of previously unaligned scholars hinges on several factors. Scholars are looking for a potentially different combination of benefits and outcomes when evaluating their next research endeavor, such as publications; funding for graduate students or post-docs; funding for lab or field expenses; recognition in their department, institution, or discipline; movement into a new research area; and intellectual satisfaction or excitement. Research development professionals help guide the conversation as collaborative relationships form, helping team members identify individual and team goals, and facilitating exchanges about strategic approaches in response to a particular grant funding opportunity that identify what is both paramount and possible within the approach, guidelines, funding amounts and restrictions of that opportunity.

RDPs can also play an important role in translating disciplinary language across transdisciplinary teams to facilitate discussions that can lead to the development of an integrated research concept. Mediating these conversations requires a research development professional to enable complex communication among experts, while also coordinating shared team knowledge with the language, mission, and expectations of the funding agency.

There are various models and tools for facilitating such team, language, and research-building meetings. In these sometimes tense scenarios, the research development professional is ideally a neutral and has enough authority in the environment to keep the process moving toward the end goal. The research development professional provides critical tools for successful meetings including the following:

- Up front expectations about team goals, standards, and ethics.
- Ample time for multiple, iterative meetings.
- Neutral space in which to meet, whether it is a physical or virtual location.
- Shared visualization tools, such as a white board, large notepads, virtual creative spaces (Google docs for example).
- Social activities, such as lunch breaks or after-hours activities. Breaks, timeouts, and non-work interactions outside of the workspace are known to promote greater collective performance on a team (Pentland 2012; Huber and Lewis 2010). These activities create the time and space for socializing and allowing team members to get to know each other on a personal, nonexpert level (Huber and Lewis 2010).

28.4 Metrics and Team Science; the Role of Research Development Professionals

Team science-related metrics have been difficult to normalize across activities or institutions. One of the challenges is definition of the phenomenon being measured; for example: metrics to evaluate collaborative research itself, metrics related to individuals' participation in team science, or metrics to evaluate the value of research development intervention (Falk-Krzesinski et al. 2011). However, developing and interrogating appropriate metrics for team science and developing a team science evaluation framework represents an important opportunity for research development professionals.

28.4.1 Teaming Process

One of the most important contributions research development professionals can likely make is in defining and measuring metrics of team processes—both summative (e.g., satisfaction surveys) and formative evaluations (e.g., social network analysis, over time; reach as well as size of a network) that illuminate effective practices

for fostering and elevating superordinate identity resulting in improved performance. In the evaluation of team science, research development professionals have generally agreed that one of the most important aspects to interrogate and measure is the process of team formation and performance. The science of team science (SciTS) research area is developing more and more data that suggests effective research teams have to have strong team processes in order to function optimally (Frey et al. 2006; Gajda 2004; Guimerà et al. 2005).

In addition, these evaluations can be both formal and informal—in fact, research development professionals can develop many summative evaluations independently from formal processes. In particular, perception evaluations can be especially valuable for the research development professional in terms of understanding team process. For example, an evaluation that focuses on the level of collaboration among team members would be an incredibly useful research development tool (Frey et al. 2006). Regardless of the results (e.g., high vs. none), reported differences in the levels of collaboration between engaged parties of a team can be indicative of the need for further investigation or intervention from research development professional. Such formative instruments can be a powerful tool for the research development professional to make midcourse corrections, evaluate progress on a quarterly or semiannual basis, or can be used as a prerequisite for faculty requesting internal institutional support.

Drawing from the literature and empirically derived tools, research development professionals can begin to evaluate the collaboration readiness of individual researchers to help guide the effective development of research teams. A newly developed tool for measuring individual collaboration readiness (Lotrecchiano et al. 2016; Mallinson et al. 2016) will soon be widely available as a team science evaluation instrument. The Motivation Assessment for Team Readiness, Integration, and Collaboration (MATRICx) is a psychometric tool for measuring individual motivation for engagement in team science that research development professionals will be able to administer to select individuals or to all members of an existing or forming team. In addition, to evaluate the sociotechnical collaboration readiness of the collective set of individuals on a new or established distributed team, research development professionals can employ the online diagnostic survey Collaboration Success Wizard (http://hana.ics.uci.edu/wizard/). The tool probes factors that may strengthen or weaken the collaboration, offering both personal and project-level reports on the social and technical aspects that guide research development professionals and team leaders to build successful and productive collaborative projects.

28.4.2 Research Outcomes

Traditional research output metrics (e.g., number of publications, citations per publication) for examining the impact of research will persist, but new metrics that focus on the impact of interdisciplinary scientific collaboration are beginning to emerge as well, and research development professionals can play a critical role in guiding their institutions' research and faculty affairs leadership to integrate these new modes of evaluation.

Science of team science researchers are developing new evaluation metrics for team science outcomes (Börner et al. 2010; Falk-Krzesinski et al. 2010; Falk-Krzesinski et al. 2011). For example, a new collaboration index has been devised to assign relative credits to coauthors of a given paper (Stallings et al. 2013). This axiomatically weighted "C-index" better captures a researcher's scientific caliber than simply counting one's total number of publications or the traditional "H-index," allowing for fairer and sharper evaluation of researchers with diverse collaborative behaviors. Another example is the RC-index and the CC-index for quantifying the collaboration activities of researchers and scientific communities based on the measures of collaboration network structure of researchers, the number of collaborations with other researchers, and the productivity index of coauthors, two new indices (Abbasi et al. 2010).

Moreover, new and more specific collaboration metrics are being used by data providers to complement traditional individual research output metrics and it is essential that research development professionals understand how to interpret these. For example, Elsevier's SciVal institutional research performance solution includes metrics related to quantify the degree of institutional collaboration on publications (intra-institutional collaboration, national collaboration, and international collaboration) and quantify collaborations with the industry sector (academic-corporate collaboration metric; Colledge and Verlinde 2014).

Another opportunity is for research development professionals to define ways to measure their contribution to the research outcomes of the scientific collaborations they support. In the absence of (potentially unethical) randomized controlled trials where subsets of faculty are given access to certain interventions and others are excluded, it will always be a challenge to identify which research development interventions are objectively effective, and, perhaps more to the point, *how much* they influence the research outcomes of the teams. However, both within and outside the research development profession, there has been increasing recognition of the subjective impacts of research development support as they relate to the culture and community of research at a given institution.

One potential framework is in the context of "knowledge brokerage"—currency familiar to the field of Integration and Implementation Science (I2S; Falk-Krzesinski 2013.)

28.4.3 Credit for Team Science

As new approaches to recognizing and rewarding individual researchers/faculty members' contributions are developed, research development professionals will serve as guides in their appropriate use for evaluation purposes.

Attempts to apply fractional ownership to publications have been fraught with challenges to appropriately represent credit. These approaches may be precise—in that they represent appropriate distribution of discrete contributors—but are not likely to be accurate representations of the *value* and extent of contributions by the individual researchers involved. Thus, a new area of focus, is attribution of researchers' full contribution to team science. The dominant recognition framework accounting for characteristics of team science is Project CRediT (Brand et al. 2015; CASRAI 2017; http://casrai.org/credit). CRediT establishes a comprehensive contributor role schema to augment traditional authorship assignment, and ultimately associated bibliometrics, including team roles related to conceptualization, review and editing, supervision, funding acquisition, and project administration, among others, and clarifies whether these roles were leading or supporting in a given project.

Unsurprisingly, components of team science metrics are beginning to play into the incentive structure for faculty, most importantly the promotion and tenure process (Klein and Falk-Krzesinski 2017). Research development professionals are well positioned to help translate new team science evaluation into information that can guide changes related to tenure policies. Specifically, research development professionals can advise on addressing changes to the promotion and tenure process across four dimensions: Policy, Process, Practice, and Perception. Policies for promotion and tenure vary vastly at scales as small as individual appointment, promotion, and tenure (APT) committees within the same department. Although many disciplines, departments, and colleges value and protect their independence in promotion and tenure policies, this independence also contributes to the opacity and apparent mystical thinking applied in many of these programs. Research development professionals can contribute to improvement of these environments by informing the process or providing guidance for how uniform and transparent team science policies might be put in place (See also Chap. 39 of this book). Then, by sharing information from the literature base, research development professionals can inform practice, assisting with on-the-ground implementation of policy. Similarly, research development professionals

can provide a context on how to train researcher leaders and researchers to engage in effective Practices throughout the Process. They are also on the front lines of faculty engagement and can gather and compile feedback for research and faculty affairs leaders about researchers' perception of the effectiveness of policies, processes, and practices.

28.5 Example from the Field: The Center for Research, Excellence, and Diversity in Team Science (CREDITS)

Recognizing that diversity on scientific teams amplifies innovation, productivity, and impact, research development professionals in California have developed team science training opportunities for faculty members and researchers in the University of California (UC) and California State University (CSU) systems. Funded by the National Science Foundation, Elsevier Foundation and UC Office of the President, the Center for Research, Excellence, and Diversity in Team Science (CREDITS) forges collaborative relationships and partnerships among diverse teams of scholars, and aims to diversify the professoriate in California. The three core activities are: (1) an annual team science leadership and team formation retreat for faculty and postdoctoral scholars; (2) a team science and institutional change training program for administrative leaders, such as Chancellors/Presidents, Provosts, Deans, Chairs, etc.; and (3) research and evaluation that builds our knowledge about team science and diversity. Training for scholars and administrators takes place in an annual intensive 3-day CREDITS Retreat that combines workshops, lectures, discussion groups, and community building activities. The program has had positive effects on participants' confidence and competencies in multiple areas, including those related to forming and managing diverse teams, and to writing successful collaborative cross-disciplinary grant proposals. More information about CREDITS can be found here: https://oru.research.ucsb.edu/teamscience/.

28.6 Example from the Field: One Research Team's Experience with Research Development and Team Science

In this section, we provide one example of the role of research development professionals in facilitating a cross-disciplinary grant proposal. According to Kyle Lewis, Chair and Professor of Technology Management at UC Santa Barbara, research development professionals played an instrumental role in developing a successful grant proposal for team science research. Research development professionals helped Lewis and her team to interpret the agency's funding opportunity, form the core research team, estimate resources and develop a provisional budget, frame and articulate the research ideas, and facilitate a rigorous internal review. Lewis credits the research development team with the smooth and timely development of a successful grant proposal.

This funding opportunity is perfectly aligned with my research! At least it seemed a perfect alignment to me, a relative latecomer to extramural funding for research. I quickly discovered that funding announcements are designed to reach as many researchers as possible, and that the "perfect fit" is a much more complicated assessment than I had imagined. I was surprised to learn that there are often many stakeholders that are involved in shaping and evaluating prospective research. Trying to parse meaning from the written announcement only (which might reflect selected stakeholders' priorities) is unlikely to reveal critical information. Fortunately, my institution's Research Development team is composed of professionals with Ph.Ds in both STEM and social science fields, all with a track record of extramurally funded research in their own right. Although they were not experts in my specific field of research, they had prior experience with my targeted funding agency, and they knew enough about interdisciplinary social science approaches to help guide my proposal strategy.

Beyond their early insights about how to interpret the call for proposals and frame my research project, they also offered the excellent advice to talk to the Program Officer in charge of the grant. In my discussions with the program officer, I gained insights about the priorities of the agency and what that might mean for our proposal. With suggestions from my research development professional, I was able to develop productive questions, along with potential insights gained, related to the history of the funding mechanism, the agency's research priorities, agency expectations for the composition of the research team, and how the proposal would be reviewed.

28.6.1 Forming the Research Team

With information gathered from the research development professionals and program officer, I started brainstorming a list of potential research teammates (who happened to be external to my institution), reached out to two, and together we developed a list of additional teammates. The research development team advised me on the likelihood that some of our prospective research team members might already be assembling into other research teams. Indeed, this was the case—although disappointing, this gave us insight into "the competition" we might be up against.

28.6.2 Provisional Resources/Budget

Experienced research development professionals know what I did not: Even seemingly large amounts of funding do not go very far. On the advice of the research development team, I got a better idea of the value/time trade-offs by creating a provisional budget. Even though the budget estimates were likely to change later, creating a provisional budget at an early point was eye opening. It required that our team consider each member's roles, time commitments, and availability, and the fair allocation of funding across team members. Ask your research development professional to help with a provisional budget template (with updated information about overhead percentages, tuition support for research assistants, etc.) Use this information to run different scenarios.

28.6.3 Developing the Research Ideas

Our team had no shortage of research ideas. The challenge was sorting through the ideas and choosing among them. At this point in our proposing process, the experience of the research development team was invaluable in helping us to gauge the scope and scale of the proposed research—were our research ideas "impactful" enough? Was the research effort (and associated outcomes) commensurate with the agency's funding target? Was our proposal in line with the agency's mission? Research development professionals worked with us to collect examples of successful past proposals, and took an active part in early team meetings, which meant our team benefited from their guidance at the earliest stages of the project. Our research development professionals also reviewed and commented on successive drafts of proposals throughout the entire process.

28.6.4 Internal Proposal Review: The Red Team

One of the most useful and impressive ways that our research development team helped with our proposal process was in organizing a *Red Team Review*. The review team was carefully curated by our research development team to include representatives from several disciplines—similar to the expected composition of the agency's review team. The most challenging part of the review was *hearing* the feedback objectively. It is hard not to be defensive when ideas are criticized or scrutinized, but our research development professionals feedback helped us to absorb the criticism by reminding us that agency reviewers will see the same "red flags" and have the same questions as the Red Team. They also helped us to distinguish between conceptual problems identified by the Red Team as opposed to writing and strategy problems in the proposal. For example, they identified when key ideas were buried in the text, or when the writing itself (especially when written by a team of people) made important con-

cepts or arguments difficult to understand. Our research team learned that rather than defend, we should ask questions—in what ways did the proposal fail to meet a reviewer's expectations? What was difficult to understand? What was clear? What are particular strengths of the proposal that could be emphasized? What should be the priorities for future edits of the proposal? Answers to these questions provided our team with clear and focused feedback that drove our final edits to the proposal.

28.6.5 The Decision

Our proposal was ranked as a finalist for the award. The feedback we received from the agency was helpful in understanding some of the strengths and weaknesses of our proposal. We learned that our team did not have the winning proposal. Of course, this was a big disappointment! There were several upsides to losing, however. First, our team members now have a good research agenda that we could implement together or in smaller subset teams. Second, the funding agency expressed interest in some of the ideas described in the proposal and requested a new proposal for a separate funding initiative. The happy ending is that we won that subsequent award. I have no doubt that the quality of our initial proposal, research team, and research development support throughout the process were important influences on the agency's decision to consider a separate award. Now, with a smaller research team, we are moving forward with our funded research.

28.7 Conclusion

The science of team science field continues to evolve as an effective evidence-based platform to help maximize the efficiency and effectiveness of scientific collaboration. In many ways, the growth in the importance of research development has been a reflection of the increasingly important role played by research discoveries around collaboration. As new metrics and reward and recognition frameworks for team science continue to rapidly emerge, research development professionals can play a very significant role in advancing the uptake and application of these new findings across all domains of knowledge. This will enable institutions to engage in more robust strategic planning for investments in cross-disciplinary scientific collaboration.

References

AAAS. Member Spotlight; 2013. http://membercentral.aaas.org/blogs/member-spotlight/jacob-levin-brings-research-money.

Abbasi A, Altmann J, Hwang J. Evaluating scholars based on their academic collaboration activities: two indices, the RC-index and the CC-index, for quantifying collaboration activities of researchers and scientific communities. Scientometrics. 2010;83:1–13.

Börner K, Contractor N, Falk-Krzesinski HJ, Fiore SM, Hall KL, Keyton J, Spring B, Stokols D, Trochim W, Uzzi B. A multi-level systems perspective for the science of team science. Sci Transl Med. 2010;2:cm24.

Brand A, Allen L, Altman M, Hlava M, Scott J. Beyond authorship: attribution, 1337 contribution, collaboration, and credit. Learned Publishing. 2015;28:151–5.

Burkhard R. Towards a framework and a model for knowledge visualization. In: Tergan SO, Keller T, editors. Knowledge visualization and information visualization – searching for synergies. London: Springer-Verlag; 2005. p. 238–55.

Campbell AG, Leibowitz MJ, Murray SA, Burgess D, Denetclaw WF, Carrero-Martinez FA, Asai DJ. Partnered research experiences for junior faculty at minority-serving institutions enhance professional success. CBE-Life Sciences Education. 2013;12(3):394–402.

Cañas A, Carff R, Hill G, Carvalho N, Arguedas M, Eskridge T, Lott J, Carvajal R. Concept maps: integrating knowledge and information visualization. In: Tergan SO, Keller T, editors. Knowledge visualization and information visualization – searching for synergies. London: Springer-Verlag; 2005. p. 205–19.

Card SK, Mackinlay JD, Shneiderman B. Readings in information visualization: using vision to think. Los Altos, CA: Morgan Kaufmann; 1999.

CASRAI (Consortia Advancing Standards in Research Administration). CRediT; 2017. p. 1355. http://docs.casrai.org/CRediT. Accessed Apr 2017.

Chung KC, Shauver M. Fundamental principles of writing a successful grant proposal. J Hand Surg Am. 2008;33(4):566–72. https://doi.org/10.1016/j.jhsa.2007.11.028.

Colledge L, Verlinde R. SciVal metrics guidebook. Amsterdam: Elsevier; 2014. https://www.elsevier.com/research-intelligence/resource-library/scival-metrics-guidebook

DeBono E. New think: the use of lateral thinking in generation of new ideas. NY: Basic Books; 1967.

Dorling H, White D, Turner S, Campbell K, Lamont T. Developing a checklist for research proposals to help describe health service interventions in UK research programmes: a mixed methods study. Health Res Policy Syst. 2014;12:12. https://doi.org/10.1186/1478-4505-12-12.

Falk-Krzesinski HJ. I2S and research development professionals: time to develop a mutually advantageous relationship. In: Bammer G, editor. Disciplining interdisciplinarity. Canberra: Australian National University Press; 2013.

Falk-Krzesinski HJ, Börner K, Contractor N, Fiore SM, Hall KL, Keyton J, Spring B, Stokols D, Trochim W, Uzzi B. Advancing the science of team science. Clin Transl Sci. 2010;3:263–6.

Falk-Krzesinski HJ, Contractor N, Fiore SM, Hall KL, Kane C, Keyton J, Klein JT, Spring B, Stokols D, Trochim W. Mapping a research agenda for the science of team science. Res Eval. 2011;20:143–56.

Finholt TA. Collaboratories as a new form of scientific organization. Econ Innov New Technol. 2003;12(1):5–25.

Fischer F, Bruhn J, Gräsel C, Mandl H. Fostering collaborative knowledge construction with visualization tools. Learn Instr. 2002;12:213–32.

Frey BB, Lohmeier JH, Lee SW, Tollefson N. Measuring collaboration among grant partners. Am J Eval. 2006;27:383–92.

Gajda R. Utilizing collaboration theory to evaluate strategic alliances. Am J Eval. 2004;25:65–77.

George JF. Groupware. Encyclopedia Information Systems. 2003;2:509–18.

Guimerà R, Uzzi B, Spiro J, Amaral L. N. Team assembly mechanisms determine collaboration network structure and team performance. Science. 2005;308:697–702.

Hall K, Feng A, Moser R, Stokols D, Taylor B. Moving the science of team science forward: collaboration and creativity. Am J Prev Med. 2008;35(2 Suppl):S243–9. https://doi.org/10.1016/j.amepre.2008.05.007.

Havermahl T, LaPensee E, Williams D, Clauw D, Parker RA, Downey B, Liu J, Myles J. Model for a university-based clinical research development infrastructure. Acad Med. 2015;90(1):47–52.

Huber GP, Lewis K. Cross-understanding: implications for group cognition and performance. Acad Manag Rev. 2010;35(1):6–26.

Huckman RS, Staats BR, Upton DM. Team familiarity, role experience, and performance: evidence from Indian software services. Manag Sci. 2009;55(1):85–100.

Kerr D, Murthy U. Divergent and convergent idea generation in teams: a comparison of computer-mediated and face-to-face communication. Group Decis Negot. 2004;13:381–99.

Klein JT, Falk-Krzesinski HJ. Interdisciplinary and collaborative work: framing promotion and tenure practices and policies. Res Policy. 2017;46:1055–61.

Laughlin P, Sigerstad AMH. The research Administrator's role in creating a supportive environment for interdisciplinary research. Res Manag Review. 1990;4(1):1–17.

Leeming J. Finding job satisfaction in research development. Blog post, Naturejobs; 2016. http://blogs.nature.com/naturejobs/2016/03/16/finding-job-satisfaction-in-research-development/.

Levin J. The Emergence of the Research Development Professional, Chronicle of Higher Education; 2011.

Lotrecchiano GR, Mallinson TR, Leblanc-Beaudoin T, Schwartz LS, Lazar D, Falk-Krzesinski HJ. Individual motivation and threat indicators of collaboration readiness in scientific knowledge producing teams: a scoping review and domain analysis. Heliyon. 2016;2:e00105.

Mallinson T, Lotrecchiano GR, Schwartz LS, Furniss J, Leblanc-Beaudoin T, Lazar D, Falk-Krzesinski HJ. Pilot analysis of the motivation assessment for team readiness, integration, and collaboration (MATRICx) using Rasch analysis. J Investig Med. 2016;Web.08:jim-2016-000173.

Mason E, Learned L. The role of "development" in a research administration office. J Res Admin. 2006;37(1):23–34.

NORDP Member Database: Lead Author's search of NORDP Membership database; 2016. www.nordp.org.

NORDP website, National Organization of Research Development Professionals. www.nordp.org.

Nov O, Jones M. Knowledge creativity and IS: a critical view. In: 38th International Conference on System Sciences 2005. Washington D.C.: IEEE Computer Society Press; 2005.

Olson GM, Olson JS. Distance matters. Human Comp Interact. 2000;15(2):139–78.

Onal Vural M, Dahlander L, George G. Collaborative benefits and coordination costs: learning and capability development in science. Strateg Entrep J. 2013;7(2):122–37.

Pan RK, Kaski K, Fortunato S. World citation and collaboration networks: uncovering the role of geography in science. Sci Rep. 2012;2

Pentland A. The new science of building great teams. Harv Bus Rev. 2012;90(4):60–9.

Perry LM. Factors influencing interdisciplinary research collaborations; 2014. ProQuest Dissertation and Theses Database.

Porter R. What do grant reviewers really want, anyway? J Res Admin. 2005;36(2):47–55.

Porter R. Can we talk? Contacting grant program officers. Res Manag Rev. 2009;17:1.

Stallings J, et al. Determining scientific impact using a collaboration index. Proc Natl Acad Sci. 2013;110: 9680–5.

Walker DM, Pandya-Wood R. Can research development bursaries for patient and public involvement have a positive impact on grant applications? A UK-based, small-scale service evaluation. Health Expect. 2015;18(5): 1474–80.

Part VIII

Facilitating Complex Team Science Initiatives

Best Practices for Researchers Working in Multiteam Systems

29

Dorothy R. Carter, Raquel Asencio,
Hayley M. Trainer, Leslie A. DeChurch,
Ruth Kanfer, and Stephen J. Zaccaro

Contents

D. R. Carter · H. Trainer
Department of Psychology, University of Georgia,
Athens, GA, USA

R. Asencio
Krannert School of Management, Purdue University,
West Lafayette, IN, USA

L. A. DeChurch (✉)
School of Communication, Northwestern University,
Evanston, IL, USA
e-mail: dechurch@northwestern.edu

R. Kanfer
School of Psychology, College of Sciences,
Georgia Institute of Technology, Atlanta, GA, USA

S. J. Zaccaro
College of Humanities and Social Sciences,
George Mason University, Fairfax, VA, USA

29.1 State of the Science: Best Practices for Working in Multiteam Systems

There is conflicting evidence about the capacity for scientific collectives (e.g., research teams, centers) to seed grand innovations. On the one hand, sociological research convincingly argues for "the dominance of teams in the production of knowledge," and in particular, in the production of *high impact* knowledge (Wuchty et al. 2007). On the other hand, research shows that many teams—especially large, interdisciplinary, and geographically distributed teams—are especially prone to underachieving in terms of publications, patents, and commercialization outcomes (Cummings and Kiesler 2005). Indeed, although team science often requires large numbers of specialized experts to work together, many large organizational groups are susceptible to weak member motivation and poor coordination. Recently, we concluded a six-year programmatic investigation into this organizational conundrum. Our research considered how best to organize and support collaboration for scientific innovation.

Specifically, our aim was to better understand how to scale up teamwork to contexts involving complex, interdisciplinary, and geographically distributed collectives focused on scientific innovation. We modeled the challenges facing today's scientific teams by connecting groups of students enrolled in different disciplinary courses (i.e., Social Psychology, Ecology, Innovation Management) at different universities in the United States and France together to form complex interdisciplinary collectives. Across eight semesters, students enrolled in these courses were required to collaborate with fellow classmates, as well as students enrolled in the other participating courses, in order to develop an innovative solution for a complex scientific problem. The problems tackled by these student groups were highly interdisciplinary, requiring the synthesis of knowledge and ideas from multiple areas of expertise. For example, in several semesters, the groups were asked to select an ecological problem within a large highly populated city (e.g., pollution), identify the human behaviors and attitudes that contributed to that problem, and devise a plan to implement a new technology that would help resolve the problem.

Throughout each semester, we collected extensive data on teamwork processes and performance in order to understand the teamwork processes that support scientific innovation. This programmatic stream of research, along with the extant literature on collaboration, teamwork, and innovation within the organizational sciences, has led us to draw three key conclusions for the management of team science.

29.1.1 Conclusion #1: Many Science Teams Are Actually "Multiteam Systems"

The first conclusion is that what is often characterized as "team" science is a bit of a misnomer. Many of today's crucial scientific challenges are not tackled by single teams working in isolation, but by collaborative entities which more closely resemble what organizational scholars term *Multiteam Systems* or "MTSs" for short (Mathieu et al. 2001). Whereas the external boundary of a single *team* is defined by the presence of one or more "team" goals requiring inputs from and interdependent interactions among all team members (Kozlowski and Ilgen 2006), MTSs are distinguishable by their more complex, *multilayered* goal structures (Mathieu et al. 2001; Zaccaro et al. 2012). Defined formally, MTSs are organizational forms comprised of two or more distinct "component" teams whose members pursue both local, "team-level" goals involving interdependencies among a subset of the system (i.e., their fellow teammates), as well as broader "system-level" superordinate goals requiring interdependent interactions among all of the component teams.

Given the increasing complexity of the problems facing twenty-first-century organizations and communities, MTSs, with their networks of specialized component teams, have caught the attention of researchers grappling with organizational challenges in domains as varied as the military, aviation, health care, disaster response, and space exploration, to name a few (e.g., DeChurch and Marks 2006; Bienefeld and Grote 2014; Healey et al. 2009; Vessey 2014). Due to exponential increases in the availability and complexity of knowledge and trends toward interdisciplinarity and interconnectivity, MTSs are increasingly prevalent in science.

In fact, the size and scope of scientific collaboration has expanded steadily over the past five decades (Wuchty et al. 2007). In response to the inherently complex "contemporary public, health, environmental, political, and policy challenges" (Stokols et al. 2008, p. S96), it is now commonplace for scientific collaborations to span the bounds of multiple institutions and laboratories. Challenges such as translational medicine (Asencio et al. 2012) or particle physics (Heidl et al. 2015) often demand contributions from multiple specialized teams, each of which provides unique intellectual contributions. For example, the construction of the Large Hadron Collider in Switzerland involved the contributions and expertise of a large system of over 10,000 personnel including physicists, engineers, computer scientists, and other professionals (LHC Study Group 1995). This project required an intricate network of teamwork processes across hundreds of universities, laboratories, and countries.

Importantly, referring to the immense interdependent system that built the Large Hadron

Collider as a science "team" may lead to incorrect conclusions about the best ways to support collaboration at this scale. Indeed, although "all team science projects, regardless of size or level of disciplinary integration, face challenges related to effectively developing and conducting a shared research agenda" (National Research Council 2015, p. 37), members of scientific collectives comprised of multiple interdependent teams may face additional challenges that are not typically considered within small science teams. For instance, Winter and Berente (2012) observed that teams from multiple, diverse fields are increasingly required to accomplish translational science goals. However, members of systems composed of individuals and teams with diverse expertise and institutional agendas often pursue multiple, and sometimes competing, goals. Conflict and collaboration breakdowns are likely when different team goals are not aligned, or when team goals are misaligned with those of the system as a whole.

Within the literature on teams, researchers have uncovered a variety of mechanisms that enable teams to be successful, such as affective (e.g., cohesion; Beal et al. 2003), behavioral (e.g., coordination; LePine et al. 2008), and cognitive (e.g., team mental models; Mohammed et al. 2010) relational states and processes. This research has yielded a number of applications. For example, following the idea that affective attachment to the team may influence how a team performs, team-building exercises have become a common intervention for new and established teams in an attempt to boost the sense of trust and cohesion among members (Salas et al. 1999). However, when we consider how teams operate in the broader context of MTSs, the objective is no longer simply optimizing outcomes for a single team. Component teams embedded in broader interconnected systems must find the right mix of internal team activities and external cross-team activities that optimize outcomes for both the team as well as the system as a whole. Yet, the push and pull of team and multiteam goals can cause internal tensions and conflicts. Sometimes, the affective, behavioral, or cognitive forces that enable the success of a team can hinder the performance of the MTS, and likewise, the forces that enable MTS success may hinder one or more of the component teams.

A process or property that results in differential effects for teams and MTSs is known as a *countervailing force* (DeChurch and Zaccaro 2013). For example, encouraging flexibility within teams and empowering members to make decisions can enhance creativity and innovative thinking within teams (Hoch 2013). However, in tightly coupled systems, flexibility within one team could equate to unpredictability and coordination decrements for the system as a whole (Lanaj et al. 2013). In this case, team flexibility and empowerment acts as a countervailing force—positively impacting team outcomes while negatively impacting system outcomes. Likewise, team-building exercises that strengthen cohesion and other affective bonds within teams can benefit team performance and satisfaction (Mullen and Cooper 1994). However, strong team cohesion can also have countervailing effects at team versus system levels. For instance strong team cohesion can sometimes limit the likelihood that team members will share information with members of other teams and could contribute to competition and conflict between teams, ultimately harming the viability of the system (DeChurch and Zaccaro 2013).

Practically, managers of scientific MTSs should take note of system characteristics such as the degree of difference between teams and the level of fluidity and flexibility within and between teams (Luciano et al. 2015) in order to determine how to strike the right balance of building strong teams versus building strong interteam bonds. For example, leaders may consider the alignment between team and multiteam goals. There may be less potential for countervailance when team and multiteam goals are closely aligned, because the resources teams need will more closely match the needs of the system. Managers may not be able to change the goals, per se, but they can ensure members clearly see the connection between team and system goals. Managers should also consider the relative weight, hierarchical arrangement, and/or the timeline for goals within and across teams. For example, the necessary emphasis of one goal over others at any given time will influence where members focus their efforts, and therefore, the outcomes they choose to optimize.

In summary, the MTS organizational form has become nearly ubiquitous in science. To organize and support grand innovations such as the Large Hadron Collider requires that we set our microscope at the right magnification (i.e., the "MTS-level"; DeChurch and Zaccaro 2010) and understand much of scientific teamwork through a multiteam lens. For example, the potential for countervailing forces to exist in MTS contexts suggests that managers of these systems cannot simply rely on interventions focused within component teams. Moreover, the development and implementation of best practices for the management of MTSs is paramount to the advancement of science and technology in today's society. The kinds of levers that optimize performance in MTSs are the subject of our next conclusion.

29.1.2 Conclusion #2: Border Processes Such as Interteam Leadership and Boundary Spanning Communication Are Key Levers for Scientific Multiteam System Effectiveness

MTS theory clarifies that the presence of shared superordinate goals means that MTS members must interact collaboratively with fellow teammates, as well members of other teams, in order to achieve their objectives (Mathieu et al. 2001). Challenging interteam collaboration, however, many scientific MTSs are comprised of component teams with different disciplinary backgrounds, areas of expertise, norms, and/or organizational memberships (Zaccaro et al. 2012). These differences can create psychological and/or practical divides between teams which can lead members to experience a much stronger sense of shared identity and cohesiveness in relation to fellow teammates than they experience in relation to members of other teams. At times, these "ingroup–outgroup" attitude structures can

limit collaborative interactions between teams, and could even lead some MTS members to act competitively toward members of other component teams (Brewer 1979; Cuijpers et al. 2016; Tajfel 1982; Tajfel and Turner 1979). Thus, our second conclusion is that a key difference between managing a scientific "team" and managing a scientific "MTS" is the need to facilitate collaboration processes at the *border* between different teams.

The two border processes with the most empirical support in the MTS literature are *interteam leadership* and *boundary spanning communication*. Boundary spanning and interteam leadership processes are key levers that help members to overcome interteam divides and facilitate multiteam collaboration and performance. These mechanisms both involve relationships that bridge the boundaries of different component teams. However, interteam leadership and boundary spanning communication often serve distinct and critical functions within MTSs.

First, in MTS contexts, boundary spanning refers to communication and/or information sharing processes connecting members of different component teams. Often, boundary spanning is undertaken by a relative few number of individuals, who, by virtue of their position in a communication network, facilitate the flow of information between teams. Boundary spanners play an important role in facilitating team and system performance in that they represent their teams to external entities, orchestrate coordinated action between teams, and import knowledge to their team (Ancona and Caldwell 1992; Marrone 2010). Furthermore, boundary spanners can be critical in times of uncertainty as they are in the ideal position to manage unforeseen problems (Kapucu 2006).

MTS research establishes that boundary spanning processes are essential to multiteam effectiveness (Hoegl et al. 2004). Boundary spanning can support the flow of information across teams and interteam coordination, help teams avoid redundancy, and help ensure that inputs from different teams can be combined into a final product. In fact, for systems composed of highly interdependent component teams, the degree to which teamwork processes involving communication and information sharing (e.g., planning, goal specification, monitoring, providing backup) span the boundaries of different teams positively predicts system performance beyond the effects of these teamwork processes occurring within teams (Marks et al. 2005).

Interteam leadership is another key boundary process that impacts MTS effectiveness (Carter and DeChurch, 2014). Whereas boundary spanning communication underpins important teamwork behaviors between teams, interteam leadership is the motivational force that allows the system to act as a coherent whole. Thus, whereas boundary spanning serves a connectivity function, leadership serves a motivational function (Kanfer and Kerry 2012). In practice, these two processes work in concert. However, because leadership and boundary spanning communication meet different functional needs, it is useful to consider them separately when designing interventions for MTSs.

In multiteam contexts, leadership involves shifting teams' attention to and from within-team activities and between-team activities, depending on the demands of the task and performance environment (Marks et al. 2005; DeChurch and Marks 2006). More effective MTSs tend to contain leaders who facilitate both strategizing and coordinating behaviors both within as well as between teams (DeChurch and Marks 2006). Without interteam leadership, component teams often struggle to integrate their contributions with those of other teams. For example, research suggests that formal leadership teams whose members assume responsibility for planning and directing the efforts of constituent teams can facilitate system performance by helping to relieve the information processing complexity that can occur in large collaborations (Davison et al. 2012; DeChurch and Marks 2006; Lanaj et al. 2013).

Organizational research clarifies that in addition to the behaviors of formal leaders (e.g., managers) *informal* leadership influence processes often emerge among organizational members (Carter et al. 2015; Contractor et al. 2012; Pearce and Conger 2003). Likewise, leadership in multiteam contexts often involves informal, as well as

formal, processes of influence. Our findings suggest that informal influence processes are highly relevant to scientific MTS innovation, particularly when informal influence spans the boundaries of different component teams. For example, our research shows that self-managing MTSs—those lacking a "formal" leadership or integration team—tend to produce more innovative outcomes when their informal leadership structures exhibit greater than average connectivity between teams (Carter et al. 2014). The emergence of more informal influence processes between teams may reflect a system where members of different teams are able to push their local agenda to other teams when necessary, but are also receptive to the needs of other teams.

To summarize, boundary spanning and formal as well as informal interteam leadership are foundational to effective collaboration. However, in MTSs, members have the complex task of managing information and maintaining member motivation to support both local as well as global goals. Practical interventions like *team charters*—explicit and documented plans for how group members will interact with one another (Mathieu and Rapp 2009)—can be adapted to suit the need for integration across component teams in MTSs. In fact, initial evidence from our research suggests that generating multiteam charters that document norms for boundary spanning communication and interteam leadership processes before members begin (or resume) their collaboration, can help facilitate multiteam innovation performance (Asencio et al. 2012). Developing a multiteam charter may help a system clarify which individuals (e.g., team members, formal leaders) should be performing specific boundary spanning and/or interteam leadership activities (e.g., sharing information, strategizing, coordinating) and when (i.e., during which project phase). Being explicit about the forms of communication and influence can be a stepping-stone toward successful collaboration.

Extant research on MTS effectiveness provides additional guidance as to which arrangements of individuals, activities, and timing may be most beneficial for MTS performance. For example, research suggests that whereas leadership activities can be shared among all members *within* component teams (Bienefeld and Grote 2014), interteam coordination is enhanced when teams designate a smaller set of members to act as boundary spanners and/or engage in interteam leadership activities between teams (Davison et al. 2012). Evidence also supports the use of MTS-level leaders (e.g., members of "MTS integration" teams; Mathieu et al. 2017) to help structure the interaction patterns across component teams. For example, DeChurch et al. (2011) conclude that MTS-level leaders are essential for setting the coordination structures and managing the flow of information between teams.

Moreover, findings from research conducted by Hoegl and Weinkauf (2005) suggest that systems need greater levels of integration across teams (e.g., in terms of boundary spanning communication and/or interteam leadership processes) during initial "concept" phases of a project as compared to later, development and/or implementation phases. When component teams interface with one another early on—clarifying their respective inputs and outputs—this helps to ensure that the teams' outputs will integrate with those of other teams during later project phases. However, Hoegl and Weinkauf (2005) also clarify that MTS-level leaders should provide guidance regarding project structuring throughout all phases of MTS performance in order to ensure members understand with whom they need to integrate and coordinate.

29.1.3 Conclusion #3: MTS Management Is a Balancing Act: Systems Require Both Integration Across and Differentiation Between Component Teams

Our third conclusion stems from our empirical investigations of MTSs in action as well as social psychological theories of groups and intergroup relations. As discussed in the previous section, a key role of multiteam leaders and boundary spanners is to connect component teams and facilitate a coordinated system of action to achieve collective goals. However, this conclusion should not be taken to mean that managers of MTSs should "over-connect" by attempting to breakdown team boundaries altogether and create a single shared identity for the entire system. In fact, our third conclusion is that *supporting multiteam collaboration is a balancing act* requiring leaders and boundary spanners to both facilitate *integrated efforts* across teams while also maintaining the *differentiation* between teams that is necessary to ensure members and teams are individually identified and motivated to contribute to the system.

Indeed, we have come to realize that attempting to create one large cohesive "team" with a single shared identity is not the best way to support multiteam performance (Asencio et al., 2013). Our group memberships helps define who we are, and thus, people strive to ensure that their own groups are unique and important (e.g., Abrams and Hogg 2010; Hogg et al. 2012; Tajfel and Turner 1979). Going back to our programmatic study of MTSs, we find support for this idea. We directly compared students working in an MTS structure, with functionally different component teams, to students working in one large interdisciplinary team. Compared to the interdisciplinary teams, students working in the MTS structure were able to focus more deeply on the disciplinary contributions of their team and ultimately contribute more effectively to MTS innovation performance. In contrast, students working in the large interdisciplinary team were more inclined to focus on managing the interface between teams throughout the project (Hoegl and Weinkauf 2005), thereby preventing a focused effort on their unique disciplinary contributions (LoPilato et al. 2016).

In fact, rather than ensuring collaboration between groups, attempting to establish strong identification across an entire MTS can exacerbate tensions between groups, especially when the different group memberships in the system (e.g., teams, institutions, areas of expertise) are important to members' sense of self (Hogg et al. 2012). A more effective strategy for a multiteam leader is to maintain the diversity of the system, allowing teams to remain specialized and unique, while also ensuring that the teams understand the importance of one another's specialized contributions to the overall goals of the system (Hogg et al. 2012). For example, leaders can strategically use rhetoric to communicate the importance of collaborating across teams, while at the same time emphasizing the team's identity by referencing the unique contributions of the team, and how these contributions connect to valued team goals (Hogg et al. 2012).

Furthermore, the natural tendency for teams to erect strong boundaries is often seen as highly problematic (Luciano et al. 2015). However, in moderation, it can actually be functional and beneficial to scientific innovation for teams to have clearly defined boundaries that prevent excessive communication between teams. On the one hand, a high volume of interactions across teams can promote a unified MTS identity and diminish perceptions that other component teams are part of "outgroups." However, a high volume of interactions across teams can also blur team boundaries, dissolving a team's own sense of identity. Therefore, cross-team communication can be a countervailing force in that it may promote the success of the MTS by building up a superordinate identity, but can hinder the success of component teams by diminishing the teams' sense of importance and specialization. Furthermore, should cross-team communication dissolve team boundaries to the point at which the system is actually functioning as a large interdisciplinary team, the system may fail to reap the benefits of specialization and differentiation across teams that promote innovation (Asencio et al. 2012).

The need for group boundaries—and a space for members of different component teams to explore different ideas—is supported by research showing *privacy* promotes local team efforts to experiment with new ideas or processes (Bernstein 2012). Likewise, in another study, Shore et al. (2015) showed that groups who exhibit a *moderately* dense structure of communication, as opposed to a highly dense communication structure, tended to engage in greater exploration for potential solutions (i.e., a critical part of innovation). This work suggests that too much integration in a group communication structure can result in overly rapid convergence in information interpretation, reducing the exploration of theories or solutions to problems, and thus, reducing innovativeness.

Thus, the need for boundary spanning communication discussed in Conclusion 2 should not be taken to mean that *all* members of component teams in MTSs should communicate and collaborate directly with all other members. Too much direct interaction between teams—especially among members of teams whose contributions are not as central to the overall goals of the system—is unnecessary and can be detrimental to system performance (Davison et al. 2012). A key caveat of the necessity for boundary spanning in multiteam contexts is that the *structure* of boundary spanning matters. Too many open communication channels can result in a chaotic communication structure, where information is lost or misinterpreted. Such chaotic structures can be especially problematic in very large systems, such as those that are prevalent in science (Stokols et al. 2008). As mentioned previously, managers in MTSs can help to structure communication within and between teams using interventions such as team charters so that ideas flow across team boundaries as required by task demands while unnecessary and/or redundant connections are avoided.

Certainly, component teams in some scientific MTSs are highly differentiated from one another with regard to features such as their areas of expertise, publishing norms, team-level goals, and/or institutional demands. Such differences might exacerbate the ingroup–outgroup attitude structures discussed previously in Conclusion 2. Thus, many MTS managers may find that balancing act of managing a MTS often requires a greater emphasis on interteam integration as opposed to interteam differentiation. However, the end game for designing MTSs is not complete integration, or at least not the way it is typically conceived.

29.1.3.1 Multiteam System Science

In conclusion, what is widely labeled *team science* (National Research Council 2015) is very often undertaken by an organizational form known as the *Multiteam System*. Many of the organizational challenges that threaten the success of scientific collectives, such as disciplinary diversity, geographic distribution, and conflicting goals, stem from their multiteam nature. Thus, interventions that are designed to build effective teams will not be optimally effective for scientific MTSs unless the interventions are adapted to reflect the multiteam nature of these complex social systems.

As an aid for designing interventions, we summarize five characteristics of effective MTSs in Table 29.1. These characteristics are

Table 29.1 Diagnostic questions for designing interventions for MTSs

Multiteam system characteristic	Diagnostic question
MTS goal hierarchy: Each MTS component team pursues subordinate team goals, while also pursuing superordinate system goals (Mathieu et al. 2001)	Do MTS members understand the goals of different teams, and how the different goals are related to one another?
Interteam interdependence: Each component team is mutually reliant on at least one other team (Murase et al. 2014; Marks et al. 2005; Mathieu et al. 2001)	Do MTS members understand the teams on whom they are most reliant? Do MTS members understand the teams who are most reliant on them?
Interteam differentiation: The boundaries of each component team are identifiable (Hogg et al. 2012)	Is each component team in the system uniquely identified? Are members aware of their distinct team-level identities, goals, and contributions to the system?
Boundary spanning communication: Communication processes that bridge a team to other teams in the MTS, and to the external environment (Ancona and Caldwell 1992; DeChurch et al. 2011; Davison et al. 2012)	Does each component team have at least one individual who serves as a boundary spanner, who continuously works to maintain and develop relationships with other teams' boundary spanners?
Interteam leadership: Influence relationships between teams that motivate members to work together toward the accomplishment of MTS goals (Carter and DeChurch 2014)	Do MTS members have a subset of individuals who provide leadership in support of multiteam goals? Are leaders facilitating connections between teams and motivating the members of all component teams to pursue team as well as MTS goals?

key *targets* for intervention strategies designed to facilitate MTS functioning. The first three are the MTS goal hierarchy, interteam interdependence, and interteam differentiation. These social architectures are defining features of an MTS. Interventions that build members' understanding of MTS goal hierarchies and interteam interdependence have been shown to promote MTS performance (e.g., Murase et al. 2014). Interventions that maintain the unique identities of different subgroups have been shown to promote innovation (Shore et al. 2015). The next two characteristics are boundary spanning and interteam leadership—social levers with a strong evidentiary basis. These social levers have been shown to promote MTS performance (e.g., Davison et al. 2012; DeChurch and Marks 2006). Interventions like multiteam charters, debriefing procedures, leader rhetoric, and structured communication patterns, can be used effectively within these systems. However, they need to be focused on creating and sustaining work processes both within component teams, as well as between them. Preserving the unique identities and subordinate goals of the different teams, while also affording a social architecture to align them, is the key to working in and supporting MTSs.

Acknowledgments This material is based upon work supported by the National Science Foundation under Grant Nos. SES-1219469, SMA-1063901, and SMA-1262474. Any opinions, findings, and conclusions or recommendations expressed in this material are those of the authors and do not necessarily reflect the views of the National Science Foundation.

References

Abrams D, Hogg MA. Social identity and self-categorization. In: Dovidio JF, Hewston M, Glick P, Esses VM, editors. The SAGE handbook of prejudice, stereotyping and discrimination. London, UK: Sage; 2010. p. 179–93.
Ancona DG, Caldwell DF. Bridging the boundary: external activity and performance in organizational teams. Adm Sci Q. 1992;37:634–65.
Asencio R, Carter DR, DeChurch LA, Zaccaro SJ, Fiore SM. Charting a course for collaboration: a multiteam perspective. Transl Behav Med. 2012;2(4):487–94.

Asencio R, Murase T, DeChurch LA, Chollet B, Zaccaro SJ. Social identity in cross-functional multiteam systems. In: DiRosa G, DeChurch LA, editors. The meaning and measurement of entitativity in complex organizational forms. Symposium Conducted at the Annual Meeting of Society for Industrial and Organizational Psychology, Houston, TX; 2013.

Beal DJ, Cohen RR, Burke MJ, McLendon CL. Cohesion and performance in groups: a meta-analytic clarification of construct relations. J Appl Psychol. 2003;88(6):989.

Bernstein ES. The transparency paradox: a role for privacy in organizational learning and operational control. Adm Sci Q. 2012;57(2):181–216.

Bienefeld N, Grote G. Shared leadership in multiteam systems how cockpit and cabin crews lead each other to safety. Human Fact. 2014;56(2):270–86.

Brewer MB. In-group bias in the minimal intergroup situation: a cognitive-motivational analysis. Psychol Bull. 1979;86(2):307.

Carter DR, DeChurch LA. Leadership in multiteam systems: a network perspective. In: Day D, editor. The Oxford handbook of leadership and organizations. Oxford, UK: Oxford University Press; 2014. p. 482–502.

Carter DR, DeChurch LA, Zaccaro SJ. Impact of leadership network structure on the creative output of multiteam systems. Acad Manag Proc. 2014;2014:1.

Carter DR, DeChurch LA, Braun MT, Contractor NS. Social network approaches to leadership: an integrative conceptual review. J Appl Psychol. 2015;100(3):597.

Contractor NS, DeChurch LA, Carson J, Carter DR, Keegan B. The topology of collective leadership. Leadersh Q. 2012;23(6):994–1011.

Cuijpers M, Uitdewilligen S, Guenter H. Effects of dual identification and interteam conflict on multiteam system performance. J Occup Organ Psychol. 2016;89(1):141–71.

Cummings JN, Kiesler S. Collaborative research across disciplinary and organizational boundaries. Soc Stud Sci. 2005;35(5):703–22.

Davison RB, Hollenbeck JR, Barnes CM, Sleesman DJ, Ilgen DR. Coordinated action in multiteam systems. J Appl Psychol. 2012;97(4):808.

DeChurch LA, Marks MA. Leadership in multiteam systems. J Appl Psychol. 2006;91(2):311.

DeChurch LA, Zaccaro SJ. Perspectives: teams won't solve this problem. Human Fact. 2010;52(2):329–34.

DeChurch LA, Zaccaro SJ. Innovation in scientific multiteam systems: Confluent and countervailing forces. In National Academy of Sciences Workshop on Science Team Dynamics and Effectiveness, Washington, DC; 2013.

DeChurch LA, Burke CS, Shuffler ML, Lyons R, Doty D, Salas E. A historiometric analysis of leadership in mission critical multiteam environments. Leadersh Q. 2011;22(1):152–69.

Healey MP, Hodgkinson GP, & Teo S. Responding effectively to civil emergencies: The role of transac-

tive memory in the performance of multi team systems. In Proceedings of NDM9 the 9th International Conference on Naturalistic Decision Making; 2009. pp. 53–59.

Heidl RA, Hollenbeck JR, Howe M, & Yu A. The impact of informal ties on the performance of individuals and teams embedded in multiteam systems in the context of large-scale collaborative science. Paper Presentation at the 75th Annual Meeting of the Academy of Management: Vancouver, CA; 2015.

Hoch JE. Shared leadership and innovation: the role of vertical leadership and employee integrity. J Bus Psychol. 2013;28(2):159–74.

Hoegl M, Weinkauf K, Gemuenden HG. Interteam coordination, project commitment, and teamwork in multiteam R&D projects: a longitudinal study. Organ Sci. 2004;15(1):38–55.

Hoegl M, Weinkauf K. Managing task interdependencies in Multi-Team projects: A longitudinal study. J Manag Stud. 2005;42(6):1287–308.

Hogg MA, Van Knippenberg D, Rast DE. Intergroup leadership in organizations: leading across group and organizational boundaries. Acad Manag Rev. 2012;37(2):232–55.

Kanfer R, Kerry M. Motivation in multiteam systems. In: Zaccaro SJ, Marks MA, DeChurch L, editors. Multiteam systems: an organization form for dynamic and complex environments. New York, NY: Routledge; 2012. p. 81–108.

Kapucu N. Interagency communication networks during emergencies boundary spanners in multiagency coordination. Am Rev Public Adm. 2006;36(2):207–25.

Kozlowski SW, Ilgen DR. Enhancing the effectiveness of work groups and teams. Psychol Sci Public Interest. 2006;7(3):77–124.

Lanaj K, Hollenbeck JR, Ilgen DR, Barnes CM, Harmon SJ. The double-edged sword of decentralized planning in multiteam systems. Acad Manag J. 2013;56(3):735–57.

LePine JA, Piccolo RF, Jackson CL, Mathieu JE, Saul JR. A meta-analysis of teamwork processes: tests of a multidimensional model and relationships with team effectiveness criteria. Pers Psychol. 2008;61(2):273–307.

LHC Study Group. The large hadron collider, conceptual design. Geneva: CERN/AC/95–05 LHC; 1995.

LoPilato A, Asencio R, DeChurch LA, Kanfer R, Zaccaro SJ. Team design and scientific innovation: A quasi-experiment. Paper accepted at the annual meeting for the Interdisciplinary Network for Group Research (INGRoup), Helsinki, Finlaend; 2016.

Luciano MM, DeChurch LA, Mathieu JE. Multiteam systems: a structural framework and meso-theory of system functioning. J Manag 2015, 014920e6315601184.

Marks MA, DeChurch LA, Mathieu JE, Panzer FJ, Alonso A. Teamwork in multiteam systems. J Appl Psychol. 2005;90(5):964.

Marrone JA. Team boundary spanning: a multilevel review of past research and proposals for the future. J Manag. 2010;36(4):911–40.

Mathieu JE, Rapp TL. Laying the foundation for successful team performance trajectories: the roles of team charters and performance strategies. J Appl Psychol. 2009;94(1):90.

Mathieu JE, Marks MA, Zaccaro SJ. Multi-team systems. In: Anderson N, Ones DS, Sinangil HK, Viswesvaran C, editors. Organizational psychology: Vol. 2. Handbook of industrial, work and organizational psychology. London: Sage; 2001. p. 289–313.

Mathieu JE, Hollenbeck JR, van Knippenberg D, Ilgen DR. A century of work teams in the journal of applied psychology. J Appl Psychol. 2017;102(3):452.

Mohammed S, Ferzandi L, Hamilton K. Metaphor no more: a 15-year review of the team mental model construct. J Manag. 2010;36(4):876–910.

Mullen B, Cooper C. The relation between group cohesiveness and performance: an integration. Psychol Bull. 1994;115:210–27.

Murase T, Carter DR, DeChurch LA, Marks MA. Mind the gap: the role of leadership in multiteam system collective cognition. Leadersh Q. 2014;25(5):972–86.

National Research Council. Enhancing the Effectiveness of Team Science. Washington. DC; The National Academies Press. 2015. https://doi.org/10.17226/19007.

Pearce CL, Conger JA. Shared leadership: reframing the hows and whys of leadership. Newcastle upon Tyne: Sage; 2003.

Salas E, Rozell D, Mullen B, Driskell JE. The effect of team building on performance an integration. Small Group Res. 1999;30(3):309–29.

Shore J, Bernstein E, Lazer D. Facts and figuring: an experimental investigation of network structure and performance in information and solution spaces. Organ Sci. 2015;26(5):1432–46.

Stokols D, Misra S, Moser RP, Hall KL, Taylor BK. The ecology of team science understanding contextual influences on transdisciplinary collaboration. Am J Prev Med. 2008;35(2 S):S96–S115.

Tajfel H. Social psychology of intergroup relations. Annu Rev Psychol. 1982;33(1):1–39.

Tajfel H, Turner JC. An integrative theory of intergroup conflict. Social Psychol Intergroup Relations. 1979;33(47):74.

Vessey WB. Multiteam systems in the spaceflight context: current and future challenges. In: Salas E, editor. Pushing the boundaries: multiteam Systems in Research and Practice. Bingley: Emerald Group Publishing Limited; 2014. p. 135–53.

Winter SJ, Berente N. A commentary on the pluralistic goals, logics of action, and institutional contexts of translational team science. Transl Behav Med. 2012;2(4):441–5.

Wuchty S, Jones BF, Uzzi B. The increasing dominance of teams in production of knowledge. Science. 2007;316:1036–9.

Zaccaro SJ, Marks MA, DeChurch L, editors. Multiteam systems: an organization form for dynamic and complex environments. New York, NY: Routledge; 2012.

Sarah J. Gehlert

Contents

Effective team functioning and performance relies to a large extent on having a shared identity across team members. This shared identity usually is based on a shared mission and goals and is greatly facilitated by the development of a shared mental model of the research endeavor. In the pages that follow, we will outline the successful development of a shared mental model in one center of a transdisciplinary team-based initiative funded by the National Institutes of Health and highlight the value of the model to the development and implementation of the research initiative.

S. J. Gehlert (✉)
College of Social Work, University of South
Carolina, Columbia, SC, USA
e-mail: SGEHLERT@mailbox.sc.edu

30.1 The Life Cycle of Transdisciplinary Team-Based Research

Hall and colleagues proposed a four-phase model to highlight the phases of development of a transdisciplinary research team, with development, conceptualization, implementation, and translational phases (Hall et al. 2012). The four-phase model is useful in breaking down the steps that lead to the final stage of translational team research, namely translating research results into real-world solutions. According to the four-phase model, the first or development phase includes the process of forging a shared mission and goals, as members begin to develop critical awareness of their team enterprise (Hall et al. 2012). This shared mission and goals then forms the basis for developing a shared mental model that integrates all of the projects during the team's implementation phase. This integrated model helped to establish the team's mental model. Two types of mental models have been frequently discussed in relation to team performance, team-related mental models and task-related mental models, e.g., (Mathieu et al. n.d.). Team-related mental models have to do with the team functioning and expected behaviors, while task-related mental models contain information regarding the materials or equipment needed for the task or the manner in which resources for achieving that task are used.

© Springer Nature Switzerland AG 2019
K. L. Hall et al. (eds.), *Strategies for Team Science Success*,
https://doi.org/10.1007/978-3-030-20992-6_30

As outlined by Hall et al., developing a shared mental model of research is critical to establishing the team communication and problem-solving skills that allow a research plan to be outlined and pursued (Hall et al. 2012). Because research funding is time limited, expedient development of a research plan allows teams more time to achieve their strategic aims. Thus, developing a shared mental model is critical to the success of transdisciplinary team-based research. Yet rather than being intuitive and inevitable, shared model construction requires actions and process. Not attending to this action and process increases the likelihood that projects will operate as separate constellations without cohesion or decrease the likelihood that a model developed to represent the contributions of all of the center's projects. In either case, group identity, and cohesion that follows will be sacrificed and teams will fail to meet their full potential.

30.2 The Center for Interdisciplinary Health Disparities Research

The Center for Interdisciplinary Health Disparities Research (CIHDR) at the University of Chicago was one of the original eight Centers for Population Health and Health Disparities (CPHHDs) funded jointly by the National Cancer Institute and the National Institute of Environmental Health Science in 2003. The impetus for CIHDR came when a larger group of investigators from across the University of Chicago campus assembled to answer the CPHHD request for proposals (RFA) on health disparities (http://grants.nih.gov/grants/guide/rfa-files/RFA-CA-09-001.html) after a faculty member invited a wide variety of health scholars from around the campus to attend. The majority of those assembled worked in cancer disparities or asthma disparities, and a number of those assembled shared an interest in the social origins of the African-American and white disparity in breast cancer mortality. One member of the assembled group, a clinician scientist who later emerged as a leader, stated her opinion that the

African-American and white disparity in breast cancer mortality would persist even after the development of an effective treatment, due to its social origins. Because of the obvious excitement around this issue, the larger group deferred to the breast cancer disparity group to take the university's lone slot to answer the RFA. The author of this chapter became the Principal Investigator and began to interview behavioral scientists on campus to complete the team, which at that point included clinical, biological, and social scientists. The first behavioral scientist interviewed agreed to participate.

Once the resulting application was funded, CIHDR investigators organized around the shared research question that emerged during the initial campus-wide meeting, and which was the centerpiece of the application, namely, how features of the social environments of African-American women contribute to the African-American and white disparity in breast cancer mortality. In preparing their applications, team members decided that the research question might best be addressed through four research projects, which were led by investigators with primary backgrounds in the social, behavioral, and biological sciences. The two biological scientists also had clinical duties as breast oncologists. Despite their disparate backgrounds, investigators' desire to answer the articulated research question united the group.

The four main projects' lead investigators represented a range of disciplines. A project using a rodent model involving Sprague-Dawley rats was led by a biopsychologist considered to be an international expert in open-cage experimentation (McClintock). A second project using an SV40 transgenic mouse model was led by a breast oncologist who is also a molecular biologist (Conzen). These two projects used rodent models that mimic human breast cancer to identify pathways by which the social environment influences an aggressive form of breast cancer. Working with animal models allowed social conditions to be manipulated and biological outcomes assessed across the life cycle of the animals. Prior work by McCintock et al. (2005) and Hermes et al.

(2009) formed the basis for how the two projects were set up.

A third CIHDR project enrolled African-American women living in neighborhood areas on Chicago's predominantly African-American South Side. Women were enrolled at the time of diagnosis with first-episode breast cancer at three South Side hospitals and tumor tissue was collected at the time of biopsy or tumor excision through a fourth CIHDR project led by Dr. Olofunmilayo Olopade. The third project was led by a social scientist (Gehlert) with expertise in community-engaged health research. She and her team followed a group of African-American women over time who were newly diagnosed with their first episode of breast cancer (Hermes et al. 2009; Gehlert 2013). These women lived on Chicago's South Side, in 15 neighborhood areas with largely African-American residence. Although geographically homogenous, the sample of women varied by socioeconomic status, from women who were homeless to those with median family incomes higher than the Chicago average. The fourth project, led by Dr. Olopade, a breast oncologist who is also an expert in the genetics of breast cancer among women of West African ancestry, gathered excess tumor tissue from these women and examined gene expression.

30.3 Developing a Shared Conceptual Model

During its developmental phase, as outlined above, the CIHDR team explored ways of knitting their projects into an articulate whole after funding was obtained from National Cancer Institute. It became clear that the four CIHDR projects had the potential to be mutually informative and that taken together, they could provide an ideal mechanism for investigating the pathways through which the social environment shapes biology and health. The group realized that their origins in a variety of disciplines gave them the unique opportunity to consider social, behavioral, and biological aspects of health using shared projects and analyses. Yet, as previously stated, the ability to take an overview of a multi-

project center is neither intuitive nor inevitable, and little guidance is available on how to achieve this broader perspective. Scientific training remains project specific.

The process of developing a shared mental model challenged the group to incorporate all four projects into a cohesive whole that would accurately represent the contribution of each project. This, in essence, meant that each project leader and investigator had to simultaneously consider her own project and the center as a whole. This mental balance of project and center depended on an investigator's ability to articulate her own project in terms that could be understood by project leaders from other disciplines and to actively listen to project descriptions by other team members.

We anticipate that our mental model is a hybrid of the team-based and task-based mental models outlined above, in which functioning, expected behaviors, resources, and equipment were decided through an iterative process that occurred after we began to merge the projects into a meaningful and coherent whole. The exercise that we conducted to integrate our individual projects produced a conceptual model. Individual investigators and project leaders participated in the exercise of model production during a prolonged session led by the PI (Gehlert) in which we used a white board and markers to iteratively produce a model into which all of the center's work fit. The outcome was that each investigator had an idea of how their work fit into the center's work as a whole. We believe that this gave each team member the opportunity to lay down a mental model that had features of both a team-based and a task-based mental model, thus affecting both team functioning and behavior and determining the materials needed to achieve the center's mission and specific aims.

The next essential step in the process, which was facilitated by team-based components of our mental model, was developing a set of group rules of engagement and style of communication that was acceptable to all. This is analogous to establishing an environment or atmosphere of psychological safety, which is also considered in the four-phase model (Hall et al. 2012). This task of facilitating the group in developing a set of rules for engagement and communication fell to the Principal Investigator. The process not only resulted in establishing a set of rules for engagement and communication, but also set the stage for group problem solving. A mutually informative, iterative approach to science emerged that was based on agreed-upon rules of communication and an evolving critical group identity. In this process, an idea was proposed in one project and explored by others to determine what it might mean for their projects. For example, McClintock et al. (2005) and Hermes et al. (2009) found that normally highly social rats that were socially isolated from the time of weaning became hyper-vigilant to novel phenomena in their cage environments and developed more malignant spontaneous mammary gland tumors at a much earlier age than their non-isolated peers. Even prior to tumor growth, both the isolated SV40 Tag transgenic mice studied by Conzen and her team (Hermes et al. 2009) and McClintock's inbred rat strains (Williams et al. 2009) developed heightened stress hormone responses to an acute stressor. Perhaps more important for the study of human psychosocial functioning was the discovery that within a group, those rats isolated from reciprocal care and support, particularly in the face of stressors, were more likely to die at an earlier age with mammary tumors than their non-isolated peers (Yee et al. 2008). Those with recip-

rocal support relationships survived the longest with mammary tumors, which may mirror discrimination among humans. McClintock's project also influenced Gehlert's projects with African-American women. After McClintock and her team determined that socially isolated rates were more likely to develop mammary tumors, Gehlert's team added measures of social isolation and loneliness to their interviews with women.

Ultimately, we refined our shared model of the research center, including its four projects and their interconnections (see Fig. 30.1). This was done in a second team-wide meeting, again using a white board and dry markers, with everyone adding to the model so that it eventually included all projects. The resulting model represents a multilevel and multifactorial approach to African-American and white cancer disparities that considers influences from within the cell to the level of society. Each CIHDR project, two of which used animal models (Projects 1 and 4) and two of which worked with African-American women living on Chicago's South Side (Projects 2 and 3), had a place in the shared model (McClintock et al. 2005; Gehlert et al. 2008).

The shared CIHDR story was one in which race for African-American women living on Chicago's South Side determined psychological functioning. Based on findings from animal modeling in Project 1 and focus groups with 503

Fig. 30.1 Center for Interdisciplinary Health Disparities Research shared mental and conceptual model of African-American and white disparities in breast cancer mortality

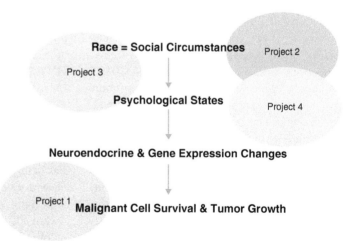

South Side residents in Project 3, we focused specifically on women's psychological reactions to social isolation. Many women in the study reported feeling lonely because family and other important social contacts lived a distance away from them, rendering contact by anything other than telephone or social media difficult. Also, crime in neighborhoods and the inability to afford safe housing caused women to spend more time at home than desired, prohibiting more casual neighborhood contacts (Gehlert et al. 2011). We found a constellation of three highly correlated social and factors, isolation, depression, and vigilance in response to crime and other threats to safety, which produced two distinct groups of women in factor analysis, one of who were depressed and lonely, and another of which women who questioned their purpose in the world or failed to understand where they fit into society (Gehlert et al. 2011).

A mutually informative, iterative approach to science developed that persisted through the 5 years of the CIHDR. This process allowed the CIHDR team to fully explore all components of their shared model, from elements of the social environment, especially features of urban neighborhoods, to psychological responses to those features, to gene and hormone expression within tumors. By giving each project equal weight, which was achieved by leveling the playing field by having CIHDR administered through the Institute for Mind and Biology, which is free standing rather than administered by any one school or division of the university, the transdisciplinary approach allowed investigators to explore hypothesized determinants of hormone and gene expression changes, as well as those changes themselves, in equal depth, without favoring any one element of the model (Gehlert et al. 2010). If CIHDR had been administered by any of the schools or divisions to which its PI and project leaders belonged, this might have privileged that unit over others.

Another essential step in the group's conceptualization phase was developing a shared lexicon that incorporated key words from individual projects. The shared CIHDR lexicon, which the Principal Investigator updated regularly and distributed to the team over the course of the center, included words such as "apoptosis" and "methylation" from Project 1, "acquired vigilance" from Projects 2 and 4, and "collective efficacy" from Project 3. The shared lexicon further cemented CIHDR's team-based mental map. Learning these terms not only allowed leaders to understand the descriptions and updates that came from other CIHDR projects, but also gave team members tangible tools for articulating CIHDR's shared story, and the shared mental model of the research endeavor, to a variety of lay and professional audiences. Leaders presented CIHDR results individually and in pairs, which added to a sense of group unity, engagement, and joint ownership. These paired presentations had the secondary benefit of informing project leaders about other projects, or the parts of the shared mental model in which they were not expert. Over time, project leaders were able to present the story of the center as a whole, based on their growing understanding of other ·projects and how they contributed to CIHDR's overall mission. It gave each investigator a better grasp of the full center's research, and the interconnections between the four projects.

30.4 Conclusions

The CIHDR team assembled around an aim of understanding the African-American and white disparity in breast cancer mortality in all of its complexity, taking a multilevel, multifactorial approach. To wit, investigators from the biological, behavioral, and social sciences came together to understand the influences of the social environments of African-American women with breast cancer on their psychological functioning and tumor biology, using both human and nonhuman animals models, in a format that was mutually informative and allowed them to test hypotheses across projects.

Although very challenging, CIHDR's successes came from the team's ability to develop a shared mental model of the research center, including the interconnections among the four center research projects, that provided them with tools for telling the broader story of how the social environmental "gets under the skin" to influence tumor biology in a way that disadvantages African-American women in terms of breast cancer outcomes like survivorship. The CIDHR model has implications for other centers and multicenter initiatives. If investigators have the will to work together as a team, the action steps followed by CIDHR, including rules for communication to create an environment of psychological safety, development of a shared lexicon for the center, development of a shared mental model of the research center, and development of shared oral presentations, provide a template for achieving unity across a variety of multi-project research enterprises.

A number of actions facilitated the development of this shared model. These included the Principal Investigator leading the group in setting a set of rules of engagement and respectful communication that were acceptable to all and reinforcing the importance of using these rules across the life span of the center. It also included maintaining an environment or atmosphere of safety that allowed all team members to speak without censure or other negative consequences.

The shared model (Fig. 30.1) articulated each project's contribution to the whole. As a tangible representation of each project's place in the work of the center as a whole, it heightened the team's sense of unity, drew attention to points of intersection between projects, and increased the overall level of team functioning.

References

Gehlert S. Turning disciplinary knowledge into solutions. J Adolescent Health. 2013;52:S98–S102.

Gehlert S, Sohmer D, Sacks T, Mininger C, McClintock M, Olopade O. Targeting health disparities: a model for linking upstream determinants of downstream interventions. Health Aff. 2008;27:339–49.

Gehlert S, Murray A, Sohmer D, McClintock M, Conzen S, Olopade O. The importance of transdisciplinary collaborations for understanding and resolving health disparities. Soc Work Public Health. 2010;25:408–22.

Gehlert S, Mininger C, Cipriano-Steffens T. Placing biology in breast cancer disparities research. In: Burton LM, Kemp SP, Leung M, Matthews SA, Takeuchi DT, editors. Communities, neighborhoods, and health: expanding the boundaries of place. New York: Springer; 2011. p. 57.

Hall KL, Vogel AL, Stipelman BA, Stokols D, Gehlert S. A four-phase model of transdisciplinary team-based research: goals, team processes, and strategies. Trans Behav Med. 2012;2:215–30.

Hermes GL, Delgado B, Tretiakova M, Cavigelli SA, Krausz T, Conzen SD, et al. Social isolation dysregulates endocrine and behavioral stress while increasing malignant burden of spontaneous mammary tumors. PNAS. 2009;106(52):22393–8.

Mathieu JE, Heffner TS, Goodwin GF, Salas E, Cannon-Bowers JA. The influence of shared mental models on team process and performance. J Appl Psychol. 200(85):273–83.

McClintock MK, Conzen SD, Gehlert S, Masi C, Olopade F. Mammary cancer and social interactions: identifying multiple environments that regulate gene expression throughout the life span. J Gerontol. 2005;60(I):32–41.

Williams JB, Pang D, Delgado B, Kocherginsky M, Tretiakova M, Krausz T, et al. A model of gene-environment interaction reveals altered mammary gland gene expression and increased tumor growth following social isolation. Cancer Prev Res. 2009;2(10):850–61.

Yee JR, Cavigelli SA, Delgado B, McClintock MK. Reciprocal affiliation among adolescent rats during a mild group stressor predicts mammary tumors and lifespan. Psychosom Med. 2008;70:1050–9.

The Value of Advisory Boards to Enhance Collaboration and Advance Science

31

Sarah J. Gehlert, Deborah J. Bowen,
Maria Elena Martinez, Robert Hiatt,
Christine Marx, and Graham Colditz

Contents

Beginning in the late 1990s, the National Cancer Institute (NCI) incentivized team science, including four multicenter initiatives, Transdisciplinary Tobacco Use Research Centers (TTURC), Centers for Population Health and Health Disparities (CPHHD), Centers of Excellence in Cancer Communication Research (CECCR), and Transdisciplinary Research in Energetics and Cancer (TREC). The impetus for this new approach to science was to accelerate the march from basic discoveries to population change by increasing connections between investigators (Colditz et al. 2016). The four initiatives were complex, each including four or more centers with three to four research projects. Initiatives and centers had a good deal of autonomy

S. J. Gehlert (✉)
College of Social Work, University of South
Carolina, Columbia, SC, USA
e-mail: SGEHLERT@mailbox.sc.edu

D. J. Bowen
Bioethics and Humanities, University of Washington,
School of Public Health, Seattle, WA, USA

Health Services, University of Washington, School of
Public Health, Seattle, WA, USA

M. E. Martinez
Department of Family and Preventive Medicine,
University of California San Diego,
La Jolla, CA, USA

R. Hiatt
Department of Epidemiology and Biostatistics,
University of California, San Francisco, CA, USA

C. Marx
Division of Public Health Sciences, Washington
University, St. Louis, MO, USA

G. Colditz
School of Medicine, Siteman Cancer Center, and
Institute for Public Health, Washington University in
St. Louis, St. Louis, MO, USA

© Springer Nature Switzerland AG 2019
K. L. Hall et al. (eds.), *Strategies for Team Science Success*,
https://doi.org/10.1007/978-3-030-20992-6_31

on how they coordinated the activities of their investigators and projects, and leaders used a variety of methods to foster collaboration. In the following pages, we report the experiences of one of the centers of the TREC initiative, the TREC at Washington University (WU TREC). The WU TREC initially set up an Internal Advisory Board and External Advisory Board to provide feedback to the team through the research process. We describe how using the two boards helped to foster increased connections and collaboration among investigators from different disciplines and among the four projects, allowing the center to move from basic science to evaluation of policies within communities. We describe how the two boards began to work together to help WU TREC team members to see ways of better collaborating so that the four projects formed a coherent whole that extended from basic laboratory science to clinical and workplace policy applications. We believe that the advisory boards were invaluable in enhancing our transdisciplinary work and increasing the impact of WU TREC science.

31.1 The Transdisciplinary Research on Energetics and Cancer Initiative

The mission of the National Cancer Institute's Transdisciplinary Research on Energetics and Cancer (TREC) initiative was to integrate diverse disciplines to find effective interventions across the life span to reduce the burden of obesity and cancer and to improve population health (Gehlert et al. 2014). Four research centers (Harvard University, the University of California San Diego, the University of Pennsylvania, and Washington University in St. Louis) and a coordination center (Fred Hutchinson Cancer Research Center) were funded from 2011 to 2016, during TREC's second cycle of funding. Over 30 academic disciplines were represented within the initiative's four research centers and coordination center (National Cancer Institute 2019; Patterson et al. 2013). Here we focus on the Washington

University TREC and authors of this chapter served as the Washington University (WU) TREC's Director,[1] Co-Director,[2] and center manager.[3]

The WU TREC's four research projects were implemented during the first months after funding. They vary in focus to address energetics and cancer from a variety of directions. The objective of Project 1 is to investigate the effect of high-fat diet and changes in metabolic bioenergetics on prostate gland development and susceptibility to prostate cancer in male offspring. The project uses an animal model of transgenerational transmission of prostate proliferation in pups from a high-fat maternal diet during pregnancy. Project 2 is a longitudinal study of the role of physical activity in prostate cancer outcomes among African-American men, specifically whether physical activity and obesity, individually and jointly, influence sexual and urinary function outcomes among men with clinically localized prostate cancer undergoing radical prostatectomy. Project 3 examines worksite wellness policy across Missouri, surveying employees to determine the role of workplace policy in shaping obesogenic behaviors of employees. Project 4 combines more traditional epidemiological methods with community-based participatory research to produce a better understanding of cancer risk. It does this by building models of the social determinants of obesity in non-Hodgkin Lymphoma and other cancers through stakeholder engagement (Colditz et al. 2016).

Although the four projects were designed to be interconnected, the IAB and EAB helped the group of investigators to realize more connections. This may have occurred because board members were not invested in the day-to-day operations of the four projects, nor were they committed to the achievement of the projects' specific aims, as was the case with project investigators. This allowed them to think more broadly and view the bigger picture rather than focusing inward to aims and procedures. They were able,

---

[1] Graham Colditz

[2] Sarah Gehlert

[3] Christine Marx

for example, to make suggestions to investigators such as exploring how workplace policy might influence pregnant workers' food choices, thus linking Project 1 and Project 3. Another such suggestion took a life span approach to obesity across generations and used the knowledge to develop educational materials for women in obstetric and gynecology clinics. This funded project linked Projects 1 and 4 and included junior investigators.

31.2 Efforts at Collaboration at the Washington University in St. Louis TREC

As has been mentioned, structural mechanisms in the form of advisory boards were initially set into place to provide feedback to the WU TREC team. The Director and Co-Director established a six-member External Advisory Board (EAB) immediately after the funding award was announced by NCI. Their philosophy in naming EAB members was to choose members with expertise in areas salient to the center's four projects, specifically animal models of cancer (Project 1), physical activity and nutrition (Project 2), policy (Project 3), and risk assessment (Project 4). In addition to content expertise, members were selected with an eye to those from around the country who were known to think broadly and creatively. To ensure that the team remained attuned to the population health implications of its work and the translation of its scientific findings, the Director of the St. Louis County Department of Health was invited to serve on the EAB and a second EAB member had significant policy experience at the national level. Two chapter coauthors served as EAB members.[4]

The EAB met one time per year for 1–1.5 days to allow ample time for meeting while accommodating travel. The basic structure of meetings across the years was a series of small and larger group sessions and opportunities for networking, followed by a debriefing session with the Director, Co-Director, and center manager. The

latter session produced a set of action steps to be completed by the next meeting. Table 31.1 provides examples of the actions suggested by EAB members during EAB meeting debriefings and the action taken by the Washington University TREC in response to those suggestions, most during the funding period. The final, fifth-year EAB meeting was held at the end of 2015.

An Internal Advisory Board (IAB) was established to provide a perspective on TREC's progress that was embedded in the culture of the university, and thus took into account the character and operations of the institution yet was external to the center itself. It included 15 Washington University faculty members from the biological, clinical, behavioral, and social sciences selected by the Director and Co-Director, none of whom participated directly in TREC projects or cores. The purpose of the IAB was to provide a more objective perspective on center functioning, for example the center's progress toward achieving its overall specific aims, while serving as a conduit for communication between TREC investigators and administrators and investigators from various units of the university. Table 31.1 also includes actions suggested by IAC members and WU TREC responses to those suggestions. These complemented and reinforced EAB suggestions, which was achieved by inviting IAB members of EAB meetings in later years. An example of convergence is the suggestion by the EAB in year 2 to begin to change the university culture toward transdisciplinary team science research, which was echoed by the IAB in year 3.

The intent for both advisory boards was for the WU TREC to make a lasting impression on the university by setting a mechanism in place that would foster and sustain transdisciplinary team science beyond the TREC initiative. They urged the Director and Co-Director to meet with the Chancellor and Provost to suggest specific mechanisms for incentivizing collaborations across disciplines. Meetings were held with the two top administrators and the Vice Chancellors for Research and Administration. The suggestions that accrued included establishing a cross-campus committee of senior faculty members with experience in transdisciplinary team sci-

---

[4]Maria Elena Martinez & Robert Hiatt

Table 31.1 Selected action steps suggested by Internal Advisory Board (IAB) and External Advisory Board (EAB) of the Washington University Transdisciplinary Energetics and Cancer Research Center

Topic	Action suggested	Action taken
Resource utilization	Year 1, EAB: Expand research to previously unused female pups in animal model project	Female pups used in other studies rather than being sacrificed
	Year 1, IAB: Build on gaps and spinoffs from existing projects and bring in clinicians, rather than focusing on adding new academic investigators	• Added a requirement (for years 3 and 4) to build on early data from at least one TREC research project or developmental project • Added clinician to Project 4 leadership
Translation	Year 1, EAB: Expect results in year 4 rather than year 5 to streamline translation	Shifted funding for developmental projects from year 5 to year 4 to encourage earlier results
	Year 2, EAB: Engage more clinicians to help move along the translational continuum; link clinicians to dissemination and implementation core resources	• Encouraged early career investigator (TREC developmental project PI and clinician) to apply for *Mentored Training for Dissemination & Implementation Research in Cancer* two-year fellowship • Added clinician to Project 4 leadership
Integration of projects and cores	Year 1, EAB: Better integrate projects and cores	• Dissemination and Implementation Core presented workshops at year 2 IAB meeting and TREC Scientific Meeting • Added a dissemination and implementation requirement for within-center developmental awards
	Year 1, EAB: Push integration of the use of measures	• Projects 2 and 3 began to share data elements • Project 2 added GIS measures
	Year 1, IAB: Each project should strive to inform new research questions in other projects	Example action: Project 1 inquiries about impact of obesity during pregnancy yielded additional questions for Project 4, which revealed a research gap in modeling obesity in pregnant women
	Year 1, IAB: Develop a common framework	Built a Center-level shared conceptual model that has since been used for multiple strategic applications, including identifying gaps and prioritizing Pilot funding
Change university culture about transdisciplinary team science	Year 2, EAB, year 3 IAB: Change the university culture about team science, allowing for better support of pre-tenure investigators to do team science	• Held conversations with university and school administrators resulting in some changes in tenure and promotion policy • Initiated TREC Transdisciplinary Cancer Prevention and Control Postdoctoral Training Program open to outside trainees
	Year 5, IAB: Hire scientific/technical writer to help in pursuing opportunities and communicating across/outside of author's discipline	No action to date
Sustainability of TREC activities and accomplishments	Year 5, EAB: Diversify pursuit of funding to include private donors/entrepreneurial science	In process

ence who could evaluate the team science efforts of junior investigators who chose to be evaluated as such. This evaluation would be then added to a tenure portfolio that included the more customary letters of recommendation for internal and external evaluators. A second suggestion led to the establishment of internal research funds for projects involving teams of investigators from different disciplines. Importantly, each of the two suggested actions sent a message that WU administrators supported the transdisciplinary team science efforts of junior investigators, and helped to establish a safe environment for this approach to science.

31.3 Advisory Board Functions and Contributions

At the first meeting of the IAB, after six months of TREC operation, project and core leaders briefly described their research questions and specific aims for feedback from IAB members. Although this general structure was repeated during each subsequent year of funding, subsequent meetings were tailored to the needs of the center at that point in time. The 2015 IAB meeting, for example, was devoted to generating ideas for perpetuating the work of the TREC and its style of scientific collaboration on the WU campus after funding ceased. This topic was first generated during the first EAB meeting in 2011 and remained a theme for subsequent EAB and IAB meetings. Meeting with the Chancellor and Provost and other top administrators was part of ensuring that WU TREC gains were sustained. By the final EAB and IAB meetings, the groups were able to generate concrete ideas for sustaining the work of TREC in terms of obesity and cancer and transdisciplinary team science in general. These included our suggestions for creating a safe environment for junior investigators who wanted to pursue transdisciplinary team science that valued their collaborative work across disciplines. Annotating their curriculum vitae to highlight their unique contribution to collaborative work is a concrete example of an action designed to change how scholarship was viewed and evaluated.

One way that EABs furthered our transdisciplinary efforts was through prioritizing cross-project connections. During the first year of WU TREC operation, project leaders expressed concern that fulfilling their specific aims was difficult enough without the additional expectations and requirements presented by center operation. They voiced concern about dividing their time between project-specific and larger center activ-

ities and needs, and this concern was raised during the first annual EAB meeting. Upon hearing these concerns during small and large group sessions with investigators, EAB members echoed the Director's and Co-Director's charge to operate as an entity rather than a series of independent research projects and challenged the group to create a shared conceptual or mental model. This model was developed during a later session to which all WU TREC investigators were invited, led by DJB, a senior visiting cancer scholar, using a method of externalizing cognition in which maps and diagrams were generated to portray how each project, and ultimately each discipline, fit into the WU TREC as a whole.

Another way that our EAB added to the project was by generating the new research ideas for each project and for the center as a whole. The WU TREC conceptual model was expanded during the second IAB meeting, which was held shortly after the group model building session. Rather than merely describing their progress toward the project's specific aims, project leaders were asked to discuss their project-specific progress in terms of its contribution to the overall WU TREC conceptual model. Immediately after that, a panel of project leaders and investigators generated a list of possible future collaborations during an interactive session facilitated by DJB. This panel discussion was fueled by the content of presentations that had been made by each project leader earlier in the meeting, as reflected by leaders of the other three projects. A number of new ideas were generated and recorded that were beyond the original goals of the projects.

Although WU was the only TREC to implement both and an IAB and an EAB, both the Harvard University and University of Pennsylvania TRECs implemented IABs. In all three cases, TREC leaders noted that their advisory boards helped prevent their research projects from focusing only inward, encouraging them toward bolder and more innovative collaborations (National Cancer Institute 2019). The leaders of these centers noted that investigators tended to regress toward monodisciplinary functioning in the absence of external encouragement to take a bigger picture and consider how their work contributed to the shared agenda of the TREC mission as a whole.

31.4   Conclusion

Although our purpose in establishing and IAB and EAB as the part of the WU TREC was simply to provide feedback to TREC investigators rather than to foster collaboration among investigators, their establishment had the unintended, positive consequence of facilitating communication, and ultimately collaboration, among projects. During their first meeting with TREC investigators, for example, IAB members suggested moving our basic science work from an exclusive emphasis on male gender to add female outcomes. This allowed the team to expand its focus to the effects of dietary factors in female pups rather than disposing of them. The outcome of forcing an expanded focus on the WU TREC as a whole rather than one specific project, which allowed the center as a whole to envision our march from basic discovery to application and the evaluation in communities.

Advisory boards are valuable in expanding the vision of research centers, and thus maximizing communication, collaboration, and the generation of new ideas. This is possible because team investigators tend, from necessity, to focus inward to their own projects, missing possible new synergies that can be seen by those who are less invested in the day-to-day operations of projects, as is the case with IAB and EAB members. EABs whose members originate outside the universities that they are advising help to force a bigger picture of a center's work that includes how the work will be translated into improved population health. IABs whose members represent various parts of a university help to challenge university structures and operations to foster transdisciplinary team science. In the case of the Washington University TREC, this included the aforementioned guidelines for promotion and tenure that supported rather than challenged team science, helping the institution to move beyond perceived impediments imposed by university policies and entrenched modes of operation.

References

Colditz GA, Gehlert S, Bowen DJ, Carson K, Hovmand PS, Moley KH. Toward a modern science of obesity at Washington University: how we do it and what is the payoff. Cancer Prev Res. 2016;9(7):503–8.

Gehlert S, Hall KL, Vogel AL, Hohl S, Hartman S, Nebeling L, Thompson B. Advancing transdisciplinary research: the transdisciplinary energetics and cancer initiative. J Transl Med Epidemiol. 2014;2(2):1033.

National Cancer Institute: Transdisciplinary research on energetics and cancer (TREC) centers. 2019. https://cancercontrol.cancer.gov/brp/hbrb/trec/index.html. Accessed 27 Mar 2019.

Patterson RE, Colditz G, Wu F, Schmitz K, Anima RS, Brownson R, Thornquist M. The 2011–2016 Transdisciplinary Research in Energetics and Cancer (TREC) initiative: rationale and design. Cancer Causes Control. 2013;24(4):695–704.

Designing and Developing Coordinating Centers as Infrastructure to Support Team Science

32

Betsy Rolland

Contents

As collaborative science increasingly becomes the norm, drawing researchers into projects from multiple sites, multiple disciplines, and multiple institutions, coordination of the people, tasks, information, and documents produced by the research has become increasingly onerous and time-consuming. Coordinating Centers (CCs), central bodies tasked with developing systems and processes to support collaborative work in order to facilitate a network's progress toward its scientific goals, emerged as a solution to this problem by centralizing critical coordination work in one designated entity responsible for

bringing together all the moving parts. Yet a dearth of research on the coordination of team science, in general, and CCs, in particular, means that CCs are developed by funding agencies and research teams with limited empirical evidence on how best to design an infrastructure that encourages and facilitates collaboration.

While there are a variety of ways of funding and forming CCs, one of the most common is represented by the NIH U-mechanism (i.e., a cooperative agreement), which funds a CC as a separate, independent entity alongside funded research sites. Networks come in many shapes and sizes, but CC-led networks generally consist of a CC, funding agency representatives, and a set of research sites. In order to understand CCs and their place in a research network, it is important to understand that such a research network functions as a system, and the CC is just one part of that system. The work of each part of that system is dependent upon and, in turn, influences the others.

Because CCs take many forms and are funded under a variety of mechanisms, it is difficult to identify how many CCs exist across the research enterprise, the amount of money being invested in this type of coordination infrastructure, or how quickly the prevalence of CCs is growing. We do know, however, that major funders are supporting CCs. For example, the National Institutes of Health (NIH) has invested

B. Rolland (✉)
Carbone Cancer Center and Institute for Clinical and Translational Research, University of Wisconsin-Madison, Madison, WI, USA
e-mail: brolland@wisc.edu

© Springer Nature Switzerland AG 2019
K. L. Hall et al. (eds.), *Strategies for Team Science Success*,
https://doi.org/10.1007/978-3-030-20992-6_32

substantial funds in CCs and other coordination mechanisms for multi-center research initiatives and research networks such as the Breast Cancer & the Environment Research Program, the Clinical Sequencing Exploratory Research program, the Childhood Cancer Survivorship Study, and the Early Detection Research Network, to name just a few. In practice, the limited availability of best practices or theoretical frameworks for CCs means that a new CC often spends precious time, energy, and resources to figure out how best to organize itself and its collaborative processes in order to help its network achieve its scientific goals.

In this chapter, I share results from my NCI-funded research on the role of CCs in collaborative, coordinated networks. The aim of this study was to describe the work a CC does, as well as to identify those aspects of the CC infrastructure that influenced how scientists collaborated and that impacted scientific outcomes of the project, in the hopes of beginning to develop necessary best practices. Drawing upon this work, as well as my own experience building and managing multiple CCs, I propose three design elements that should be addressed as funding agencies and research teams consider how best to design, develop, and evaluate coordinated networks for maximum collaboration, efficiency, and effectiveness: (1) clarity of roles and responsibilities; (2) a funding structure that requires collaborative work; and (3) the inclusion of a scientific role for the CC.

32.1 Research Background and Methods

My research focused on two NCI-funded CCs: the Biomarker Network and the Screening Network (Network names are pseudonyms). The goal of the Biomarker Network was to identify and validate biomarkers of cancer, while the goal of the Screening Network was to characterize the screening process for several cancers in order to identify potential areas of improvement. The Biomarker Network was in its third funding

cycle, while the Screening Network was at the beginning of its first funding cycle, as I began my research. What is most interesting about these two CCs is that they were run, primarily, by the same group of PIs and staff at one institution, which, in theory, should have resulted in a straightforward application of the CC's skills, processes, and systems developed for the Biomarker Network to the Screening Network. Unfortunately, this was not the case, and the Screening Network struggled to achieve its scientific goals, while the Biomarker Network continued its strong scientific progress. Analysis of our qualitative data, collected in over 95 h of observation and 17 interviews, revealed striking differences in the design of the infrastructures of the two networks.

32.2 What Does a Coordinating Center Do?

The types of work done by a CC are highly dependent on the scientific objectives of the network being coordinated, generally ranging from administrative and operational tasks like organizing conference calls through more advanced scientific work such as developing protocols and conducting statistical analyses. CCs are most frequently led by PhD-level scientists, especially by biostatisticians, and staffed with a variety of positions that may include project managers, computer programmers, data managers, clinical coordinators, and administrative assistants, depending on the needs of the specific projects undertaken by the network. While the scientific objectives of the network will determine exactly what tasks fall to the CC, there are categories of work in which most CCs commonly engage. Drawing upon the literature and my own research on CCs, I developed a typology of work practices in a CC-enabled network [1]:

1. *Structural work*: those activities that shape the official rules of the network and dictate its organizational structure, once funded and instantiated;

2. *Collaboration development work*: the extra work scientists participating in a network do to elevate the disparate groups of individuals and institutions toward a functioning whole, or, in the words of many of our participants, to make the consortium "greater than the sum of its parts";

3. *Operational work*: the administrative and technological tasks done in support of the network's scientific objectives;

4. *Data work*: work focused on the generation of the highest possible quality data for collaborative projects.

Again, to understand what a CC does, it is necessary to view that work in the context of the network it is coordinating, as part of the larger system. Examples of each type of work for each network participant type (CC, research center, funding agency representative) are included in Table 32.1; further details on each type of work and more examples can be found in Rolland (2013). This list is not exhaustive and similar tasks may be performed by different participants. The table is meant simply to give shape to the types of work being done by the network, as a whole, and to emphasize the interdependence of the tasks. While these tasks may not all be unique to a coordinated network, it is the way in which the tasks must function together as a whole that makes the work of designing a coordinating center uniquely challenging. Furthermore, ensuring that each type of participant understands not only its own role but also the role of the other entities is critical to the success of the network, as discussed below.

Table 32.1 Typology of work practices in a CC-enabled network

Type of work practice	Example CC tasks	Example research site (Grantee) PI tasks	Example funding agency representative tasks
Structural	• Negotiating revisions to scientific objectives in case of unexpected funding changes	• Submitting grant proposal • Agreeing to accept funds and follow FOA	• Writing the FOA • Making funding changes • Revising scientific objectives as needed
Collaboration development	• Deciding how to interpret FOA in practice (with Funding Agency) • Negotiating questions of roles and responsibilities • Prioritization of projects in view of limited resources	• Participating in committees and working groups • Fulfilling role in network • Attending meetings	• Deciding how to interpret FOA in practice (with CC) • Evaluating grantee progress, reviewing progress reports • Ensuring network moving toward scientific objectives
Operational	• Organizing meetings and conference calls • Programming data entry system • Coordinating protocol development • Management of IRB approvals	• Sending questions to CC • IRB documentation submission to CC • Registering for meetings	• Creating agendas for meetings • Scheduling site visits
Data	• Distilling scientific questions to specific data points for collection • Statistical analyses • Protocol development and study design	• Data extraction to produce network-requested datasets • Running assays or experiments according to agreed-upon network protocols	• Representing interest of Funding Agency in protocol development • Reviewing analysis results

32.3 How Does the CC Infrastructure Design Impact the Scientific Outcomes of a Project?

Three design elements emerged from this research as critical to ensuring that the CC's infrastructure supported, instead of discouraged, collaboration: (1) clarity of roles and responsibilities; (2) a funding structure that required collaborative work; and (3) the inclusion of a scientific role for the CC. Each of these elements, individually, had the potential to impact the CC's ability to help the network achieve its scientific aims.

32.3.1 Clarity of Roles and Responsibilities

The division of labor in the network was especially important to the work of the CC. Because the role of a CC is often defined in vague terms (*supports*, *coordinates*, *facilitates*), a CC may end up responsible for any work that does not fit neatly into one of the other roles described in the funding announcement. Furthermore, if the roles of the CC, the research sites, or the funding agency are poorly defined or understood, network members may spend substantial time discussing how to divide the work. This was observed in the Screening Network, in which the CC and NCI program representatives were out of synch in their understanding of each other's roles as well as the role of the research sites. In practice, this meant weekly meetings spent hashing out who would do what instead of strategic discussions of how to achieve the group's scientific objectives. This disconnect had two main impacts. First, it slowed down the group's work. Second, the disconnect sparked conflict between the CC and the research sites, which were being asked to do work they thought fell under the purview of the CC. The group members' trust in one another quickly declined. The Biomarker Network, on the other hand, established very clear roles and responsibilities from the beginning, and I observed no conflict in this area.

Establishing clear roles and responsibilities is a design element that must be addressed at the earliest stages of designing the network. The funding announcement can help, laying out as much detail as possible for the grantees, while leaving flexibility for the network to evolve. As the network grows and changes over the funding period, participants benefit from ongoing, collaborative conversations about what work must be done, how it moves the group toward its scientific objectives, and who should do it. The CC can take a leadership role by facilitating and tracking such discussions, and regular meetings of a steering committee can serve as a neutral venue for holding them. Having CC staff and PIs trained in conflict resolution, strategic planning, and meeting facilitation can help this work go well.

32.3.2 Funding Structure

A second key design element is the network's funding structure, which is set by the funding agency in the funding announcement. In the Biomarker Network, a large portion of the overall funding was reserved for collaborative work across multiple sites. Furthermore, each research site was required to spend a portion of its own budget for collaborative work with other sites, a requirement which was strictly enforced and monitored. The Biomarker Network also had annual evaluation criteria that explicitly measured and assessed how collaborative each site had been during the previous year based on how they had spent those funds, among other criteria. By doing so, the funding structure actually *required* collaborative work rather than simply encouraging it in name alone. The Screening Network, on the other hand, did not have funds reserved exclusively for supporting collaborative work and research sites were encouraged to use the funds earmarked for cross-network projects to cover shortfall in their budgets caused by unexpected cuts.

These different approaches to funding structure resulted in different mindsets in the two networks about working on cross-network projects, and, really, different cultures of collaboration. A strong, positive culture of collaboration and openness led to successful projects, which led to even more collaboration and openness, resulting in a virtuous cycle. Multi-site collaboration is challenging for a number of reasons, but when funds are reserved for collaborative work as required by the funding announcement, and rules for collaboration are enforced, it ensures that researchers participate in multi-site collaborations, despite the challenges. In a network where funds have not been reserved for collaborative work in the original funding announcement, it is still possible for participants to decide to use their own funds to support collaborative work. Here, the CC can help negotiate the rules of engagement for such cross-network projects, perhaps even identifying additional funding sources and facilitating applications for new projects.

32.3.3 A Scientific Role for the CC

Finally, designing a scientific role for the CC encourages collaboration by both integrating the CC as a scientific partner—instead of simply an administrator—and increasing the CC's investment in the quality of the network's scientific work. It is also key to attracting top scientific talent to run the CC. In the Biomarker Network, the biostatisticians leading the CC developed novel methods for identifying and validating promising biomarkers. In order to do this work, the CC needed data of the highest possible quality, so they invested resources in their data systems. The CC PIs and staff were also viewed as strong scientific collaborators, because their work enhanced the work being done by the research sites. In fact, the research sites routinely consulted the Biomarker Network CC with their most difficult statistical questions, another area of strength among the CC staff members. In the Screening Network, the work being done by the CC was, at first, primarily operational. The collaborative work did require guiding the discussions about which data to collect in a network-wide database, which is an important scientific work; however, this work was delayed by the budget cuts discussed above and by a lack of expertise in some of the key scientific areas.

Responsibility for this design element falls primarily to the funding agencies who design the funding announcements, and we urge those designing such announcements to think about not only the logistics of organizing a network, but also of the skills and knowledge needed to facilitate the network's scientific progress. As neutral third parties, CCs can focus on the overall mission of the network while also helping each individual site achieve its own objectives. Within the structure and mission set out by the funding agency, the CC must also ensure that it has the necessary scientific expertise to address the scientific breadth of the network; for a CC to be a *scientific facilitator* instead of simply an *administrative coordinator* requires experience and knowledge in the network's area of scientific focus.

32.4 Conclusion

A research network is a system, and a systems-thinking and user-centered design approach are required to design, develop, and evaluate networks for maximum collaboration, efficiency, and effectiveness. The design elements discussed above are just three areas where decisions made by funding agencies and researchers in designing and running networks are too important to be left to chance or historical precedent. The way in which a network is coordinated impacts the speed and quality of its scientific progress, but little research exists that can be used to guide decision-makers in this design process. There have been relatively few evaluations specifically focused on CC operations, and we know little about what makes a CC high- or low-performing or how different CCs, with different structures, roles, and other characteristics, have impacted the scientific outcomes of their network. In order to create a *science of coordination*, these questions must be explored and hypotheses tested. As collaborative research continues to increase its reach, we must invest in developing the knowledge needed to craft strong CCs to support their collaborative networks.

Reference

Rolland B. Greater than the sum of its parts: coordinating centers as facilitators of network-level work in cancer epidemiology coordinating center enabled networks (Doctoral dissertation). 2013. https://digital.lib.washington.edu/researchworks/handle/1773/22888.

Part IX

Education, Training, and Professional Development for Cross-Disciplinary Team Science

Training to Be a (Team) Scientist

33

Stephen M. Fiore, Catherine Gabelica,
Travis J. Wiltshire, and Daniel Stokols

Contents

The original version of this chapter was revised.
The correction to this chapter is available at
https://doi.org/10.1007/978-3-030-20992-6_46

S. M. Fiore (✉)
Cognitive Sciences, Department of Philosophy,
University of Central Florida,
Orlando, FL, USA

Cognitive Sciences Laboratory, Institute for
Simulation and Training, University of Central
Florida, Orlando, FL, USA
e-mail: sfiore@ist.ucf.edu

C. Gabelica
Human Resources Management, IÉSEG School of
Management, Paris, France

T. J. Wiltshire
Department of Cognitive Science and Artificial
Intelligence, Tilburg University, Tilburg, Netherlands

D. Stokols
Department of Urban Planning and Public Policy, and
Department of Psychological Sciences, School of
Social Ecology, University of California Irvine,
Irvine, CA, USA

33.1 Introduction

In the early twenty-first century, many have lamented the lack of a sufficient scientific workforce capable of contributing to the modern knowledge-intensive economy (AACU 2007; NRC 2015). At the same time, others have noted the lack of a scientific workforce capable of collaborating across scientific disciplines (NRC 2005, 2014, 2015). More and more it is recognized that the science and technology workforce is being inadequately prepared for careers in the coming century (Crow and Dabars 2015; Duderstadt 2000). In the study of workforce preparation, reports have identified gaps between the knowledge, skills, and attitudes (KSAs) employers are seeking and those held by graduates (HRA 2015; NRC 2017). This includes not just skills in, for example, data analysis and problem solving, but also teamwork and interpersonal skills (e.g., communication across professions), attitudes and abilities to collaborate with non-academic partners and colleagues spanning multiple cultures, geographic regions, and time zones (Brint et al. 2009; Brown et al. 2010; Karlin et al. 2017; Olson and Olson 2014; Stokols 2018). Furthermore, according to a report on career preparation recently commissioned by the Association of American Colleges and Universities, college graduates' "self" perceptions of KSAs are divergent from employer assessment (HRA 2015). For example, nearly 2/3 of college graduate believe they can effectively work in a team whereas only approximately 1/3 of managers stated college graduates demonstrate this competence. Similarly, over half of college graduates felt they are able to work with those possessing different backgrounds but only less than 1/5 of managers saw this as the case.

The combination of these factors leads to a need to better prepare the scientific workforce for participation in the larger collaborative scientific enterprise and contribute to the needs of society more broadly (Fiore et al. 2018). In service of this, recent reviews describe the rich body of research on teamwork and our understanding about collaboration as it relates to structural (e.g., technology, virtuality; Olson et al. 2008) and compositional features (e.g., ability, faultlines) as well as mechanisms (e.g., conflict, motivation) mediating process and performance (Bezrukova et al. 2009; Mathieu et al. 2017). Still others focus on training to document how researchers have developed a deep understanding of how trainee characteristics and training design influence learning and performance outcomes (Bell et al. 2017). In this chapter we focus on a somewhat narrow aspect of this research—that having to do with training and education where knowledge is diverse and members collaborate to address significant societal and scientific problems. We draw from the aforementioned literatures to distill key ideas about teamwork competencies identified as being foundational to effectiveness for the scientific workforce.

Our overarching point is that we must move beyond traditional forms of learning and education that seek only to train discipline-specific content (e.g., methods, processes, concepts). Rather, we argue that, to successfully meet the scientific workforce need of the twenty-first century, we must also understand how to improve learning and professional development focused on improving collaboration across disciplines and professions. In support of this argument, recent reports from the National Academies of Science noted that there is an increased need to emphasize interdisciplinary and transdisciplinary approaches to learning with more focus on experiential and problem-based learning—whether in the laboratory or in internships and apprenticeships (NRC

2015, 2017). This presents a significant challenge for research on learning in that it illustrates two fundamentally different, but now integrated, learning objectives. One is the acquisition of knowledge sufficient to be an expert in a field, yet sufficiently knowledgeable enough about other disciplines to work collaboratively on complex problems. The other is learning the kinds of teamwork competencies supporting collaboration with others on such problems (see also Nurius and Kemp 2019 in this volume for additional discussion of team science competencies).

The former need has long been recognized as a challenge for interdisciplinary education (Klein 1996). But the latter need is an important part of the new field called the "Science of Team Science (SciTS)," a field dedicated to understanding and improving scientific teamwork (Borner et al. 2010; Fiore 2008; Hall et al. 2008; Stokols et al. 2008; Hall et al. 2018). Considering these in combination, teamwork in science requires both knowledge from multiple disciplines and also collaboration across disciplines and professions. Those engaged in such work often have advanced degrees, creating collaborations among professionals with deep knowledge and experience. Thus, problem solving in such contexts requires not just the application of knowledge from diverse areas, but the teamwork competencies necessary to successfully integrate said knowledge.

Considering this in light of the policy needs previously mentioned, we compare this with traditional definitions of teams—that is, "interdependent collections of individuals who share responsibility for specific outcomes for their organizations" (Sundstrom et al. 1990, p. 120). This concept of interdependence has been foundational to the study of teams, as has been the need for coordination across clearly articulated roles to meet specifically defined and explicit goals (e.g., Swezey and Salas 1992). As such, it aligns well with the context of scientific collaboration. But we argue that, to truly address science and technology workforce needs, definitions of teams must add the concept of interdisciplinarity.

Definitions of interdisciplinary research vary (cf., Repko et al. 2017), but one of the early distinctions was put forth by the Organization for Economic Cooperation and Development in 1972 (see also NRC 2005). The OECD report in 1972 outlined a set of the core ideas that have been used in many definitions of interdisciplinary, noting that such research involves: "The interaction among two or more different disciplines. This interaction may range from simple communication of ideas to the mutual integration of organizing concepts, methodology, procedures, epistemology, terminology, data, and organization of research and education in a fairly large field ... a common effort on a common problem with continuous intercommunication among the participants from the different disciplines" (pp. 25–26). Overall, then, we can see the complementarity between teamwork and interdisciplinary research in that they both involve coordination and communication among those with specialized knowledge and clearly defined roles, for the purposes of addressing a shared problem.

At issue is that the science workforce has been, and is still predominantly trained, in a way at odds with an interdisciplinary perspective to collaboration. They have been socialized within a discipline to learn, not just content knowledge but the norms and cultures of a discipline. Furthermore, they receive little, if any, training on how to function as a member of a team. This produces a myriad of problems for scientific teamwork—from terminology differences and challenges with communicating across disciplines, to divergent epistemologies about how to pursue knowledge—often resulting in failures of the scientific team. In short, to train the next-generation workforce, we must understand how to overcome traditional learning and education practices that have narrowly focused on content knowledge and move towards a more interdisciplinary learning environment (cf., Bosque-Perez et al. 2016; Chang et al. 2005). Here, learning would involve not just acquisition of knowledge from varied disciplines, but also the ability to collaborate with those from different fields. For workforce preparation, we argue that science education and professional development must focus on learning how to be a "team" scientist.

Towards this end, in this chapter we draw from the literature on interdisciplinary education and training that has evolved to support changes in scholarship and collaborations across disciplines and professions. The chapter is divided into two main sections. In the first half, a brief review of the literature on learning and training for interdisciplinary science is provided. Here we outline the various educational and professional development programs developed by universities and/or supported by the federal government. In general, these programs have been developed to address science and technology workforce needs via identification of various competencies necessary for success and how to train teams for complex scientific and societal problem solving. The second half provides an integration of ideas from the organizational sciences that serves as conceptual scaffolding for learning how to engage in team science. This is meant to provide some coherence to the varied forms of educational and professional development programs that have identified a myriad number of competencies thought to be needed for interdisciplinary teamwork. We conclude this section with a brief description of notional approaches for training these competencies. These were derived from the literature on team training but adapted for consideration in the context of scientific collaboration and S&T workforce preparation. Our goal is to lay the foundation for research on interdisciplinarity in support of scientific workforce development and helping to produce the next generation of team scientists.

33.2 Interdisciplinary Learning

33.2.1 A Brief History of Interdisciplinary Learning

Although much attention was paid to interdisciplinary education in the latter part of the twentieth century, thinking on this topic started surprisingly earlier in the "modern" academy. In one of the earliest mentions of interdisciplinary research, Brozek and Keys (1944) described how Yale University was developing interdepartmental research programs such as the "Yale Institute of Human Relations" in the 1930s to study complex social and scientific issues. They referred to this as a natural result of disparate academic units recognizing their similar interests and the value of pursuing them cooperatively. They cite the pioneering and prescient vision of Yale's president, James Rowland Angell, who had pronounced in 1930 that the purpose of such centers was to "correlate knowledge and coordinate technique in related fields, [such] that greater progress may be made in the understanding of human life from the biological, psychological and sociological viewpoint" (p. 509). What Brozek and Keys (1944) were suggesting is that interdisciplinary research, and its focus on cooperating to solve societal problems, needed to be an accepted form of practice when learning to be a scientist. They argued that such environments are better able to nurture an appreciation for social problem solving via the integration of broad perspectives while still pursuing fundamental scientific knowledge. Specifically:

"There are two very serious reasons why the inclusion of this new research form should be a part of graduate schools: Numerous problems of a fundamental theoretical character which require a cooperative approach are not likely to be studied by industrial laboratories, the very existence of which often depends upon immediate, practical results. The second reason is still more important. Industrial organizations only very rarely will provide the time and personnel to carry out a training program of high academic standards. There must be a genuine interest in acquainting the student with the full breadth and depth of the interdisciplinary research problems, which implies a full freedom to explore aspects other than those which belong to the student's immediate field of specialization. The most adequate 'climate' for the training of graduate students in cooperative research is a place in which such an approach is actually practiced, because there is no substitute for the method of learning by doing. At the same time, the institution in charge of the training program must be well aware of its scientific and social responsibilities and must provide stimulating supervision which is or should be a distinguishing feature of student-teacher relationship on the graduate level" (p. 509, Brozek and Keys 1944).

Not only was this thinking ahead of its time from the standpoint of interdisciplinarity, it also foresaw what is now an important component of action research; that is, a blurring of the distinction between basic and applied science (see Stokols 2014). As such, these ideas clearly resonate with current perceptions of interdisciplinary learning and training. Further, by trying to do away with the juxtaposition between basic and applied research, they are strikingly similar to ideas in science policy over 50 years later. In his landmark work, *Pasteur's Quadrant*, Stokes (1997) illustrated how important scientific gains were often due to this blending of basic and applied research. Stokes used Louis Pasteur as the model for what he labels *use-inspired basic science* showing how Pasteur's groundbreaking and significant studies in microbiology always had a consideration for use (i.e., disease prevention), yet still produced fundamental gains in understanding. Using such examples, Stokes suggests that both science and science policy can benefit from considering research that has a quest for fundamental understanding and a consideration of use. Others have taken a similar tack when arguing for science as societal problem solving. Based upon the writings and actions of one of our nation's founders, Holton and Sonnert (1999) argued along analogous lines to propose a model of *Jeffersonian Science*. Here, research has as its motivation a particular social problem in which we are scientifically ignorant. As Holton and Sonnert (1999) explain, the purpose is "to remove that basic ignorance in an uncharted area of science and thereby to attain knowledge that will have a fair probability--even if it is years distant--of being brought to bear on a persistent, debilitating national (or international) problem" (p. 62).

We have used this brief historical account on interdisciplinarity and this thinking on science policy to call out a simple yet important point. For these accounts illustrate that the tension identified nearly ¾ of a century ago, is still problematic when discussing interdisciplinary research. They bring to the fore the barriers that rise when training tries to teach a learner to think beyond traditional disciplinary boundaries or consider how knowledge can be applied to solve problems. If we are to successfully solve the significant scientific and societal problems of the twenty-first century, and better prepare the scientific workforce, we must overcome these challenges and understand the processes necessary for learning how to be a team scientist. With this cautionary note as our precursor, we now turn to a discussion of interdisciplinary learning as it was explored in latter part of the twentieth century.

33.2.2 Interdisciplinary Education in the Twentieth Century

Interest in, and attention to, interdisciplinary education waxed and waned in the postwar era (see Klein 1990 for a full discussion). But serious attention to developing interdisciplinary programs began, in earnest, in the health sciences in the 1960s (Lavin et al. 2001). It was at this time that interdisciplinary educators began to develop courses that maximized the learning of broad skills while minimizing discipline-specific skills. Such efforts were not fully accepted as they led to concerns about the shallowness of the educational training. Nonetheless, they are relevant to our focus on team science because it was here that we see initial acknowledgement of *interpersonal competencies*. Scholars studying interdisciplinary education started to discuss the types of communication and group process challenges such as conflict and role ambiguity that can emerge when students from different disciplines are brought together (Hohle et al. 1969). From this, interdisciplinary internships and fellowships began with the goal of teaching students how to communicate when working with other disciplines (Lupella 1972). Others focused on analogous challenges and the need for groups to develop collaboration skills when working with other disciplines (AACU 2007; Brint 2009; Jacobson 1974). As noted by Fiore (2008), in the ensuing decades, while interdisciplinarity increased in popularity, knowledge of how to support it remained relatively static. Specifically, "although interdisciplinary research swelled, there were not proportional changes in the understanding or training of interpersonal issues. But we did see the beginning of minimum competencies being identified as interdisciplinary course-

work began to become more prevalent. That is, as interdisciplinary coursework began to pull students in many different directions, curriculum committees and professional organizations began to mandate the minimum level of understandings students within particular disciplines had to master" (p. 264). This illustrated a movement more towards the focus on disciplinary content and the minimum levels of knowledge that should be learned as opposed to the interpersonal factors that arise when working across disciplines.

As training and education research and theory began to evolve in the 1990s, scholars also started to focus on macro-level issues such as how organizations could better support interdisciplinarity (Lavin et al. 2001). Klein (1996) was one of the first to articulate a coherent conceptualization of interdisciplinary learning at this broader institutional and organizational scale. In discussing how departments, centers, and institutes could form a foundation for supporting interdisciplinarity, she described the hurdles that needed to be overcome to address traditional perspectives on practice. Interdisciplinary education requires organizational-level support, minimally, for professional development (e.g., training faculty) as well as protection from disciplinary norms (e.g., tenure reviews that punish work outside one's discipline). Even better, such support can include, for example, mentoring, physical space for collaborations, and cross-disciplinary training. From this, an environment can be nurtured that creates a norm for interdisciplinarity. This includes research and teaching that encourages a broader perspective on problems as well as communication across departmental boundaries. Furthermore, in order for such practices to be sustained, institutional support must be consistent and embedded within the university culture (see Canadian Academy of Health Sciences 2017; Klein 2010; Klein and Falk-Krzesinski 2017; The Academy of Medical Sciences 2016; Vogel et al. 2019).

In sum, there has been a significant amount of attention paid to understanding and improving interdisciplinary learning. But, despite this interest in interdisciplinarity, a notable gap remained. Specifically, little, if any, discussions addressed interdisciplinary *teams*. The majority of this literature considered the intellectual aspects of interdisciplinarity but did not attend to collaboration more specifically. At most, the focus was on the individual who would work in a collaborative environment, rather than on the actual collaborative context. From this arose attention to interpersonal factors required for teamwork. As such, this represented an important development in the context of learning and education for the scientific workforce; that is, the need to teach competencies associated with interdisciplinary collaborations.

As these approaches were evolving to include competencies, another challenge emerged. In brief, there are many different competencies associated with interdisciplinarity, and early discussions in this literature lacked the conceptual clarity necessary to develop educational content and pedagogy. First, there is a level of competency one has to have regarding *disciplinary content* (e.g., how much foundational knowledge in biology must one acquire). But there is also competency required for thinking *across disciplinary content* (e.g., if one wants to understand biophysics, on what should their coursework focus to help them understand how to conceptualize related factors crossing these disciplines). Finally, there is also a set of competencies associated with one's ability to engage in *interdisciplinary teamwork* (e.g., how to address conflict that might arise when working with someone with different disciplinary norms). But discussions in this early literature would often conflate these very real and very important differences.

We return to this problem in the concluding section and offer some theoretical clarity to move our understanding of interdisciplinary learning forward. But we next describe some of the work that sought to more precisely identify the varied types of competencies necessary for interdisciplinary teamwork. This is broken out into two sections. The first focuses on research examining interdisciplinary programs where learning was designed to cover content from multiple disciplines. The second focuses on programs specifically developed by federal organizations to support education and training for the next generation of the scientific workforce.

33.2.3 Educating Individuals for Interdisciplinary Collaboration

Reflecting on what is necessary for success in the twenty-first-century workplace, we can minimally state that interdisciplinary collaborations differ in the degree to which they require teamwork as well as the integration and application of knowledge; that is, from understanding how to work with people and methods from other disciplines/professions, to synthesizing concepts and theories to produce actionable knowledge (Nash 2008; Repko et al. 2017). In the modern workforce, the challenges of interdisciplinarity are often dealt with on an ad hoc basis where leaders or managers address conflict or communication problems as they emerge. Although this might succeed in the short term, more is required to ensure a scientific workforce capable of addressing complex scientific and societal challenges (Brown et al. 2010; Crow and Dabars 2015, 2019; Stokols 2018). What is needed is not only sufficient training for collaboration across disciplines, but also consideration of how the competencies necessary for effectiveness in teams could be instilled through educational experiences. This includes interdisciplinary experiential learning that comes through both coursework (e.g., group projects) and internships at the undergraduate, graduate, and post-graduate levels, to produce what Stokols (2014) referred to as "an enduring intellectual orientation among students and scholars" (p. 58). The goal is developing the intellectual and interpersonal capacity for effective collaboration on interdisciplinary work.[1]

In this section we provide discussion of the types of programs that have been embedded in educational practice to meet the aforementioned goals. Our review includes those efforts that

---

[1] Note that Hirsch Hadorn et al. (2008), Rosenfield (1992), Stokols (2018), and others have written extensively about transdisciplinary education and research. For example, Misra et al. (2015) developed and tested a scale for assessing attitudinal, behavioral, and intellectual dimensions of scholars' "transdisciplinary orientation." Because many of the concepts and approaches are relevant to interdisciplinary education and training, this distinction is not addressed in this chapter.

target both graduate and undergraduate students and range from individual courses to curriculum-wide efforts. We focus on studies of interdisciplinary learning that examined the types of competencies supporting interdisciplinarity. Although much has been written about interdisciplinary education, our selection is driven by studies that have provided at least some form of quantitative summary of their findings. A notable gap is that there have been few field studies of interdisciplinary collaboration (see Hall et al. 2008, Stokols et al. 2005, and Vogel, 2012 for examples), with the majority of research on interdisciplinary learning relying on surveys, interviews, and archival analyses.

Perhaps one of the earliest recognitions of the need to delineate the competencies associated with interdisciplinary education and practice came from Stokols (1998). In discussing interdisciplinarity in the context of "Social Ecology," Stokols (1998) identified the "knowledge, skills, and attitudes" (KSAs) necessary for effective collaboration. These ideas were built upon and expanded in a comprehensive review of KSAs necessary for cross-disciplinary educational programs, with emphasis on preparation for work in the health and medical sciences (Nash et al. 2003). By drawing from Stokols' observations, Nash and colleagues linked these with theorizing on interdisciplinarity more generally, and graduate school pedagogy, in particular, to categorize competencies for scientific collaboration. It was here that we begin to see important distinctions being drawn between the varied types of interdisciplinary competencies. Furthermore, Nash et al. suggested how these could be developed through the use of particular methods available in graduate school. For example, it was suggested that attitudinal competencies, such as valuing collaboration across disciplines, or risk taking to venture outside one's discipline, could be instilled through activities such as coursework, seminars and workshops, mentoring, and the institutional environment. Knowledge competencies, such as understanding core theories and methods from other disciplines, could be learned through the above-mentioned activities as well as from group work such as journal clubs. Skill-based compe-

Table 33.1 Primary set of interdisciplinary competencies identified by Lattuca et al. (2013a)

Interdisciplinary competence	Defined
Interdisciplinary skills	Ability to consider and apply perspectives from outside one's own discipline and to more generally make connections across varied disciplines
Reflective behavior	Ability to recognize when general approach to thinking about an issue needs to be altered or when specific problem-solving approach may need reconsideration
Recognizing disciplinary perspectives	Understanding content, methods, and boundaries of disciplinary knowledge and how these can be differentially applied dependent upon situational needs

tencies such as taking a methodologically pluralistic approach could be learned through all of the above (see Table 33.1, adapted from Lattuca et al., 2013a).

Others have similarly examined the issue of competencies, but have done so via the perspective of experts experienced in interdisciplinary collaboration. Using a consensus study of expert opinion, Holt (2013) identified what are seen as critical individual competencies for effective performance in these environments. Similar to earlier analyses of competencies, Holt found that experts viewed as important, *Intra*personal Competencies (e.g., broad intellectual curiosity, recognize personal strengths and weaknesses with regard to interdisciplinary research), Disciplinary Awareness and Exchange (e.g., awareness of assumptions of own discipline, engage colleagues from outside disciplines), Processes of Integration (e.g., develop shared interdisciplinary vision, modify work based upon influence of others), Teamwork, Management, Leadership (e.g., build communication strengths, manage conflict, trusting value of teammates), and Competencies of Fruition (e.g., presenting research at interdisciplinary conferences, partner with those in other disciplines on proposals).

Research also provides a more in-depth analysis of particular graduate programs designed to foster interdisciplinary learning. For example, University of California-Irvine's "School of Social Ecology" offers a doctoral seminar specifically developed to expose students to a broad range of disciplines relevant to this field and in preparation for working in this area. In order to examine how such coursework led to a broader perspective on the integration of disciplines, Mitrany and Stokols (2005) conducted a content analysis of doctoral dissertations produced by the school. This involved, for example, analyzing the range of methods and concepts within the dissertations and their integration, and showed that students in this program demonstrated an interdisciplinary orientation in their scholarship. Further, department size and diversity had an influence on the degree of interdisciplinary learning. When students came from smaller departments made up of diverse faculty, the dissertations were rated higher on interdisciplinary factors. They suggest that this more intimate collegial context provided an environment supportive of such research, noting that "collaboration on the basis of shared interests rather than shared institutional affiliations is perhaps more readily achieved in smaller and more diverse departments" (p. 446).

Mentors have also been found to play an important role in interdisciplinary learning and the development of the attributes fostering collaboration competence. Mentors, or even supervisors, who encourage learners to acquire and synthesize knowledge from a broad base, help them acquire skills and attitudes supportive of interdisciplinary work. Furthermore, in line with the idea that interdisciplinarity often blurs the distinction between basic and applied research (cf. Stokes 1997), research suggests that, when trained in institutions that take a problem-focused approach to scholarship (e.g., a center for research on environmental sustainability), learners are come to "avoid the conceptual biases associated with *disciplinary chauvinism* and the *ethnocentrism* of traditional academic departments" (p. 66, Stokols 2014; cf., Campbell 1969).

As noted at the onset, teamwork in the modern scientific workforce requires collaboration across disciplines and professions. This includes teamwork consisting of those with a range of education and training. Because such teamwork often involves employees without post-graduate degrees, research has also examined interdisciplinary learning at the undergraduate level. For example, some have studied the effects of student exposure to not just the scientific and technical content, but also the broader societal context of the problems in which their profession would eventually work (Lattuca et al. 2013a). These initiatives focus not just on learning science content, but also on the larger social, environmental, and economic perspectives in which scientific and technical problems are embedded. Echoing the words of Brozek and Keys decades earlier, Lattuca et al. argued that this required students understand theory and concepts from outside their own disciplines in order to collaborate with team members from varied professions. Towards this end, they set out to identify the nature of the competencies necessary for students to manage interdisciplinary collaborations. Based upon a large-scale study of over 5000 undergraduate students across over 30 institutions, they identified three overall categories of interdisciplinary competencies (see Table 33.1 for a description).

Relevant to understanding effective outcomes from interdisciplinary collaboration, Lattuca et al. identified an additional distinction that needs to be taken into account. Specifically, in their review of the literature on interdisciplinary learning, they found that the field often conflates the distinction between interdisciplinary *processes* and interdisciplinary *products*. For example, an interdisciplinary process could be something devised to help the learner comprehend how to integrate varied concepts from disciplines to create a new product or solve a particular societal problem. An interdisciplinary product is some artifact (whether it be material or conceptual) that has effectively synthesized ideas from varied disciplines (e.g., a conceptual model that draws from, and integrates, varied disciplines to solve some problem).

As an exemplar for disentangling interdisciplinary processes and products, the University of

California-Irvine's "Interdisciplinary Summer Undergraduate Research Experience" program (ID-SURE) was developed to combine coursework and research fellowships to cultivate the kinds of skills that support conceptual integration. In a study of the program's effectiveness, Misra et al. (2009) examined the relationship between the curriculum strategy and transdisciplinary processes and products and how the transdisciplinary orientation of the mentor influenced these. Curricular strategies included activities like team projects, laboratory research, and journal club meetings and products included projects, papers, and grades. Process measures encompassed attributes such as interdisciplinary perspectives, behaviors relating to collaborative activities, and participation in team projects. Results showed that the program increased scientific appreciation and transdisciplinary perspectives, as well as increased the amount of interdisciplinary collaborative activities in which the students engaged. Further, team-focused projects were found to be instrumental to these changes.

In a similar vein, others have studied whether interdisciplinary programs produce changes in cognitive processes as the learner progresses through the curriculum. For example, Lattuca et al. (2013b) studied the influence of interdisciplinary programs on a set of learning outcomes relevant to thinking across disciplines. In a longitudinal study of about 200 students, they compared students majoring in traditional disciplinary programs with those in interdisciplinary programs. In looking for changes in scores measuring critical thinking, need for cognition, and attitudes towards learning, they found no real differences that could be attributed to either a particular major or the structure of the program. But their data suggest there are already selection biases occurring at the undergraduate level. Specifically, students in the interdisciplinary majors showed the lowest change scores in the need for cognition measure and attitudes towards learning. What's important here, then, is that students choosing interdisciplinary programs may already be predisposed to prefer complex and abstract thought and appreciate learning across disciplines.

Finally, Stokols (2014) complements the focus on training competencies with a discussion of cultivating a more general intellectual orientation. This moves us from discussions of just coursework or educational activities. And it speaks more broadly to the need for developing a rich interdisciplinary experience that fosters a culture for nurturing one's intellect and the application of interpersonal competencies in service of team science. Stokols argues that a well-developed intellectual orientation enables one "to communicate more effectively with fellow team members who represent diverse disciplinary and philosophical perspectives, and to identify more readily with the collaborative and integrative goals of the team" (p. 61). In this vein, he explicated a set of attributes that characterized an intellectual orientation ideal for collaborations that span multiple disciplines (see Table 33.2). In the context of preparing the scientific workforce, this distinction is important in that we can think of the aforementioned competencies outlined by Nash et al. (2003) as specific targets for instruction while Stokols (2014) provides us with strategic goals for interdisciplinary education more broadly.

Table 33.2 Attributes of an intellectual orientation suited for collaboration across disciplines (adapted from Stokols 2014; see also Stokols' 2018 and Misra et al.'s 2015 discussion of a transdisciplinary orientation)

Attributes	Description
Values	The values that motivate one to acquire knowledge from other disciplines that are relevant to scientific problem solving
Attitudes	The attitudes that predispose one to integrate knowledge from a varied set of disciplines
Beliefs	The beliefs that such efforts are necessary and can lead to effective outcomes
Skills and knowledge	The skills and knowledge that are critical to think across disciplines in order to synthesize varied concepts and theories
Behaviors	The behaviors that support activities for integrating perspectives and working with others outside one's discipline

In sum, the key points that need to be considered from this brief review of the literature on interdisciplinary education are as follows. First, when assessing interdisciplinary learning, researchers need to clearly delineate between processes and products. This will help better understand and measure the pedagogical practices designed to teach "how" to integrate across disciplines and "what" the outcomes of such practices should be. Second, research must work to identify the particular competencies that support this. Researchers have begun to delineate the variety of competencies that support interdisciplinary collaborations, but such studies are still the exception. Furthermore, we still have little empirical evaluation of which learning activities are best suited for particular competencies. Finally, research must help more fully examine the developmental trajectory of these competencies. From this, we can better determine when and how to implement programs differentially devised to target particular interdisciplinary processes and outcomes and better prepare the scientific workforce.

33.2.4 Federal Programs in Support of Interdisciplinary Education

In addition to programs that evolve out of interest within universities, other educational initiatives are created more strategically to meet national workforce needs. In this vein, the National Science Foundation developed a funding mechanism specifically aimed at interdisciplinary learning in science and engineering. The NSF Integrative Graduate Education and Research Traineeship (IGERT) program was created to support university efforts aimed at producing scientists who can engage in teamwork that crosses disciplinary borders. Although this program has been in existence for a number of years, relatively few systematic studies of its efficacy have been done. To redress that gap, and in order to examine the degree to which funded projects aligned with existing pedagogy on developing interdisciplinary scholars, a qualitative study of proposals was undertaken (Borrego and Newsander 2010). This

examined the learning outcomes that were explicitly articulated across 130 successfully funded proposals. This involved studying the narratives provided by proposers and categorizing how they characterized their graduate training.

First, although IGERTs are, by definition, interdisciplinary, 50% of proposers still stated that graduate student trainees would gain grounding in a specific, or "traditional" discipline. What is important about this finding is the recognition of the continuing challenge of breadth versus depth in interdisciplinary training. As described by Borrego and Newsander (2010), one proposal explained this issue quite well: "It is not feasible to expect tomorrow's scientists to have expertise in both social and aquatic systems, but what is feasible is to create an appreciation of the intellectual challenges faced by the respective disciplines, the methodology used to pursue these challenges, and the ability to formulate and solve interdisciplinary problems effectively" (p. 73).

Second, 30% of proposers argued that their graduate programs would encourage integration and broad perspective on scientific challenges. This was described as a form of systems thinking where graduate student trainees would be taught to take a broader view on the scientific challenge while still working to integrate concepts from relevant disciplines. This aligns with arguments that solving complex problems requires one to adapt a systems theory approach for integrating multiple levels of analysis to build a more thorough understanding of science collaborations. But this perspective also moved beyond scientific borders as 24% of proposers noted that they would encourage students to take perspectives encompassing societal and global issues. This type of graduate training, then, complements what some consider as an important element of action research—that of including stakeholders and pursuing translational outcomes (something argued in early discussions of interdisciplinary research; see Brozek and Keys 1944).

Third, 41% of proposers stated that their center would create a culture of teamwork. This was found to be the most clearly articulated learning outcome. As described by Borrego and

Newsander (2010), one proposal specifically noted that they wanted to train a generation of scholars who are able to "communicate with researchers from other disciplines, and to work collaboratively, creatively, and productively together" (p. 75). Finally, 24% of proposers noted that their projects would emphasize the importance of interdisciplinary communication. This included both an understanding of the language and concepts from participating disciplines and the ability to communicate complicated concepts to nonscience audiences.

Relevant to consideration of the need for the modern scientific workforce to work across both disciplines *and* professions, an important finding from this research is how "integration," as a learning outcome, is viewed differently between scientists and engineers and those in the humanities. In particular, while integration across disciplines was a commonality, those in the humanities additionally considered "critical thinking" as crucial while those in science and technology considered "teamwork" as fundamental. Borrego and Newsander argued that critical reflection on disciplinary inconsistencies and limitations was a particular strength that could be put to use when solving complex problems. They suggested that, if the sciences incorporated the humanities conception of critical awareness, it could greatly extend how science and engineering conceives of interdisciplinarity. Specifically, they stated that, although "engineering and science faculty members avoid criticism of disciplinary structures, they would certainly say they value graduate students' critical thinking about the problem at hand and the value of various disciplinary approaches to it" (p. 78). Overall, though, what we see in this analysis is specific articulation of a need to train collaborative competencies. That is, while all noted the grounding in disciplinary education, just as important was the need to cultivate the particular competencies that supported integration of ideas across disciplines.

While programs such as the IGERT target training at the graduate level, other federal programs consider how training should be developed at that post-graduate level when students are entering the scientific workforce. Such efforts are created to support complex research while also fostering the collaboration competencies necessary for success. As an example of how such programs have been systematically devised, the National Cancer Institute's Transdisciplinary Research on Energetics and Cancer I (TREC I) initiative set out to develop competencies enabling teamwork. These centers supported a variety of training activities converging on the goal of enhancing interpersonal and intrapersonal competencies along with training scientific competencies (Vogel et al. 2012).

Activities ranged from transdisciplinary research courses, journal clubs for members, and writing retreats to develop skills in collaborative writing and research. They also included not just traditional mentoring, but co-mentoring and multi-mentoring to expose trainees to multiple disciplinary perspectives. These programs also worked to strengthen collaboration across centers. Here, a coordinated effort was created to support professional development activities (e.g., visiting mentors at other centers), learning across centers (e.g., Internet-based seminars), and thematically related workshops at annual meetings.

An analysis of training effectiveness for the TREC centers, using a cross-sectional design, found changes in attitudes towards working across disciplines (i.e., enhanced transdisciplinary orientation), improved ability to work across disciplines (i.e., intrapersonal/interpersonal competencies for collaboration), as well as increased scientific competency to work with other disciplines (i.e., development of scientific skills for transdisciplinary research). Importantly, there were also changes in scientific output with increases in scholarly productivity for trainees affiliated with TREC as measured by number of publications/presentations and number of collaborative authors. Multi-mentoring experiences were also associated with greater transdisciplinary orientation and positive perception of one's center (Vogel et al. 2012).

Federal programs have also focused more specifically on developing sophisticated mentoring strategies to foster the development of interdisciplinary career paths. NIH's "Building Interdisciplinary Research Careers in Women's

Health" (BIRCWH) program is designed for junior faculty interested in advancing research in women's health. Through establishment of mentoring teams, the BIRCWH program provides participating scholars with multiple perspectives on a range of scientific and career issues. One indicator of success in such programs is idea generation in the form of grants submissions in the area of women's health. A study of the program showed that a majority of scholars applied for competitive grants after completing the training and that approximately half were successful (Nagel et al. 2013). More detailed analyses of the program identified the need to develop written contracts between participants to manage mentoring expectations (Guise et al. 2012). Also important was the need to clearly articulate roles for the mentoring team such that some focus on career issues while others focus on scientific content. Comparative analysis shows that scholars participating in the BIRCWH program have a grant-funding rate of 38% compared to the NIH average of 29% (see also Guise et al. 2017).

Nonetheless, while mentoring has consistently been identified as a crucial component of interdisciplinary education and training, it is too often lacking for scholars. In a recent survey on the "Global State of Young Scientists," the unavailability of mentoring was one of the top four career obstacles identified (see Friesenhahn and Beaudry 2014). Similarly problematic is the lack of training junior scientists receive on "how" to engage in training and supervision of students and post-docs. This was likened to parenting in that it was never explicitly taught in their graduate education; rather, it is something reported as being learned along the way (Friesenhahn and Beaudry 2014).

In sum, a small number of university curricula and federal programs have examined learning and education for interdisciplinarity. Many have identified the kinds of competencies necessary for success in the scientific workforce. Further, some have delineated between learning scientific content from various disciplines and learning how to work on a team with those from other disciplines. Nonetheless, rigorous empirical research on the efficacy of such programs is still lacking. More problematic, though, is that nothing is known about the success of such programs to the scientific enterprise, overall. This includes a lack of longitudinal studies on the graduates of such programs and a comparison of their interdisciplinary scholarship to other scientists. But it also includes a lack of research on how the introduction of such programs has influenced the production of knowledge, overall. This points us to a significant gap in understanding when it comes to learning how to be a team scientist and what this means for the success of the scientific workforce. In the next section we discuss a way forward for research on interdisciplinary learning and training in the context of scientific teamwork.

33.3 Addressing the Challenge of Interdisciplinary Teamwork

Fully addressing the challenging dimensions of interdisciplinary science requires that we go beyond the extant literature. While much can be gained by directly adopting some of what has been studied, either in education or in training research, there are still notable gaps when it comes to understanding how these methods can be used to improve the performance of science teams. What is also lacking, though, is conceptual grounding in how to understand the relationship between the various educational and professional development programs devised for interdisciplinary learning. In the final half of this chapter, we redress this gap and provide conceptual and theoretical guidance that can be used to more precisely develop and study learning and training approaches supporting interdisciplinary collaboration. First, we discuss the lack of conceptual clarity in terminology used in the literature on education and training for interdisciplinary scholarship. Second, we provide a framework integrating the varied competencies that have come out of the study of interdisciplinarity. Third, we review notional training approaches that fit within various facets of this competency framework. Our goal is to provide a form of conceptual scaffolding that provides both short-term and long-term guidance for training the next-generation scientific workforce on how to become a team scientist. In the short term, existing approaches for interdisciplinary learning can be improved through a more rigorous adoption of concepts from the organizational sciences. In the long term, research that builds from these suggestions could make a significant contribution to our understanding of how performance improves across the life span of science teams and how this affects the scientific enterprise.

33.3.1 Coming to Terms with Terms

What is clear from the review of interdisciplinary learning programs is the fuzziness of terminology used to describe the education and training. Specifically, education and training are two general terms that are too often used with little specification as to what is meant. While the context of the discussion can often be used to discern a given meaning, the tremendous variety of settings in which education and training can take place still leaves much room for error. Training can be used to describe an hour-long presentation on a given scientific topic or a method for managing conflict within one's team. It can also be used to describe a workshop spanning hours or days where one receives more intense exposure to, for example, new methods for visualizing complex data, or how to lead and manage members of a scientific team. Education might be used when discussing a guest lecture from a noted scholar, or to describe a particular course developed to teach team-based projects for working with students from different disciplines. It might also be used when broadly discussing a curriculum centered on interdisciplinary learning.

These examples are meant to illustrate two fundamental distinctions that emerge and must be accounted for when trying to bring some coherence to discussions of training and education for team science. First is the content of the material to be learned. The examples above were purposely dichotomized to illustrate a fundamental distinction made in the literature on team training and one to which we return at the conclusion of this chapter. Specifically, when team training research began to evolve, it was recognized that an important distinction needed to be made between taskwork and teamwork (Salas et al. 1992). Taskwork is a label for the activities in which one engages that are pertinent to achieving the goals and objectives for which the team is formed (e.g., running a procedure for data collection, completing a particular statistical analysis). Teamwork describes the activities involved in interacting with members of one's team and that are necessary for success (e.g., communication; back-up behaviors). Second is the duration of the learning activity. The literature on training and education might discuss short courses lasting hours or days or entire curricula that might span months or years. Table 33.3 provides a rudimentary illustration of this breakdown. While it is certainly possible for an educational or training experience to teach both taskwork and teamwork, our point here is that it is important not to conflate these as the content has a direct bearing on the pedagogical approach.

An additional complicating factor is the context in which the term is being used. When in academic settings, the term training is most often used to describe any learning experience that occurs outside of the classroom, while education is the term typically used to describe in class learning experiences. This distinction may seem relatively simple and somewhat robust when

Table 33.3 Illustrative breakdown of content and duration of learning experience

		Nature of the content	
		Taskwork	Teamwork
Duration	Short	A one-day workshop teaching a specific statistical test	A weekend retreat teaching methods for conflict management
	Long	A course teaching attendees methods for conducting network analyses	A course utilizing group projects to teach attendees how to collaborate in science teams

talking about students. For example, doctoral seminars are clearly educational and guidance by one's adviser in a laboratory is construed of as graduate training. But, what do we label the experience when doctoral students attend a colloquium describing a new finding that has a significant bearing on their research? Is this still labeled "education" even when not in a classroom? If so, how is it described if a post-doc is attending? Since they have completed their Ph.D. program, do we now label it "training?"

To answer this, perhaps we might fall back on the recently developed term of "continuous learning." This term has come to mean a form of education where professionals are acquiring new knowledge, but which is, in reality, coursework that would be considered training by others. Thus, this distinction loses clarity depending upon where one is in their career. It is problematic in that the difference between education and training might merely depend upon where one is in their career. Or, perhaps we can adopt what some in organizational psychology suggest; that is, we could state that education is generally used to describe more general exposure to content whereas training is used to describe exposure to specific content. While this scheme might be useful when discussing professionals (i.e., those no longer in school), the fuzziness, again, becomes apparent when applied in academia. For example, students taking a short course on a particular statistical technique might have the experience labeled as education, whereas a postdoc or faculty member in the same course might view it as training.

Our point is that the use of the terms education and training can sometimes be arbitrary in the literature and dependent upon the scholar conducting research in this area and/or where the research gets published. This discussion is not mere semantics or academic wordplay but something that must be addressed in light of the policy challenges associated with developing the scientific workforce. Specifically, the clarity with which such terms are used has a direct bearing on how programs around them are designed, how processes and outcomes are measured, and how funding around them is allocated. As such, this has a bearing on the design of scientific curricula, the development of training for scientists, and on the development of science policy. Despite these important distinctions, for the sake of order to the literature, in this chapter, we use the terms adopted by the papers being reviewed. But we stress that the above distinctions need to be kept in mind so that some degree of coherence can be developed for team science in both science policy and science practice.

33.3.2 Understanding Team Competencies for Science Teams

What is also clear is the wide variety of competencies thought to be needed for effective performance in interdisciplinary collaborative environments. In this section we discuss how a competencies framework developed in the organizational sciences can be used as a theoretical framework for classifying these competencies. Specifically, Fiore (2008) built off earlier theorizing to suggest a competency framework that could be adapted to support training research in science teams. He argued that more careful consideration of the knowledge, skills, and attitudes supporting teamwork is necessary for team science. This, he suggested, can be accomplished through the use of the competency framework put forth by Cannon-Bowers et al. (1995). Within this framework, collaborative competencies can be decomposed into a 2 × 2 framework whereby they vary in the degree to which they are teamgeneric or team-specific and task-specific or taskgeneric. As shown in Table 33.4, by combining these, four types of competencies are produced

Table 33.4 Types of team competencies (Cannon-Bowers et al. 1995)

Team competencies		Relation to task	
		Specific	Generic
Relation to team	Specific	Context-driven	Team-contingent
	Generic	Task-contingent	Transportable

(i.e., context-driven, team-contingent, task-contingent, transportable).

We suggest that, when considering learning and training for the scientific workforce, the situational and environmental context needs to drive the determination of which competencies are necessary for a given team (cf. Bowers et al. 2000). In particular, Fiore (2008) argued that this breakdown can provide a nuanced understanding of the training requirements for differing science teams depending upon their experience with each other and the type of scientific problem on which they are working. Furthermore, attending to these distinctions can help us precisely classify the variety of university developed and federally sponsored interdisciplinary learning programs just discussed. For example, context-driven competencies are those required by a particular task and team involved on a specific scientific problem. Teams that have stable membership and perform a small range of tasks that are similar in their nature tend to require these types of competencies. Team-contingent competencies are team-specific but are applicable across a wide variety of tasks. This would be the case for a laboratory team who know each other well, but who are working on a variety of scientific problems. Task-contingent competencies are specific to a particular task, but transportable across teams (i.e., not dependent on the particular make-up of the team). This is the case when considering a scientific problem, irrespective of makeup of a team. Finally, transportable competencies are both team- and task-generic (i.e., they apply across a wide range of teams and collective tasks). These are the general kinds of competencies that benefit all forms of scientific teamwork. In short, this framework provides an important foundation for understanding how to conceptualize the competencies to be trained for scientists more generally, and for specific teams in particular. But it additionally helps us to understand how differing educational and professional development programs—ranging from workshops to seminars to entire curricula—can be developed in support of targeting particular collaborative competencies.

Within this competency framework, we can go further and delineate the knowledge, skills, and attitudes (KSAs) attributed to science teams.

From this, learning outcomes for science team training can be better specified. For example, when thinking about KSAs for scientific teams, knowledge can be construed of as long- and short-term memory that is drawn on to recognize and utilize environmental information supporting the scientific problem at hand. In the domain of training for team science, this effectively refers to any stored or dynamically obtained information that is required by the team. But this can be broken down further using the taskwork and teamwork dimensions. For science teams, task-relevant knowledge can be specific to a particular context (e.g., a given laboratory), or generically related to a given goal (e.g., experimental procedures). Team-relevant knowledge can also be specific to a particular scientific context (e.g., understanding the idiosyncrasies of members in a given laboratory), or generically related to a given team goal (e.g., roles played on differing scientific teams). If knowledge represents the information that individuals and teams require to perform tasks, skills are the means by which they do so; that is, "how" to do something (Cunningham 2008). Skills are developed both generally and in-context, and are acquired through practice and training (Ericsson 2004). For a science team, task-relevant skills can similarly be context-specific as well as generically related to a given goal. Team-relevant skills can also be context-specific or -generic for teamwork. Finally, attitudes pertain to the values and individual differences pertinent to a team and their task (Cunningham 2008). In relation to a task, attitudes refer to how a scientist views, for example, a particular methodology (e.g., surveys vs. interviews). In relation to the team, they can pertain to how one feels about working on a scientific team (e.g., collaborative orientation). Task-relevant attitudes might be specific to a particular context (e.g., pursuing a given laboratory's methodological approach), or generically related to a given goal (e.g., values associated with doing applied research). Team-relevant attitudes can also be specific to a particular context (e.g., how one feels about working on an interdisciplinary team), or generically related to teamwork (e.g., collective orientation).

In sum, this approach moves beyond current conceptions of science team competencies by clearly distinguishing between generic and specific team and task competencies and delineating the particular KSAs associated with these. This can help to better address the training challenges arising from complex scientific teamwork (cf. Cummings and Kiesler 2005). In particular, the interdisciplinary nature of modern science teams necessitates we better understand the competencies required for effective teamwork. By specifying the form of the competency required for a given team, we are able to target particular challenges faced by teams. But it is not always the case that such specific training need be developed. The above framework helps us to more broadly conceptualize education and training initiatives and determine when these varied forms of training may be helpful. To that end, in Table 33.5, we provide representative examples of the varied types of KSAs that can exist in science teams, but categorized using the generic versus specific team and task breakdown (Fiore and Bedwell 2011).

Note that these competencies have to do with what we see as teamwork in the context of complex problem solving as in science. A gap in the literature, though, has to do with the kinds of competencies necessary for multi-team systems. In the study of teams in organizations, a multi-team system (MTS) describes a set of interdependent "component" teams that are collaborating towards some common goals (Marks et al. 2005). Asencio et al. (2012) discussed MTS in the context of science collaborations and what are the particular challenges they face in terms of collaboration and coordination. But what is additionally needed is specification of any unique competencies required for MTS. For example, the challenges of participating in a MTS would seem to require an additional, "trans-team" set of competencies. This could be something such as effective boundary work among the leaders and members of the various teams that comprise the system. This is like Obstfeld's (2005) concept of the "tertius iungens" scholar who is able to effectively link the members from multiple teams. In addition to the boundary-spanning competencies of effective MTS members, there is also the ability to share leadership roles among those who lead the component teams within the systems (DeChurch and Marks 2006). This could include, for example, behavioral and interpersonal competencies associated with shared versus singular leadership roles.

Building on this, Fiore (2013) argued that interdisciplinary collaborations would benefit by learning and education programs targeting the quadrant labeled "transportable" team competencies. In the organizational sciences, these are often referred to as interpersonal competencies but they are often used without precise operationalization, leading to conceptual confusion. To address this problem, findings from a number of papers on interpersonal training were synthesized to develop taxonomy of competencies (Klein et al. 2006). At the most general level, these were

Table 33.5 Types of KSAs associated with science team competencies

Representative science team competencies		Relation to task	
		Specific	Generic
Relation to team	Specific	Context-driven	Team-contingent
		• Knowledge—team objectives and resources	• Knowledge—teammate characteristics
		• Skills—particular analyses	• Skills—providing teammate guidance
		• Attitudes—collective efficacy	• Attitudes—team cohesion
	Generic	Task-contingent	Transportable
		• Knowledge—procedures for task accomplishment	• Knowledge—understanding group dynamics
		• Skills—problem analysis	• Skills—communication and assertiveness
		• Attitudes—trust in technology	• Attitudes—interdisciplinary appreciation

defined as goal-directed behaviors, including communication and relationship-building competencies, that are employed during interaction episodes. These interactions are characterized by a need for complex perceptual and cognitive processes, dynamic verbal and nonverbal exchanges, and diverse roles, motivations, and expectancies (Klein et al. 2006). When considering scientific workforce development needs, these align quite well with a number of the competencies discussed earlier. Fiore (2013) adapted this approach for consideration within interdisciplinary education. He described how they can be used as learning objectives for educational and professional development designed to support interdisciplinary science teams (refer to Table 33.6).

Note that these competencies only address interpersonal factors associated with teamwork in scientific collaboration. A notable gap in the literature is specifying what are the intellectual capacities needed in team science partnerships. This could be the ability to conceptualize problems systemically and at multiple scales (e.g., accounting for genome × exposure interactions in health science). This could also be associated with competencies needed to bridge disparate "knowledge cultures" (e.g., Brown et al. 2010). For example, in the widely divergent world views of science and society, these need to be carefully negotiated and navigated in translational partnerships among scholars, lay citizens, community professionals, elected officials, policymakers, etc. Stokols (2018) referred to this as "transepistemic," a particular type of transdisciplinary action research necessitating integration of knowledge and world views held by scientists and a variety of stakeholders. As such, we must address the competencies needed to help science teams deal with the challenges of not only doing inter- or transdisciplinary integration across different academic fields, but also linking academic and non-academic knowledge cultures.

Table 33.6 Interpersonal competencies applied to science teams

Communication competencies	
Active listening	• Carefully attending to what is said
	• Asking other party to explain exactly what is meant
	• Requesting that ambiguous ideas or statements are repeated
	In interdisciplinary learning, this competency targets "listening to learn and understand" and "listening to contribute and integrate to problem solving"
Oral and written communication	• Sending verbal and written messages clearly
	• Speaking/writing constructively
	• Speaking/writing critically in appropriate ways
	In interdisciplinary learning, this competency targets the ability to "express yourself clearly to others outside one's discipline" (e.g., avoiding jargon) and "effectively conveying intended meaning of other disciplinary perspectives"
Assertive communication	• Directly expressing one's ideas and opinions
	• Addressing conflict purposely and openly
	• Addressing differences without intimidation
	In interdisciplinary learning, this competency targets the ability to "propose ideas," to "defend one's disciplinary values/methods" and to "be directive and appropriately assert your needs and views"
Relationship management competencies	
Coordination	• Understanding how to work with others as a team
	• Being mindful of interdependencies and how to pace activities
	• Offering help/back-up as needed
	In interdisciplinary learning, this competency targets understanding importance of "awareness of shared scientific goals" and "monitoring and feedback"

(continued)

Table 33.6 (continued)

Interdisciplinary appreciation	• Appreciating differing disciplinary theories and concepts
	• Respecting varied disciplinary methods
	• Encouraging input from across disciplinary perspectives
	In interdisciplinary learning, this competency targets learning "acceptance of, and openness to new ideas" and "sensitivity to disciplinary perspectives"
Collaborative orientation	• Predisposition to provide help to others
	• Intellectual curiosity in service understanding others
	• Building rapport with others
	In interdisciplinary learning, this competency targets the ability to "elicit ideas for purpose of understanding" and "offer solutions in support of problem solving"

33.3.3 Learning and Training for Team and Task Competencies

In the final section, we provide representative examples of the kinds of training that can be used for developing these varied forms of competencies. Although these have not specifically been conceptualized within the aforementioned competencies framework, their approach aligns well with each quadrant. Furthermore, even though not all have been tested in the context of science teams, the approaches are generalizable to numerous contexts. As such, we offer these as notional interventions that can be introduced for educational or professional development in support of training the next generation of team scientists.

33.3.4 Training for Context-Driven Competencies

As described earlier, context-driven competencies are those required by a particular task and team involved on a specific scientific problem.

Problem-based learning (PBL) is a method that is optimal for these competencies. In PBL, facilitators or tutors are used to guide small group learning (Barrows 1996) on specific problems. With the use of problems derived from the actual domain to be learned and representative or real-world situations (i.e., "authentic problems"), students are first encouraged to produce their naïve understanding of the problem, identify similarities across the group, and generate potential hypotheses and solutions (Gijselaers 1996). A key part of this process is that students discuss any lack of understanding they have and what knowledge needs to be acquired to solve the problem. From this, learning goals are identified and students work in and out class to gather and integrate the knowledge necessary to produce a solution. Finally, a reflective component is built into the process where students debrief on what they have learned. Although some debate exists as to the specifics of the strategies employed within PBL (Dochy et al. 2003; Hmelo-Silver 2004, for reviews), meta-analyses find that small group learning was related to academic achievement (Norman and Schmidt 2000), and that group debate improved the development of shared knowledge and problem solving (Hmelo-Silver 2004). But these reviews suggest that there be a flexible amount of self-direction dependent upon where in the learning trajectory students are (Hmelo-Silver 2004; Vermunt and Verloop 1999). Perhaps most important were the outcomes contrasting knowledge acquisition versus application. First, traditional classroom-based instruction, when compared to PBL, showed some benefits on factual knowledge and standardized tests (Vernon and Blake 1993). But PBL showed some benefit for knowledge application and retention (Dochy et al. 2003).

33.3.5 Training for Team-Contingent Competencies

As noted, team-contingent competencies are team-specific but are applicable across a wide variety of tasks. Fitting with this is an approach coming out of research in philosophy. The

Toolbox project was developed to overcome the communication challenges experienced by scientists working across disciples (O'Rourke and Crowley 2013). This relies on probing statements that participants complete before and after a Toolbox workshop. These are devised to elicit fundamental assumptions team members have about science, particularly from the perspective of their own discipline. During the workshop, these are used to guide discussion about the views scientists hold and share them with team members so that differences can be made explicit. This forces members to reflect on their idiosyncratic epistemologies as well as the values they bring to the science team. As such, it uses a form of philosophical dialogue to target development of the knowledge, skills, and attitudes supportive of interdisciplinary communication. Studies of workshop participants find that, after engaging with the Toolbox facilitators, there is an increase in awareness about the varied scientific approaches pursued by other team members and that this process enhances their appreciation for diversity in research (Schnapp et al. 2012).

33.3.6 Training for Task-Contingent Competencies

As described, task-contingent competencies are specific to a particular task, but transportable across differing teams. Training research on knowledge building is well suited for this competency. Knowledge building is foundational to complex problem-solving as it is critical to solution generation (Fiore et al. 2010). It is particularly important when teams consist of members with varied forms of knowledge and expertise. Interdisciplinary science teams are, by definition, made of members holding diverse forms of knowledge. When collaborating, these members must integrate that knowledge to generate solutions to complex problems. This is challenging because performance problems emerge when team members do not share task mental models. Furthermore, research finds that teams rarely discuss information held uniquely, and, rather, tend to communicate only about the knowledge they

share (Wittenbaum and Park 2001). In order to address these problems, Rentsch et al. (2010) conducted a study explicitly focused on team training for knowledge building. This consisted of a schema-enriched communication (SEC) component as well as a knowledge object component. For the SEC component, team members were trained to engage in communicative processes that elicit the structure and organization of their knowledge, as well as the assumptions, meaning, rationale, and interpretations associated with each member's knowledge. The knowledge object component consisted of utilizing an external representation (i.e., an information board) that allowed for team members to post and organize their knowledge in a common space that allows them to visually manipulate that knowledge, more easily remember it, as well as to draw attention to specific information as appropriate. This has been used to test the effectiveness of knowledge building training on a problem-solving task requiring resource allocation. Results show that knowledge building training improves knowledge transfer (i.e., the exchange of knowledge from one team member to another), knowledge interoperability (i.e., knowledge that multiple team members are able to recall and use), cognitive congruence (i.e., an alignment or matching of team member cognitions), and higher overall team performance on the task (Rentsch et al. 2010; Rentsch et al. 2014).

33.3.7 Training for Transportable Competencies

As noted, transportable competencies are applicable across a wide range of teams and tasks, that is, generic to both the team and the task. Team reflexivity training has evolved to provide a robust approach for training general team competencies. Team reflexivity training requires that members engage in some form of reflection on prior performance episodes. This reflection encompasses focusing on the objectives that were or were not met, the strategies used, and the group processes engaged. The goal is to adapt team processes to improve future interaction

(Gabelica et al. 2016; Gurtner et al. 2007). Although individual methods of reflexivity interventions may differ, the general procedure includes the following steps after a team performance episode: (1) reviewing the task performance of the group (e.g., "How did you ask for information? How did you pass on information? How was the team organized?"; Gurtner et al., p. 132), (2) thinking about potential improvements in the processes and methods used to complete the task (e.g., "Are there alternatives to your chosen task performance procedures, and if so, what are they?"; p. 132), and, (3) creating suggestions for future work such that the next time the task is done the processes and outcomes are improved. Gurtner et al. found that teams trained using the above steps had interaction mental models more similar as compared to a control. Furthermore, the reflexivity intervention had a direct effect on SMMs and was also partially mediated by the commander's communication of strategies. Additionally, SMMs influenced strategy implementation, which then impacted performance. The study demonstrated that shared mental models can be improved by reflecting on what work has been accomplished so far and reflecting on how performance could be improved in the future. Van Ginkel et al. (2009) found that reflexivity training also improved team shared task understanding and decision quality.

33.3.8 Summary

These strategies represent examples of the form of training that can support learning to be a team scientist. But much empirical work needs to be done in the field (i.e., in actual classroom and work settings), to determine the effectiveness of these methods for the scientific workforce. In support of this, we next identify core features of training for teams, adapted from Gabelica and Fiore (2013), that need to be more systematically integrated across these. From this, we can better understand how to implement these core elements in a coherent way and test if and how they improve individual and group learning (see Table 33.7).

Table 33.7 Core features needed to examine the effectiveness of learning approaches for competencies training

- Use small groups
- Provide immediate and regular feedback (from instructors, peers, or professional guests)
- Use formative assessment allowing for refinements and adjustments of ongoing work
- Ensure regular communication of ongoing work
- Use complex and real-world problem solving
- Support meta-discussions (via metacognitive techniques)
- Ensure multi-interactions among learners and instructors
- Provide explicit training of problem-solving skills
- Use scaffolding/modeling from the trainer

Finally, what is also necessary is more consistent usage of assessment measures that tap teamwork. To achieve this, we suggest there be a more systematic integration of methods from the organizational sciences on team training with the educational and professional development programs devised for training scientists to work in teams. More importantly, such research must adopt and integrate existing measures of taskwork *and* teamwork into curricula for team science to better understand and assess how differing KSAs are acquired and used. This includes consideration of self-ratings of soft skills (Kantrowitz 2005), and peer- and self-ratings like that found in the Comprehensive Assessment of Team Member Effectiveness measure (Ohland et al. 2012). This latter assessment includes general categories of team member involvement like contribution to the team's work, keeping the team on track and appropriately interacting with teammates. Also recommended is implementation of measures using behavioral observation scales that focus on observable skills and use behavioral referents assess interpersonal skills like collaborative problem solving and conflict resolution as well as self-management processes like planning and task coordination (Taggar and Brown 2001). In short, our goal is to help integrate research on team training and team competencies with research on interdisciplinary learning to examine the efficacy of these interventions focused on learning to be a team scientist.

33.4 Conclusions

We began this chapter with a discussion of the pressing needs for scientific workforce development and the apparent failure to adequately train for teamwork and communicating and collaboration across scientific and professional disciplines. Although educational programs supporting interdisciplinary learning have been developed in a number of universities, empirical assessment of their efficacy is lacking. Similarly, federal research organizations have instituted various programs devised to support educational and professional development for interdisciplinary science. But robust assessment of their effectiveness is also lacking. Furthermore, there is little, if any, understanding on how these are affecting the scientific ecosystem overall. Across all of these, though, is lack of attention to "teaching" teamwork with little emphasizing the KSAs that could improve collaboration.

Despite these limitations, we focused on research examining interdisciplinary learning and education and the particular competencies identified as necessary for success in scientific teamwork. An important similarity to our review of educational practices and interdisciplinarity is that training research has also focused on KSAs as learning outcomes. Drawing from the decades-long tradition of learning research in psychology and education, Kraiger et al. (1993) were some of the first training researchers to argue for a taxonomical breakdown of learning outcomes along the lines of knowledge, skills, and attitudes. This provides a conceptually meaningful framework that is also at a useful level of granularity for developing both interventions and assessments. We adapted this for science teams and added the team/task, generic/specific competencies framework coming out of the training literature.

We also reviewed methods of training showing promise in helping scientists to acquire the collaborative competencies necessary for interdisciplinary teamwork. These interventions approach learning in complementary ways. Some focus on helping team members understand how to learn through reflection and provide feedback for them to diagnose what processes led to effective and ineffective outcomes. Others focus on learning the specific forms of communication that ensure teams share the information most relevant to their task needs. These meet the needs for successful science, in that teams must understand not just how to do their tasks, but must also know how to collaborate. We suggest that, for knowledge-intensive organizations to succeed, greater emphasis must be placed on the combination of these competencies in the educational pipeline and into professional development. In this way, we can understand how to augment education and training so that learning is not simply about acquisition of knowledge for developing task competencies. Additionally, we can include methods devised to foster interdisciplinary collaboration, that is, education for learning how to be a team scientist.

Acknowledgments The writing of this paper was partially supported by Grant NNX16AO72G from the National Aeronautics and Space Administration. The views, opinions, and findings contained in this article are the authors and should not be construed as official or as reflecting the views of the University of Central Florida or the National Aeronautics and Space Administration.

References

AACU. College learning for the new global century. Washington, DC: Association of American Colleges and Universities; 2007.

Asencio R, Carter DR, DeChurch LA, Zaccaro SJ, Fiore SM. Charting a course for collaboration: a multiteam perspective. Transl Behav Med. 2012;2(4):487–94.

Academy of Medical Sciences. Improving recognition of team science contributions in biomedical research careers. London (UK): Academy of Medical Sciences; 2016.. http://www.acmedsci.ac.uk/more/news/collaborating-on-large-science-projects-must-not-harm-careers/

Barrows HS. Problem-based learning in medicine and beyond: a brief overview. In: Wilkerson L, Gijselaers WH, editors. New directions for teaching and learning, 1996(68). San Francisco, CA: Jossey-Bass Publishers; 1996. p. 3–11.

Bell BS, Tannenbaum SI, Ford JK, Noe RA, Kraiger K. 100 years of training and development research: what we know and where we should go. J Appl Psychol. 2017;102(3):305–25.

Bezrukova K, et al. Do workgroup faultlines help or hurt? A moderated model of faultlines, team identification, and group performance. Organ Sci. 2009;20(1):35–50.

Borner K, Contractor N, Falk-Krzesinski HJ, Fiore SM, Hall KL, Keyton J, et al. A multi-level systems perspective for the science of team science. Sci Transl Med. 2010;2(49):1–5.

Borrego M, Newsander LK. Definitions of interdisciplinary research: toward graduate-level interdisciplinary learning outcomes. Rev High Educ. 2010;34(1):61–84.

Bosque-Perez NA, et al. A pedagogical model for team-based, problem-focused interdisciplinary doctoral education. Bioscience. 2016;66(6):1–12.

Bowers CA, Jentsch F, Salas E. Establishing aircrew competencies: a comprehensive approach for identifying CRM training needs. In: O'Neil HF, Andrews D, editors. Aircrew training and assessment. Mahwah, NJ: Erlbaum; 2000. p. 67–84.

Brint SG, Turk-Bicakci L, Proctor K, Murphy SP. Expanding the social frame of knowledge: interdisciplinary, degree-granting fields in American colleges and universities, 1975–2000. Rev High Educ. 2009;32(2):155–83.

Brown VA, Harris JA, Russell JY, editors. Tackling wicked problems through the transdisciplinary imagination. London (UK): Earthscan; 2010.

Brozek J, Keys A. General aspects of interdisciplinary research in experimental human biology. Science. 1944;100:507–12.

Campbell DT. Ethnocentrism of disciplines and the fish-scale model of omniscience. In: Sherif M, Sherif CW, editors. Interdisciplinary relationships in the social sciences. Chicago, IL: Aldine Press; 1969. p. 328–48.

Canadian Academy of Health Sciences (CAHS). Academic recognition of team science: how to optimize the Canadian academic system. Ottawa, ON: The Expert Panel on Academic Recognition of Team Science in Canada, CAHS; 2017.

Cannon-Bowers JA, Tannenbaum SI, Salas E, Volpe CE. Defining team competencies and establishing team training requirements. In: Guzzo R, Salas E, editors. Team effectiveness and decision making in organizations. San Francisco, CA: Jossey-Bass; 1995. p. 333–80.

Chang S, et al. Adapting postdoctoral training to interdisciplinary science in the 21st century: the cancer prevention fellowship program at the national cancer institute. Acad Med. 2005;80(3):261–5.

Crow MM, Dabars WB. Designing the new American university. Baltimore, MD: Johns Hopkins University Press; 2015.

Crow MM, Dabars WB. Restructuring research universities to advance interdisciplinary collaboration. In: Hall KL, Vogel AL, Croyle RT, editors. Strategies for team science success: handbook of evidence-based principles for cross-disciplinary science and practical lessons learned from health researchers. New York, NY: Springer; 2019.

Cummings JN, Kiesler S. Collaborative research across disciplinary and institutional boundaries. Soc Stud Sci. 2005;35(5):703–22.

Cunningham I. Are "skills" all there is to learning in organizations? The case for a broader framework. Development and Learning in Organizations. 2008;22(3):5–8.

DeChurch LA, Marks MA. Leadership in multiteam systems. J Appl Psychol. 2006;91(2):311–29.

Dochy F, Segers M, Van den Bossche P, Gijbels D. Effects of problem-based learning: a meta-analysis. Learn Instr. 2003;13(5):533–68.

Duderstadt JJ. A university for the 21st century. Ann Arbor, MI: University of Michigan Press; 2000.

Ericsson KA. Deliberate practice and the acquisition and maintenance of expert performance in medicine and related domains. Acad Med. 2004;79(10):S70–81.

Fiore SM. Interdisciplinarity as teamwork: how the science of teams can inform team science. Small Group Res. 2008;39(3):251–77.

Fiore SM, Rosen MA, Smith-Jentsch KA, Salas E, Letsky M, Warner N. Toward an understanding of macrocognition in teams: predicting processes in complex collaborative contexts. Hum Factors. 2010;52(2):203–24.

Fiore SM, Bedwell W. Team Science Needs Teamwork Training. In: Presented at the Second Annual Science of Team Science Conference, Chicago, IL; 2011.

Fiore SM. Overview of the science of team science. In: Presented at the National Research Council's Planning Meeting on Interdisciplinary Science Teams, January 11, Washington, DC; 2013. http://tvworldwide.com/events/nas/130111/ppt/Fiore%20FINAL%20SciTS%20Overview%20for%20NRC.pdf. Accessed May 2014.

Fiore SM, Graesser A, Greiff S. Collaborative problem solving education for the 21st century workforce. Nat Hum Behav. 2018;2:367–9. https://doi.org/10.1038/s41562-018-0363-y.

Friesenhahn I, Beaudry C. The global state of young scientists–project report and recommendations. Berlin: Akademie Verlag; 2014.. http://www.raje.es/en/wpcontent/uploads/2014/01/GYA_GloSYS-report_webversion.pdf

Gabelica C, Fiore SM. What can training researchers gain from examination of methods for active-learning (PBL, TBL, and SBL). In: Proceedings of the Human Factors and Ergonomics Society Annual Meeting. September 2013, 57(1):1,462-1,466. 2013. http://pro.sagepub.com/content/57/1/462.refs.

Gabelica C, Van den Bossche P, Fiore SM, Segers M, Gijselaers WH. Establishing team knowledge coordination from a learning perspective. Hum Perform. 2016;29(1):33–53.

Gijselaers WH. Connecting problem-based practices with educational theory. New Dir Teach Learn. 1996;1996:13–21. https://doi.org/10.1002/tl.37219966805.

Guise JM, Nagel JD, Regensteiner JG. Best practices and pearls in interdisciplinary mentoring from building interdisciplinary research careers in women's health directors. J Women's Health. 2012;21(11):1114–27.

Guise JM, Winter S, Fiore SM, Regensteiner JG, Nagel J. Organizational and training factors that promote team science: a qualitative analysis and application of theory to the national institutes of health's BIRCWH career development program. J Clin Transl Sci. 2017;1(2):101–7.

Gurtner A, Tschan F, Semmer NK, Nägele C. Getting groups to develop good strategies: effects of reflexivity interventions on team process, team performance, and shared mental models. Organ Behav Hum Decis Process. 2007;102(2):127–42.

Hall KL, Feng AX, Moser RP, Stokols D, Taylor BK. Moving the science of team science forward: collaboration and creativity. Am J Prev Med. 2008;35(2):S243–9.

Hall KL, Vogel AL, Huang GC, Serrano KJ, Rice EL, Tsakraklides SP, Fiore SM. The Science of Team Science: a review of the empirical evidence and research gaps on collaboration in science. Am Psychol. 2018;73(4):532–48.

Hart Research Associates. Falling short? College learning and career success. Washington, DC: Association of American Colleges and Universities; 2015.

Hirsch Hadorn G, et al., editors. Handbook of transdisciplinary research. Dordrecht (London): Springer; 2008. https://doi.org/10.1007/978-1-4020-6699-3.

Hmelo-Silver CE. Problem-based learning: what and how do students learn? Educ Psychol Rev. 2004;16(3):235–66.

Hohle BM, McInnis JK, Gates AC. The public health nurse as a member of the interdisciplinary team. Nurs Clin North Am. 1969;4(2):311–9.

Holt VC. Graduate education to facilitate interdisciplinary research collaboration: identifying individual competencies and developmental learning activities. In: Poster Session Presented at the Meeting of the SciTS 2013 Conference Session on Learning and Training for Team Science, Evanston, IL. 2013. http://www.scienceofteamscience.org/2013-sessions%2D%2Dlearning-and-training-for-team-science. Accessed May 2014.

Holton G, Sonnert G. A vision of Jeffersonian science. Issues Sci Technol. 1999;16(1):61–5.

Jacobson SR. A study of interprofessional collaboration. Nurs Outlook. 1974;22:751–5.

Karlin B, et al. The role of the university: engaged scholarship in the anthropocene. In: Matthew R, et al., editors. The social ecology of the anthropocene: continuity and change in global environmental politics. Hackensack (NJ): World Scientific Publishers; 2017.

Kantrowitz TM. Development and construct validation of a measure of soft skills performance (Unpublished dissertation). Atlanta, GA: Georgia Institute of Technology; 2005.

Klein JT. Interdisciplinarity: history, theory, and practice. Detroit, MI: Wayne State University Press; 1990.

Klein JT. Crossing boundaries: knowledge, disciplinarities, and interdisciplinarities. Charlottesville, VA: University of Virginia Press; 1996.

Klein JT. Creating interdisciplinary campus cultures: a model for strength and sustainability. San Francisco, CA: Jossey-Bass; 2010.

Klein C, DeRouin RE, Salas E. Uncovering workplace interpersonal skills: a review, framework, and research agenda. In: Hodgkinson GP, Ford JK, editors. International review of industrial and organizational psychology, 21. New York: Wiley & Sons, Ltd.; 2006. p. 80–126.

Klein JT, Falk-Krzesinski HJ. Interdisciplinary and collaborative work: framing promotion and tenure practices and policies. Res Policy. 2017;46(6):1055–61.

Kraiger K, Ford JK, Salas E. Application of cognitive, skill-based, and affective theories of learning outcomes to new methods of training evaluation. J Appl Psychol. 1993;78(2):311–28.

Lattuca LR, Knight D, Bergom I. Developing a measure of interdisciplinary competence. Int J Eng Educ. 2013a;29(3):726–39.

Lattuca, L.R., Knight, D.B., Seifert, T., Reason RD, Liu Q. The influence of interdisciplinary undergraduate programs on learning outcomes. In: Presented at the 94th Annual Meeting of the American Educational Research Association, San Francisco, CA. 2013b.

Lavin MA, Reubling I, Banks R, Block L, Counte M, Furman G, Miller P, Reese C, Viehmann V, Holt J. Interdisciplinary health professional education: a historical review. Adv Health Sci Educ. 2001;6(1):25–47.

Lupella RO. Postgraduate clinical training in speech pathology-audiology: experiences in an interdisciplinary medical setting. Am J Speech Lang Hearing Assoc. 1972;14(11):611–4.

Marks MA, DeChurch LA, Mathieu JE, Panzer FJ, Alonso A. Teamwork in multiteam systems. J Appl Psychol. 2005;90(5):964–71.

Mathieu JE, Hollenbeck JR, van Knippenberg D, Ilgen DR. A century of work teams in the Journal of Applied Psychology. J Appl Psychol. 2017;102(3):452–67. https://doi.org/10.1037/apl0000128.

Misra S, et al. Evaluating an interdisciplinary undergraduate training program in health promotion research. Am J Prev Med. 2009;36(4):358–65.

Misra S, Stokols D, Cheng L. The transdisciplinary orientation scale: Factor structure and relation to the integrative quality and scope of scientific publications. J Collab Healthcare Transl Med. 2015;3(2):1042.

Mitrany M, Stokols D. Gauging the transdisciplinary qualities and outcomes of doctoral training programs. J Plan Educ Res. 2005;24(4):437–49.

Nagel JD, Koch A, Guimond JM, Galvin S, Geller S. Building the women's health research workforce: fostering interdisciplinary research approaches in women's health. Global Adv Health Med. 2013;2(5):24–9.

Nash JM. Transdisciplinary training: key components and prerequisites for success. Am J Prev Med. 2008;35(2):S133–40.

Nash JM, Collins BN, Loughlin SE, Solbrig M, Harvey R, Krishnan-Sarin S, Unger J, Miner C, Rukstalis M, Shenassa E, Dube C, Spirito A. Training the transdisciplinary scientist: a general framework applied to tobacco use behavior. Nicotine Tobacco Res. 2003;5(Suppl. 1):S41–53.

National Research Council. Facilitating interdisciplinary research. Committee on facilitating interdisciplinary research and committee on science, engineering, and public policy. Washington, DC: The National Academies Press; 2005.

National Research Council. Convergence: facilitating transdisciplinary integration of life sciences, physical sciences, engineering, and beyond. Washington DC: The National Academies Press; 2014.

National Research Council. Enhancing the effectiveness of team science. Washington DC: National Academies Press; 2015.

National Research Council. Building America's skilled technical workforce. Washington DC: The National Academies Press; 2017. https://doi.org/10.17226/23472.

Norman GR, Schmidt HG. Effectiveness of problem-based learning curricula: theory, practice and paper darts. Med Educ. 2000;34(9):721–8.

Nurius PS, Kemp SP. Individual level competencies for team collaboration with cross-disciplinary researchers and stakeholders. In: Hall KL, Vogel AL, Croyle RT, editors. Strategies for team science success: handbook of evidence-based principles for cross-disciplinary science and practical lessons learned from health researchers. New York, NY: Springer; 2019.

Obstfeld D. Social networks, the tertius iungens orientation, and involvement in innovation. Adm Sci Q. 2005;50(1):100–30.

OECD. Interdisciplinarity: problems of teaching and research in universities. Paris: Organization for Economic Cooperation and Development; 1972.

O'Rourke M, Crowley SJ. Philosophical intervention and cross-disciplinary science: the story of the toolbox project. Synthese. 2013;190(11):1937–54.

Ohland MW, Loughry ML, Woehr DJ, Bullard LG, Felder RM, Finelli CJ, Layton RA, Pomeranz HR, Schmucker DG. The comprehensive assessment of team member effectiveness: development of a behaviorally anchored rating scale for self- and peer evaluation. Acad Manag Learn Educ. 2012;11(4):609–30.. http://amle.aom.org/content/11/4/609.full.pdf+html

Olson JS, Olson GM. Working together apart: collaboration over the internet. San Rafael, CA: Morgan & Claypool Publishers; 2014.

Olson GM, Zimmerman A, Bos N. Scientific collaboration on the internet. Cambridge, MA: MIT Press; 2008.

Rentsch JR, Delise LA, Salas E, Letsky MP. Facilitating knowledge building in teams: can a new team training strategy help? Small Group Res. 2010;41(5):505–23.

Rentsch JR, Delise LA, Mello AL, Staniewicz MJ. The integrative team knowledge building strategy in distributed problem-solving teams. Small Group Res. 2014;45(5):568–91.

Repko AF, Szostak R, Buchberger MP. Introduction to interdisciplinary studies. Los Angeles, CA: Sage Publications; 2017.

Rosenfield PL. The potential of transdisciplinary research for sustaining and extending linkages between the health and social sciences. Soc Sci Med. 1992;35(11):1343–57.

Salas E, Dickinson TL, Converse SA, Tannenbaum SI. Toward an understanding of team performance and training. In: Swezey RW, Salas E, editors. Teams: their training and performance. Norwood, NJ: Albex; 1992. p. 3–29.

Schnapp LM, Rotschy L, Hall TE, Crowley S, O'Rourke M. How to talk to strangers: facilitating knowledge sharing within translational health teams with the toolbox dialogue method. Transl Behav Med. 2012;2(4):469–79.

Stokes DE. Pasteur's quadrant: basic science and technological innovation. Washington DC: Brookings Institution Press; 1997.

Stokols D. The future of interdisciplinarity in the School of Social Ecology. In: Paper Presented at the Social Ecology Associates Annual Awards Reception, School of Social Ecology, University of California, Irvine. 1998. https://eee.uci.edu/98f/50990/Readings/stokols.html.

Stokols D. Training the next generation of transdisciplinarians. In: O'Rourke M, Crowley S, Eigenbrode SD, Wulfhorst JD, editors. Enhancing communication and collaboration in interdisciplinary research. Los Angeles, CA: Sage Publications; 2014. p. 56–81.

Stokols D. Social ecology in the digital age—solving complex problems in a globalized world. London, UK: Academic Press; 2018.

Stokols D, Hall KL, Taylor BK, Moser RP. The science of team science: overview of the field and introduction to the supplement. Am J Prev Med. 2008;35(2):S77–89.

Stokols D, Harvey R, Gress J, Fuqua J, Phillips K. In Vivo studies of transdisciplinary scientific collaboration: lessons learned and implications for active living research. Am J Prev Med. 2005;28(2S2):202–13.

Sundstrom E, DeMeuse KP, Futrell D. Work teams: applications and effectiveness. Am Psychol. 1990;45(2):120–33.

Swezey RW, Salas E, editors. Teams: their training and performance. Westport, CT: Ablex Publishing; 1992.

Taggar S, Brown TC. Problem-solving team behaviors: development and validation of BOS and a hierarchical factor structure. Small Group Res. 2001;32(6):698–726.

Van Ginkel W, Tindale RS, van Knippenberg D. Team reflexivity, development of shared task representations, and the use of distributed information in group decision making. Group Dyn Theory Res Pract. 2009;13(4):265–80.

Vermunt JD, Verloop N. Congruence and friction between learning and teaching. Learn Instr. 1999;9(3):257–80.

Vernon DT, Blake RL. Does problem-based learning work? A meta-analysis of evaluative research. Acad Med. 1993;68(7):550–63.

Vogel AL, Feng A, Oh A, Hall KL, Stipelman BA, Stokols D, Okamoto J, Perna FM, Moser R, Nebeling L. Influence of a National Cancer Institute transdisciplinary research and training initiative on trainees' transdisciplinary research competencies and scholarly productivity. Transl Behav Med. 2012;2(4):459–68.

Vogel AL, Hall KL, Klein JT, Falk-Krzesinski HJ. Broadening our understanding of scientific work for the era of team science: implications for recognition and rewards. In: Hall KL, Vogel AL, Croyle RT, editors. Strategies for team science success: handbook of evidence-based principles for cross-disciplinary science and practical lessons learned from health researchers. New York, NY: Springer; 2019.

Wittenbaum GM, Park ES. The collective preference for shared information. Curr Dir Psychol Sci. 2001;10(2):70–3.

Continuing Professional Development for Team Science

34

Bonnie J. Spring, Angela Fidler Pfammatter, and David E. Conroy

Contents

34.1 Introduction

Increasing numbers of funding announcements call for research that involves collaboration across several scholarly disciplines. Yet many senior scientists were trained at a time when cross-disciplinary and team-based work were

B. J. Spring (✉) · A. F. Pfammatter
Department of Preventive Medicine, Northwestern University Feinberg School of Medicine, Chicago, IL, USA
e-mail: bspring@northwestern.edu

D. E. Conroy
Department of Kinesiology, College of Health and Human Development, The Pennsylvania State University, University Park, PA, USA

much less common and, indeed, often discouraged. When the lead author was in graduate school, standard wisdom from senior mentors was to dig deep and specialize with the aim of mastering a narrow, focused domain of knowledge over which the mentee could eventually claim greater knowledge than anyone else. Even co-publication was discouraged to the extent possible, since individual intellectual contributions to the work might be questioned during promotion and tenure review. Now fast forward to the present when scientists from all generations are expected to collaborate not only with people from their own discipline, but also with others who were trained in unfamiliar branches of science. This circumstance creates a great need for professional development opportunities in team science that cut across multiple disciplinary backgrounds and experience levels. To address this need, our group previously developed the www.teamscience.net learning modules as a free online experiential training resource for team scientists (NIH UL1TR001422) (Aronoff and Bartkowiak 2012; Hall et al. 2008; Hesse 2011). In this chapter, we illustrate the use of the modules in conjunction with an in-person workshop to address initial challenges to the launch of a newly funded, interdisciplinary, geographically distributed team involving health professionals and computer scientists. Team-based learning principles (Kumar et al. 2015; Michaelsen and Sweet 2008) were applied to

© Springer Nature Switzerland AG 2019
K. L. Hall et al. (eds.), *Strategies for Team Science Success*,
https://doi.org/10.1007/978-3-030-20992-6_34

create a workshop designed to jump start communication among diverse members of the collaborative group.

34.2 Bridging Technical and Content Expertise: The MD2K Project

The Mobile Big Data to Knowledge (MD2K) Center is a $10.8 million Big Data Center of Excellence funded by the National Institutes of Health (U54 HG008073) (Michaelsen et al. 2008). Aims of the MD2K Center are to: (1) develop novel hardware and software to analyze health data generated by wearable sensors, and (2) examine the ability of these tools to prevent two adverse health events: relapse to smoking among recently quit smokers, and re-hospitalization among recently discharged heart failure patients (Michaelsen et al. 2008). The research team assembled to accomplish the work includes experts from several disciplines (computer science, engineering, medicine, behavioral science, and statistics) who also happen to be distributed across 11 universities spanning four time zones in the United States.[1] To conserve budget for the research, MD2K investigators hold only one face-to-face meeting annually, augmented by regular conference calls. Anticipating that the varied backgrounds and lack of prior collaboration among the co-investigators could create communication challenges, MD2K's lead investigators chose to devote part of their first in-person meeting to team science training.

---

[1]Universities that collaborate on the MD2K Study included Cornell Tech, New York, NY; Georgia Tech, Atlanta, GA; Northwestern University Feinberg School of Medicine, Chicago, IL; Ohio State University, Columbus, OH; Rice University, Houston, TX; University of California, Los Angeles, CA; University of California, San Diego, San Diego, CA; University of California, San Francisco, San Francisco, CA, University of Massachusetts Amherst, MA; University of Memphis, Memphis, TX; and University of Michigan, Ann Arbor, MI.

34.3 Team Science Training Workshop: MD2K Team Launch

A customized team science training experience developed by our group was offered to 68 attendees of the first annual MD2K all-hands meeting held at the University of Memphis in October 2014. All of the materials needed to conduct this team training workshop appear in Table 34.1. Collaborating investigators, postdoctoral fellows, and graduate student trainees all were invited to participate. The workshop had three goals, to: (1) introduce participants to the benefits and challenges of conducting interdisciplinary team science, (2) expose some potentially confusing differences in terminology, research methods, and assumptions that health scientists and computer scientists might expect to encounter during the course of collaboration, and (3) examine different reward structures across disciplines.

34.3.1 Pre-Workshop Training Activity

Prior to arriving at the workshop, attendees were asked to complete the Science of Team Science Module (Team Science 101), the first of four online team science training modules available at www.teamscience.net (Aronoff and Bartkowiak 2012; Hall et al. 2008; Hesse 2011). This initial interactive module provides a comprehensive introduction to team science concepts, including communication strategies, facilitators and barriers to collaboration, and evaluation of team functioning. Since the team science knowledge base is new to most participants, and since no strong contingencies are implemented to enforce completion of the pre-work, it is assumed that some participants will complete the learning modules, and others will not. This disparity in preparation introduces variability into the knowledge base that members bring to group exercises, mimicking real-world group dynamics that arise from member differences in expertise and conscientiousness.

Table 34.1 Preparing for each component of a team science training workshop

Workshop component	Purpose	Lessons learned	Materials
Pre-workshop online training	Provide foundational knowledge for discussions	Compliance is limited and reflective of conscientiousness	Email, personal computer or mobile device access, account (free) on www.teamscience.net
Opening workshop activity	Create opportunity to experience team performance advantage	Need be prepared to draw out any whose scores match or surpass team level so that social reinforcement offsets subsequent risk of disengagement due to low benefit	Large open room with movable meeting tables for small groups Quiz 1: Team Science 101 Knowledge (see Box 34.1) Response feedback system (IF-AT scratch off cards keyed to quiz answers)
Core workshop activity	Create opportunity to unmask and discuss team disciplinary differences in vocabulary, perspective, assumptions	Prior discussion with team members representing different disciplines helps to make quiz items effectively evocative	Large open room with movable meeting tables for small groups Quiz 2: Project-specific team science challenges (prepared for each project individually; see Box 34.2) Response feedback system (inexpensive option: color paddles; high-tech options: clickers or real-time SMS polling)

34.3.2 Opening Workshop Activity: Experiencing the Team Performance Advantage

Upon arrival at the workshop, participants were seated at tables in groups of eight. Each table included a mixture of research scientists and trainees from both the behavioral/medical sciences and computer science/engineering. Workshop leaders distributed a 13-item multiple-choice quiz about the Science of Team Science module and asked each participant to complete the quiz individually. Questions for this first quiz (see Box 34.1) are deliberately crafted to be challenging and somewhat ambiguous, eliciting differences of opinion. After participants had approximately 10 min to complete the quiz, one group co-leader collected them for scoring, while another distributed a single blank copy of the same quiz and an immediate feedback assessment technique (IF-AT) answer form to each Table. IF-AT answer forms (available from Epstein

Educational Technologies: info@epsteineducation.com) display four covered response options corresponding to the four multiple-choice answers for each question. Prior to receiving any feedback about their individual quiz scores, the group seated at the table was asked to discuss and to reach consensus about the answer to each question. Having reached consensus, the group scratched off the coating that covered their response choice to see whether they received a star—immediate feedback that their answer was correct. If their first choice was correct, participants gave themselves credit for that quiz item. If not, the group chose and scratched off another response option, and so on until they selected the correct answer. After answering all the questions, the team totaled the score they achieved when working as a team. Workshop facilitators then returned the scored quizzes that participants had taken as individuals, so that participants could compare the two scores. In our experience, the test score achieved by the group almost always surpasses that achieved by most, if not all, individual team members. Hence, engaging in this exercise gives participants a direct, compelling personal experience of the performance advantage they can gain by working as a team.

Box 34.1 Quiz 1: Team Science 101 Knowledge Quiz

1. In network science, an echo chamber is a situation in which
   (a) one member dominates and repeatedly says the same thing
   (b) everyone speaks but no one listens to anyone else
   (c) group members voice the same opinions *
   (d) group members listen only to those who agree
2. Micro-finance (the policy of making small loans to impoverished women without collateral) emerged from a collaboration among a Bengali economist, a Chicago Bank, and the Ford Foundation. The Bengali economist was awarded a Nobel Prize in recognition of the work. Which type of science does this collaboration illustrate?
   (a) Interdisciplinary
   (b) Unidisciplinary *
   (c) Multidisciplinary
   (d) Transdisciplinary
3. You are an untenured junior investigator planning to submit an NIH research grant. The budget has sufficient funds to support 20% effort from you and one other investigator. Which of the following should you invite to be your co-investigator?
   (a) Senior investigator at a higher status institution *
   (b) Senior investigator at a same status institution
   (c) Supportive senior colleague at your own institution
   (d) Junior colleague at your institution with whom you've collaborated effectively
4. A senior biochemist is planning a major new research program and trying to decide whom to invite to join the project team. Which of the following is preferable?
   (a) 7 senior colleagues—4 of them prior collaborators
   (b) 1 new senior colleague and 7 junior colleagues—5 of them prior collaborators
   (c) 2 senior colleagues—both prior collaborators, and 1 new junior colleague
   (d) 5 senior and 3 junior scientists—6 of them prior collaborators *
5. Which of the following is a disincentive for a senior faculty member to become engaged in transdisciplinary team science research?
   (a) Experts who usually review his/her grant proposals may not understand and may not fund the new work.
   (b) Unique team science skills may be called upon by university leadership, creating administrative burdens.
   (c) Evaluators' difficulty in assigning ownership for the work may impede tenure consideration.
   (d) All are disincentives. *
6. What good advice can a mentor offer a junior research scientist about team science?
   (a) If your main research questions cross disciplinary boundaries, strongly consider going ahead
   (b) Consider your tenure review timeline: teams usually take longer to complete projects
   (c) Evaluate the team leader's prior collaborations to see if the individual seems trustworthy
   (d) All are correct *
7. What would be the strongest research design to evaluate the impact of a solo science versus a team science approach to research?
   (a) Use an intermittent time series design. Start one group of scientists working

(continued)

Box 34.1 (cont.)

      alone; shift them to working in teams. Start a different group working in teams; shift them to working alone. See whether performance is better in teams or alone.

  (b) Conduct bibliometric studies comparing the citation impact of single-authored versus multi-authored papers (excluding self-citations).

  (c) Perform case studies within the same university of scientists who work alone versus in teams. See which is more productive.

  (d) Randomly assign one group of scientists to work on a research project alone and another group to work in teams. See which group does better.

8. How often should team members meet face to face?
  (a) Weekly
  (b) Every 6 months
  (c) At least once a year
  (d) Monthly

9. What proportion of very large team science projects fail?
  (a) Large team science and solo small science projects both usually succeed and in similar proportions.
  (b) A majority of large team science projects succeed.
  (c) A majority of large team science projects fail.
  (d) Large team science and solo small science projects both usually fail and in similar proportions.

10. What is the most frequent type of team science conflict?
  (a) Conflict about order of authorship
  (b) Conflict about data interpretation and conclusions
  (c) Conflict between mentor and mentee
  (d) Conflict about free riding

11. Which of the following is NOT very important to discuss before beginning a team science project?
  (a) Expectations and policies about authorship
  (b) What will happen if an investigator leaves the institutions
  (c) Who will hold the copyright to published articles
  (d) Who will do which parts of the work

12. Which of the following statements about leadership is true?
  (a) An effective leader minimizes conflict to the extent possible.
  (b) Supportive leaders are most effective for extroverted teams.
  (c) Charismatic leaders are most effective for introverted teams.
  (d) There is no single best type of leader.

13. What did Tuckman consider to be the natural sequence of stages in team formation?
  (a) Storming, forming, norming, performing
  (b) Forming, storming, norming, performing
  (c) Norming, performing, storming, reforming
  (d) Forming, performing, norming, storming

34.3.3 Core Project-Related Workshop Activity: Eliciting Diverse Disciplinary Vocabulary and Points of View

Once the groups had experienced the benefits of teamwork while working on a novel topic (team science), their next activity applied what they had learned to solving problems more directly related to their research problem (mobile health). Workshop leaders gave the group seated at each table a single copy of a new quiz containing 11 multiple-choice items. These items were designed to elicit differences in the terminology, methods, and priorities that health scientists versus computer scientists/engineers apply to their work (see Box 34.2).

Box 34.2 Quiz 2: MD2K Team Science Quiz

1. An interdisciplinary team has come together to develop and refine a sensor system and algorithms that automatically determine how many calories a person consumes. Which of the following signifies that the initial phase of the project has been completed?
   (a) The research has many artifacts.
   (b) Team members agree on whether they still want to work together.
   (c) The budget has been spent.
   (d) The research has no artifacts.

2. Multiple regression analysis of data from your study show that the number of calories someone ate for breakfast accounts for 75% of the variance in how many calories they later eat for lunch. Which of the following phenomena does this illustrate?
   (a) Prediction
   (b) Explanation
   (c) Correlation
   (d) Compensation

3. You want to design a system that predicts in real time when a smoker will begin to smoke. What should you do first?
   (a) Develop a sensor that detects smoking.
   (b) Create a theoretical or conceptual model of factors that influence when someone smokes.
   (c) Develop a model from a dataset that includes physiological data from smokers when they are smoking and not smoking.
   (d) Interview smokers and ask what they do just before they smoke.

4. You have taken 1000 photographs of a college campus. Now you train a machine learning algorithm to detect pictures that include food. You apply the algorithm to a new set of 1000 photographs and find 97% correct classification of food photographs. What should you do next?
   (a) Build an app that uses smart vision to help dieters stay away from food.
   (b) Speak to clinicians about how they can use your discovery.
   (c) See what proportion of the photographs included food.
   (d) Analyze what physical features the algorithm is using to classify food vs. not food.

5. When evaluating a new sensor system to predict 5-day risk of congestive heart failure, which is the most important outcome metric?
   (a) Whether the system's predictions are accurate.
   (b) Whether patients will wear the sensors consistently.
   (c) Whether physicians find the information useful.
   (d) All of these are similarly important.

6. Which is most professionally valuable?
   (a) A publication in *Nature* (h5 median = 495).
   (b) A presentation at the IEEE Conference on Computer Vision and Pattern Recognition, CVPR (h5 median = 167).
   (c) A publication in *New England Journal of Medicine* (h5 median = 495).
   (d) The value of each depends on your profession.

7. Which is the most desirable authorship position?
   (a) Second
   (b) Last
   (c) Second to last
   (d) First

8. A multi-disciplinary team is studying the skin microbiome. The leaders of the collaborating team are a physicist, a computer scientist, and a physician. The research is funded by a grant from NIH on which the physician is PI, a grant from NSF on which the computer scientist is PI, and a grant from DOD on

(continued)

Box 34.2 (cont.)

which the physicist is PI. The NIH grant is the largest, followed by the DOD grant, followed by the NSF grant. The computer scientist develops a new sensor that reads the skin microbiome. The physician applies the sensor to patients newly exposed to ebola. The physicist discovers a characteristic network structure in the microbiome of individuals who develop ebola. Where should the team publish the first paper about this work?

   (a) In a medical journal because the physician's NIH grant is the largest.

   (b) Wherever the team's "prenuptial" collaboration agreement stipulated.

   (c) In the physicist's choice of journal because her discovery of the new network structure is the main innovation.

   (d) The team should write three papers: one first authored by the physicist and published in a basic science journal, another first authored by the physician and appearing in a medical journal, and the third first authored by the computer scientist and presented at a CS conference.

9. What role does a theory (or conceptual model) play in research on mobile big data to knowledge?

   (a) Theory informs what should be measured.

   (b) Theory is developed after the data are modeled to explain how the model works.

   (c) Theory informs what should be measured and predicts how the measures should interrelate.

   (d) Theory informs what should be measured and how and why the measures should interrelate, and theory should be evaluated and refined on the basis of how well the computational modeling works.

10. In a medical school, the strongest positive influences on tenure and promotion are

   (a) Federal grants

   (b) Interdisciplinary collaborations

   (c) Publication in high-impact specialty journals

   (d) Punctuality and professional appearance

11. Interdisciplinary research collaborations

   (a) are usually helpful for academic tenure and promotion

   (b) are helpful for senior faculty but not junior faculty

   (c) take more time to accomplish than unidisciplinary collaborations are as helpful for junior faculty as for senior faculty

Each group completed this quiz together as a team; no scratch off sheets were provided and no individual performance feedback was given. After giving the groups 15 min to select their answers, the workshop leader led a 45-min discussion of the responses. The leader read each question and response option aloud and then counted down from 3. On the count of 1, a representative from each table held up a color-coded paddle revealing their choice of answer. Many attendees were shocked by the diversity of answers chosen. The leader then called upon a group that had selected the correct response and a group that chose the most frequently selected incorrect alternative, inviting each to explain their choice of answer. Considerable debate and group discussion ensued.

The animated dialogue during this activity revealed great differences of opinion about the correct answers to questions. Health scientists accustomed to considering "artifacts" as problems reflecting experimental error were perplexed about why computer scientists wished to accumulate as many artifacts as possible (because computer scientists use the term "artifact" to designate software products). Differences of opinion surfaced about the role and importance of theory in research, the most problematic types of research error, the appropriate priority to be given to data exploration versus hypothesis-testing, the best venues to disseminate findings, and optimal operational criteria to recognize high-impact work. Many attendees expressed surprise that others interpreted the questions so differently. The emergent dialogue directly reflected different disciplinary perspectives, vocabulary, and reward structures that were just beginning to become evident within the project team and that continued to resurface in subsequent years. Often it was trainees who helped to translate between the discrepant viewpoints of senior faculty in the health and engineering sciences, an experience they described as highly empowering. Trainees are in a unique position by virtue of their relative newness to their respective fields. While faculty often feel compelled to demonstrate their professional prowess publicly, the trainee role allows greater latitude to acknowledge lack of understanding. Hence, trainees can voice the "dumb questions" that many faculty feel they couldn't ask without losing face, and that need to be addressed to help team members begin to grasp another discipline's unfamiliar modes of thought.

34.3.4 Workshop Evolution: Beyond Team Assembly to Launch and Maturation

Feedback about the MD2K pilot workshop was positive, with attendees reporting new awareness of challenges and opportunities associated with working in interdisciplinary teams. Many stated that the workshop heightened their favorable attitudes about collaborating across disciplines. Some reported feeling surprised to learn that team science challenges are so commonplace, but also hopeful because the facilitated discussion demonstrated that resolution is often possible through communication. An outgrowth of the workshop was that several participating institutions contracted with our group to coach their newly forming interdisciplinary teams. Experience with MD2K and other team science projects we support suggests that new challenges and incentives for interdisciplinary collaboration emerge as a cross-disciplinary team evolves. Hence, our current practice is to offer teams a sequence of several workshops, tailored to address their differing needs as they progress from team assembly to launch and then through increasing stages of maturation. In MD2K, for example, the great complexity of the technology that urgently needed to be developed caused work flow to proceed initially in a primarily multidisciplinary, sequential fashion, with each discipline independently developing its own fairly refined prototype before handing it off to the disciplinary counterpart (Spring et al. 2012). Technical conference papers and NSF grants were the main professional incentives during this phase. Once the health scientists began to deploy the technology with study participants, the collaboration transitioned to become interdisciplinary (Spring et al. 2012). Now the scientists needed to work jointly, albeit each group from its own disciplinary perspective, having the frequent dialogue necessary to problem solve new usability problems and bugs that emerged once technology-naïve patients used the new systems. Closer contact among the computer science and health science members of the team made the scientific dialogue richer, but also introduced more opportunities for misunderstanding and conflict (e.g., based on the appraisal that the technology team was behaving dismissively or that the health science team was imposing unreasonable, perfectionistic performance demands). The discomfort and resource burdens needed to address these issues can easily prompt teams functioning at an interdisciplinary or even transdisciplinary level to retreat to less effortful multidisciplinary or even unidisciplinary modes of operation, unless regularly reminded of professional rewards (real-world application, health journal publications, NIH grants) that can be attained only by sustaining interdisciplinary collaboration.

34.4 Summary

The present observations demonstrate that team science training is feasible for a large cross-disciplinary group. The approach taken to train the MD2K project team combined structured online learning with hands on, in-person group activities. Workshop activities were designed to demonstrate experientially the benefits of teamwork and to unmask disciplinary variation in terminology, approach, and assumptions. Pre-workshop homework and an opening workshop activity laid groundwork for a core activity designed to elicit engaged discussions regarding project-specific challenges. Although the interpretation must be offered cautiously because of the absence of formal evaluation with a control group, we believe the MD2K team's ability to progress from multidisciplinary to interdisciplinary collaboration was facilitated by its exposure to the initial MD2K team science launch workshop. Our subsequent in-person training activities with teams have incorporated two additional features. First, all trainings now incorporate formal evaluation, and we are also exploring features (linguistic, social connectivity) that mark the evolution of collaboration. Second, we now deploy sequential trainings to address several stages of team maturation. A first workshop focuses on project organization, administration, and logistics; a second on developing and refining a collaboration agreement; a final workshop focuses on conflict and reward management and envisions the team's and the project's future.

Acknowledgement Research reported in this publication was supported, in part, by the National Institutes of Health's National Center for Advancing Translational Sciences, Grant Number UL1TR001422 and by a Big Data Center of Excellence funded by the National Institutes of Health (U54 HG008073). The content is solely the responsibility of the authors and does not necessarily represent the official views of the National Institutes of Health.

References

Aronoff DM, Bartkowiak BA. A review of the website TeamScience.net. Clin Med Res. 2012;10(1):38–9. Clinical Medicine & Center of excellence for mobile sensor data-to-knowledge (MD2K). Journal of the American Medical Collaboration and Creativity. American Journal of Preventive Medicine. 2008;35(2 Suppl): S243-S249.

Hall KL, Feng AX, Moser RP, Stokols D, Taylor BK. Moving the science of team science forward: health professions education: a guide to using small groups for improving learning. Sterling, VA: Stylus; 2008.

Hesse B. COALESCE: CTSA online assistance for leveraging the science of collaborative effort. J Am Med Assoc. 2011;306(17):1925–6. https://doi.org/10.1001/jama.2011.1593.

Kumar S, Abowd GD, Abraham WT, al'Absi M, Beck JG, Chau DH, Wetter DW. Center of excellence for mobile sensor data-to-knowledge (MD2K). JAMIA. 2015;22(6):1137–42. https://doi.org/10.1093/jamia/ocv056.

Michaelsen LK, Sweet M. The essential elements of team-based learning. New Dir Teach Learn. 2008;116:7–27.

Michaelsen LK, Parmelee DX, McMahon KK, Levine RE. Team-based learning for Research. 2008; 10(1): 38–39.

Spring B, Hall KL, Moller AC, Falk-Krzesinski HJ. An emerging science and praxis for research and practice teams. Transl Behav Med. 2012;2(4):411–4.

Training for Interdisciplinary Research in Population Health Science

35

Christine Bachrach, Stephanie A. Robert, and Yonette Thomas

Contents

The original version of this chapter was revised. The correction to this chapter is available at https://doi.org/10.1007/978-3-030-20992-6_46

C. Bachrach (✉)
Maryland Population Research Center, University of Maryland, College Park, MD, USA
e-mail: chrisbachrach@gmail.com

S. A. Robert
School of Social Work, University of Wisconsin-Madison, Madison, WI, USA

Department of Population Health Science, University of Wisconsin-Madison, Madison, WI, USA

Y. Thomas
Maryland Population Research Center, University of Maryland, College Park, MD, USA

American Association of Geographers, Washington, DC, USA

35.1   Introduction

How do you create a cadre of scientists who can work across disciplines to produce an integrative understanding of the mechanisms—from the biological to the sociological—through which health and health disparities are produced? The need for these inter- and transdisciplinary scientists has never been greater. A host of factors have coalesced to inspire rapidly rising demand for "upstream" solutions to address health and health disparities to complement traditional investments in medical care. Despite massive investments in medical care, the U.S. trails other advanced economies on most measures of health and in gains to life expectancy (NRC and IOM 2013). We have made limited progress in addressing disparities in health across race and ethnicity and between rich and poor. At the same time, scientists have amassed compelling evidence to demonstrate the impact of upstream or contextual determinants such as economic conditions, housing, community cohesion, food environments, and nonhealth policies on health and health disparities.

"Population health" approaches to improving health complement medical care by addressing the multiple causes of health that operate at different levels—with an emphasis on how social and physical environments impact health directly and indirectly through their effects on cognition, behavior, and biology.[1] Population health *science* provides the foundation for population health strategies. It integrates knowledge, theory, and tools from multiple disciplines to develop a broad understanding of the multifactorial pathways that produce health and health disparities and the cascade of mechanisms through which health and health disparities are produced.[2] For example, a population health study might involve a team of scientists studying the contributions of early childhood education policies to health differentials in adulthood across different communities. Such a study could investigate the social, economic, cognitive, and behavioral sequelae of policy differences and the pathways through which these sequelae influence the development of chronic diseases (e.g., diabetes, cardiovascular disease). It could draw on the expertise of endocrinologists, developmental psychologists, education researchers, economists, sociologists, and cognitive scientists. In short, population health science is often team science—a team science that fully embraces cross-disciplinary[3] collaboration and integration.

The integration of the basic social sciences alongside the basic biological, clinical, and behavioral sciences is essential to population health science. Many health-focused sciences treat social contextual determinants as "exposures" rather than processes endogenous to the living systems they are studying.[4] By addressing

the processes that drive social systems and produce "social exposures," processes of stratification, economic cycles, political movements, migration, diffusion, and institutional change, the social sciences can greatly enrich and deepen the understanding of social determinants and the avenues for addressing their effects on health. Conversely, social scientists need to work more closely with biological scientists to understand how social factors "get under the skin" to affect health.

Training in population health science faces several challenges. The first is the location and structure of training programs. Schools of public health are a natural site for population health training. After all, public health and population health are closely related concepts, and schools of public health are expected to create a cross-disciplinary environment. Because of the importance of a full range of disciplines to population health, however, there are few schools of public health that can both meet the requirements of professional public health training and provide a full range of exposure to disciplines relevant to population health training. For example, although coursework in social and behavioral sciences is required for public health training, most schools cannot provide a full range of theory and methodology needed to study social systems without bringing in expertise from liberal arts campuses. At many universities, liberal arts campuses also often host the local expertise in population dynamics, which is crucial to population health.

Although schools of public health are natural sites for building population health training, there are other potential sites and options, as we discuss later. But no matter the model or location, bridging across health and liberal arts campuses is necessary but not easy. Scientists in schools of medicine and public health tend to be divided from social scientists and other scientists in the liberal arts not only by scientific approach and

---

[1]Kindig and Stoddart (2003) define population health as "the health outcomes of a group of individuals, including the distribution of such outcomes within the group." However, typical usage also implicates the upstream approaches that may be used to improve aggregate health, and we adopt this usage here. See Kindig (2012) for yet another meaning, more appropriately called "population medicine."

[2]Population health science acknowledges a close relationship to public health, but extends traditional scholarship and training in public health to better incorporate the full range of disciplines that contribute to population health knowledge, including the basic social sciences.

[3]In past work, the authors have used "interdisciplinary" to describe the integrative nature of population health science. In deference to the editors' desire for a common taxonomy in this volume, we adopt "cross-disciplinary" here to refer to multi-, inter-, and trans-disciplinary work.

[4]The problem with this approach can be illustrated with an

extreme example: one might say that a death was caused by exposure to a bullet, neglecting a larger and more useful explanation that took into account the relationship of social and economic conditions, environmental stressors and stress response pathways, patterns of social interaction, and public policies to the firing of the bullet.

discipline-based incentive structures but also by institutional boundaries, geography, and weak network connections.

A second challenge is that, in order to offer effective strategies for improving health, population health science must embrace the full range of basic to translational and implementation science. This requires another dimension of cross-disciplinarity in training programs, linking scientists pursuing highly theoretical questions to those seeking evidence to inform policy, and linking applied scientists to leaders in nonscience sectors such as business, education, and government who have the ability to effect change in upstream conditions.

Finally, sustained funding for population health training is limited. Most universities tend to focus on disciplinary programs. Although funding from federal agencies has spurred many universities to offer cross-disciplinary programs related to health, few of these produce cross-disciplinary population health scientists.[5] Foundation support for science training is dwindling. The Robert Wood Johnson Foundation began funding an exemplary fellowship program in population health science in 2002, but closed the program in 2016 to pursue other goals. Across all funding sources, opportunities for new training programs are highly constrained.

As a result, training programs that build the skill base for population health science are in short supply. Although most health scientists recognize the importance of cross-disciplinarity, training in cross-disciplinary science has not necessarily followed. In a recent study of public health programs in Canada, over three quarters endorsed the value of interdisciplinary, multidisciplinary or cross-disciplinary training opportunities, but only one-third (32%) provided them (Mishra et al. 2011).

35.2 A Model: Robert Wood Johnson Health & Society Scholars

The Robert Wood Johnson Foundation launched the Health & Society Scholars (HSS) program in 2003 with the goal of training cross-disciplinary scientists to investigate the effects of contextual factors on behavior and biology and to strengthen the knowledge base supporting population-wide interventions. The program was designed to bring disciplinary scientists into conversation with the issues in population health and health disparities and with the insights, methods, and contributions of other disciplines relevant to those questions.[6]

At each of six university sites, faculty representing diverse disciplines relevant to population health designed a program that both exposed trainees to a broad range of disciplinary approaches and also engaged them in cross-disciplinary exchange and research. Faculty made the final selection of the six trainees at each site (three new trainees each year for 2 years) with an eye toward creating small group environments composed of people with complementary and synergistic disciplinary expertise. These trainees interacted continuously with each other, with a set of cross-disciplinary core faculty, and with faculty from departments across the university. Scholars were required to move beyond their own disciplinary backgrounds, learn from other disciplines, and engage with other disciplines to conduct population health research.

The program offered intensive group-level and individual mentoring on skills needed to conduct cross-disciplinary research and navigate future career challenges as a cross-disciplinary scientist. Trainees worked with mentors from multiple disciplines. The program provided financial support for mentoring by program fac-

---

[5]A review of NIH training grants funded in 2013 identified 70 with potential relevance to population health training. While many were interdisciplinary, few engaged social science and few explicitly targeted the development of interdisciplinary skills. Foundation support leadership programs (e.g., Kaiser Permanente, Robert Wood Johnson Foundation) and some federally funded programs address policy leadership (e.g., a fellowship program under the Satcher Health Leadership Institute). The National Science Foundation supports interdisciplinary training under its NSF National Research Traineeship Program (formerly IGERT), but not in population health science.

[6]For further information on RWJF Health & Society Scholars, see http://www.healthandsocietyscholars.org/

ulty. Scholars received training in leadership skills and the translation of knowledge to policy and practice through modeling, mentoring, experience-based learning, and/or direct instruction.

The program promoted collaboration across sites. Through annual conferences, it created a community of scholars, alumni, faculty, and advisory committee members that supported learning and collaboration.

The HSS program also sought to strengthen cross-disciplinary cultures and the concept of population health at participating universities. Program faculty at each site spanned at least two schools within the university, and in one case bridged across different universities. Each site was provided a pool of funds that could be used flexibly to support not only scholar research but also projects that would engage nonprogram faculty in cross-disciplinary population health research. In some cases, these funds supported cross-sectoral efforts—bringing researchers and knowledge users together to create projects that both examined and addressed population health problems.

To assess the program's success in producing interdisciplinary population health scientists, alumni from five early scholar cohorts (2004–2008) were compared with a sample of program finalists who had not participated. Outcomes, including indicators of professional experience, productivity, leadership, and engagement in population health research, were assessed during the period 2011–2015. At the time of application, there were no differences between scholar and finalist samples in background characteristics or indicators of qualifications and fit for the program.[7] By 2001–2015, both groups had achieved significant career success, but, compared to finalists, scholars had published significantly more, had higher publication impact scores, and were more likely to be engaged in interdisciplinary population health research (Realmuto et al. 2017; Bachrach et al. 2017).

35.3 A Vision for Future Training in Cross-disciplinary Population Health Science

The decision by RWJF to close all of its site-based training programs, including HSS, prompted efforts to assess lessons learned from the program and apply them in envisioning future training in population health science. On June 1–2, 2015, scientists, educators, and practitioners met at the Institute of Medicine in Washington DC to reflect on future priorities for training in cross-disciplinary population health science.[8] The goal of the meeting was to develop a vision for the production of outstanding scientists who can integrate knowledge, theory, and methods from diverse disciplines and participate effectively in cross-disciplinary teams to address complex population health issues. Participants included scientists working in fields contributing to population health research, leaders in academic training in population health science and/or cross-disciplinary training in related areas, health care and public health professionals, and representatives from scientific associations, foundations, and the National Institutes of Health.

Meeting participants reviewed goals and principles, existing models, and best practices in population health science training. Recommendations[9] focused on the key competencies needed by population health scientists, elements of training critical for providing those competencies, and the institutional supports needed to ensure the support of training programs. They also addressed the types of training useful at each stage of the educational process (undergraduate to postdoctoral) to produce a pipeline of skilled cross-disciplinary scientists. Finally, meeting participants proposed a model for future pre- and postdoctoral

---

[7]Measured by ratings given by the program's National Advisory Committee to each applicant.

[8]The meeting received support from the IOM Roundtable for Population Health Improvement, the NIH Office of Behavioral and Social Sciences Research, the National Institute on Minority Health and Health Disparities, and the Robert Wood Johnson Foundation Health & Society Scholars program.

[9]A full report of the meeting is available on the Roundtable's website.

training in cross-disciplinary population health science.

35.3.1 Key Competencies

What does it take to produce outstanding scientists who can integrate knowledge, theory, and methods from diverse disciplines and participate effectively in cross-disciplinary research to address complex population health issues? Three core competency domains are particularly salient: *knowledge acquisition, cross-disciplinary collaboration skills, and knowledge translation and exchange.* Many additional competencies contribute to creating strong scientists *in general* (e.g., research ethics, general leadership skills), but these are not discussed here.

Training in broad population health *knowledge* has the aim of increasing the creativity and scope of the population health scientist, improving the scientist's ability to contribute effectively in a cross-disciplinary team, and enabling a scientist to produce rigorous population health research alone or in teams. Because population health science is not a discipline, it does not have a defined "core" of knowledge, theory, and principles. The relevant knowledge derives from multiple disciplines and (1) addresses health broadly; (2) includes a multilevel focus on the determinants of health (including, but not limited to, social determinants); (3) addresses population-level health including both across- and within-population disparities, and (4) often engages a developmental or life course perspective. Specific examples of competencies in the *knowledge acquisition* domain are given in the full report.

Broad exposure to multidisciplinary knowledge provides a common foundation for members of cross-disciplinary teams seeking to integrate diverse theory and methods to address population health problems. A strong population health scientist will have both depth and breadth in knowledge. No one trainee will master all existing literatures, metrics, methods, and design strategies, but all should have a broad awareness of and respect for diverse contributions and approaches.

Training in *cross-disciplinary collaboration skills* prepares scientists to effectively lead and/or work with others who have different approaches to or expertise in population health topics. When working with people from other disciplines and sectors (e.g., business, government, the public), population health scientists must learn to communicate their knowledge in ways that others can understand and to develop an appreciation and understanding of the language and approaches of others. Developing this mutual understanding and respect is difficult without also acquiring collaborative skills. Examples of competencies include fostering and maintaining working relationships among individuals who differ in their perspectives, beliefs, and approaches; establishing shared norms and clear roles and responsibilities within a group; fostering group cohesion; problem-solving and conflict resolution, leadership; and communication. A further skill involves the design of cross-disciplinary teams based on the characteristics of a problem and guiding those teams to sound integrative research designs.

These skills are sometimes developed in disciplinary approaches to scientific training, but are rarely <u>explicitly</u> addressed.[10] Yet they are imperative for future population health scientists to work effectively with people from other disciplines and sectors. Moreover, for the growing proportion of the population health science workforce who expects to work outside of academia, these cross-disciplinary and team skills are often crucial. In fact, academia is chastised by nonacademic employers who sometimes find new scientists unprepared to work in team environments with people from different disciplines and sectors.

The third domain of competencies is skills and expertise in *knowledge translation and exchange.* There is growing consensus that population health scientists should be concerned not only with producing rigorous science, but also with taking an active role in ensuring that the science they produce can contribute to improving population health.

---

[10]See also Canadian Academy of Health Sciences 2005 for a similar call for training in interdisciplinary skills.

Knowledge translation and exchange incorporates "*push*," "*pull*," and "*exchange*" approaches to the communication and application of scientific findings. In the first, the scientist pushes or disseminates knowledge out to user communities in various formats such as media coverage, clinical guidelines, and policy briefs (Grimshaw et al. 2012; Lavis et al. 2003; CHSR 1999; Lomas 2007). In the second, the users of knowledge pull information from knowledge producers, develop capacity for digesting new knowledge, and apply knowledge effectively in decision-making. An understanding of these processes helps scientists better understand when and how to disseminate their research to user communities. "*Exchange*" approaches refer to the development of bidirectional collaborative relationships between the producers and users of knowledge that promote the exchange of ideas over time. Exchange relationships can improve the relevance of the research produced and the efficiency of take-up of the new research by the users of evidence.

Relevant competencies in this domain[11] include: (1) an understanding of where one's work fits along the translational continuum from basic science to application, and how one can effectively move one's science forward along that continuum; (2) skill in engaging knowledge brokers and other avenues for communicating research to practitioners, policy-makers, and the media; (3) skills for framing and communicating research findings as appropriate for different audiences; (4) an understanding of different theories of or approaches to knowledge translation and exchange; (5) knowledge of how potential user communities (e.g., scientists, practitioners, and/or policy-makers) can access and use research findings and the barriers and incentives they experience in doing so; (6) skills in developing and maintaining relationships with user communities over time to enhance exchange of information; and (7) the ability to engage user communities in the design of research.

Depending on their scientific emphases, training programs will inevitably vary in the extent to which all of these competencies are addressed. However, the benefits of helping trainees understand the newest approaches, options, and dilemmas regarding knowledge translation and exchange and encouraging them to develop impactful research agendas—agendas that are tailored to more directly inform efforts to improve health and reduce disparities—cannot be overstated. Even better, practical experience in knowledge exchange with community members or practitioners working to improve population health can both inform the development of new research agendas and also provide skills in collaborating across sectors to develop evidence-based interventions and strategies.

35.3.2 Critical Elements of Training

These competencies can be achieved through a combination of mechanisms, but three are noteworthy for their importance in future population health science training. These include: (1) mentoring (using a multiple mentor model) in scientific areas, knowledge exchange, cross-disciplinary skills, and professional development domains; (2) experience as part of a cross-disciplinary research team; and (3) immersion of trainees in a cross-disciplinary environment. Of course, other training practices are also useful: cross-disciplinary courses, interactive seminars, mentored study, and group-based experiential learning opportunities such as organizing conferences or engaging policy-makers or community members in population health projects.

Mentorship plays a critical role in helping trainees in the sciences to achieve successful academic trajectories (Bland et al. 2009; Pfund et al. 2014). Mentorship is especially important in cross-disciplinary population health training because the field encompasses such a broad range of content, disciplinary approaches, and career pathways. As a result, individual training trajectories may (and perhaps should) be highly individualized, and experienced mentorship is required to help trainees devise and stay on their course. Mentorship is needed in all three of the competency areas discussed above: knowledge

---

[11]A full list of competencies in this domain is included in the report.

acquisition, cross-disciplinary skills, and knowledge translation and exchange, as well as in career challenges such as choosing disciplinary or cross-disciplinary publication venues, negotiating authorship expectations, securing academic or other positions, and promotion.

While ideally mentors would be experienced cross-disciplinary scientists who have mastered these competencies themselves (Nash 2008), the relative youth and diversity of this cross-disciplinary field means that such faculty may be in short supply. As a result, new training programs in cross-disciplinary population health science need to consider a range of methods of mentoring trainees. Having multiple mentors or a team of mentors who can support the trainees in various aspects of their independent research and professional development is essential (Guise et al. 2017). Providing team research opportunities that gather multiple mentees and mentors in a cross-disciplinary research endeavor for colearning and training is another key strategy. Team research projects can facilitate "vertical" mentoring strategies which incorporate trainee-to-trainee mentoring among undergraduates, predocs, and postdocs as well as traditional faculty mentoring.

Mentoring is most effective when adequately managed and supported. Training directors must have the experience to help trainees work effectively with multiple mentors. Faculty time for mentoring activities should be compensated. Unlike traditional disciplinary science where faculty members are compensated by the skilled labor that mentees may provide to a mentor's project, cross-disciplinary science requires mentorship less closely tied to faculty projects. As such, the lack of compensation in NIH T32 grants represents a major challenge for training in population health science. Finally, evidence-based mentor training for both mentors and mentees can improve the effectiveness of mentoring investments.[12]

As suggested above, involvement in a *cross-disciplinary research team* provides trainees with multiple opportunities. It complements didactic training by allowing trainees to apply their growing knowledge and skills to real research problems. It hones skills in research design: for example, in the cross-disciplinary context, skill in analyzing concepts and methodologies from multiple disciplines in formulating questions and approach. It also develops competence in navigating the many decision points involved in research, from fieldwork problems to questions about publication and translation. Joining or forming a cross-disciplinary team provides the trainee an opportunity to observe and build cross-disciplinary skills as the trainee has to navigate the different perspectives and styles of multiple disciplines and personalities and learn how to move complicated projects forward.

Learning to be a cross-disciplinary scientist requires more than just participation in a cross-disciplinary team science project, however. It requires that individuals gain a deep understanding of how their science informs the solution of complex problems across different contexts and the confidence to infuse their knowledge in a team environment in which they may be a junior partner. This requires *sustained immersion* in an environment that fosters the development of these strengths. The concept of immersion goes beyond team experience to making cross-disciplinarity the way of life within a training program. This means designing projects, seminars, and classes to include a diverse trainee group and to require participants to manage and transcend disciplinary boundaries in all problem-solving activities. It means providing ongoing opportunities and incentives for building scholarly networks across cross-disciplinary boundaries. It means providing mentoring in cross-disciplinary values and skills. It also means providing many opportunities for modeling the behaviors and strengths of faculty who demonstrate cross-disciplinary and leadership skills as well as successful strategies for career success as a cross-disciplinary scientist. There is no quick substitute for programs that require trainees to disengage from disciplinary structures and

---

[12] See information on the new NIH-funded National Research Mentoring Network (NRMN) for information about various mentor and mentee training options.

engage peers, teachers, and role models from different disciplines over an extended period of time.

At a minimum, creating such an environment requires several kinds of resources—the ability to select trainees based not only on (essential) scientific credentials but also the ability to "play well with others;" the ability to create small-group settings that are large enough to provide disciplinary variability but small enough to force cross-disciplinary exchange[13]; time for sustained interactions that can produce cross-disciplinary understanding and commitment; and a faculty engaged in and committed to cross-disciplinary research. It requires disciplinary diversity at the faculty and trainee level and incentive structures that promote engagement with the program by individuals and programs with relevant expertise.

Disciplinary diversity within programs often depends on the institutional structures, geography, social networks, and incentives in place at a university. Epidemiology, sociology, medical geography, psychology, and demography are common participants in population health science, but programs should diversify more broadly. Finding ways to incentivize biologists to participate in cross-disciplinary population health endeavors is one challenge; integrating clinical scientists (e.g., physicians, nurses) and individuals from other sectors involved in population health practice and policy (e.g., industry, government, education, social work) in population health research teams is another.

35.3.3 Institutional Contexts and Resources

For even the best-designed training program with carefully specified goals, a diverse and supportive institutional context is essential for success. Population health science draws on disciplines typically distributed across many segments of a university. Ideally, trainees need to have access to top-notch social science, public health, allied health, and medical school departments, and often schools of business, education, public policy, social work, architecture, and more. Access to government, public health, and clinical settings can also benefit training by providing hands-on experience with knowledge translation and exchange. Even at universities where all of these resources are available, however, linkages between different campuses and schools are often weak or nonexistent.

Both universities and funding organizations play an important role in strengthening these linkages. While some universities are able to provide special funding to promote cross-disciplinary research among their faculty, often it is the infusion of external funds that stimulates and supports these efforts. Examples include NIH and NSF funding that supports training programs and research centers[14] and foundation support for programs like HSS. Finding ways to extend these efforts is not only essential for building effective training programs in population health science, but also offers important benefits for universities, the development of scientific knowledge, and the public good.

University leaders and external funders also could do much to align incentive structures and funding supports with the needs of cross-disciplinary training in population health science. One key challenge that many universities are now tackling is the need to reform promotion and tenure criteria to explicitly address the value of cross-disciplinary work and to set standards for documenting relevant contributions. Another relevant target may be joint appointments that, while offering junior scholars the opportunity to do innovative work across disciplines, may also double their service commitments and thereby

---

[13] In the RWJF Health & Society Scholars program, sites found that having six trainees in place at a given site was an optimal number, allowing for both rich interdisciplinary interaction and strong mentoring.

[14] For example, the National Institute on Minority Health and Health Disparities supports Centers of Excellence to address health disparities through interdisciplinary research, research training and education, and community engagement. The National Science Foundation supports the NSF Research Traineeship Program which promotes interdisciplinary training.

impede their progress to tenure. Addressing structural barriers, such as physical distance, departmental philosophical silos, and lack of financial incentives for team teaching, mentoring, and cross-disciplinary course development, is also essential (Canadian Academy of Health Sciences 2005). Changing existing practices requires not only new guidelines and procedures, but also the breaking down of long-standing academic cultures that privilege disciplinary contributions. Funders can play an important role in promoting such change through prioritizing cross-disciplinary research. Funders can also do much to increase the incentives for talented junior scientists to obtain cross-disciplinary training by increasing stipends and supporting travel to multiple conferences.

35.3.4 Diversity

Achieving diversity within training programs is essential to ensure a robust and diverse workforce for population health science and action. Several types of diversity are relevant, such as racial, ethnic, socioeconomic, and regional background; interests related to research across the continuum from basic science to application; and goals for working in academic vs. practice settings.

Attracting students from minority and disadvantaged backgrounds is a critical challenge for training in population health science. At the graduate level, minorities and disadvantaged groups are underrepresented in the fields that comprise population health, including the social, behavioral, and basic biological sciences (Darity et al. 2009; Crisp et al. 2009; Chang et al. 2008).[15] Reaching out early in the pipeline—during college or even high school—may be an important step.

Attracting trainees with interests and goals that span the continuum from basic science to

---

[15]From 1975–2000, interdisciplinary majors thrived especially at "large, wealthy, arts and sciences-oriented universities on the East or West coasts" (Brint et al. 2009: 175). As such, undergraduate programs may have produced and maintained inequalities in the population health science pipeline.

application is another critical challenge. Although those who matriculate in PhD programs often anticipate careers in academia, recent data suggest that half of PhDs in the sciences do not take academic jobs (National Science Foundation 2014). The field of population health needs both individuals who are well grounded in scientific theory and methods *and* individuals who understand on-the-ground opportunities and constraints that affect how problems in population health can be addressed. Diversity, both within and across training programs, in the interests and goals of recruited trainees is needed to meet the workforce demands and strengthen the movement of knowledge "from bench to curbside."

35.3.5 The Training Pipeline

There is no single path to becoming a population health scientist. Some individuals do not discover the concepts and approaches of population health until they are already in graduate school; increasingly, some may do so during their undergraduate years.

In today's world, training in population health should be conducted at all levels. Exposure to population health concepts should start early, through investments at the high school and college levels. However, the greatest current need is for advanced scientific training at the doctoral and postdoctoral levels. Summer programs, midcareer, and senior-level sabbaticals can also contribute to an integrated strategy.

Offering a variety of entry points can cast the widest net for individuals who can contribute to population health science. In addition, offering training at all levels not only helps to recruit and train future population health scientists, but also can expose a broader range of trainees to population health ideas. Such exposure can create a mass of people who are more effective contributors to population health knowledge and action through the range of careers that they may engage in, not to mention through their actions as well-informed citizens.

Training at the high school and college levels provides early exposure to population health concepts, engages students' interest, and lays a foundation of basic skills and competencies. In high school, curricula can introduce students to complex thinking about the multiple determinants of and solutions to population health issues.[16] At the undergraduate level, they can introduce students to population health science and orient them towards cross-disciplinarity. Cross-disciplinary majors for undergraduates are growing rapidly: from 1970 to 2000, the total number of cross-disciplinary majors at U.S. colleges and universities grew by nearly 250%, outstripping an 18% increase in college and university enrollments (Brint et al. 2009). However, access to these programs tends to be concentrated at elite colleges and resource constraints often limit what programs can offer. Cross-disciplinary programs in population health at the undergraduate level are also increasing; most fit one of three models: interdepartmental majors, undergraduate public health majors, and cross-disciplinary health and society majors.[17]

While graduate training in cross-disciplinary population health science is essential to build a cadre of trained researchers, there is no agreed-upon ideal sequence. Some experts believe that achieving mastery of a discipline at the predoctoral level provides an essential foundation for expanding into cross-disciplinary work as a postdoctoral fellow, while others argue that deferring cross-disciplinary training at the predoctoral level is a mistake.[18] In light of this, a diversity of training opportunities—cross-disciplinary doctoral programs in population health science, predoctoral programs that supplement disciplinary training, and postdoctoral training—should be available to accommodate the many pathways individuals may take to becoming a population health scientist.

A limited, but diverse, set of doctoral programs in the U.S. leads to a cross-disciplinary

degree in population health.[19] The focus of these programs differs depending on where the programs are housed. Some programs are clinically focused while others reflect traditional public health models. While many of these programs explicitly aim to produce cross-disciplinary scientists, the extent to which they emphasize cross-disciplinary and transdisciplinary, as contrasted with multidisciplinary, population health education and research is unclear.

An alternative approach to population health training at the graduate level is to offer students enrolled in traditional disciplinary or clinical doctoral programs supplementary training in cross-disciplinary population health science. These programs recruit predoctoral fellows from different departments and schools and provide knowledge, skills, and experience relevant to cross-disciplinary population health science. Minors and certificate programs expose trainees to knowledge about population health through courses outside of his/her field. Cross-disciplinary population health training programs (typically funded by an NIH T32), by contrast, assemble a cohort of scholars who learn from each other over time, gather faculty from different disciplines, and provide opportunities for cross-disciplinary research projects.

Many population health scientists view postdoctoral fellowships as the ideal setting in which to bring skilled researchers together with researchers from other fields to train them to conduct inter- or transdisciplinary research. By the time of the postdoc, trainees have established themselves as experienced researchers with strong research skills. Most have developed an understanding of disciplinary cultures and have the maturity and breadth of perspective that allows them to engage across fields. The Robert Wood Johnson Foundation HSS program, discussed previously, was the only postdoctoral program explicitly devoted to training in population

---

[16] An NIH program that develops and distributes science curricula supplements for grades K-12 could provide a useful mechanism for promoting this.

[17] Based on a review by Sara Shostak and colleagues at Brandeis University; see the full report for details.

[18] See full report for a detailed discussion of these issues.

[19] Based on a search conducted by Tiffany Green and colleagues at Virginia Commonwealth University for doctoral programs that use the term "population health." The search identified 25 program in the U.S., but few conformed to the vision for population health training advanced here.

health, but a number of other programs still pursue related goals.[20]

35.3.6 A Recommended Model

Participants in the June 2015 meeting developed a recommended model for future training in cross-disciplinary population health science at the pre- and postdoctoral levels. The proposed model has the following features:

- It consists of a set of *center-based* training programs. This reflects strong agreement that cross-disciplinary training requires immersing a diverse, critical mass of trainees in cross-disciplinary networks and research over an extended period of time. A center-based model provides trainees the opportunity to engage in ongoing research with faculty from different backgrounds, and to learn from other trainees-in-residence who are from diverse backgrounds but who are similarly committed to learning how to collaborate to produce creative and impactful population health research. This model implies funding training at the institutional (program) level rather than at the individual level, to enable institutions to assemble appropriate diversity among trainees, faculty, and training resources.
- Participating centers represent *three types of strengths:*
  - capacity to conduct state-of-the-art cross-disciplinary population health research;
  - capacity to engage with and address population health problems in underserved and/

or high-need geographic areas and population groups; and
  - capacity to recruit diverse and underrepresented trainees.
- Because many centers will not have strength in all of these areas, an optimal strategy would be to recruit centers with diverse strengths, involving not only well-established centers in elite research universities but also new centers located in institutions with strengths in community engagement and the ability to address population health problems facing local or regional underrepresented communities.
- As discussed earlier in this chapter, each center should engage a *critical mass* of trainees in hands-on, *experiential research training,* through involvement in *problem-focused* research teams that are *cross-disciplinary and/ or multisectoral.*
- Each center designs its own curriculum to complement learning gained from participating in a research team. The training curriculum would draw on tools such as regular seminars, coursework, and independent study to ensure that trainees develop basic competencies in population health knowledge, metrics, methods, research design, and knowledge translation and exchange. The appropriate curricular offerings are likely to depend on the program goals, the stage of training, and the existing skills, knowledge, and goals of each trainee.
- *Each center designs an intensive, multidisciplinary mentoring system.* Each trainee should have a primary mentor who ensures that broad competencies are achieved, guides the trainee towards a focused research agenda, facilitates access to resources and expertise the trainee needs to advance that agenda, and provides a sounding board and resource for trainee concerns. In addition, trainees will need multiple mentors with expertise in relevant disciplines, knowledge exchange, and other competencies. The primary mentor would help navigate the challenges of a multiple-mentor or team mentor model.
- The overall set of center-based programs *captures broad heterogeneity* in the types of pop-

---

[20]As one example, the Cancer Health Disparities Training Program at the University of North Carolina, Chapel Hill, trains public health researchers in the competencies needed to address health disparity issues in cancer using a socio-ecological model of health. The program involves faculty from six departments and two centers involved in interdisciplinary research teams. The program is sited in a school of public health and does not advertise expertise in social science.

ulation health problems addressed as well as specific approaches to program design and curricula. At the same time, mechanisms are put in place to promote *networking, exchange, and synergies* among the individual programs, so that gaps in any single program can be balanced by the ability of the larger program to address a broad range of population health issues.

The proposed model has similarities to and differences from the RWJF HSS. Like HSS, it is grounded in immersion in a cross-disciplinary environment, training and mentoring in cross-disciplinary (and other) skills, and the networking of programs to promote collaboration and exchange. It moves beyond HSS in requiring trainees to participate in a cross-disciplinary, problem-based team research experience and in emphasizing training in knowledge translation and exchange. While requiring a complex set of resources, the model flexibly leverages existing resources to build a cost-effective strategy for advancing training in cross-disciplinary population health science.

The goal of constructing such a program creates opportunities for collaboration between traditional funders in health science training such as the NIH and other interested federal, nonfederal, and private organizations. Within the NIH, a partnership across the many institutes and offices that have a stake in population health science could provide the necessary scientific foundation for the program. However, without modification, traditional NIH T32 mechanisms, for example, may not suffice to fully support the different facets of this training model. The model's focus on an integration of science and translation opens the door to broader collaborations: with other federal agencies with a stake in, or a potential impact on, population health (e.g., the Centers for Disease Control and Prevention, Centers for Medicare and Medicaid Services, Health Resources and Services Administration; Department of Housing and Urban Development, Department of Education, Environmental Protection Agency); with accountable care organizations and the health care finance industry; with other industries seeking to improve employee health; and with private foundations.

35.4   Conclusion

As noted early in this chapter, training programs that produce scientists with the competencies needed for population health science are in short supply. Some related programs have emerged within schools of public health, public policy, health professional schools, and liberal arts programs, but most are limited in cross-disciplinary range, health outcomes considered, and in attention to cross-disciplinary skills and skills for knowledge translation and exchange. The one postdoctoral program explicitly targeted to produce population health scientists closed in 2016.

At the same time, complex global health challenges and soaring health care costs, persistent health disparities, and lagging health indicators for the U.S. have triggered a rapidly increasing demand for population health science and the solutions it can offer for improving population health. The recommendations and model training program advanced by a distinguished group of scientists and practitioners provide a foundation for moving forward. This vision provides a path for ensuring that training in cross-disciplinary population health science not only remains available, but also benefits from lessons learned in earlier programs and becomes increasingly responsive to the needs of knowledge users. Through building creative partnerships around this vision, we can ensure a robust future pipeline of leaders with the scientific and translational skills to improve the health of our population.

Acknowledgement This chapter is based on a report on future needs for interdisciplinary training in population health science commissioned by the Institute of Medicine Roundtable on Population Health Improvement (Bachrach et al. 2015).

References

Bachrach CA, Robert S, Thomas Y. Training in interdisciplinary population health science: current successes and future needs. Washington DC: Institute of Medicine Roundtable on Population Health Improvement; 2015. http://nationalacademies.org/hmd/~/media/Files/Agendas/Activity%20Files/PublicHealth/PopulationHealthImprovementRT/

Commissioned%20Papers/Training%20 Population%20Health%20Science%20final.PDF

Bachrach C, Moody J, Sheble L, et al. Effects of an inter-disciplinary postdoctoral program on interdisciplinary science. In: Science of Team Science (SciTS) 2017 Conference. Clearwater Beach, FL; 2017. http://www. scienceofteamscience.org/2017-scits-conference.

Bland CJ, Taylor AL, Shollen SL, Weber-Main AM, Mulcahy PA. Faculty success through mentoring. Lanham, MD: Rowman & Littlefield Education; 2009.

Brint SG, Turk-Bicakci L, Proctor K, Murphy SP. Expanding the social frame of knowledge: inter-disciplinary, degree-granting fields in American col-leges and universities, 1975–2000. Rev High Educ. 2009;32(2):155–83.

Canadian Academy of Health Sciences. The benefits and barriers to interdisciplinary research in the health sci-ences in Canada: framework document. 2005.

Chang MJ, Cerna O, Han J, Saenz V. The contradictory roles of institutional status in retaining underrepre-sented minorities in biomedical and behavioral sci-ence majors. Rev High Educ. 2008;31(4):433–64.

Canadian Health Services Research Foundation. Issues in linkage and exchange between researchers and decision makers. 1999. http://www.cfhi-fcass.ca/migrated/pdf/ event_reports/linkage_e.pdf. Accessed 29 Mar 2015.

Crisp G, Nora A, Taggart A. Student characteristics, pre-college, college, and environmental factors as predic-tors of majoring in and earning a STEM degree: an analysis of students attending a Hispanic serving insti-tution. Am Educ Res J. 2009;46(4):924–42.

Darity WA, Sharpe RV, Swinton OH. The state of blacks in higher education. 2009. http://mpra.ub.uni-muenchen. de/34411/1/MPRA_paper_34411.pdf. Accessed 28 Mar 2015.

Grimshaw JM, Eccles MP, Lavis JN, Hill SJ, Squires JE. Knowledge translation of research find-ings. Implement Sci. 2012;7:50. https://doi. org/10.1186/1748-5908-7-50.

Guise JM, Geller S, Regensteiner JG, Raymond N, Nagel J, Building Interdisciplinary Research Careers in Women's Health Program Leadership. Team mentoring for interdisciplinary team science: les-sons from K12 scholars and directors. Acad Med. 2017;92(2):214–21.

Kindig D. Is population medicine population health? Improving population health: policy, practice, research. 2012. http://www.improvingpopulation-health.org/blog/2012/06/is-population-medicine-pop-ulation-health.html. Accessed 14 Nov 2013.

Kindig DA, Stoddart G. What is population health? Am J Public Health. 2003;93:380–3.

Lavis JN, Robertson D, Woodside JM, McLeod CB, Abelson J. How can research organizations more effectively transfer research knowledge to decision makers? Milbank Q. 2003;81:221–2.

Lomas J. The in-between world of knowledge brokering. BMJ. 2007;334:129–32.

Mishra L, Banerjee AT, MacLennan ME, Gorczynski PF, Zinszer KA. Wanted: interdisciplinary, multidis-ciplinary, and knowledge translation and exchange training for students of public health. Can J Public Health. 2011;102(6):424–6.

Nash JM. Transdisciplinary training: key components and prerequisites for success. Am J Prev Med. 2008;35:S133–40.

NRC, IOM. U.S. health in international perspective: shorter lives, poorer health. Washington, DC: The National Academies Press; 2013.

National Science Foundation. Survey of doctorate recipients, 2013. Alexandria, VA: National Center for Science and Engineering Statistics; 2014.. http:// ncsesdata.nsf.gov/doctoratework/2013/

Pfund C, House SC, Asquith P, Fleming MF, Buhr KA, Burnham EL, Eichenberger Gilmore JM, Huskins WC, McGee R, Schurr K, Shapiro ED, Spencer KC, Sorkness CA. Training mentors of clinical and transla-tional research scholars: a randomized controlled trial. Acad Med. 2014;89(5):774–82.

Realmuto L, Daniel S, Weiss L, Moody J, Sheble L, Bachrach C. The Robert Wood Johnson Foundation Health and Society Scholars: A structured evalua-tion. Report to the Robert Wood Johnson Foundation, February 17. 2017.

Cross-Disciplinary Team Science with Trainees: From Undergraduate to Postdoc

36

William M. P. Klein

Contents

36.1 Introduction

When one thinks about a conventional cross-disciplinary scientific team, the image that might come to mind is a group of seasoned researchers with disparate backgrounds, perhaps with one or more junior faculty members in the mix. Indeed, that is often the constitution of a scientific team, and such teams can produce stellar research ideas and outcomes. I have greatly enjoyed participating on teams having some approximation of this profile and am fortunate in my current role at the National Cancer Institute to have well-heeled research collaborators in fields such as epidemiology, medicine, public health, and health policy as well as in areas of psychology and behavioral

W. M. P. Klein (✉)
Division of Cancer Control and Population Sciences,
National Cancer Institute, Bethesda, MD, USA
e-mail: Kleinwm@mail.nih.gov

science outside my home field of social psychology.

Nevertheless, because of the nature of my career, most of the scientific teams on which I have participated have not looked like this at all. I spent my first eleven post-PhD years on the faculty at Colby College, a small Northeastern liberal arts college. Although I collaborated some with researchers at other institutions, a good many of my research collaborations were with my undergraduate students. I then moved to the University of Pittsburgh, where I collaborated a great deal with graduate students—both those I was mentoring and others—as well as with undergraduates. After seven years there, I moved to my current position at the National Cancer Institute, where I direct the institute's Behavioral Research Program. In this role, I end up collaborating extensively with postdoctoral fellows. In the aggregate, then, a significant proportion of my collaborative, cross-disciplinary ventures have been with trainees along multiple stages of the career continuum. In addition to being exceptionally rewarding, these collaborations have taught me a lesson or two about optimizing them for all concerned.

In truth, it was well before any of this that I came to appreciate the value of team-based, cross-disciplinary research. As an undergraduate, I participated in a program at Northwestern University called Mathematical Methods in the Social Sciences. The program was essentially a mathematics major, yet with heavy application to the social sciences; we talked about game theory in the context of negotiations, and network analysis in the context of social movements. Students were required to double major in a social science of their choice—I chose psychology—and complete a senior thesis (in collaboration with a faculty member) that integrated the two majors. As it turns out, my coursework in social psychology had whetted my interest in judgment and decision-making, an area well aligned with an understanding of statistics and probability. This integration of two disciplines led to my graduate work at Princeton University on the psychology of risk perception—the topic of my dissertation and the grist for fruitful collaborations with my graduate advisor, Ziva Kunda (Klein and Kunda 1993, 1994) and researchers in many other fields over the years.

36.2 Team Science with Undergraduates

Following graduate school, I marched off to Colby College with a host of ideas about how to pursue my research interests in risk perception. I was intrigued about why and when people underestimate their risk, the extent to which they resist changes to their risk perceptions, the way in which social comparison influenced risk perception, and how the answers to any of these questions might inform the development of impactful risk messages. But how was I to move forward with these ideas? Although I was able to explore some of these questions with colleagues at other institutions like Neil Weinstein, a physical chemist who became interested in risk underestimation (e.g., Weinstein and Klein 1995), and Isaac Lipkus, a psychologist working in a cancer center (e.g., Lipkus et al. 2001), some of the best possible collaborators were sitting right in front of me in the courses I was teaching. I invited many of them to join my research laboratory and worked closely with them—often in small teams. For example, it was with my students that I was able to explore

how threatening feedback influences the construction of risk perceptions (Klein et al. 2001) and how self-serving biases in risk perception might have unfortunate consequences (Radcliffe and Klein 2002).

Despite these examples, I made some mistakes that seemed entirely avoidable with the benefit of 20/20 hindsight. Perhaps the most significant one was the criterion I used to decide whom I might invite from my classes to join my laboratory. It was a simple one—I chose the A students. Such a strategy seemed entirely prudent; they were, after all, the top students in the class, so it seemed reasonable to assume that they would also be stellar research collaborators. Sometimes they were, but not always. I came to believe that some A students may be gifted test-takers who say and do the right things in a traditional course setting, but who do not thrive in a team-based research setting. My sense is that cross-disciplinary team research is at its best with individuals who are creative, intellectually flexible, do not despair in the face of ambiguity, and work seamlessly and selflessly in a team with others who may have different motives and work styles. Students who have determined the formula for getting a good grade may or may not have these attributes, and I found that it was important to glean what I could about these attributes when reflecting on who might thrive as a research collaborator in my laboratory. Of note, this lesson translated later on to the recruitment of new graduate students into my laboratory at the University of Pittsburgh.

I learned two other lessons working on research teams with undergraduates. First, undergraduates do not really have a home discipline yet—they do declare majors but are taking courses in many areas inside and outside their major fields. Also, taking 8–12 courses in a field does not seem enough to have a professional identity in that field. Collaborating with bright undergraduates, then, is probably about as cross-disciplinary as it gets. Although their training can limit their contributions to a scientific team in some ways, it enhances those contributions in others. Undergraduates can provide a fresh perspective and ask difficult but important and tractable questions about the assumptions we make in our research. They can also provide some correction to the sometimes inevitable effects of investigator bias on the framing and testing of research questions. Moreover, when doing research on issues that matter to them personally, their input becomes essential. My research on norm perceptions and risk perceptions regarding undergraduate alcohol use was greatly informed by the discussions we had in my upper level seminars and laboratory meetings (e.g., Klein et al. 2007).

The second lesson is that our students are not our clones. Of course, that is a good thing for all kinds of reasons, not the least of which is that our research benefits from a diversity of opinions and perspectives. What I wish to note here, though, is that our students sometimes have very different career trajectories than the ones we chose ourselves. As a psychology professor, it was important for me to acknowledge that very few of my students would go off and get their graduate degrees in psychology and become professors like me. Some of them were headed to medical or law school, others to education, others to graduate school in other areas of passionate interest, others to entrepreneurial and other unforeseen opportunities. That presented an interesting challenge for me—to make our research collaborations maximally engaging for scientific team members who would not be moving on to the next grant, manuscript, or research project after finishing our team project. Indeed, they were more likely to be moving on altogether. As a social psychologist, I was keenly aware that creativity and engagement are maximized when one feels a high degree of autonomy and involvement (Amabile and Pillemer 2012). Thus, I learned that I needed to mold and pitch my research ideas in such a way that my students could grab hold of them in ways that aligned with their own future goals. Fortunately, my interest in health risk perception was not a stretch for students interested in medical school, counseling, and other careers in mental and physical health.

36.3 Team Science with Graduate Students

Moving from a liberal arts college to a major research university provided the opportunity to infuse the talents and perspectives of graduate students into my laboratory. Graduate students are often on a different trajectory than undergraduates, given that they have made an explicit decision to obtain an advanced degree in a particular discipline. From the very beginning of their studies they develop expertise and an identity in a particular field—usually their mentor's home discipline—placing them in the position of learning how to collaborate and conduct team science at the same time that they are learning their new discipline. As a mentor, it was clear to me that this was a critical time to model good team behavior—taking all perspectives into account, openly acknowledging different incentive structures and career goals when making decisions about team member roles and authorship, providing feedback on drafts respectfully and in a timely manner, and practicing honesty and selflessness. Leading a research team as a senior investigator with junior colleagues such as graduate students means paying as much attention to process as to content.

My research teams have benefited in numerous ways from the inclusion of graduate students. For example, many of the graduate students I have worked with or advised over the years have been on dual training streams in which they are learning clinical skills (e.g., clinical psychology, genetic counseling) concurrently with research skills. I have found that the clinical experiences they glean from their clinical training provide countless opportunities to enrich the quality and nature of our research together. To be sure, risk perceptions and decision-making take on a new meaning when construed and explored in the context of people making real and consequential decisions about their health, such as choosing to receive the results of genetic tests. Graduate students are also likely to be learning the latest statistical and methodological tools in their coursework, which can then be applied to the work they conduct in their research teams. By virtue of taking courses in their own and other departments around campus, they bring new ideas to the table that are, by definition, cross-disciplinary.

Teaching students from other research groups in advanced courses, and serving on their committees, can lead to many rewarding collaborative opportunities. As an example, Jennifer Phillips, a student of Stephen Manuck's with an interest in effects of socioeconomic status (SES) on health outcomes, co-authored a paper with me based on her comprehensive exam in which she integrated her understanding of SES effects with the health cognitions she was learning about in my courses. In particular, she leveraged these disparate literatures to argue that cognitions such as self-efficacy could help explain the link between SES and cardiovascular disease (Phillips and Klein 2010). My own graduate students were particularly effective at stretching my interests into new areas; for example, Jennifer Cerully was one of the first to help me think about how emotions might influence risk perceptions—a product of her master's thesis (Cerully and Klein 2010)—an interest I continue to pursue.

My positive experience working with graduate students was also imbued with many lessons about how to do good team science while being a good mentor. In addition to the aforementioned role modeling, I found it important to think explicitly about how to weigh the needs of a team research project against the career and personal needs of my students. Large cross-disciplinary team projects often require extensive time, funding, and a healthy dose of faith that all of the investment in these projects will ultimately bear fruit. Those attributes often do not align with the time-delimited nature of graduate education. Yet there are ways to address this discrepancy. One can be thoughtful, for example, about having graduate students add survey items, modules, or additional arms (in the case of a randomized controlled trial) to large projects so that they can use a portion of the data for their theses and possible publications. Doing so permits opportunities for them to collect primary data within the context of a larger project, given that many programs require

the collection of primary data for thesis work. The demands of team science can also be incompatible with personal needs and decisions such as having children or managing health issues. It behooves the senior investigator to be sufficiently aware of all aspects of a team project in order to be able to step in and maintain progress while making it possible for students involved in the project to step off and attend to their personal, educational, and family needs.

Then there are more logistical and operational issues to consider. Graduate students eventually leave the nest—as they should. If they have played a principal role in a team project, their role might need to change appreciably upon beginning the next stage of their career. Thinking about this eventuality in advance can reduce unnecessary and demoralizing delays in the progress of a team-based research project. If they managed the data set, it would be useful to know where the files are and how to use them. If they handled IRB approvals and amendments, all of that information needs to be accessible. These days, sharing laboratory files on a network or cloud can facilitate such sharing, but it still helps to teach good filing and organizational skills when managing a large research project so that the "hand-off" is as seamless as possible.

Finally, research teams can be derailed by conflict, social comparisons, and many other social and group processes. Evidence suggests that people compare their ideas, performance, and attributes with those of others nearly automatically (Gilbert et al. 1995), and that such comparisons can influence a group's creativity and performance (Dugosh and Paulus 2005). People are affected by comparisons even when more diagnostic, objective information is available (Klein 1997). Graduate students are sometimes low on the chain of influence, so their concerns about their own performance—and how it compares to that of peer graduate students on a team project—can be amplified. In my view, mentors and senior collaborators on a project need to be aware of this dynamic and address it by giving individualized encouragement and feedback, and by creating a nonevaluative team environment.

36.4 Team Science with Postdoctoral Fellows

One of the great joys of my current position at NCI is that I get to work with bright, talented, energetic, and collaborative postdoctoral fellows having a wide variety of disciplinary backgrounds such as public health, psychology, health policy, and genetics. NCI possesses a one-of-a-kind program (the Cancer Prevention Fellowship or "CPF" program) in which PhDs from many areas earn a Masters of Public Health (MPH) funded by NCI and then spend up to three years in residence at NCI conducting research with staff—usually in cross-disciplinary research teams. Postdocs also join NCI on other training streams such as our Cancer Research Training Award (CRTA) mechanism. Although these positions may be somewhat different than more traditional postdoctoral positions at universities where an individual may be heading up one major project or directing a laboratory, they are similar in that they are defined as research positions for newly minted PhDs to establish their professional identity.

My work on risk perception, risk communication, and decision-making has gone in many exciting directions due largely to my collaborations with postdocs such as Erin Ellis, Rebecca Ferrer, Stephanie Fowler, Jada Hamilton, Paul Han, Annette Kaufman, Amber Koblitz, David Portnoy, Elise Rice, Megan Roberts, Cendrine Robinson, Jennifer Taber, Chan Thai, Erin Turbitt, Erika Waters, and Kara Wiseman, among others. Jennifer Taber and Rebecca Ferrer have joined me in collaborating with behavioral scientists and geneticists at the National Human Genome Research Institute (NHGRI) on a study of 600+ people who have had their genomes sequenced and completed surveys measuring a variety of health cognitions such as risk perception, affective forecasting, and information avoidance. This highly cross-disciplinary project has led to several publications (e.g., Ferrer et al. 2015; Taber et al. 2015). Moreover, this and other projects have led us to rethink how we measure and conceptualize risk perception (e.g., Ferrer et al. 2016; Taber and Klein 2016).

I have found that postdocs are excited about the opportunity to work on research teams, as it exposes them to new ways of addressing research questions and involves them in projects that can make more than just an incremental contribution to the literature. If anything, the challenge is not to convince them of the value of such research, but rather to help guide them to make prudent decisions about where to devote their time and energy given the wealth of opportunities available to them. As a mentor, I find it important to help postdocs prioritize efforts in such a way that they have projects along all stages of the research continuum (from generating new ideas to polishing up manuscripts), and that they build a "brand" that might be easily conveyed in an elevator speech or a job interview. Doing so may or may not cohere with the needs of a team project, which necessitates flexibility in assigning roles and responsibilities. Looking out for a postdoc might also mean arranging opportunities to lead some projects and be secondary on others to maximize publication and other opportunities. Moreover, it may mean involving them on scientific teams that can provide networking opportunities which can, in turn, lead to employment options down the road.

36.5 Concluding Thoughts

Cross-disciplinary scientific teams often include students and trainees of all stripes. They can make important contributions to the progress and success of these teams; at the same time, the motives undergirding those contributions and the benefits these individuals accrue may be different than they are for other, more established members of the research team. In my experience, undergraduates are usually unfettered by assumptions and disciplinary norms and biases, bring new perspectives to the table, and express enthusiasm about their first experiences as researchers. Selecting the "ideal" undergraduates to maximize collaborations is not as easy as it may look, and one must acknowledge their disparate career trajectories and interests (and quick departures).

Graduate students bring even more experience to the team, complemented by advanced and often state-of-the art statistical and methodological expertise as well as knowledge of other disciplines from their varied coursework. But they are also people—with career needs and personal needs—and these needs must be considered to maximize the benefit of team research projects to them. Finessing large research projects and research programs in ways that offer graduate students opportunities for primary and secondary data collection and authorship on resulting manuscripts can enhance the yield of those projects and programs as well as facilitate the careers of the graduate students involved. This is also the case for post-doctoral fellows, who are still building a curriculum vitae and professional identity and looking at possible career options around the corner. Fortunately, postdocs have moved beyond the course requirements and high level of evaluation endemic to graduate study, and can stretch their wings to explore new areas of inquiry with more independence and without much administrative or teaching burden. Thus, they can be ideal collaborators on a team research project.

Not all teams include students and trainees, and some probably should not. But those that do have a great deal to gain. Perhaps most importantly, experiences in cross-disciplinary team research early in one's career provide a foundation for later engagement in—and leadership of—such research endeavors. If the students and trainees in our cross-disciplinary team research go on later to participate in and lead high impact team science projects, I contend that we will have succeeded not only as scientists but as dutiful citizens of science.

References

Amabile TM, Pillemer J. Perspectives on the social psychology of creativity. J Creat Behav. 2012;46(1):3–15.

*Cerully JL, Klein WMP. Effects of emotional state on behavioral responsiveness to personal feedback. J Risk Res. 2010;13(5):591–8.

Dugosh KL, Paulus PB. Cognitive and social comparison processes in brainstorming. J Exp Soc Psychol. 2005;41(3):313–20.

Ferrer RA, Klein WMP, Persoskie A, *Avishai-Yitshak A, Sheeran P. The tripartite model of risk perception (TRIRISK): distinguishing deliberative, affective, and experiential components of perceived risk. Ann Behav Med. 2016;50(5):653–63.

Ferrer RA, *Taber JM, Klein WMP, Harris PR, Lewis KL, Biesecker LG. The role of current affect, anticipated affect, and spontaneous self-affirmation in decisions to receive self-threatening genetic risk information. Cognit Emot. 2015;29(8):1456–65.

Gilbert DT, Giesler RB, Morris KA. When comparisons arise. J Pers Soc Psychol. 1995;69(2):227–36.

Klein WM. Objective standards are not enough: affective, self-evaluative, and behavioral responses to social comparison information. J Pers Soc Psychol. 1997;72:763–74.

Klein WMP, *Blier HK, *Janze AM. Maintaining positive self-evaluations: reducing attention to diagnostic but unfavorable social comparison information when general self-regard is salient. Motiv Emot. 2001;25:23–40.

Klein WMP, *Geaghan TR, MacDonald TK. Unplanned sexual activity as a consequence of alcohol use: a prospective study of risk perceptions and alcohol use among college freshmen. J Am Coll Heal. 2007;56:317–23.

Klein WM, Kunda Z. Maintaining self-serving social comparisons: biased reconstruction of one's past behaviors. Personal Soc Psychol Bull. 1993;19:732–9.

Klein WM, Kunda Z. Exaggerated self-assessments and the preference for controllable risks. Organ Behav Hum Decis Process. 1994;59:410–27.

Lipkus IM, Klein WMP, Rimer BK. Communicating uncertainty about breast cancer risk. Cancer Epidemiol Biomarkers Prev. 2001;10:895–8.

*Phillips JE, Klein WMP. Do social cognitive factors mediate the association between socioeconomic status and coronary heart disease risk? Soc Personal Psychol Compass. 2010;4:704–27.

*Radcliffe NM, Klein WMP. Dispositional, unrealistic, and comparative optimism: differential relations with knowledge and processing of risk information and beliefs about personal risk. Personal Soc Psychol Bull. 2002;28:836–46.

*Taber JM, Klein WMP. The role of conviction in personal risk perceptions: what can we learn from research on attitude strength? Soc Personal Psychol Compass. 2016;10(4):202–18.

*Taber JM, Klein WMP. The role of conviction in personal risk perceptions: what can we learn from research on attitude strength? Soc Personal Psychol Compass. 2016;10(4):202–18.

Weinstein ND, Klein WM. Resistance of personal risk perceptions to debiasing interventions. Health Psychol. 1995;14:132–40.

Restructuring Research Universities to Advance Transdisciplinary Collaboration

37

Michael M. Crow and William B. Dabars

Contents

Whether the context for knowledge production and innovation is the set of major research universities, system of government agencies and federal laboratories, or the research and development efforts of industry, transdisciplinary collaborative engagement is essential in addressing the complex challenges that confront society. Although research teams sometimes comprise researchers from within a single disciplinary field (Hall et al. 2008), interdisciplinary collaboration is generally a requisite for effective team science (Fiore 2008, 251), or, more broadly, team research—collaborative discovery, creativity, and innovation undertaken by researchers and practitioners from across the spectrum of disciplinary and interdisciplinary fields. This chapter thus examines the accommodation of inter- or transdisciplinarity within the set of American research universities relevant to the advancement of team research. The chapter concludes with a brief case study of the restructuring of academic organization and operations undertaken in part to advance transdisciplinary collaboration—and thus team research—at Arizona State University (Crow and Dabars 2015).[1]

---

[1]The discussion of interdisciplinarity in this chapter contains revised passages from our coauthored book, *Designing the New American University* (Baltimore: Johns Hopkins University Press, 2015), and various texts we have either coauthored or authored singly on this topic, including our coauthored book chapters "Interdisciplinarity and the Organizational Context of Knowledge in the American Research University," in *The Oxford Handbook of Interdisciplinarity*, second ed., edited by Robert Frodeman, Julie Thompson Klein, and Roberto Carlos Dos Santos Pacheco (Oxford: Oxford University Press, 2017), and "Interdisciplinarity as a Design Problem: Toward Mutual Intelligibility among Academic Disciplines in the American Research University," in *Enhancing Communication and Collaboration in Interdisciplinary Research*, edited by Michael O'Rourke et al. (Los Angeles: Sage, 2013).

M. M. Crow
Office of the President, Arizona State University, Tempe, AZ, USA

W. B. Dabars (✉)
School for the Future of Innovation in Society, Arizona State University, Tempe, AZ, USA
e-mail: dabars@asu.edu

© Springer Nature Switzerland AG 2019
K. L. Hall et al. (eds.), *Strategies for Team Science Success*,
https://doi.org/10.1007/978-3-030-20992-6_37

The National Research Council (NRC) Committee on the Science of Team Science characterizes transdisciplinarity as research that "aims to deeply integrate and also transcend disciplinary approaches to generate fundamentally new conceptual frameworks, theories, models, and applications" (NRC 2015, 5–6). Our usage of the term connotes knowledge production construed as integrative—transcending the spurious dichotomy between research characterized as either fundamental or applied (Shneiderman 2016)—as well as collaborative, which may include researchers from multiple disciplines as well as from outside the academy (Gibbons et al. 1994; Frodeman 2014). Because the university is no longer invariably the predominant locus of knowledge production, the criteria for the evaluation of quality in research and scholarship are increasingly no longer exclusively disciplinary, but social, political, and economic as well (Weingart 2010, 12). Collaboration across transdisciplinary, transinstitutional, and transnational frameworks maximizes the potential to advance knowledge production and innovation in real time and at the scale necessary for the attainment of desired social and economic outcomes.

"Team research leads to higher quality outcomes and higher impact, compared to individual research," Ben Shneiderman contends. "Teams often produce higher quality research than an individual can because they bring complementary knowledge, skills, and attitudes, take on more ambitious projects, apply diverse research methods, and have larger networks" (2016, 157–58). But the transdisciplinary collaboration characteristic of team research requires optimally configured institutional frameworks as well as an academic culture oriented toward innovation. Despite broad consensus regarding the imperative for such collaboration, however, disciplinary acculturation continues to shape successive generations of scientists, scholars, and practitioners while the traditional correlation between disciplines and departments persists as the basis for academic organization (Abbott 2001, 126–128). Disciplines are epistemological, administrative, and sociocultural modes of organization (Wallerstein 2003) that continue to structure

institutional frameworks as well as mediate knowledge production and diffusion. Disciplinary partitioning represents one of the most pernicious design limitations to the further evolution of knowledge production in the American research university (Crow and Dabars 2013, 2015).

Similarly, inimical to the advancement of transdisciplinary collaboration is the assumption that research and scholarship are primarily solitary endeavors and that optimal outcomes inevitably emerge from the amalgamation of individual contributions. Entrenchment in discipline-based departments mirrors an academic culture that prizes individualism over teamwork and the discovery of specialized knowledge over problem-based collaboration. The imperative for the restructuring of academic organization in this context is attested by the rapid growth in the percentage of publications contributed by two or more authors (Wuchty et al. 2007). Across all scientific fields, single-author research papers have declined from 30% in 1981 to 11% in 2012. In some fields, scientific papers now average five authors (Voosen 2013). By 2013, 90% of papers in science and engineering journals were written by teams (NRC 2015, 19). Although coauthored contributions need not be interdisciplinary, assessments of coauthorship patterns attest to increasing heterogeneity in disciplinary affiliation (Porter et al. 2007).

Because academia places greater value on the discovery of new knowledge by individual scientists, less prestige attaches to problem-based collaboration undertaken in a context of real-world application and accountability to constituencies outside the academy (Sarewitz 2016). The same is true for collaborative execution of projects that advance knowledge through assimilation, synthesis, implementation, and application (Nelson et al. 2010). In this sense, the collaboration characteristic of research teams sometimes follows patterns of technological development that are the product of recombinant innovation, which refers to the combination or recombination of existing ideas, products, and processes (Arthur 2009, 21). Recent analysis of nearly 18 million scientific papers confirms the extent to which new knowledge derives from novel insights into existing knowledge. According to Brian Uzzi and colleagues, "The highest-impact science is primarily grounded in exceptionally conventional combinations of prior work yet simultaneously features an intrusion of unusual combinations." Their assessment suggests that the interdisciplinary collaboration found in team science is especially conducive to innovation and impact: "Teams are 37.7% more likely than solo authors to insert novel combinations into familiar knowledge domains" (Uzzi et al. 2013, 468).

Among the six items specified in the charge to the Committee on the Science of Team Science in the report *Enhancing the Effectiveness of Team Science* is the question: "What types of organizational structures, policies, practices, and resources are needed to promote effective team science in academic institutions, research centers, industry, and other settings?" (NRC 2015, 3). A decade earlier the National Academies report *Facilitating Interdisciplinary Research* emphasized the essential correlation between interdisciplinary collaboration and applied research initiatives that depend for their effectiveness on team efforts. Such large-scale initiatives comprise "scientists, engineers, social scientists, and humanists... addressing complex problems that must be attacked simultaneously with deep knowledge from different perspectives." The report contends that there can be "no question about the productivity and effectiveness of research teams formed of partners with diverse expertise" and recommends "substantial alteration of the traditional academic structures or even replacement with new structures and models to reduce barriers" to interdisciplinary collaboration (CFIR 2005, 17). Consistent with its call for new structural models, the report underscores the importance of supportive institutional policies: "Whatever their structure, interdisciplinary projects flourish in an environment that allows researchers to communicate, share ideas, and collaborate across disciplines" (CFIR 2005, ix, 172).

Because "deep knowledge integration" is among the principal challenges that confront science teams (NRC 2015, 5), the concept of convergence is especially relevant in this context. Convergence refers to the increasing integration of the life sciences, physical sciences, mathematical and computational sciences, and fields of engineering, as well as the behavioral and social sciences and arts and humanities. As formulated by a committee convened by the National Research Council, convergence is an approach to research that engenders "comprehensive synthetic frameworks that merge areas of knowledge from multiple fields to address specific challenges." The development of partnerships requisite to scientific investigation is essential to the integration of essential "subsets of expertise" (NRC 2014, 17). An earlier National Science Foundation assessment, for example, considered the unification of scientific disciplines and convergence of technologies with reference to the integration and synergistic recombination of the four domains of nanoscience and nanotechnology; biotechnology and biomedicine, including genetic engineering; information technology, including advanced computing and communications; and, cognitive science, including cognitive neuroscience—collectively termed "NBIC," i.e., nano-bio-info-cogno (Roco and Bainbridge 2002).

37.1   Institutional Design to Accommodate Transdisciplinarity and Team Research

Reconceptualizing and restructuring a knowledge enterprise as complex as a major research university—to accommodate transdisciplinary collaborative endeavor, or with any other objective in mind—represents a process often as deliberate and precise as scientific research or technological invention (Simon 1966/1996, 1–24). The design process offers the potential for colleges and universities to reconceptualize their missions and goals and restructure and recalibrate their organization and standard operating procedures to advance chosen objectives and initiatives, including the transdisciplinary collaboration characteristic of team research. Novel transdisciplinary configurations represent institutional experiments that can recalibrate the course of inquiry and enhance both discovery and the application of research. If academic structures adequate to the resolution of a problem do not exist, new units must be purpose-built. A new aggregation may at its inception simply represent a best-guess strategic amalgamation, but such reconfigurations may lead to unexpected discoveries through serendipity (Merton and Barber 2004).

Insight into the social construction of knowledge production notwithstanding (Giddens 1984; Goldman 1999), the tacit assumption persists that institutional frameworks have historically somehow been optimally configured to facilitate both the discovery and dissemination of knowledge. Indeed knowledge production is situated—"in part a product of the activity, context, and culture in which it is developed and used" (Brown et al. 1989, 33)—and in part path-dependent, which is to say, shaped by a previous sequence of decisions (Peacock 2009). But the implications of this reflexive interdependence are too often dismissed as adventitious to discovery and innovation and minimized as merely perfunctory administrative distractions (Brown and Duguid 1991).

An institution as complex as the American research university must continuously evolve to keep pace with the proliferation of new knowledge (Wilson 2010), but structural inertia impedes organizational change (Hannan and Freeman 1989). Resistance to novel institutional arrangements exacerbates the tendencies toward routine, standardization, and inertia that have been identified as hallmarks of bureaucracies (Downs 1967, 8). But the bureaucratic mind-set pejoratively associated with large impersonal public agencies that perform standardized and repetitive tasks is not normally conducive to discovery, creativity, and innovation (Crow and Dabars 2015). Isomorphism describes the paradoxical tendency for organizations and institutions operating within a given sector to emulate one another and become increasingly homogeneous but not necessarily more efficient. The outcome of the competition for power and legitimacy that produces dominant organizational models is not differentiation but isomorphic conformity (DiMaggio

and Powell 1983, 147–149). Filiopietism, or the excessive veneration of tradition, moreover encourages adherence to historical models long after their relevance or usefulness has diminished (Crow and Dabars 2015).

37.2 Historical Perspective on the Relevance of Inter- and Transdisciplinarity to Team Research

The contemporary context for a theoretical appreciation of interdisciplinarity was established during the first international conference on the topic at the University of Nice in September 1970, which was organized by the Centre for Educational Research and Innovation (CERI) in collaboration with the Organization for Economic Cooperation and Development (OECD) (Apostel et al. 1972). But recognition of the potential for enhanced productivity and creativity inherent in the collaboration among disciplines characteristic of scientific teamwork and, more broadly, team research preceded by decades the explication of interdisciplinarity of the OECD conference (Bush and Hattery 1956).

An historical assessment of knowledge production in this context lies outside the scope of the present discussion, but an appreciation for antecedents to our contemporary approaches to team research could arguably begin with the growth in federal investment in scientific research associated with World War II, beginning with the formation of such large-scale multidisciplinary research and development efforts as the MIT Radiation Laboratory, active between 1940 and 1945, and the Manhattan Project, active between 1942 and 1946, and followed by the development of the system of national laboratories, where the "pursuit of large multidisciplinary programs put a premium on… the team approach" (Westwick 2003, 28, 65). Basic scientific research conducted in contexts of technological application—the industrial research and development operations at AT&T Bell Labs in the mid-twentieth century, for example (Sarewitz 2016)—encouraged disciplinary integration and collaborative endeavor.

Shneiderman cites the invention of the transistor in this context: "Team research is the source of some of the great breakthroughs of all time, such as the 1947 invention of the transistor. It took the complementary skills of an applied researcher, Walter Brattain, a basic researcher in quantum theory, John Bardeen, and the solid-state physicist William Shockley" (2016, 157).

As the central nodes of an integrative discovery and commercialization network, research universities have served as the key institutional actors in the national system of innovation, a concept which embraces the economic, political, and social institutions relevant to knowledge production (Crow and Bozeman 1998). The growth in organized research units (ORUs)—interdisciplinary research centers and institutes established by universities to advance basic and applied research distinct from academic departments—following World War II has been integral to the ascent to global dominance of the postwar American scientific research enterprise (Geiger 1990). The impetus toward interdisciplinary collaboration has by one estimate led to the establishment of nearly three thousand research centers presently active at 25 leading major research universities (Jacobs 2013, 91).

More recently, differentiated institutional configurations spanning disciplinary boundaries attest to the potential for alternative academic platforms to advance collaborative engagement. An interdisciplinary think tank modeled on the Institute for Advanced Study in Princeton, the Zentrum für interdisziplinäre Forschung (ZiF), or Center for Interdisciplinary Research, for example, serves as the nucleus of Universität Bielefeld in Germany, which was established in 1969 and conceived interdisciplinarily from its inception. To cite but a single example of an independent interdisciplinary research institute spanning the natural and social sciences, the Santa Fe Institute, established in 1984, has brought together a community of scholars that has produced groundbreaking theoretical approaches to the study of complex adaptive systems. In the twenty-first century, a number of major research institutions, including University College London, have sought to reconfigure their research enterprises based on transdisciplinary "grand challenge" themes.

37.3   Further Perspective on Transdisciplinarity and Team Research

The transdisciplinary dimension of team science is inherent in the shift from disciplinary research, which Michael Gibbons and colleagues associated with Mode 1 knowledge production, to research that is predominantly collaborative and applied, associated with Mode 2 (Gibbons et al. 1994). Consistent with the practice of team science, the new paradigm of knowledge production is "socially distributed, application-oriented, trans-disciplinary, and subject to multiple accountabilities" (Nowotny et al. 2003, 179). The transinstitutional dimension of transdisciplinary collaboration—and thus team science—is modeled in the "triple helix" of innovation described by economist Henry Etzkowitz (2003). The collaboration between academic, industry, and government partners comprises intersecting knowledge networks that leverage input from diverse multi- and interdisciplinary perspectives. Etzkowitz makes the important point that the Mode 2 paradigm, which embraces both fundamental and applied research, represents the foundational platform for science institutionalized during its formative period in the early modern era (2008, 141–142).

The proliferation of academic research on interdisciplinarity often neglects relevant literature on teams and teamwork available from such fields as organizational theory and cognitive and social psychology. As cognitive psychologist Stephen Fiore puts it: "To the degree that we can equate interdisciplinary research with team research, we can consider the implementation of principles from teamwork and team training to improve interdisciplinary research and the practice of team science" (Fiore 2008, 253). But theoretical discussions of interdisciplinarity often overlook organizational models heuristically relevant to team science. Knowledge networks and knowledge-centric social formations, including invisible colleges, communities of practice, epistemic communities, and firms construed as knowledge-centric, represent viable models for interdisciplinary team engagement. The concept of invisible colleges derives from the early modern period and refers to any collaborative engagement of scholars and scientists focused on similar or related problems (Price 1986). Communities of practice and epistemic communities are knowledge-based social networks (Wenger 1998). The recognition that firms may be understood as knowledge-centric is implied by their correlation to academic, and especially scientific, research groups (Etzkowitz 2003). Indeed firms have been modeled as epistemic communities wherein competitive advantage is a function of collaborative contextual conceptualization of intellectual capital, both explicit and tacit (Håkanson 2010, 1804, 1809). As one organizational theorist characterizes the role of communication in this context: "The essence of the firm is its ability to create, transfer, assemble, integrate, and exploit knowledge assets" (Teece 2003).

Research teams have been conceptualized as nodes in knowledge networks and interdependent constituent agents that transcend individual limitations in complex adaptive systems (Miller and Page 2007). Science teams exhibit in their aggregate behavior the characteristics of complex adaptive systems, including nonlinearity, self-organization, and emergence (Kozlowski and Klein, 2000, cited in NRC 2015, 54). The distributed cognition in epistemic cultures posited by Karin Knorr Cetina (1999) and crowdsourcing and "cognitive surplus" described by Clay Shirky (2010) are relevant in this context. The coordination of effort by team practitioners, moreover, facilitates opportunities for the transmission of tacit knowledge and the application of existing knowledge. Collaborative engagement leverages the tacit dimension to knowledge production, referring to the exchange of inherent practical understanding of given research problems and methods and associated technologies based on direct experience. While explicit knowledge is readily standardized, codified, and diffused, tacit

knowledge is more effectively transmitted through the direct interpersonal communication characteristic of teams (Von Hippel 1994). The cognitive diversity inherent in teams, moreover, correlates with enhanced performance and outcomes (Hong and Page 2004).

Knowledge is a product of negotiation and consensus, a collaborative process that Jürgen Habermas terms "communicative rationality" (1987). Indeed, Julie Thompson Klein points out, Habermas contends that the integration of disciplinary vernaculars has the potential to "generate a new common understanding through reciprocal comprehension and consensus" (2013, 14). The team collaboration integral to knowledge networks such as invisible colleges hence promotes the flow of knowledge—as opposed to its accumulation or maintenance within stocks of knowledge. The inverse correlation between the proverbial silo mentality of conventional disciplinarity and the synergies unleashed during interdisciplinary exchange is self-evident. Organizational theorists contend that the value of stocks of knowledge is diminishing even as the knowledge base must be continually replenished through participation in relevant networks (Hagel et al. 2010, 7, 11, 73).

Invisible colleges represent a historical prototype for the "academic leagues" that Jonathan Cole envisions. Because such leagues represent collaboration within networks of scientists and scholars, the approach is relevant to team science. In order to add value, these *de facto* alliances—rather than formal mergers—coordinate top complementary programs, especially from different fields. Cole cites the example of the Earth Institute at Columbia University leading an interdisciplinary consortium of 15–20 universities worldwide to advance sustainability. And whereas most such collaboration is spurred by the objective of research, Cole recommends the development of "quasimergers" for teaching and joint degree programs. Although such programs may be cost effective, he cautions that the requisite new structural relationships could threaten perceptions of institutional autonomy (Cole 2016, 171–183).

37.4 A Case Study in the Reconceptualization of a Major Research University

Among the various interrelated and interdependent dimensions to the reconceptualization and restructuring of the academic organization of Arizona State University (ASU) is the advancement of inter- and transdisciplinarity intended to promote collaborative engagement among researchers and practitioners. The reconfiguration of academic departments and frequent recombination of disciplinary and interdisciplinary fields must be appreciated within the broader context of the comprehensive reconceptualization of the entire institution. The advancement of interdisciplinarity has been one of eight interdependent "design aspirations" associated with the reconceptualization of the youngest major research institution in the United States and, with more than one hundred ten thousand undergraduate, graduate, and professional students enrolled in fall 2018, the largest university in the nation governed by a single administration. Of this number, more than 37,000 students are enrolled through ASU Online. The reconceptualization was conceived with the objective of establishing a foundational prototype for an alternative model for a subset of public research universities. The New American University model developed by Michael M. Crow during his presidency of the university combines accessibility to an academic platform underpinned by discovery and a pedagogical foundation of knowledge production, inclusiveness to a broad demographic representative of the socioeconomic diversity of the region and nation, and maximization of societal impact (Crow and Dabars 2015, 7–8, 62).

The reconfiguration of academic organization proceeded through the development of a federation of unique and differentiated academic units, including transdisciplinary departments, research centers, institutes, schools, and colleges—organizational constructs henceforth generally referred to as "colleges and schools," with colleges representing a particular amalgamation of schools. Following reconceptualization some core disciplines remain departmentally based while others were reorganized into new and explicitly interdisciplinary configurations. Although administrative efficiency is sometimes cited as an objective, the reconfiguration generally aligned with the intent to facilitate teaching and research or, more narrowly, to promote collaboration among researchers to better address societal challenges. The reorganization of the life sciences faculties that preceded the comprehensive reconceptualization suggests the momentum of the shift toward interdisciplinarity. In July 2003, the biology, microbiology, and plant biology departments and the program in molecular and cellular biology merged to form the new ASU School of Life Sciences (SOLS). Within a framework of seven faculty groups, more than one hundred life scientists, engineers, philosophers, social scientists, and ethicists continue to self-organize into teams around key societal and environmental challenges.

The collaborative "design process" empowered relatively autonomous faculty committees, or design teams, to restructure the academic framework through an inclusive bottom-up approach enabled by top-down and center-out empowerment of faculty teams. Organizational theorists thus envisage optimal institutional change driven not by an administrative elite but rather by "passionate individuals distributed throughout and even outside the institution, supported by institutional leaders who . . . realize that this wave of change cannot be imposed from the top down" (Hagel et al. 2010, 7, 11, 73). The approach could be likened to the "design-build" process. A concept borrowed from the architectural profession and construction industry, design-build refers to the integration of conception and execution by a single team. The process may be likened to a sequence of charettes, which the *Oxford English Dictionary* defines as a "period of intense (group) work, typically undertaken in order to meet a deadline. Also: a collaborative workshop focusing on a particular problem or project." In some cases, the relative autonomy of design teams assumed the tenor of a "skunkworks," an industry term that in broad usage specifies an informal and autonomous group often working in isolation. Retrenchment to the proverbial drawing board permitted teams to assume a "blank slate" standpoint conducive to thought experiments. The architectonic metaphors enlisted in this context suggest the imperative for structural change as well as continuous adaptation and recalibration through repeated course corrections (Crow and Dabars 2015, 247).

Among the new transdisciplinary schools operationalized during the past 15 years are the School of Earth and Space Exploration (SESE); School of Human Evolution and Social Change (SHESC); School of Politics and Global Studies; School of Social Transformation; School of Historical, Philosophical, and Religious Studies (SHPRS); and School for the Future of Innovation in Society (SFIS), which originated in the Consortium for Science, Policy, and Outcomes (CSPO). Both the school and consortium are dedicated to the interdisciplinary examination of the societal and cultural context within which science is conducted and seek to enhance the contributions of science and technology to an improved quality of life, with particular attention to responsible innovation and distributional impacts—questions of who is likely to benefit from public investments in knowledge production and innovation. The Julie Ann Wrigley Global Institute of Sustainability (GIOS), which incorporates the School of Sustainability (SOS), brings together scientists, engineers, and humanists with government policy makers and industry leaders to develop solutions to the challenges of environmental, economic, and social sustainability.

The School of Earth and Space Exploration epitomizes efforts to institutionalize transdisciplinary collaboration. Established through an amalgamation of the former Department of Geological Sciences and the astronomy, astrophysics, and cosmology faculties of the former Department of Physics and Astronomy—thereafter the Department of Physics—SESE includes theoretical physicists, systems biologists, biogeochemists, and engineers who advance the development and deployment of critical scientific instrumentation. Transdisciplinary fluidity facilitates collaboration among more than 60 faculty members and 100 research scientists, engineers,

and postdoctoral scholars. Subfields within astrophysics and cosmology, for example, include computational astrophysics; physics of the early universe; and the formation of galaxies, stars, and planetary systems. The broad theme of exploration represents a transdisciplinary conceptualization of the quest to discover the origins of the universe and expand our understanding of space, matter, and time (Crow and Dabars 2015, 280–281).

The set of new schools complements existing academic units reconceptualized to facilitate interdisciplinary collaboration. The Ira A. Fulton Schools of Engineering, for example, have evolved from a single conventional college of engineering and applied sciences to comprise five distinct research-intensive transdisciplinary schools: the School of Biological and Health Systems Engineering; School of Computing, Informatics, and Decision Systems Engineering; School of Electrical, Computer, and Energy Engineering; School for Engineering of Matter, Transport, and Energy; and School of Sustainable Engineering and the Built Environment. A sixth school, the Polytechnic School, focuses on use-inspired translational research and offers students interested in direct entry into the workforce an experiential learning environment. Within these six schools, more than two dozen research centers advance transdisciplinary collaboration, including the Security and Defense Systems Initiative, which addresses national and global security and defense challenges through an integrative systems approach; Flexible Display Center, a cooperative agreement with the U.S. Army to advance the emerging flexible electronics industry; and LightWorks, an endeavor in renewable energy fields, including artificial photosynthesis, biofuels, and next-generation photovoltaics.

The Biodesign Institute, a premier transdisciplinary research center advancing biologically inspired design, addresses global challenges in health care, sustainability, and national security. By fostering a convergence of broad scientific fields of biology, nanotechnology, informatics, and engineering under one roof, the institute advances our understanding in human health and the environment through research in such areas as personalized diagnostics and treatment, infectious diseases and pandemics, national security threats, and renewable sources of energy.

As one of only a small cadre of institutions that have embraced a mandate for fundamental transformation, ASU has recognized the imperative to scale to support vanguard research on problems that will be solved only through large-scale collaborative inter- and transdisciplinary efforts. The intent to pioneer vanguard research and development capabilities represents a significant departure from the traditional model of individual investigator-initiated initiatives and required Biodesign researchers to predict the trajectory of advances in the biosciences and establish large-scale collaborative and convergent programs in spaces not occupied by peers.

Among the 15 constituent research centers of the Biodesign Institute are the Center for Innovations in Medicine, dedicated to the improvement of medical diagnostics and the treatment and prevention of disease; ASU-Banner Neurodegenerative Disease Research Center, a research alliance to advance the treatment of Alzheimer's, Parkinson's, and other neurodegenerative diseases; the Virginia G. Piper Center for Personalized Diagnostics, where research teams seek to identify and test new biomarkers associated with biological subtypes of diseases like cancer to improve treatment outcomes and survivability; and the Center for Mechanisms of Evolution, which focuses on mechanisms of organismal adaptation across all the genetic, cellular, and phenotypic levels and role of random genetic drift and recombination across populations.

Biodesign teams moreover collaborate with researchers from Mayo Clinic Scottsdale. In collaboration with Mayo Clinic, ASU has established joint degree programs in law, business, and nursing, collaboration in bioengineering and bioinformatics research, and innovative health solutions pathways with the potential to educate 200 million people about healthcare; engage 20 million people in online healthcare delivery; and enhance treatment for two million patients. Students who attend Mayo Medical School will have the opportunity to participate in a number of dual degree programs, including ASU's Master's of Healthcare Delivery. A joint team science program is advancing high impact projects with near-term clinical translation potential in biomedical engineering, sensing, and functional restoration.

In a sense, each of the Biodesign Institute research centers represents a discrete albeit interrelated team—or set of teams, which frequently include researchers from academic units throughout the university as well as industry and government partners. Team collaboration is behind the success of a new effort in synthetic biology to demonstrate how the biological information contained within ribonucleic acid (RNA) can be adapted to create logic circuits capable of performing computations; development of a diagnostic platform called ImmunoSignature, which with a single drop of blood can detect diseases that involve an immune response, including cancer, autoimmune, infectious, metabolic, and neurological diseases; and a project to enable large-scale cultivation of microalgae—species of microscopic single-cell organisms that can be used to produce renewable biofuels that recycle carbon dioxide from the atmosphere. The Atmospheric Carbon Dioxide Capture and Membrane Delivery project, undertaken to assist the U.S. Department of Energy (DOE) in its efforts to promote the advancement of clean and renewable energy, brings together teams of researchers from the Swette Center for Environmental Biotechnology, Center for Negative Carbon Emissions, and Center for Applied Structural Discovery (CASD)—constituent research centers of the Biodesign Institute—with physicists and civil, environmental, and sustainability engineers from the School of Sustainable Engineering and the Built Environment (Caspermeyer et al. 2015/2017).

New transdisciplinary research centers that span the humanities and social sciences include the Institute for Humanities Research; Center for the Study of Religion and Conflict, which promotes research on the dynamics of religion in contemporary society with the objective of seeking solutions and informing policy; Complex

Adaptive Systems Initiative (CASI), a collaborative effort to address global challenges in health, sustainability, and national security; and Global Security Initiative (GSI), an interdisciplinary hub for global security research that addresses emerging challenges characterized by complex interdependencies and uncertainties and seeks to advance societal openness and inclusiveness as well as connections to the global defense, development, and diplomacy communities.

Team science indisputably contributes to the momentum of interdisciplinary collaboration at ASU, which may in part be attested by the growth in the number of active sponsored projects involving investigators from different academic departments. Such collaborative endeavors rose by 182% between FY 2003 and FY 2018, outpacing projects involving researchers in single departments, which increased by only 27%. The total value of active sponsored projects from single units during this timeframe increased 106%, while the value of projects involving more than one unit increased 367%.

More broadly, the New American University model demonstrates that research excellence and broad accessibility are not necessarily mutually exclusive. ASU has succeeded in advancing both the academic rigor and diversity of our student body, which increasingly includes more and more students from socioeconomically disadvantaged and historically underrepresented backgrounds, including a significant share of first-generation college applicants. As a consequence of the new model, soaring enrollment growth has been accompanied by unprecedented increases in freshman persistence, degree production, learning outcomes, minority enrollment, academic success, and all measures of quality of graduates. Corollary achievements include growth in research infrastructure and sponsored expenditures, which since 2004 have made the ASU research enterprise the fastest growing in the United States. As a consequence of the ambitious expansion of the research enterprise, research-related expenditures over the period FY 2002 to FY 2018 have grown by more than a factor of five—without significant growth in the size of the faculty—reaching a record of $618 million in FY 2018, up from $123 million in FY 2002.

37.5 Toward the Institutional Accommodation of Transdisciplinarity and Team Science

The restructuring of academic organization to facilitate inter- and transdisciplinary collaboration—and thus team science—is a process that for each institution must necessarily be *sui generis*. The sequence of deliberations and decisions associated with the design process cannot be codified into a lexicon of strategies applicable to other institutional contexts. Moreover, the corollary challenge remains for institutions to produce students who are adaptive master-learners empowered to integrate a broad array of interrelated disciplines and negotiate the changing workforce demands of the knowledge economy.

If the academy is to advance collaborative innovation, the debate must engage a broad community of disciplines as well as the wisdom and expertise developed in commerce, industry, and government. The maintenance of strict disciplinary boundaries undermines our impetus to initiate a conversation with those outside our own sphere of disciplinary expertise (Crow 2007). Scientists, scholars, and practitioners from disparate domains of knowledge must cultivate "interlanguages" intelligible to other disciplines—not unlike the pidgins or creoles through which different subcultures negotiate trading zones (Galison 1997, 48). Literary scholar Stefan Collini aptly frames this imperative as the "intellectual equivalent of bilingualism," which he defines as a "capacity not only to exercise the language of our respective specialisms, but also to attend to, learn from, and eventually contribute to, wider cultural conversations" (1998, lvii). Our collective survival as a species may be contingent on our capacity to collaborate across disciplinary boundaries, which assumes the continued evolution of knowledge enterprises optimally designed to foster mutual intelligibility among academic disciplines and interdisciplinary fields (Crow and Dabars 2015, 205–207).

References

Abbott A. Chaos of disciplines. Chicago: University of Chicago Press; 2001.

Apostel L, Berger G, Briggs A, et al., editors. Interdisciplinarity: problems of teaching and research in universities. Paris: Organization for Economic Cooperation and Development; 1972.

Arthur WB. The nature of technology: what it is and how it evolves. New York: Free Press; 2009.

Brown JS, Duguid P. Organizational learning and communities-of-practice: toward a unified view of working, learning, and innovation. Organ Sci. 1991;2(1):40–57.

Brown JS, Collins A, Duguid P. Situated cognition and the culture of learning. Educ Res. 1989;18(1):32–42.

Bush GP, Hattery LH. Teamwork and creativity in research. Administrative Science Quarterly. 1956;1(3):361–372.

Caspermeyer J, Harth R, Kullman J. News releases. 2015/2017. Tempe, AZ: Biodesign Institute, Arizona State University.

Cole JR. Toward a more perfect university. New York: Public Affairs; 2016.

Collini S. Introduction to C. P. Snow, The two cultures. Cambridge: Cambridge University Press; 1998.

Crow MM. None dare call it hubris: the limits of knowledge. Issues Sci Technol. 2007;23(2):29–32.

Crow MM, Bozeman B. Limited by design: R&D laboratories in the U.S. national innovation system. New York: Columbia University Press; 1998.

Crow MM, Dabars WB. Designing the new American university. Baltimore: Johns Hopkins University Press; 2015.

Crow MM, Dabars WB. Interdisciplinarity as a design problem: toward mutual intelligibility among academic disciplines in the American research university. In: O'Rourke M, Crowley S, Eigenbrode SD, Wulfhorst JD, editors. Enhancing communication and collaboration in interdisciplinary research. Los Angeles: Sage; 2013. p. 294–322.

DiMaggio PJ, Powell WW. The iron cage revisited: institutional isomorphism and collective rationality in organizational fields. Am Sociol Rev. 1983;48(2):147–60.

Downs A. Inside bureaucracy. Boston: Little Brown; 1967.

Etzkowitz H. Research groups as quasi-firms: the invention of the entrepreneurial university. Res Policy. 2003;32:109–21.

Etzkowitz H. The triple helix: university-industry-government innovation in action. New York: Routledge; 2008.

Fiore SM. Interdisciplinarity as teamwork: how the science of teams can inform team science. Small Group Res. 2008;39(3):251–77.

Frodeman R. Sustainable knowledge: a theory of interdisciplinarity. Basingstoke: Palgrave Macmillan; 2014.

Galison P. Image and logic: a material culture of physics. Chicago: University of Chicago Press; 1997.

Geiger RL. Organized research units: their role in the development of the research university. Journal of Higher Education. 1990;61(1):1–19.

Gibbons M, et al. The new production of knowledge: the dynamics of science and research in contemporary societies. London: Sage; 1994.

Giddens A. The constitution of society: outline of the theory of structuration. Berkeley: University of California Press; 1984.

Goldman AI. Knowledge in a social world. Oxford: Oxford University Press; 1999.

Habermas J. The theory of communicative action, vol. 2: reason and the rationalization of society. Trans. Thomas McCarthy. Cambridge, MA: MIT Press; 1987.

Hagel J, Brown JS, Davison L. The power of pull: how small moves, smartly made, can set big things in motion. New York: Basic Books; 2010.

Håkanson L. The firm as an epistemic community: the knowledge-based view revisited. Ind Corp Chang. 2010;19(6):1801–28.

Hall KL, et al. Moving the science of team science forward: collaboration and creativity. Am J Prev Med. 2008;35(2S):S243–9.

Hannan MT, Freeman J. Organizational ecology. Cambridge, MA: Harvard University Press; 1989.

Hong L, Page S. Groups of diverse problem solvers can outperform groups of high-ability problem solvers. Proc Natl Acad Sci. 2004;101(46):16385–9.

Jacobs JA. In defense of disciplines: interdisciplinarity and specialization in the research university. Chicago: University of Chicago Press; 2013.

Klein JT. Communication and collaboration in interdisciplinary research. In: O'Rourke M, Crowley S, Eigenbrode SD, Wulfhorst JD, editors. Enhancing communication and collaboration in interdisciplinary research. Los Angeles: Sage; 2013. p. 11–30.

Knorr Cetina K. Epistemic cultures: how the sciences make knowledge. Cambridge, MA: Harvard University Press; 1999.

Kozlowski SWJ, Klein KJ. A multilevel approach to theory and research in organizations: contextual, temporal, and emergent processes. In: Klein KJ, Kozlowski SWJ, editors. Multilevel theory, research, and methods in organizations: foundations, extensions, and new directions. San Francisco: Jossey-Bass; 2000, 3–90.

Merton RK, Barber E. The travels and adventures of serendipity: a study in sociological semantics and the sociology of science. Princeton: Princeton University Press; 2004.

Miller JH, Page SE. Complex adaptive systems: an introduction to computational models of social life. Princeton, NJ: Princeton University Press; 2007.

National Academies, Committee on Facilitating Interdisciplinary Research (CFIR) and Committee on Science, Engineering, and Public Policy (COSEPUP). Facilitating interdisciplinary research. Washington, DC: National Academies Press; 2005.

National Research Council. Convergence: facilitating transdisciplinary integration of life sciences, physical sciences, engineering, and beyond. Washington, DC: National Academies Press; 2014.

National Research Council. Enhancing the Effectiveness of Team Science. Washington, DC: The National Academies Press. 2015. https://doi.org/10.17226/19007.

Nelson RR, et al. How medical know-progresses. Res Policy. 2010;40:1339–44.

Nowotny H, Scott P, Gibbons M. Mode 2 revisited: the new production of knowledge. Minerva. 2003;41:179–94.

Peacock M. Path dependence in the production of scientific knowledge. Soc Epistemol. 2009;23(2):105–24.

Porter AL, et al. Measuring researcher interdisciplinarity. Scientometrics. 2007;72(1):117–47.

Price DJ d S. Little science, big science, and beyond. New York: Columbia University Press; 1986.

Roco MC, Bainbridge WS, editors. Converging technologies for improving human performance: nanotechnology, biotechnology, information technology, and cognitive science. Washington, DC: National Science Foundation; 2002.

Sarewitz D. Saving science from itself. The New Atlantis: A Journal of Technology and Society (Spring/Summer). 2016.

Shirky C. Cognitive surplus: creativity and generosity in a connected age. New York: Penguin; 2010.

Shneiderman B. The new ABCs of research: achieving breakthrough collaborations. Oxford: Oxford University Press; 2016.

Simon HA. The sciences of the artificial, 3rd ed. 1966/1996. Cambridge, MA: MIT Press.

Teece DJ. Knowledge and competence as strategic assets. In: Holsapple CW, editor. Handbook on knowledge management, vol. 1. Berlin: Springer Verlag; 2003.

Uzzi B, et al. Atypical combinations and scientific impact. Science. 2013;342(October 25):468.

Von Hippel E. Sticky information and the locus of problem solving: implications for innovation. Manag Sci. 1994;40(4):429–39.

Voosen P. Microbiology leaves the solo author behind. Chronicle of Higher Education (November 11). 2013.

Wallerstein I. Anthropology, sociology, and other dubious disciplines. Curr Anthropol. 2003;44(4):453–65.

Weingart P. A short history of knowledge formations. In: Frodeman R, Klein JT, Mitcham C, editors. The Oxford handbook of interdisciplinarity. Oxford: Oxford University Press; 2010. p. 3–14.

Wenger E. Communities of practice: learning, meaning, and identity. Cambridge: Cambridge University Press; 1998.

Westwick PJ. The national labs: science in an American system, 1947–1974. Cambridge, MA: Harvard University Press; 2003.

Wilson A. Knowledge power: interdisciplinary education for a complex world. London: Routledge; 2010.

Wuchty W, Jones BF, Uzzi B. The increasing dominance of teams in production of knowledge. Science. 2007;316:1036–9.

Building a Cross-Disciplinary Culture in Academia Through Joint Hires, Degree Programs, and Scholarships

38

Sandra A. Brown, Margaret S. Leinen, and Steffanie A. Strathdee

Contents

38.1 Introduction 489

38.2 Strategic Planning for Team Science
Topics 490

38.3 Joint Faculty Hire Framework 491

38.4 Joint Degree Programs 492

References 494

S. A. Brown, PhD (✉)
Office of Research Affairs and Departments of
Psychology and Psychiatry, University of California
San Diego, La Jolla, CA, USA
e-mail: sandrabrown@ucsd.edu

M. S. Leinen, PhD
Scripps Institution of Oceanography, and School of
Marine Sciences, University of California,
San Diego, La Jolla, CA, USA

S. A. Strathdee, PhD
Division of Infectious Diseases & Global Health
Sciences, and Department of Medicine, University of
California San Diego School of Medicine, La Jolla,
CA, USA

38.1 Introduction

The University of California San Diego has problem-focused, multidisciplinary research and training embedded in its development since Roger Revelle launched the idea of an experimental campus in the University of California (UC) system in 1960. With a limited number of departments and a plethora of programs, institutes and centers, working in thematic and problem-focused teams became common at UC San Diego.

In this brief chapter, we summarize several design and implementation aspects of the team science approach that has resulted in the rapid ascendency of UC San Diego into a top-tier research university with a research portfolio of over one billion dollars per year. In particular, we will highlight our strategic framework to promote training and research experience in team science, which includes costly new faculty hiring and time-consuming Joint Doctoral Training Program infrastructure commitments, as well as inexpensive and flexible student scholarships efforts. In each case, we describe advantages and inherent challenges these types of structures and processes produce for the academic community.

© Springer Nature Switzerland AG 2019
K. L. Hall et al. (eds.), *Strategies for Team Science Success*,
https://doi.org/10.1007/978-3-030-20992-6_38

38.2 Strategic Planning for Team Science Topics

As noted in the National Academy of Sciences (NAS) comprehensive review, the impact of team science efforts is optimized if aligned with the strategic priorities of the university (National Research Council 2015). In 2014, UC San Diego embarked on its first-ever strategic planning process. Under Chancellor Pradeep Khosla, who wanted to go beyond interdisciplinarity as a characteristic of a UC San Diego approach to specifying themes on which the university would focus. A series of Town Hall meetings were conducted including students, faculty, and staff that resulted in *Defining Our Future: UC San Diego's Strategic Plan* (UC San Diego 2014).

Based on information from these meetings and open web forum input, Academic Senate and Office of Research Affairs (ORA) leadership designed four thematic workshops that included nearly 1400 faculty and students. At each workshop, faculty gave presentations on specific interdisciplinary research ideas to enrich understanding of each themes thereby honing the narrative for each strategic research initiative. The themes are very broad to allow a variety of focus areas to emerge within each from continued discussions as the implementation plan was developed. The four university-wide research initiatives are:

- Understanding and protecting the planet
- Enriching human life and society
- Exploring the basis of human knowledge and creativity
- Understanding cultures and addressing disparities in society

38.2.1 Team Science Scholarships

The launch of the UC San Diego strategic plan in 2014 initiated an annual set of student scholarships for cross-disciplinary research to promote creative new efforts in UC San Diego priority areas. Each fall, faculty respond to a request for proposals to fund 100 undergraduate, 80 graduate and 20 postdoctoral trainees through the Frontiers of Innovation Scholarship Program (FISP). The program is administrated by ORA and senior Academic Senate faculty committees review each proposal. Committees are jointly appointed by ORA and Academic Senate leadership to ensure diverse perspectives and disciplines bear on proposal assessment. Each proposal must articulate a specific project and value relevant to at least one of the four strategic themes. Given the modest stipend level and higher training needs for undergraduate scholarships, trainees at this level work under the supervision of a single faculty member on a multidisciplinary research project. Graduate and postdoctoral trainees are supervised by at least two faculty from different disciplines on a new project in one of the four strategic research areas. The focus on innovative scholarship encourages novel, creative ideas and simultaneously supports the research need for pilot studies in fruitful future grant and publication areas. The FISP application is, by design, kept brief (two pages) to encourage even senior faculty to engage, and the applications are sorted by research initiative areas and disciplines to ensure a broad set of new studies and research experience for students. The review process is standardized with each review committee providing numerical scoring to quickly rank applications with the top 200 of 400–500 submissions recommended for funding. A final, joint review is conducted by Academic Senate leadership and the Vice Chancellor for Research to ensure a diversity of discipline and focus in the award process. In addition to direct research experience, all trainees are provided professional training opportunities over the course of the academic year. Awardees participate in a conference highlighting his or her multidisciplinary work and prepare a one-page summary of their learning and accomplishments. The training and progress are monitored by the administrators (Vice Chancellor for Student Affairs, Dean of the Graduate Division, Office of Postdoctoral and Research Scholar Affairs) using predetermined metrics of success. Objective impact such as professional presentations, manuscript publications, grant applications and continued career success (acceptance into graduate, postdoctoral programs, research-related career placements) are monitored over a 2-year period. Subjective reports of the values, knowledge, and skills obtained are also monitored to determine personal impact.

38.2.2 Challenges

Since the focus of the FISP scholarships is to promote novel, creative multidisciplinary research, it is a challenge to ensure sufficient diversity among faculty reviewing proposals to provide full appreciation for all innovative science proposed. Further, given the considerable variety in the proportion of high-quality applications across divisions and strategic research initiatives, the rankings require an administrative review to ensure all areas of campus benefit from the opportunity. An important program evaluation challenge is to ensure evaluative metrics reflect relevant qualitative and quantitative enhancement beyond current training opportunities on campus. Evaluation involves multiple administrative structures and extensive follow-ups with student scholars. Finally, this approach accelerates innovation and risk. As such, it is important to have domains and metrics included in the academic personnel review process that afford credit to such mentorship team science and new professional products. UC San Diego has articulated additional products common to new forms of team science (e.g., national database, software, scientific leadership in national programs) into the academic review process.

38.3   Joint Faculty Hire Framework

Our UC San Diego interdisciplinary joint faculty hire initiative has its roots in the strategic plan. Soon after the strategic plan was completed, Chancellor Khosla launched the joint-tenure faculty hires program to support the strategic research initiatives. These faculty have joint appointments in two different departments of the university, preferably in different divisions, with the intention to enhance targeted research areas and academic interactions across departments. Faculty have 50% assignments in each department, and departments share start-up costs, teaching commitments, and space to ensure new faculty have an intellectual home in both departments. Based on the assumption that the newer generation of scholars are more willing to engage in emergent multidisciplinary research, preference was given to early career (pre-tenure) applicants. To provide an incentive for faculty mentoring, if at the time of the tenure decision, the faculty member was tenured by one department, the faculty appointment would move exclusively to the tenuring department.

Deans embraced the joint appointment concept and agreed to provide additional faculty slots so that more faculty could be hired in each thematic area to provide a more robust cohort of joint hires.

38.3.1   Process for Multi-department Hires

The process for determining the focus of joint appointments is exemplified by the Understanding and Protecting the Planet (UPP) research initiative. An initial call for proposals from faculty and departments for specific hires in UPP resulted in about 25 proposals that were reviewed by the Chancellor and Vice Chancellors. A dominant focus on adaptation to climate change was evident and a university-wide faculty committee was formed to identify the specific topical areas and criteria for faculty recruitment. The committee identified four areas from which recruitment ensued:

- Hazards from climate impacts in the natural and built environment
- Biological and ecological systems and climate change
- Human health climate impacts and adaptation
- Measurements, sensors, and platforms

A Chancellor's Oversight Committee developed principles to be applied to all joint hires and a separate Oversight Committee managed the joint hires in each research initiative area. Joint faculty hires employ a Memorandum of Understanding between the cooperating departments to specify the responsibilities of each department of the new faculty member. The Chancellor's Oversight Committee reviewed each recommended candidate to ensure that individuals selected met the spirit of the focus and requirement of the position.

38.3.2 Challenges

There are several unique challenges to the multi-department joint hire process. Cultural differences between fields (e.g., nature of scholarship considered in tenure decisions), demanding requirements of classes with integrated scholarship, and increased communication needed for this type of research can challenge early-career faculty during a time when they are trying to establish credentials for promotions and demonstrate independence.

Practical challenges also emerged in the hiring process, such as need to accommodate differing recruitment timelines of diverse fields. Consequently, maintaining good communication between the Deans, departments, search committees and Oversight Committee is critical to academic hiring success.

The requirements that candidates meet with search committee members and individual faculty within each department is taxing for faculty and candidates.

38.4   Joint Degree Programs

A unique framework of cross-disciplinary and cross-institution training has been a standard at UC San Diego. Such joint doctoral programs (JDPs) build on the strengths of the participating campuses to generate programs that could not otherwise be realized, combining the complementary assets of faculty and facilities at both institutions. JDPs are independently reviewed, and approved by each university system to ensure that educational offerings are of high quality and do not duplicate existing degree programs.

UC San Diego and San Diego State University (San Diego State) currently offer 20 JDPs, with three examples described here in more detail. All three of these JDPs are led by joint steering, admissions and curriculum committees comprised of equal numbers of faculty from both campuses, ensuring that program decisions are made jointly and by mutual agreement between UC and CSU. Students enrolled in the JDPs are selected according to specific concentration areas or tracks, with each campus appointing a co-director for each track. Students complete course work and conduct research at both institutions—typically alternating semesters or terms each year between San Diego State and UC San Diego. Equal numbers of faculty from each campus serve on advisory and dissertation committees, providing students with extensive exposure to experts with varied interests, and the student's primary advisor and external dissertation committee can be based at either campus. Since UC San Diego and San Diego State are only 20 minutes apart, faculty from both universities often teach classes on either campus.

38.4.1 Clinical Psychology

This JDP in Clinical Psychology represents a primary partnership between the Department of Psychiatry at UC San Diego and San Diego State's Department of Psychology although faculty from other departments are involved. Founded in 1988, this program offers specialization in behavioral medicine/health psychology, neuropsychology, and experimental psychopathology. Since this JDP is consistently ranked first in the country, its annual acceptance rate is usually <5%. Each year, twelve to fifteen students are selected from a pool of 275–350 applicants. The gender ratio of currently enrolled students is over 80% female and 33% underrepresented minorities (URM). The program aims to provide research skills and approaches to human problems for students training in clinical psychology, who are being employed in increasingly diverse settings encompassing teaching, research, consultation, program evaluation, and program design and implementation science, in addition to the more traditional diagnostic and treatment responsibilities. The program is based on the scientist-practitioner model, leads to a PhD in Clinical Psychology, and provides students with integrated training in clinical and research skills. This program is designed to be completed in five, 12-month academic years. Most of the core curriculum is presented during the first 2 years, with increasing specialization in the following 3 years. Clinical practica and therapeutic training activities are coordinated with each student's progression through courses and research activities, and with advice from a guidance committee comprised of at least one faculty member from each campus. The core curriculum builds a strong background in: (a) empirical psychology, including biological, social, cognitive-affective, and individual bases of behavior; (b) conceptualizations of personality and psychopathology; (c) theory and techniques of psychological assessment; (d) empirically supported therapeutic interventions; and (e) research methods while stressing cultural competence. Training in the specialty areas after the second year includes advanced coursework and extensive research and clinical experience under faculty supervision. Students are encouraged to begin research in their first 2 years and to complete their dissertations in their fourth year. The fifth year is devoted to a clinical internship in an American Psychological Association (APA) accredited facility. Most graduates are currently in highly competitive academic, academic-related, or research positions.

38.4.2 Public Health

The JDP in Public Health was established between the Division of Epidemiology in the Department of Family Medicine and Public Health at the School of Medicine at UC San Diego, and the Graduate School of Public Health (GSPH) at San Diego State. Founded in 1980, GSPH is one of four nationally accredited schools of public health in California. The JDP in Public Health began offering a PhD with a concentration in Epidemiology in 1990 and added tracks in Health Behavior and Global Health in 2002 and 2007, respectively. Across the three tracks, the gender ratio is 65% female with 27% URM.

In response to the growing need for academics and health practitioners with global health experience, the global health track was the first of its kind in the University of California system, and one of the first in the country. Global health relates to health issues and concerns that transcend national borders, class, race, ethnicity, and culture (Koplan et al. 2009), stresses the commonality of health issues and calls for a collective, partnership-based action to resolve these issues. Accordingly, emphasis is on preparing graduates with the fundamental knowledge, and specific skills necessary to become public health researchers and professional leaders in global health settings. Proximity to the U.S./Mexico border and expertise of many current faculty support a focus on infectious diseases (e.g., HIV, TB, STDs) and health of migrant populations, although students are expected to develop other areas of specialization such as chronic/infectious disease surveillance and prevention, environmental health, maternal and child health, health policy or methodological areas such as quantitative, qualitative, and spatial research applied to address significant global health problems. In addition to didactic classes, students are expected to meet specific cultural competencies relative to the overall field of global public health and to their dissertation area, and to complete an international field practicum. Graduates of the program are competitive for research, teaching, and service positions in academic institutions, governmental and nongovernmental organizations, and businesses with global health interests within and outside of the U.S.

38.4.3 Interdisciplinary Research on Substance Use

Founded in 2015, the JDP in Interdisciplinary Research on Substance Use is the first doctoral program of its kind in the country and is uniquely positioned to respond to the growing addiction crisis in the United States (Dart et al. 2015). This program is offered through the Division of Global Public Health in UC San Diego's School of Medicine and School of Social Work at San Diego State. This JDP was designed to prepare the next generation of leaders in substance use research with the knowledge and skills to advance evidence-based and applied substance use interventions, programs, and policies. The program has a decidedly public health perspective and focuses on multisystem addiction research, preventing use and misuse of alcohol and illicit drugs, treatment, and associated biomedical, social and economic consequences. The JDP leadership also introduces students to policy-driven, systems-level intervention approaches (e.g., needle exchange programs and community-based facilities), as well as the theory and policy debates surrounding such programs. Students acquire skills and knowledge in theory, current research methods, and analytic approaches related to substance use and related problems. Courses include etiology, pharmacology, and epidemiology of substance use and its related problems, as well as the effectiveness and efficacy of interventions (including programs and policies) designed to ameliorate such problems. Financial support and tuition remission will be covered for four PhD students per year; 16 PhD students at steady state. Based on market research, graduates are expected to be highly sought after in academic units in medicine, social work and public health as well as research firms and governmental health departments.

38.4.4 Challenges

While some challenges are unique to individual JDPs, they have programmatic and logistical challenges in common. First, there are considerable administrative challenges inherent to developing new degree programs across two university systems. The lengthy review process typically begins with curriculum committees at each university's sponsoring school or college,

followed by graduate councils and the Academic Senate, and finally the system-wide degree granting approval processes, each which involve extensive and detailed review. This process typically requires several years, although adding new concentration areas within existing JDPs does not require system-wide approvals and affords flexibility for training programs with emergent science.

A financial challenge of each JDP is the commitment to full financial support for a minimum of 3 years, and in some cases, up to 5 years for each student. Faculty wishing to mentor a newly admitted JDP student commit to supporting them, usually from federal or state grants. In some cases, JDPs receive funding from their departments, school, or scholarships. Each JDP is affiliated with at least one NIH training grant.

JDP students also face logistical challenges in navigating two university systems; however, they report benefiting from the richness and diversity of the faculty, and the freedom of selecting dissertation committees at both institutions.

In summary, UC San Diego has built into its research infrastructure an academic development approach and training design that develop the culture of team science. By building all three components in alignment with the strategic plan, the university is well poised to answer the most challenging scientific questions of the future, and train those necessary to seek the answers.

References

Dart RC, Surratt HL, Cicero TJ, Parrino MW, Severtson SG, Bucher-Bartelson B, Green JL. Trends in opioid analgesic abuse and mortality in the United States. N Engl J Med. 2015;372(3):241–8.

Koplan JP, Bond TC, Merson MH, Reddy KS, Rodriguez MH, Sewankambo NK, Wasserheit JN. Towards a common definition of global health. Lancet. 2009;373(9679):1993–5.

National Research Council. Enhancing the Effectiveness of Team Science. Washington, DC: The National Academies Press. 2015. https://doi.org/10.17226/19007.

University of California, San Diego. Defining our culture: UC San Diego strategic plan. San Diego, CA: UC San Diego; 2014.

Broadening our Understanding of Scientific Work for the Era of Team Science: Implications for Recognition and Rewards

39

Amanda L. Vogel, Kara L. Hall, Holly J. Falk-Krzesinski, and Julie Thompson Klein

Contents

39.1 Introduction

The archetype of the lone scientist working independently to achieve a scientific breakthrough has had a powerful influence on how we understand the nature of scientific work. Yet how scientific work is performed, and how breakthroughs are produced, often are quite different from this model. Since the mid-twentieth century, team-based approaches have outpaced solo work across disciplines and fields (Wuchty et al. 2007; Jones et al. 2008). Most scientists now regularly participate in a mix of solo and team-based research, or exclusively team-based research.

In order to address the multifactorial dimensions of complex scientific problems, many science teams also are increasingly cross-disciplinary

K. L. Hall
Division of Cancer Control and Population Sciences,
National Cancer Institute, Bethesda, MD, USA

H. J. Falk-Krzesinski
Global Strategic Networks, Elsevier Inc., New York,
NY, USA

Philanthropy and Nonprofit Fundraising Program,
School of Professional Studies, Northwestern
University, Chicago, IL, USA

J. T. Klein
Department of English, Wayne State University,
Detroit, MI, USA

Transdisciplinarity Lab, ETH-Zurich, Switzerland

A. L. Vogel (✉)
Clinical Monitoring Research Program Directorate,
Frederick National Laboratory for Cancer Research
sponsored by the National Cancer Institute,
Frederick, MD, USA
e-mail: vogelal@mail.nih.gov

© Springer Nature Switzerland AG 2019
K. L. Hall et al. (eds.), *Strategies for Team Science Success*,
https://doi.org/10.1007/978-3-030-20992-6_39

in nature. Cross-disciplinary team science, also referred to as convergence science and integrative science, aims to accelerate scientific advances by bringing to bear and integrating a range of relevant approaches and methods from across disciplines and fields. In doing so it aims to produce science that is more holistic, and therefore has the potential to answer scientific questions more comprehensively and produce more effective solutions to complex real-world problems (Hall et al. 2012; NRC 2014; Vogel et al. 2014). As such, it has been widely recognized as essential to advancing innovation and developing solutions in today's scientific enterprise (NRC 2014; 2015).

Taken together, increases in team science and cross-disciplinary approaches underscore the need to rethink assumptions about the range of ways that effective scientific work is done, and closely related, what scientific activities should be recognized and rewarded. Specifically, there is a need to expand widely held conceptualizations of scientific work to include a range of activities that may be absent from single investigator-driven research but are essential to the success of team science, particularly cross-disciplinary team science. Likewise, there is a need to expand recognition and reward systems to acknowledge these essential scientific activities.

This book highlights a wide range of activities that are essential to success for small to large team science initiatives. Examples of scientific leadership activities unique to team science, which are highlighted in this book, include providing scientific vision for team-based research endeavors (e.g., the chapters by Berger 2019; Christen and Levine 2019; Salazar et al. 2019); composing teams that are of the right size and include collaborators with the right mix of expertise to effectively pursue the scientific goals (e.g., the chapters by Berger 2019; Hendren and Ku 2019; O'Rourke et al. 2019; Salazar et al. 2019; Twyman and Contractor 2019); facilitating the development and maintenance of shared scientific goals among collaborators from many different disciplines and fields (e.g., the chapters by Berger 2019; Jain and Klein 2019; Kozlowski and Bell 2019; Gehlert 2019; Pohl and Wuelser 2019); and leading development of a conceptual model of the scientific work that reflects the unique contributions of each of the involved disciplines and fields (e.g., the chapters by Kozlowski and Bell 2019; Hendren and Ku 2019). Authors in this book also address essential facilitative, administrative, and managerial activities for team science. These include facilitating communication across participating disciplines and fields, often involving development of shared terminology and shared understanding of key theories, concepts, and methods (the chapters by O'Rourke et al. 2019; Pohl and Wuelser 2019); and managing task coordination among team members (the chapter by Kozlowski and Bell 2019); and managing scientific and interpersonal conflict among team members (the chapter by Bennett and Gadlin 2019). These also include securing a range of resources to enable execution of the science, including training of team members in competencies for team science and, as needed, cross-disciplinary subject matter (the chapters by Fiore et al. 2019; Nurius and Kemp 2019; Spring et al. 2019); IT infrastructure for scientific collaboration including for data sharing and integration and collaborative data analysis; and scientific equipment and laboratory space (the chapters by Bennett et al. 2019; Hall et al. 2019).

The more complex the team science initiative, the more complex these tasks will be, the more skill, focus, and time they will require, and the more influence they are likely to exert on the scientific outcomes of a particular initiative (Hall et al. 2018). For example, a small team science project involving only two or three collaborators likely will require a more modest investment of time and expertise in each of the aforementioned activities than a large team science initiative involving dozens or hundreds of members (e.g., research centers, networks, or consortia) (National Research Council 2015). But whether the collaborative initiative is large or small, skillful implementation of these activities enhances effective team functioning, ultimately contributing to the quality of the scientific outcomes. Following suit, whether the team science initiative is large or small, these scientific activities deserve consideration in recognition and reward systems.

39.2 Shifting the Culture of the Scientific Enterprise to Align with Cross-disciplinary and Team Science Approaches

Recognition and reward systems, and particularly promotion and tenure policies, are essential influences on the use of cross-disciplinary and team science approaches to advance science (Falk-Krzesinski 2013; Klein and Falk-Krzesinski 2017). However, on the whole, promotion and tenure policies have been slow to change to reflect the growth of these scientific approaches. Concerns about a lack of recognition and reward for cross-disciplinary collaborative initiatives were first raised in the mid- to late twentieth century (Stone 1969 and McEvoy 1972). A survey conducted by the US National Academies in 2004 highlighted that provosts (as well as all other respondents) identified promotion and tenure criteria as a top impediment to cross-disciplinary research (Institute of Medicine 2005). Recommendations for greater recognition followed. Yet a decade later, the National Research Council report *Enhancing the Effectiveness of Team Science* (2015) reported that most US universities continued to lack comprehensive and explicit criteria for evaluating individual contributions to team-based research.

Changes to fundamental policies and procedures, such as promotion and tenure, typically are slow to occur due to the size and complexity of academic systems. In addition, academic institutions are part of a system of factors that both shape and are shaped by changes in the culture of the broader scientific enterprise. These changes occur in different contexts, including not only universities, but funding agencies and professional organizations, at different rates, and with different drivers.

A few recent examples of the variety of contexts, actors, approaches, and activities influencing advances in team science help to elucidate this point. In the academic context, one large-scale "experiment" in institutional restructuring at a major US research university, involving the partial dismantling of discipline-based departments and creation of new cross-disciplinary units, has been driven in large part by visionary leaders, including the university president (Crow and Dabars 2019, this book). At a number of major research institutions, as new buildings have been built in the past few years, leaders have taken advantage of the opportunity to support the design of physical work spaces that aim to facilitate collaboration, for example, at the Janelia Research Campus of the Howard Hughes Medical Institute and the Broad Institute of M.I.T. and Harvard (for more on this topic, see Owen-Smith 2013; Bennett et al. 2019, this book). In addition, governments, driven by complex scientific and societal goals, have invested in shared scientific infrastructure to be used by cross-national teams and multi-team systems, such as biobanks, the Human Genome Project, and the Large Hadron Collider. Government funding agencies, meanwhile, have created new funding opportunities for team science initiatives that integrate knowledge across disciplines, fields, and levels of analysis, and engage community partners. Examples include the US National Institutes of Health's Centers for Population Health and Health Disparities initiative (Warnecke et al. 2008) and Transdisciplinary Research in Energetics and Cancer initiative (Schmitz et al. 2016; Gehlert 2019, this book). They have also advanced data sharing and data integration requirements for awardees. Examples include the US National Cancer Institute's Cohort Consortium and the Patient-Centered Outcomes Research Institute's Policy for Data Management and Data Sharing.

Government agencies also have raised the profile of team science by developing resources that offer evidence-informed guidance for effective team science and by showcasing team science successes. The US National Academies has played a leading role in raising awareness of the value of cross-disciplinary team science and strategies for success through its consensus studies, *Facilitating Interdisciplinary Research* (NASEM 2005), *Convergence: Facilitating Transdisciplinary Integration of Life Sciences, Physical Sciences, Engineering, and Beyond* (National Research Council 2014), and *Enhancing the Effectiveness of Team Science*

(National Research Council 2015). The US National Science Foundation has launched a project to develop reports that "put a face on team science …[and] give us an insight into the way science increasingly is conducted today" (National Science Foundation, 2018). In addition, the National Cancer Institute created the Team Science Toolkit,[1] an online wiki-based platform comprising thousands of resources to help users lead, manage, participate in, facilitate, support, evaluate, and/or study team science initiatives (Vogel et al. 2013).

39.3 Revising Promotion and Tenure Policies to Recognize Scientific Activities Essential to Team Science

Within this broad context, over the past decade a range of government agencies and professional organizations have encouraged revisions to promotion and tenure policies to adapt to, foster, and reward team science as well as cross-disciplinarity and community-engaged scholarship. The aforementioned reports of the National Academies on interdisciplinary research, convergence science, and team science have addressed this topic (NASEM 2005; National Research Council 2014, 2015). A recent report by the Canadian Academy of Health Sciences entitled *Academic Recognition of Team Science: How to Optimize the Canadian Academic System* (2017) outlines 12 recommendations to facilitate appropriate recognition of individual contributions to team science "to help promote the full participation of Canada in global team science." These recommendations address adaptations of academic culture and behavior, and approaches for review committees to both measure and assess team science contributions. In addition, a report of the UK Academy of Medical Sciences (2015) entitled *Improving Recognition of Team Science Contributions in Biomedical Research Careers* likewise finds that perceived lack of recognition of researchers' contributions is a major deterrent to participation in team science and offers ten related recommendations. These include: "all research outputs and grants should include open, transparent, standardized and structured contribution information"; "the use of 'key' positions on publications and grants as the primary indicator of research performance, leadership and independence in team science projects should be replaced by transparent, fair processes"; and "researchers should drive change through their crucial roles as team members, peer reviewers and participants on recruitment, promotion and funding panels."

The US National Institutes of Health has provided support for revising promotion and tenure policies through its Clinical and Translational Science Award (CTSA) program. The CTSA program supports translational and clinical research and aims to foster innovation in research methods, training, and career development. Since 2014, the CTSA funding opportunity announcement (FOA) has emphasized the need to revise promotion criteria to advance new scientific approaches. The 2018 FOA stated that awarded CTSA sites "must advance team science and develop academic promotion criteria that help create a viable career path for translational scientists."[2] The FOA went on to state, "Applicants should devise ways to identify best practices in team science, and to implement successful models. A major obstacle to team science in academic health centers is the traditional promotion and tenure process, which is focused on individual accomplishment. Therefore, applicants should describe how team scientists will be evaluated in the academic promotion process, as well as consideration of how such individuals will be professionally recognized and thus incentivized to engage in collaborations."

Professional organizations also have issued white papers offering recommendations for revisions to recognition and reward systems to address team science in the context of their disciplines, fields, or professions. For example, the American Psychological Association (APA) published a report on merit review considerations for faculty involved in multidisciplinary team

---

[1] www.teamsciencetoolkit.cancer.gov

[2] Clinical and Translational Science Award (U54 Clinical Trial Optional), PAR-18-940, 2018

science (2014) which provided guidelines for dossier preparation and review, such as "clearly describe the researcher's role in driving the project(s) forward"; describe how the contribution is "essential for the overall success of the project" and influenced "the overall outcome/direction of the project," and state whether the contribution was original or a reproduction of the work of others "(e.g., was the software developed with novel, original features that will be used by others in the field, or did the scientist merely modify existing software to make it compatible with the workflow of the project)."

In addition, professional organizations have proposed revision of hiring, promotion, and tenure policies to address cross-disciplinary scholarship (c.f., Pfirman 2011; Pollack 2008) and community-engaged scholarship (c.f., Jordan 2007). For example, the Council of Environmental Deans and Directors of the National Council for Science and the Environment and the Computing Research Association each have produced recommendations for interdisciplinary hiring, promotion, and tenure (Pfirman 2011; Pollack 2008). Community-Campus Partnerships for Health's Community-Engaged Scholarship for Health (CES4Health) Collaborative has produced guidance for navigating promotion and tenure review for community-engaged scholars, who often engage in team science with community partners (Jordan 2007).

These reports, white papers, and guidelines aim to accelerate the evolution of promotion and tenure policies toward more effectively recognizing participation in team science and cross-disciplinary science, by introducing new indicators of scientific contributions. They aim to remedy the traditional model of promotion and tenure review which typically looks to a limited set of indicators—including first authorship, principal investigator roles, and contributions within a disciplinary area of expertise—as evidence of scientific contributions. Participation in team science poses challenges to the effectiveness of these traditional indicators to fully and adequately reflect scientific contributions. As team size grows, the probability of first authorship is reduced, even though one may have an essential role in the team (e.g., as the only

member of the team with a particular knowledge base or methodological skill that is essential to the initiative). As demand increases for an individual's unique skill set (e.g., conceptual, theoretical, methodological, or technical skills; ability to integrate or bridge multiple participating disciplines), as reflected in participation in multiple teams, the number of PI roles the individual can take on is necessarily more limited. In addition, the products of, and publication outlets for, cross-disciplinary team science initiatives may fall outside of one's home discipline, and colleagues therefore may not know how to judge the value of this scholarship.

Under these conditions, early career investigators are in many cases encouraged to limit their involvement in team science and cross-disciplinary inquiry, or steer clear of it entirely for a period of time, to focus on achieving what is needed for their professional advancement within traditional promotion and tenure systems. This may preclude early career investigators from contributing to teams addressing scientific problems for which their skill sets may be ideally suited, and may discourage them from pursuing highly ambitious and potentially highly fruitful scientific questions simply because these questions require team collaboration and/or do not fall within the scholarship of a single discipline.

One potential effect of these patterns is to forestall the growth of meaningful and possibly understudied or newly emerging areas of science, as well as cross-disciplinary research avenues with a decidedly translational bent. A common pattern is the senior investigator who takes on a leadership position for a large team science initiative or transitions into cross-disciplinary scholarship only after having achieved tenure on a traditional discipline-centered independent investigator model. This helps to draw into relief the critical importance of adjusting promotion and tenure policies to recognize and reward a broader range of scientific activities that are essential to cross-disciplinary and/or team science, if we are to develop a workforce that is equipped to apply these approaches when they are the most appropriate approach for a particular scientific goal.

39.4 The Range of Key Scientific Activities for Effective Team Science

A potentially helpful starting point for revision of promotion and tenure policies is careful consideration of long held assumptions about what constitute the key activities of scientists, and the best indicators of these activities. Another potentially fruitful approach is consideration of activities that are not included in our current conceptualization but are essential to the success of team-based and cross-disciplinary science, and the best indicators of these activities. These approaches are the focus of the current section of this chapter.

Traditional indicators of independent scholarly contributions, namely first author publications (or, in the case of some disciplines, last author publications), principal investigator roles, and discipline-based contributions, reflect assumptions about underlying scientific activities. These include, for example, developing the scientific vision for an initiative, gathering and leading a staff to implement the science, making essential contributions to the conduct of the science, producing work that makes a meaningful

scientific contribution, and disseminating scientific findings. These same scientific activities occur in the context of science teams but may require other indicators in order to be captured adequately. In addition, other activities occur in the context of team science that are essential to its success, and it must be captured.

A taxonomy of key scientific activities for team science enables us to elucidate the variety of essential scientific activities required for this approach and consider how these can be documented and assessed in promotion and tenure reviews. Table 39.1 provides examples of such activities. Some of the activities included in the table are common to both single investigator-driven research and team science, such as providing vision for the research and making essential contributions to its conduct. Other activities in the table are entirely absent from single investigator-driven research, for example, those that are specific to team formation, communication, and coordination. (For a thorough discussion of approaches for successfully planning and carrying out each activity, see the concluding chapter in this book, authored by Hall et al. 2019. For an in-depth discussion of how these activities map to phases in the life cycle of a cross-

Table 39.1 Key scientific activities for effective team science

Scientific goals	Key scientific activities
Conceptualize the team science initiative	• Identify the scientific problem space and the disciplines and fields needed to address it/ advance it in desired direction(s)
Create the science team	• Identify and recruit team members with the specific disciplinary, field-based, professional, policy, and/or other expertise needed to address the scientific problem • Compose a team of the right size and mix of expertise to successfully pursue the scientific goals • Obtain the necessary institutional commitments (across universities, government agencies, etc.) to enable team members to participate with full institutional recognition
Engage in cross-disciplinary and cross-field collaboration	• Enable communication across team members from different disciplines and fields by facilitating development of shared terminology, and if needed, conceptual, theoretical, and methodological knowledge specific to the initiative
Develop a shared scientific goal among team members	• Enable scientific exchange among all team members to develop shared scientific goals for the initiative • Contribute unique expertise to influence the development of the scientific goals, as well as research questions and methods, within the context of the team science initiative • Facilitate development of a shared mental model of the science (e.g., conceptual model) including how each discipline or field represented by members of the team makes a unique contribution toward the scientific goal

(continued)

Table 39.1   (continued)

Scientific goals	Key scientific activities
Implement the science	• Contribute unique conceptual, theoretical, or methodological expertise rooted in a particular discipline • Contribute unique skills in bridging disciplines and/or fields • Contribute specialized technical skills, such as designing data collection and storage systems specifically for the data generated in the project, which may include unique complexities such as bridging levels of analysis, geographic sites, etc., and/or developing new laboratory techniques, experimental resources, and/or data analytic software essential to carrying out the science • Facilitate the development, and revision/maintenance as necessary, of a shared mental model of how team members interact to implement the science and, as relevant, how they interact to develop and implement translational applications • Develop and maintain communication and task coordination systems to support team collaboration, including systems that cross boundaries such as institutions and time zones • Manage scientific and interpersonal conflict among team members • Engage team members in trainings and or reflective activities (e.g., debriefings) that enhance team collaboration • Secure a range of resources (e.g., equipment, software, funding, staffing) necessary to fully and successfully carry out the planned science
Engage in cross-center initiatives, networks, and multi-team systems	• Collaboratively develop shared leadership model • Coordinate goals and activities across collaborating entities • Develop communication and coordination systems that function across collaborating entities • Develop data sharing, data integration, and collaborative data analysis platforms as needed across collaborating entities that conform to the technological limitations and standards in place in said entities • Develop practices and procedures (e.g., operating manuals) for addressing key issues in a collaboration, including data sharing, data ownership, patent rights, order of authors, etc.
Advance the science along the translational continuum	• Identify and engage scientist and nonscientist collaborators to advance the science along the translational continuum • Revisit processes to develop shared goals, shared mental model of the contributions of each represented area of expertise, and shared mental model of team members' contributions and task coordination, given new team composition • Contribute unique skills in bridging scientific disciplines/fields with policy/programmatic approaches/goals/applications

disciplinary team science initiative, and scientific benchmarks of progress, see Hall et al. 2012.)

To recognize many of these essential team science activities in promotion and tenure policies, new indicators need to be adopted. One example is essential contributions to the design, implementation, and ultimate success of the science that was carried out. Sources of evidence may include annotation within the dossier in which, for articles where one is not first author (or, to reiterate, for some disciplines, last author), the individual's contributions to the science are described with an eye toward explicating the unique scientific contributions that were made, and how these were necessary for the advancement of the work. Another recommended source of evidence is letters from collaborators that explain one's contributions to a particular research initiative, and in what ways these were essential to the success of the initiative.

A key component that is complementary to the above is the value of the scholarship produced by the team initiative. When the scholarship is not within one's department/home discipline, letters from third-party recommenders rooted in other relevant disciplines can describe the value of the work, including, for example, how it contributes to advancing the science in other disciplines or fields, or how it addresses the interstices among disciplines and fields by bridging or integrating knowledge. A complementary indicator is disciplinary spread of citations, demonstrating the audience for the scholarship, and its influence, across disciplines and fields. Ongoing research in the SciTS field will continue to build our understanding of key scientific activities for effective team science, the impact of these activities on scientific outcomes, and indicators of these activities' quality and impact.

The recommendations provided here fall within a broader movement to develop indicators of scientific contributions that go beyond traditional documentation. For example, peer review journals increasingly are requiring the inclusion of brief statements concerning each author's role. The CASRAI CRediT (Contributor Roles Taxonomy) taxonomy of 14 different scientific activities typical of coauthors of scientific scholarship (CASRAI 2018) has been adopted by over 100 journals worldwide (Academy of Medical Sciences 2019) to help inform development of statements of author contributions. It has been endorsed by the UK Academy of Medical Sciences as an approach "to attribute recognition for a wider range of contributions than might have been traditional in single principal investigator (PI)-led teams" (Academy of Medical Sciences 2019). Another model is the OpenVIVO Contribution Role Ontology (Ilik et al. 2018), with 60 contribution roles available for post-publication annotation to allow researchers to select the exact role(s) they had on each of their scholarly works, including but not limited to peer review publications. Other examples include journals that publish peer reviews online with attribution, which are considered contributions to the published science (Hesse 2014); websites that track contributions to the science in the form of peer reviews; digital object identifiers (DOIs) for scientific products such as software and data sets to enable them to be directly cited and thereby recognized; and citable manuscripts describing data sets, also called "data papers" (Rolland 2016).

The burgeoning interest in expanding recognition and reward systems to address recent changes in how science is performed means that recommendations for new indicators of scientific contributions continue to be developed (Moher et al. 2018). For example, O'Carroll et al. (2017) propose evaluation criteria to assess open science activities and products. Examples address for example, scientific leadership (e.g., driving policy and practice in open science) and research implementation (e.g., risk management related to open sharing of data sets) that are unique to open science. The Next-Generation Metrics Group of the Open Science Policy Platform highlights the need for metrics that reflect the quality, value, and potential impact of research outputs in a way that incentivizes open science (Hormia-Poutanen et al. 2017). What these efforts—whether for team science or for open science—have in common is the ultimate goal of recognizing and rewarding scientific behaviors of collaboration, transparency, and inclusiveness that are now understood by many as essential to advancing scientific discovery.

39.5 Implications for Recognizing a Range of Scientific Roles in Team Science

The activities highlighted in Table 39.1 and additional key scientific activities for team science may be carried out by principal investigators, science team members, academic administrators, and project managers. For small science teams, the principal investigator may be able to carry out all of the leadership, coordination, and communication activities described in the table. But in larger team science initiatives, including research centers, consortia, and networks, these activities are complex and require specialized knowledge and skills, not to mention significant time investments, to be carried out effectively.

As a result of the increasing prevalence of large team science initiatives, new professional roles are emerging in which PhD trained scientists are taking on the specialized scientific activities involved in facilitating effective team processes in these initiatives. These individuals have specialized knowledge in the composition, leadership, management, and administration of large teams/multi-team systems, and often have additional expertise in cross-disciplinary and cross-field integration. They may be employed full- or part-time on one or more initiatives simultaneously, with the express aim of successfully advancing collaborative processes in order to optimize the success of the science. For a detailed discussion of these emerging professional roles in team science, also called "skills specialists," see the chapters in this volume by Hendren and Ku 2019 and by Carter et al. 2019, highlighting such roles as the Interdisciplinary Executive Scientists and the Research Development Professional. Also see the chapter in this volume by Rolland (2019), highlighting the role of Coordination Centers to facilitate cross-site coordination and collaboration in multi-site research initiatives. Rolland discusses both the organizational structures and professional roles involved in these centers.

Many scientists in these specialized roles find that traditional promotion and tenure criteria are poorly suited to capturing their scientific contributions, although colleagues in team science initiatives may see their work as essential to the quality of the scientific products. Reflecting this reality, the UK Academy of Medical Sciences recommends in its most recent report on team science (2019) that "clear career paths and development opportunities should be provided for researchers outside of the 'PI track' who play key roles in (and provide key competencies to) team science, such as skills specialists," to incentivize participation in these career paths.

While some have placed these roles outside of the tenure system (e.g., Canadian Academy of Health Sciences 2017; Hall 2018), current trends point to the benefits of a more flexible approach. The activity-based approaches to promotion and tenure review proposed in this chapter help to illuminate the similarity of scientific activities across roles, including principal investigators and skills specialists. Distinction versus overlap in such activities across roles may vary depending on the size and scale of a project. For instance, in large projects some activities (e.g., management, coordination activities) may be clearly divided across multiple individuals with distinct roles, such as the principal investigator and a skills specialist, whereas in smaller projects the principal investigator may be responsible for all of these activities. The activity-based approach to assessment of scientific contributions shifts the focus of review from roles (e.g., first author, last author, principal investigator, and specialized roles such as the Interdisciplinary Executive Scientists) to scientific activities, regardless of one's professional title. This approach enables individuals in specialized roles to participate either inside or outside of tenure systems at their institutions.

39.6   Broader Implications

When the full range of scientific activities that are key to success in team science is comprehensively considered and accounted for in promotion and tenure review, the contributions of all researchers engaged in team science can be robustly and effectively recognized. This level of acknowledgement would interact with other mutually reinforcing scientific trends described in this chapter to advance cross-disciplinary team science approaches in the scientific enterprise.

As part of this system of interacting influences, changes in promotion and tenure policies likely would lead to related changes. These are likely to include increased recruitment of faculty with expertise in cross-disciplinarity and team science, and enhancements to undergraduate and graduate training to prepare trainees for team science. These interrelated changes are, in fact, already underway in some academic institutions.

A focus in hiring, promotion, and tenure policies on scientific activities and their value to the science enterprise also would help to provide greater understanding of the critical contributions of skills specialists such as the Interdisciplinary Executive Scientists and Research Development Professional. In addition, it might help to inform ongoing efforts to develop training opportunities and career development opportunities specific to these roles (Hendren and Ku 2019, this book; Hendren 2014).

Recognition of the value of non-principal investigator scientists is already being translated into practice by funding agencies. For example, in 2018 the US National Cancer Institute introduced a new funding mechanism, called the NCI Research Specialist Award, that encourages the development of stable research career opportunities for staff scientists. It provides direct salary support so these individuals are not solely dependent on NCI grants held by others for career continuity.

In addition, recognition of the range of essential activities for team science in promotion and tenure criteria would work in consort with current trends at US federal funding agencies that require that investigators describe capabilities and resources underlying successful implementation of the science. One example is the project co-leadership plans now required in funding applications for multiple principal investigator awards from the National Institutes of Health (National Institutes of Health). Another example is recent interest from multiple federal funding agencies in collaboration plans, which may be submitted with grant applications and provide detailed plans for the successful implementation of a large team science initiative. (For more on this topic, see the concluding chapter in this book by Hall et al. 2019.)

Together, the proposed changes to promotion and tenure policies explored in this chapter, and their probable ripple effects, would contribute to a scientific workforce with a more diverse skill set—one that includes the skills needed for both independent and team-based research as well as both unidisciplinary and cross-disciplinary research. They also would enable the use of team science whenever it is the approach that is best suited to addressing a particular scientific problem.

Of course, additional changes in academia will be needed to fully achieve this vision. These include changes to administrative and budgetary systems (e.g., shared indirect costs) and norms that enable cross-departmental and team-based research. Such changes might include mapping of budgets to support key activities, including staffing (e.g., an Interdisciplinary Executive Scientist as a full-time member of a large team, center, or network), communication and coordination infrastructure, consultants as needed (e.g., for facilitated quality improvement-oriented reflection on team processes), and other resources necessary for effective team collaboration (e.g., resources related to data harmonization and database integration). They might also include academic restructuring as well as reorganization of the physical workplace, as mentioned earlier in this chapter.

This discussion is particularly relevant to scientists working in academia. However, it is also relevant to scientists operating in a broad range of contexts, including government and industry, who engage in a wide range of activities, such as setting research agendas at federal agencies, leading scientific initiatives, and serving as board members of private companies. They, too, are influenced by their institutions' systems for recognition and reward. In addition, they may have their hand on potential levers of change in promotion and tenure policies, for example, as funders who can require collaboration plans in funding applications that explicitly lay out staff capabilities and team plans around the activities represented in Table 39.1, and who can develop funding opportunities that provide financial support for these key activities.

39.7 Summary and Conclusions

To maximize the beneficial use of team science, including cross-disciplinary team science, toward solving scientific and societal problems, we must consider all influences on the adoption and success of these approaches. Promotion and tenure policies are a key influence that have been slow to evolve to reflect the growing prevalence of team science.

This chapter described the rationale for revising promotion and tenure policies, including the limitations of the current system to adequately capture the range of scientific activities involved in team science. It then highlighted a range of related changes in the culture of the scientific enterprise that influence change in promotion and tenure policies. It summarized key points from a number of white papers and reports that make the case for revisions to promotion and tenure policies and provided examples of specific recommendations and guidelines.

The chapter then proposed a wide-ranging set of scientific activities that contribute to success in team science that can be used to undergird revisions to promotion and tenure policies in order to comprehensively account for and assess the quality of an individual's scientific contributions to team science. Such a framework shifts the focus of promotion and tenure review from scientific roles to scientific activities. This shift reflects the reality of significant overlap in activities across professional roles in many team science initiatives, including across investigators and specialized roles for team science, with implications for how scientists working in specialized roles are recognized and rewarded. This shift also has potential implications for hiring, training, and establishment of new career pathways. Finally, it has broad implications for how scientific activities specific to team science are reflected in budgets, academic structures, funding, and the culture of scientific research organizations.

In closing, the time is ripe for efforts focused on the revision of promotion and tenure policies to more effectively recognize scientific contributions made in the context of team science. These efforts, in conjunction with efforts to recognize and reward related approaches, including cross-disciplinarity, community engagement, and open science, together reflect and will help to facilitate the future of science in the twenty-first century: one that leverages collaborative, cross-disciplinary, open, and reproducible science to most effectively achieve our scientific and related societal goals.

Acknowledgement This project has been funded in whole or in part with federal funds from the National Cancer Institute, National Institutes of Health, under Contract No. HHSN261200800001E. The content of this publication does not necessarily reflect the views or policies of the Department of Health and Human Services, nor does mention of trade names, commercial products, or organizations imply endorsement by the US Government.

References

Academy of Medical Sciences. Improving recognition of team science contributions in biomedical research careers. 2015. https://acmedsci.ac.uk/file-download/38721-56defebabba91.pdf. Accessed 30 Dec 2018.

Academy of Medical Sciences. From innovation to implementation: team science two years on. 2019. https://acmedsci.ac.uk/file-download/29694340. Accessed 15 Feb 2019.

American Psychological Association Board of Scientific Affairs. Appointment, tenure, promotion, and merit review considerations for psychologists with joint faculty appointments and involvement in interdisciplinary/multidisciplinary research and scholarship: a resource document. 2014. https://www.apa.org/science/leadership/bsa/interdisciplinary-joint-appointments.pdf. Accessed 30 Dec 2018.

Bennett M, Gadlin H. Conflict prevention and management in science teams. In: Hall KL, Vogel AL, Croyle RT, editors. Strategies for team science success: handbook of evidence-based principles for cross-disciplinary science and practical lessons learned from health researchers. New York, NY: Springer; 2019. p. 774.

Bennett M, Nelan R, Steeves B, Thornhill J. The interrelationship of people, space, operations, institutional leadership, and training in fostering a team approach in health sciences research at the University of Saskatchewan. In: Hall KL, Vogel AL, Croyle RT, Strategies for team science success: handbook of evidence-based principles for cross-disciplinary science and practical lessons learned from health researchers. New York, NY: Springer. 2019

Berger NA. How leadership can support attainment of cross-disciplinary scientific goals. In: Hall KL, Vogel AL, Croyle RT, Strategies for team science success: handbook of evidence-based principles for cross-disciplinary science and practical lessons learned from health researchers. New York, NY: Springer. 2019

Canadian Academy of Health Sciences. Academic recognition of team science: how to optimize the Canadian academic system. Ottawa (ON): The Expert Panel on Academic Recognition of Team Science in Canada, CAHS. 2017. https://www.cahs-acss.ca/academic-recognition-of-team-science-how-to-optimize-the-canadian-academic-system/? Accessed 30 Dec 2018.

Carter S, Carlson S, Crockett J, Falk-Krzesinski HJ, Lewis K, Endemano Walker B. The role of research development professionals in supporting team science. In: Hall KL, Vogel AL, Croyle RT, editors. Strategies for team science success: handbook of evidence-based principles for cross-disciplinary science and practical lessons learned from health researchers. New York, NY: Springer; 2019.

CASRAI. CRediT. n.d.. https://casrai.org/credit. Accessed 18 Dec 2018.

Christen SP, Levine AJ. Facilitating cross-disciplinary interactions to stimulate innovation: stand up to cancer's matchmaking convergence ideas lab. In: Hall KL, Vogel AL, Croyle RT, editors. Strategies for team science success: handbook of evidence-based principles for cross-disciplinary science and practical lessons learned from health researchers. New York, NY: Springer; 2019.

Crow MM, Dabars WB. Restructuring research universities to advance interdisciplinary collaboration. In: Hall KL, Vogel AL, Croyle RT, editors. Strategies for team science success: handbook of evidence-based principles for cross-disciplinary science and practical lessons learned from health researchers. New York, NY: Springer; 2019.

Falk-Krzesinski HJ. Team science rewards: a collaborative study on promotion & tenure policy. In: Keynote Presentation at the 2013 Annual International Science of Team Science Conference. Chicago, IL, USA. 2013.

Fiore SM, Gabelica C, Wiltshire T, Stokols D. Training to be a (team) scientist. In: Hall KL, Vogel AL, Croyle RT, editors. Strategies for team science success: handbook of evidence-based principles for cross-disciplinary science and practical lessons learned from health researchers. New York, NY: Springer; 2019.

Gehlert S. Developing a shared mental model in the context of center initiative. In: Hall KL, Vogel AL, Croyle RT, editors. Strategies for team science success: handbook of evidence-based principles for cross-disciplinary science and practical lessons learned from health researchers. New York, NY: Springer; 2019.

Hall KL. Science of team science: informing strategic institutional support. In: Virtual presentation to the California state university system annual science deans meeting, Los Angeles, CA. 2018.

Hall KL, Vogel AL, Crowston K. Comprehensive collaboration plans: practical considerations spanning across individual collaborators to institutional supports. In: Hall KL, Vogel AL, Croyle RT, editors. Strategies for team science success: handbook of evidence-based principles for cross-disciplinary science and practical lessons learned from health researchers. New York, NY: Springer; 2019.

Hall KL, Vogel AL, Stipelman B, Stokols D, Morgan G, Gehlert S. A four-phase model of transdisciplinary team-based research: goals, team processes, and strategies. Transl Behav Med. 2012;2:415–30.

Hall KL, Vogel AL, Huang GC, Serrano KJ, Rice EL, Tsakraklides SP, Fiore SM. The science of team science: a review of the empirical evidence and research gaps on collaboration in science. Am Psychol. 2018;73(4):532–48.

Hendren CO. "Inreach" and the Interdisciplinary Executive Scientist: The missing puzzle pieces for effective interdisciplinary research. Blog post on the Team Science Toolkit. 2014. https://team-sciencetoolkit.cancer.gov/Public/ExpertBlog.aspx?tid=4&rid=1838. Accessed 30 Dec 2018.

Hendren CO, Ku S. The interdisciplinary executive scientist: connecting scientific ideas, resources and people. In: Hall KL, Vogel AL, Croyle RT, editors. Strategies for team science success: handbook of evidence-based principles for cross-disciplinary science and practical lessons learned from health researchers. New York, NY: Springer; 2019.

Hesse BW. Can principles of effective team science promote more robust and reproducible research? 2014. https://teamsciencetoolkit.cancer.gov/Public/ExpertBlog.aspx?tid=4#callout. Accessed 18 Dec 2018.

Hormia-Poutanen K, Kristiansen E, Lawrence R, Leonelli S, Manola N, Méndez E, Rossel C, Vignoli M, Agostinho MD. Recommendations of the OSPP on next-generation metrics. A report of the altmetrics working group of the open science policy platform. 2017.

Ilik V, Conlon M, Triggs G, White M, Javed M. Open VIVO: transparency in scholarship. Frontiers in Research Metrics Analysis. 2018;1:1–11.

Institute of Medicine. Facilitating interdisciplinary research. Washington, DC: The National Academies Press; 2005. https://doi.org/10.17226/11153.

Jain P, Klein D. Precollaboration framework: academic/industry partnerships: mobile and wearable technologies for behavioral science. In: Hall KL, Vogel AL, Croyle RT, editors. Strategies for team science success: handbook of evidence-based principles for cross-disciplinary science and practical lessons learned from health researchers. New York, NY: Springer; 2019.

Jones BF, Wuchty S, Uzzi B. Multi-university research teams: shifting impact, geography, and stratification in science. Science. 2008;322(590S):1259–62.

Jordan C (Editor). Community-engaged scholarship review, promotion & tenure package. In: Peer Review Workgroup, Community-Engaged Scholarship for Health Collaborative, Community-Campus Partnerships for Health. 2007. https://www.ccphealth.org/wp-content/uploads/2017/10/CES_RPT_Package.pdf. Accessed 18 Dec 2018.

Klein JT, Falk-Krzesinski HJ. Interdisciplinarity and collaborative work: framing promotion and tenure practices and policies. Res Policy. 2017;46:1055–61.

Kozlowski SWJ, Bell BS. Evidence-based principles and strategies for optimizing team functioning and performance in science teams. In: Hall KL, Vogel AL, Croyle RT, editors. Strategies for team science success: handbook of evidence-based principles for cross-disciplinary science and practical lessons learned from health researchers. New York, NY: Springer; 2019.

McEvoy J III. Multi-and interdisciplinary research- problems of initiation, control, integration and reward. Policy Sci. 1972;3(2):201–8.

Moher D, Naudet F, Cristea IA, Miedema F, Ioannidis JPA, Goodman SN. Assessing scientists for hiring, promotion, and tenure. PLoS Biol. 2018;16(3):e2004089.

NASEM (National Academy of Sciences, National Academy of Engineering, and Institute of Medicine). Facilitating interdisciplinary research. Washington, DC: The National Academies Press; 2005. https://doi.org/10.17226/11153.

National Institutes of Health. Multiple principal investigators. n.d.. https://grants.nih.gov/grants/multi_pi/. Accessed 18 Dec 2018.

National Research Council. Convergence: facilitating transdisciplinary integration of life sciences, physical sciences, engineering, and beyond. Washington, DC: The National Academies Press. 2014. https://www.nap.edu/catalog/18722/convergence-facilitating-transdisciplinary-integration-of-life-sciences-physical-sciences-engineering. Accessed 18 Dec 2018.

National Research Council. Enhancing the Effectiveness of Team Science. Washington, DC: The National Academies Press. 2015. https://www.nap.edu/catalog/19007/enhancing-the-effectiveness-of-team-science. Accessed 30 Dec 2018.

National Science Foundation. Profiles in team science. n.d.. http://depts.washington.edu/teamsci/welcome.html. Accessed 30 Dec 2018.

Nurius PS, Kemp SP. Individual level competencies for team collaboration with cross-disciplinary researchers and stakeholders. In: Hall KL, Vogel AL, Croyle RT, editors. Strategies for team science success: handbook of evidence-based principles for cross-disciplinary science and practical lessons learned from health researchers. New York, NY: Springer; 2019.

O'Carroll C, Rentier B, Valdes CC, Esposito F, Kaunismaa E, Maas K, Metcalfe J, McAllister D, Vandevelde K. Evaluation of research careers fully acknowledging open science practices: rewards, incentives and/or recognition for researchers practicing open science. In: Report of the European commission directorate-general for research and innovation working group on rewards under open science. 2017.

O'Rourke M, Crowley S, Laursen B, Robinson B, Vasko SE. Disciplinary diversity in teams: integrative approaches from unidisciplinarity to transdisciplinarity. In: Hall KL, Vogel AL, Croyle RT, editors. Strategies for team science success: handbook of evidence-based principles for cross-disciplinary science and practical lessons learned from health researchers. New York, NY: Springer; 2019.

Owen-Smith J. Workplace design, collaboration, and discovery. In: Paper commissioned by the National Research Council Committee on the Science of Team Science. 2013. https://sites.nationalacademies.org/cs/groups/dbassesite/documents/webpage/dbasse_085437.pdf. Accessed 30 Dec 2018.

Pfirman S (Eds). Interdisciplinary hiring, tenure and promotion: guidance for individuals and institutions. In: The Council of Environmental Deans and Directors of the National Council for Science and the Environment. 2011. https://s3.amazonaws.com/academia.edu.documents/37064690/Intedisciplinary_Hiring_Report_FINAL.pdf? Accessed 30 Dec 2018.

Pohl C, Wuelser G. Methods for co-production of knowledge among diverse disciplines and stakeholders. In: Hall KL, Vogel AL, Croyle RT, editors. Strategies for team science success: handbook of evidence-based principles for cross-disciplinary science and practical lessons learned from health researchers. New York, NY: Springer; 2019.

Pollack M. Best practices in promotion and tenure of interdisciplinary faculty. Computing Research Association Memo. 2008. https://www.teamsciencetoolkit.cancer.gov/Public/TSResourceBiblio.aspx?tid=3&rid=2201. Accessed 30 Dec 2018.

Rolland B. Data sharing and reuse: expanding our concept of collaboration. 2016. https://teamsciencetoolkit.cancer.gov/Public/ExpertBlog.aspx?tid=4#callout. Accessed 18 Dec 2018.

Salazar M, Widmer K, Doiron K, Lant TK. Leader integrative capabilities: a catalyst for effective interdisciplinary teams. In: Hall KL, Vogel AL, Croyle RT, editors. Strategies for team science success: handbook of evidence-based principles for cross-disciplinary science and practical lessons learned from health researchers. New York, NY: Springer; 2019.

Schmitz KH, Gehlert S, Patterson RE, Colditz GA, Chavarro JE, Hu FB, Neuhouser ML, Sturgeon KM, Thornquist M, Tobias D, Nebeling LC. TREC to WHERE? Transdisciplinary research on energetics and cancer. Clin Cancer Res. 2016;22(7):1565–71.

Spring B, Pfammatter A, Conroy DE. Continuing professional development for team science. In: Hall KL, Vogel AL, Croyle RT, editors. Strategies for team science success: handbook of evidence-based principles for cross-disciplinary science and practical lessons learned from health researchers. New York, NY: Springer; 2019.

Stone AR. The interdisciplinary research team. J Appl Behav Sci. 1969;5(3):351–65.

Twyman M, Contractor N. Team assembly. In: Hall KL, Vogel AL, Croyle RT, editors. Strategies for team science success: handbook of evidence-based principles for cross-disciplinary science and practical lessons learned from health researchers. New York, NY: Springer; 2019.

Vogel AL, Hall KL, Fiore SM, Klein JT, Bennett LM, Gadlin H, Stokols D, Nebeling L, Wuchty S, Patrick K, Spotts EL, Pohl C, Riley WT, Falk-Krzesinski HJ. The team science toolkit: enhancing research collaboration through online knowledge sharing. Am J Prev Med. 2013;45(6):787–9.

Vogel AL, Stipelman BA, Hall KL, Stokols D, Nebeling L, Spruijt-Metz D. Pioneering the transdisciplinary team science approach: lessons learned from national cancer institute grantees. The Journal of Translational Medicine and Epidemiology. 2014;2(2):1027.

Warnecke RB, Oh A, Breen N, Gehlert S, Paskett E, Tucker KL, Lurie N, Rebbeck T, Goodwin J, Flack J, Srinivasan S, Kerner J, Heurtin-Roberts S, Abeles R, Tyson FL, Patmios G, Hiatt RA. Approaching health disparities from a population perspective: the national institutes of health centers for population health and health disparities. Am J Public Health. 2008;98(9):1608–15.

Wuchty S, Jones BF, Uzzi B. The increasing dominance of teams in production of knowledge. Science. 2007;316:1036–9.

The Interrelationship of People, Space, Operations, Institutional Leadership, and Training in Fostering a Team Approach in Health Sciences Research at the University of Saskatchewan

40

L. Michelle Bennett, Rachel Nelan, Brad Steeves, and Jim Thornhill

Contents

40.1 Introduction

In the mid-2000s, the University of Saskatchewan in Saskatoon, Saskatchewan Canada, decided to integrate a collaborative research and teaching approach into its Health Sciences enterprise. It was envisioned that an interdisciplinary approach would attract research funding, help maximize the research impact of the science performed and conducted, enhance clinical research, and additionally, increase opportunities for research trainees in all programs and at all levels of training (undergraduate, graduate, post-doctorate, health professional students, residents, and fellows).

With the successful award of a \$350+M grant from the Provincial government in 2005, the University embarked on an ambitious project to build an Academic Health Sciences Complex (AHSC) based on a team science approach. The newly envisioned AHSC would address eight core teaching, research, and service objectives; one of which was *the promotion of health/biomedical/clinical research through the establishment of collaborative research teams (clusters) in* areas of need, pulling together existing strengths of the University and Province.

Senior administrators were confident that a collaborative team research approach would also greatly enhance the "One Health" (advancing the health of the interrelated systems of humans, animals, and environment) multidisciplinary opportunities for faculty and students that were being developed across campus. A number of research disciplines would be included under the "One

L. M. Bennett (✉)
Center for Research Strategy, National Cancer Institute, Bethesda, MD, USA
e-mail: LMBennett@nih.gov

R. Nelan
Flad Architects, Madison, WI, USA

B. Steeves
Operations, Academic Health Sciences Center, University of Saskatchewan, Saskatoon, Canada

J. Thornhill
College of Medicine, University of Saskatchewan, Saskatoon, Canada

© Springer Nature Switzerland AG 2019
K. L. Hall et al. (eds.), *Strategies for Team Science Success*,
https://doi.org/10.1007/978-3-030-20992-6_40

509

Health" umbrella including multidisciplinary projects originating from the nursing, medical, dental, veterinary, pharmacy, nutritional, physical therapy, and clinical psychology health colleges/programs on campus as well as the new Schools of Public Health and Public Policy. The AHSC would also greatly complement the more than $1 billion investment over the last 20 years on health research infrastructure, including the Canadian Light Source Synchrotron with over 17 beamlines, a cyclotron for medical and research isotopes, the Vaccine and Infectious Disease Organization, and the Intervac level 3 biocontainment facility, as well as the Canadian Centre for Health & Safety in Agriculture (CCHSA). To fulfill the collaborative research goals of the AHSC, many new strategic initiatives would be developed and implemented. In parallel, new additions and renewals to the existing laboratory facilities would be built to provide the physical environment in which team science could thrive.

Organizationally, the University of Saskatchewan planned to transform from research aligned within five Basic Science Departments in the College of Medicine and in the nondepartmentalized College of Pharmacy and Nutrition to eight interdisciplinary biomedical health clusters from these units. These clusters were aligned and designated by leadership based on common thematic areas of research, anticipating synergies among them. They were balanced as much as possible with respect to research, teaching, and clinical responsibilities—recognizing that it would take time to achieve the desired equilibrium.

Two primary goals of this project were the enhancement of Inter-Professional Health Education and Inter-Disciplinary Health Research. This goal had a dual mission: to ensure that the graduate Health Science professionals were better prepared to deliver health care to the province to achieve better patient outcomes by working across disciplines, and second, to build a culture of collaborative Team Science to attract greater levels of research funding that would also ultimately contribute to better patient outcomes.

As the University of Saskatchewan leadership moved this vision forward, it was keenly mindful of five interacting dimensions: people, space, operations, institutional leadership, and training.

40.2 People

40.2.1 Working with the Faculty to Embrace a Team Science Culture

Faculty reaction to the impending move and the associated changes demonstrated both enthusiasm and apprehension. The expressions of apprehension were not synonymous with resistance or opposition. Instead, they were indicators of a realistic stance toward the move. Recognizing change is necessarily disruptive helps prepare people to adjust to and take responsibility.

Collaboration is a threat to one's power, status, and autonomy; even those most enthused about collaboration. These issues could be addressed using a multi-pronged approach including individual interactions, discussions within clustered groups, through shared experiences over time and through visible success.

The individuals who voiced concerns about the move could be loosely divided into three groups. The first group of scientists successfully worked autonomously and was worried how the new arrangements might disrupt what they are doing and impede their continued success. The second group of scientists was already quite successful in working collaboratively, although with colleagues other than those with whom they may be clustered in the future. This group was worried that their current successful collaborations would be disrupted or there would be pressure to collaborate with others in their cluster, taking time and energy away from their current successful collaborations. The third group included individuals who had a primary teaching mission and for whom the overall shift to a collaborative research emphasis was a threat to their current identity and place in the university.

Throughout this process, from its announcement in 2005 through planning and construction to occupancy, the faculty were all equivalent in terms of their potential to participate in the restructured program. Expectations for the different groups needed to be outlined as well as how the vision and communication strategy would align for each.

When shifting the organization to a team science research emphasis, there were many organizational questions to be addressed. The answers to the following questions could not all be answered immediately, yet they did provide a framework for being mindful of the evolution of faculty concerns and working with them over time as roles and responsibilities were refined and expectations were put in place.

- Funding levels differed between colleges. What did this mean when they come together to collaborate? Is parity important in a research cluster model?
- Some colleges needed new hires to fill teaching gaps—as opposed to having the luxury of hiring to fill research needs. What impact would this have?
- Some faculty members had very heavy teaching loads—how would this be balanced with research? And reviewed and rewarded?

40.2.2 Communicating a New Research Paradigm with the Faculty

As part of the overall process, it was important for the University to develop a communications plan grounded in the strategic plan and overall vision. Clear messages about the organizational vision were vital so everyone could understand their role. In addition, articulation of the strategy being undertaken was important so those individuals involved could be active participants in the process. It was also critical to clearly outline processes, procedures, and to set expectations so all knew what was expected of them as well as what they could expect from leadership. Mechanisms for enhancing communication included, but were not limited to, short presentations by leadership to the entire community with time for questions; meetings with cluster leaders to create two-way channels of communication and to provide clarity about expectations, roles, and responsibilities as well as what power they do and do not have in this role; sharing information broadly; and empowering individuals to participate in the overall effort.

In order for the organizational leadership to communicate clearly with the community, they needed to establish evaluation metrics to assess success. Basically, how will the future state of the organization be evaluated? The University needed to establish a baseline understanding of where the academic community was with respect to how time was divided among research, teaching, and service; and how to assess the degree of collaboration in research productivity through grant success; publication success; and technology transfer accomplishments. These metrics needed to be tracked into the future so that progress toward the goals could be noted, measured, and reported.

40.2.3 Faculty Recognition and Reward in a Team Environment

Creating a new culture that valued collaboration and team science required assuring the community that the review and reward structure would be aligned with University expectations and messages. If expectations existed for collaborative work, the review and reward system needed to recognize independent achievement in the context of collaborative efforts.

One way the University has embraced the rewards and recognition challenge of team science is by establishing a University Steering Committee to write a concept paper regarding rewards and recognition for faculty contributions to collaborative research projects. This concept paper has been developed following a university-wide survey of all faculty asking their views about the barriers for conducting collaborative research on campus and the metrics used for assessing collaborative research for promotion, tenure, and merit decisions. The survey process included follow-up group discussions with tenured and untenured faculty in departmentalized and nondepartmentalized colleges, as well as senior administrators (Department Heads, Associate Deans and Deans of Colleges, and University Vice Presidents). An extensive literature search of how other academic institutions are currently rewarding faculty involved with collaborative research projects was conducted, as well. The analysis of these three datasets (research, surveys, and discussion groups) formed the basis of a report back to the entire institutional community. The report included 12 Departmental, College, and University recommendations for evaluating current promotion, tenure, and merit guidelines for objectively recognizing and rewarding individual faculty contributions in the context of collaborative research endeavors. Recommendations included, for example, asking units if the use of MOUs, annotated CVs, and/or internationally known guidelines of authorship were helpful tools in properly assessing collaborative research work? Or, should the university faculty assessing collaborative scholarship undergo some level of competency training? Pilot studies are currently underway in several Colleges to determine if and how the recommendations might be applied to their specific disciplines. This project emphasizes the message from University leadership that team science is important, valued, and expected to be part of the academic culture.

During the Rewards and Recognition project, it has been important to keep in mind that in reviewing and rewarding faculty for their academic activities they have differences in their balance of time for teaching and research. It will be important for the committees formed to understand they will have a tremendous responsibility for modeling the behavior of future Departmental and College reviewers, through the development of new guidelines so committees can objectively assess individual accomplishments of faculty in the future, working within collaborative settings.

40.2.4 Setting Research Expectations in a Team Environment

Implementing an organizational wide effort in team science and collaboration is a huge undertaking. There are many people involved with any decision made on a daily basis. Not all decisions can be, or should be, made at the highest levels of the organization, especially if there is an interest to ensure the community is engaged and participative. Pushing decision-making and cluster-

specific strategies for operations and functioning to the lowest levels of the organization frees up time for administrative leadership, empowers clusters and teams, and provides roles and responsibilities to individuals at many different levels of the organization. In addition to top-down communication, strategies were needed for both bottom-up and cross-organizational interactions.

During times of change, people look for certainty, predictability, and clarity. From an institutional perspective, it is useful, as much as possible, to make the uncertain, certain (even if it is one small step at a time), to provide clarity about expectations so people can plan, and to assure there is understanding about the new rules and how they apply to the individual. These activities can help build and establish trust at the organizational level.

There are many moving parts at an institution engaged in shifting its culture to one that embraces and promotes collaborative research. For the University of Saskatchewan, there was an opportunity to put staff in place whose explicit role was to tend to the individual, cluster, training, and institutional needs surrounding this cultural evolution. Several functional roles were put in place to meet needs at multiple levels. For example, lab coordinators/managers were to help integrate the laboratories when the clusters were brought together, and operational committees were developed to help with assimilation into the new culture. In addition, interdisciplinary research training programs for graduate students and continued education for post-docs and faculty were high priorities.

40.3 Operations

40.3.1 Aligning Researcher Cluster Requirements in Open Labs Designed to Encourage Sustained Collaboration

The project began as a major investment in new infrastructure for the Health Sciences. The existing infrastructure was old, hard to adapt to meet the ever-changing research demands, had code and regulatory challenges and was "assigned" to academic departments which over time had increased their faculty/researcher complement, making space allocation problematic within the "assigned space boundaries."

Due to the above issues, plus the never-ending renovations of existing spaces to accommodate the next researcher coming in the door, the University wanted to modernize their approach to building new research labs. The open concept lab design was investigated.

At the same time, due to a new funding program for research group grants through the Saskatchewan Health Research Foundation (SHRF), work began in 2003 through the Vice President Research office and the Health Science Colleges on gathering researchers together that appeared to have commonalties in their research. Out of these discussions several thematic research groups or clusters were formed. Work began to bring these groups together through seminars and retreats to get a better understanding of the research potential in the various areas. Out of this work, several new research groups applied for funding and received group grants through SHRF.

This work, although not initially intended to inform the design and occupancy of the building, became the foundation for the information gathering that was required to begin the planning and design of the new buildings. As consultants began the design, representatives from each of these thematic research groups met with the consultants and influenced the design of the various lab floors. While a large portion of each lab was generic from floor to floor, each of the groups/clusters required some unique design aspects in the support rooms in each lab block.

40.3.2 Lab Managers at the Center of a New Operational Framework to Support Team Science

As the design proceeded, other groups began to develop the operational budget, which would include the additional resources required to operate such a building. Since the building was designed to be operated along research themes and not academic departments/units, it was deemed that a different type of support structure would also be required. In addition, the Provost, the executive sponsor for the project, clearly stated that this complex was to be for all the health sciences colleges/units and collectively they would be required to operate the building.

The concept of institutionally funded lab manager positions was created to support these research clusters in their new open concept laboratories (not attached to an academic unit). In addition, rationalization of other support services would be required in order for the faculty to access appropriate support services (e.g., glassware washing, decontamination of biowaste, animal care, ordering, and distribution of materials and supplies).

As this activity gained momentum, and even though the project was to be transformational for the Health Sciences, attention to the impact this change would have on the researchers was somewhat neglected. In spite of the creation of new modern facilities, there was anxiety within the research community. Budgets were set for many operational changes and of course for the physical infrastructure but there was no assigned budget to specifically address change management with the faculty/researchers and their staff.

40.4 Space

40.4.1 Planning a Facility to Foster Team Science

The planning and design of a building to facilitate team science requires the development of, and alignment with, guiding principles. The principles are set forth by the Deans, researchers, university administration, and other participants in articulating the vision for the future. For the AHS, principles were established that support enhanced interprofessional health education and interdisciplinary health research. The principles included proximity among researchers (both faculty to faculty and faculty to students), flexibility of shared research space to reduce operational costs and be adaptable for the evolving research clusters, transparency for both safety and to create a visually and physically connected environment (maximizing natural light for occupant comfort and to reduce artificial lighting loads), and to increase space for students and provide opportunities for academic collisions, both planned and unplanned.

The individual and collective spaces programmed for the AHSC were planned in parallel with the discussions and considerations for how the people would interact and collaborate to enable successful research outcomes. Academic research and teaching space can serve to support and inspire the best in faculty, students, and visitors. The tangible and intangible benefits for the University are many and can be characterized as responses to the primary goals at the inception of the project. The goals as articulated to the Provincial Government are described in the introduction to this chapter and were strategically aligned with the creation of facilities responses to ensure the best opportunity for the University to deliver on the expectations.

The physical location of the planned project was ideally aligned to meet this goal with a physical connection to the Royal University Hospital and adequate site capacity to develop both research and education space. The development of the AHSC on this site provided the added benefit of reinvigorating a campus precinct that lacked both consistent character and connections to the more prominent and historic heart of the campus.

The project was planned and implemented as three distinct but integrated projects: the research addition consisting of five floors with two large shared lab blocks per floor for interdisciplinary research clusters; an addition to enhance education, social, and population health research consisting of two floors of highly engaging student learning, study, dry lab, and amenity spaces; and a major renovation of the existing AHS building.

40.4.2 Enhancing Interdisciplinary Health Research

The goals of enhancing Inter-Professional Education and Inter-Disciplinary Health research were met specifically through the model described above by developing connected, modern, and shared spaces to aid in recruiting new faculty and students and to inspire the best in each. There are numerous opportunities for users (faculty, clinicians, health professionals, biomedical, social and public health undergraduate students, graduate students, post-doctorate fellows, medical residents, and visitors) to access, interact, and learn from each other in a variety of formal and informal spaces created in the new development and in the spaces between existing and new.

In talking with the researchers and other users about their new space, all were generally enthusiastic, understood in broad strokes why the team approach was being promoted, were excited about new collaborative opportunities, could see new possibilities, and were interested in participating. The anxiety they had was most tightly linked to uncertainty about many of the logistical elements related to the process of moving, lack of clarity about roles and responsibilities, and feeling like they were not receiving the communications and information needed to make the "uncertain" certain. It was important for the leadership to recognize that there was worry, even among those who embraced the new scheme and its opportunities.

40.4.3 Shared Research Laboratories

The need to provide modern research space was evident, as the existing research labs were poorly performing, 50-year-old spaces; planned on the concept of small, two module labs dedicated to a researcher, they would not support the transformational shift toward collaborative research.

To improve success in recruiting and retention of faculty and students and to support modern team research efforts with better research results, a large shared lab capable of housing as many as 40 individuals was developed as shown in Fig. 40.1. Each person had dedicated office space outside the lab and was allocated a five-foot-long bench within the lab. These large, open labs were complemented with a 1:1 ratio of lab support space.

The lab support space served numerous functions. These smaller rooms could be dedicated to a researcher for special work or instruments with special requirements such as dark space for microscopy. This was valuable to offset researcher anxiety about losing control of their primary lab space when moving to a shared lab environment. The support space also housed shared research assets per floor such as cold rooms, lab autoclaves, and were centrally located within the floorplate for ready access from both lab wing blocks making up each floor.

The large, open labs were designed to be expandable or contractible; meaning a research cluster could "earn" additional bench space through enhanced grant success or downsize their lab area if their program reduced in size. The restructured governance body overseeing the assignment of space would monitor and reassign space to research clusters as required.

Additionally, the large labs were planned for adaptability to accommodate shifts in research needs through accessible infrastructure backbones located in the ceiling space as seen in Figs. 40.2 and 40.3, and flexibility to support cluster or individual researcher needs at the bench through movable and adjustable casework.

Core facilities development was a priority to provide broader access to specialized program functions such as the research animal vivarium and the neuroscience behavioral testing suites. The vivarium was located at the basement level and is planned as a series of suites that enable a variety of rodent, aquatics, exotics, and large animal species to be housed for research and clinical education needs. This represents a significant paradigm shift over the existing culture of researchers transporting animals to their labs, and will streamline animal care and health maintenance while reducing exposure risks of building occupants to animal allergens. The researcher anxiety over this loss of control was addressed by providing a series of shared procedure rooms within the vivarium that can be "checked out" short-term or long-term for researchers to set up dedicated experiments.

In an important move toward broader collaborations, such as One Health work between the College of Medicine and the College of Veterinary Medicine to solve common disease and zoonotic disease threats that cross the human/animal divide, a full large animal surgical suite was included. This provides three operating rooms as seen in Fig. 40.4, and induction, recovery, scrub, and equipment staging and sterilization space. The ORs are connected via full wall-sized sliding doors, enabling the entire operating theater to be opened to one large space for teaching larger groups. This One Health approach to veterinarians and human medical providers working collaboratively is leading to the ability to solve some of the world's grand challenges around disease transmission, using common disease models.

40.4.4 Student/Faculty Interactions

Implicit to the success of interprofessional education and research are strong bonds between faculty and students. This was not inspired by the former aged facility and culture of the AHS colleges. The existing spaces did not support students with spaces to sit, study, or meet casually. Further, faculty offices were widely distributed throughout the complex and included solid doors, so there was little opportunity for students to know where to seek out faculty or know if they were in their office.

Rigorous planning for the new complex included faculty offices at the ends of the large lab blocks, in transparent office suites with glass front office doors. Faculty are located per floor, so the vitality of activity that comes with students and faculty meeting and working together is evident throughout the building. Student offices are shared and located as close to their lab as possible and in the same location adjacent to the atrium per floor—so everyone knows where the students are and with a visual line of sight to their labs.

Two atria were developed in the research facility; both take advantage of the "space between" new and existing construction. These community

Collaboration Areas per Floor

Lab Support is Shared and / or Dedicated at each end of lab block

Shared Offices access daylight from Atrium and have line of sight to labs

Research Clusters share large, open, flexible labs per floor

Atrium provides natural light from skylight to labs, offices, and corridors

Faculty offices are close to grad students and labs, and distributed per floor

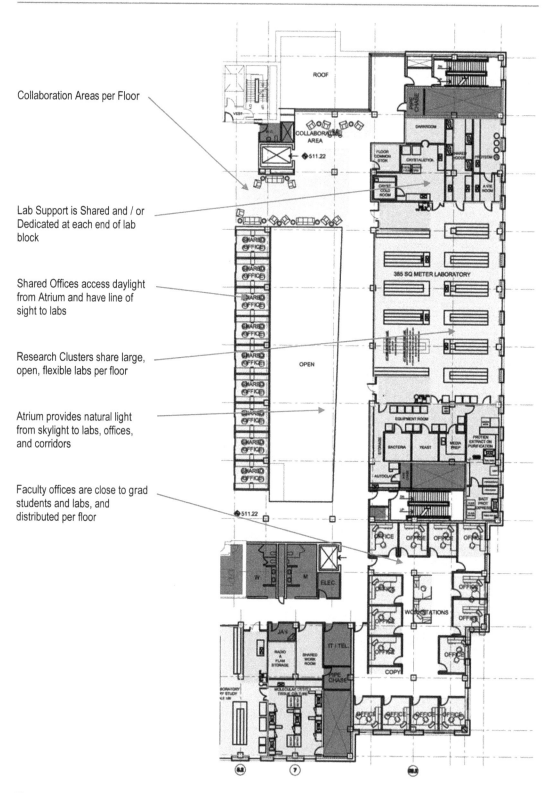

Fig. 40.1 Typical lab

Fig. 40.2 Modularity and movable components provide adaptable research space

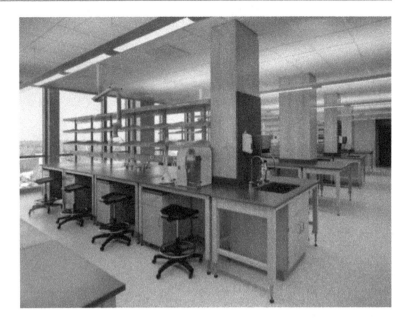

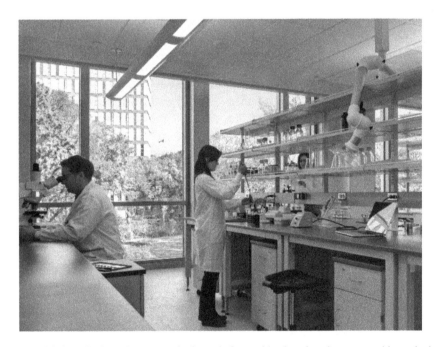

Fig. 40.3 The social side of science in a research cluster is fostered in shared environments with ample daylight and visibility within the lab

spaces serve as the primary horizontal and vertical circulation elements within the complex that also provide daylight and views deep within the floorplate. Ends of atria, landings, widenings of the corridor, and ground floor gathering spaces have all been used to provide numerous spaces at a variety of scales for students to use individually, with faculty, or with larger groups as shown

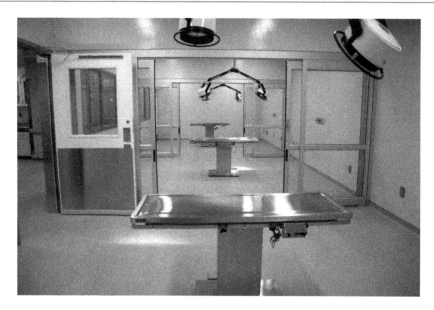

Fig. 40.4 Large animal operating rooms with full visibility through the suite can be used individually or together for larger group training

in Figs. 40.5 and 40.6. These areas have proven very successful in bringing people together in a welcoming, safe, and collegial environment; they are being used much more broadly than AHS to support the entire campus.

The community-building success of the shared research blocks, the connectedness from the research wing to the education wing and the teaching hospital, is also extended to the building exterior and beyond to engage campus networks. The new research wing wraps the existing AHS building façade, a 1960s-era facility that departed in both architectural character and material, from the original AHS wing built in the 1940s with locally quarried stone. The façade of the new research addition marks a return to the use of regional field stone and Tyndall Stone as well as traditional detailing consistent with the original academic quad (Fig. 40.7). Using the newest in building and systems technology, the addition is energy efficient, welcoming, and sensitive to its campus setting. Site development at adjacent buildings is ongoing, with a goal to build strong physical and visual connections above and below grade to the entire campus.

40.5 Institutional Leadership

40.5.1 Aligning Processes, Procedures, and Policies with the Message That Team Science Is Valued

From the early stages of planning the project, it was evident the existing governance for the ownership, assignment, reassignment, and use of space for the AHS would not support a team science model. The existing governance gave ownership and all control over use, configuration, assignment, renovation, or re-use of labs, lab support, and offices, to individual College Deans. Colleges with higher funding levels had more space, better space, and more autonomy than Colleges with lower funding levels.

A new governance model (Fig. 40.8) placed all space with a Council of seven Health Science Deans, whose role was to collectively define what space is in a Team Science environment, how it can be assigned in a way that is mutually beneficial to all the colleges, and how its use should be monitored to ensure the fullest utilization

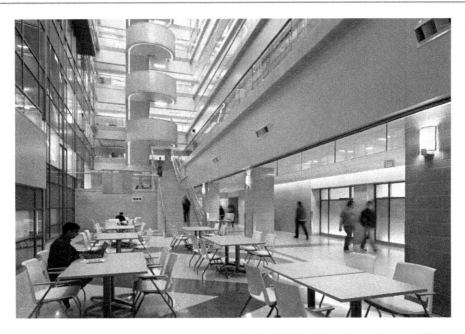

Fig. 40.5 The atrium at ground level is moderately scaled with flexible furnishings for use by many different groups. The space is a resource for the entire campus

based on funding levels and initiatives of various colleges. This approach can be broadly described as a shift from a "My Space" model to an "Our Space" model. The benefits of this to an individual or research cluster are improved operational efficiency and access to better (but shared) instruments where possible, giving them more time to focus on their research.

Institutional support was built into this model in the form of a new Lab Manager position, with the responsibility for assisting the research clusters. The Lab Manager takes on some of the day-to-day activity such as ordering shared consumables; chemical ordering and inventory; training; organizing and managing storage; and retrieval. The right individual in this role can become a trusted ally of both the research clusters and the Health Sciences Deans, to provide assurance that research spaces and equipment are running both efficiently and effectively.

After operating under the initial governance structure 4 years and while the support services were functioning quite well, the governance model needed to be refreshed (Fig. 40.9). The academic issues resulting from the new model of space utilization needed attention, and it became

problematic for consensus to be achieved and/or decisions to be made on space utilization and expansion of additional shared services under the shared governance model. Therefore, a new structure was proposed jointly by the Vice President of Research and the Provost. This new structure requires input from the Health Sciences Deans; however, decisions reside with the Vice Provost, Health and the Assistant Vice Provost, Health. Implementation of these decisions is achieved through the Director of Interdisciplinary Health Research (IDHR) or the Director of Interprofessional Education (IPE), working with the Director of Operations. Both the Director of IDHR and IPE are faculty positions, which have been hired or seconded into these new roles.

40.6 Training and Education: An Essential Element for Moving into the Future

The University of Saskatchewan has learned a lot over the last decade of how team or collaborative science for health science research at our University can be achieved. The University

Fig. 40.6 The atrium as seen in the middle of the building serves as a visual and physical connector between new and existing parts of the complex. The two atria function as primary gathering spaces for students, faculty, and visitors

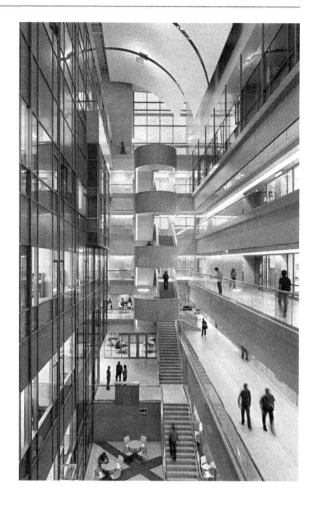

recognizes there is still much to be understood and implemented regarding research collaboration so that health research success within the Academic Health Science Complex can be maximized. To reach its true capacity to conduct Team Science health research, the effort will lie in the continued training of the researchers (students, staff, and faculty), research administrators (Department Heads, Associate Deans of Research within Colleges), and senior administrators (Deans, Health Science Council, Offices of the Provost, and the Vice President Research) to fully understand the value of collaborative health research to the campus and importantly, what is needed to maximize the potential of the research space that the new Academic Health Science

Complex (AHSC) provides to escalate the research programs for all health researchers.

With the development of research space policies within the AHSC, there is a need to continue training faculty and leaders of each research cluster on how the research space within their footprint is best allocated and used, based on faculty-approved metrics of research productivity of each health research team. Ongoing training is necessary for all existing research clusters and evolving research clusters on how best to develop a research cluster and sustain it; or alternatively, how best to dissolve the research cluster when appropriate. Research clusters need to appoint/elect research leaders with the institution, providing proper financial and administra-

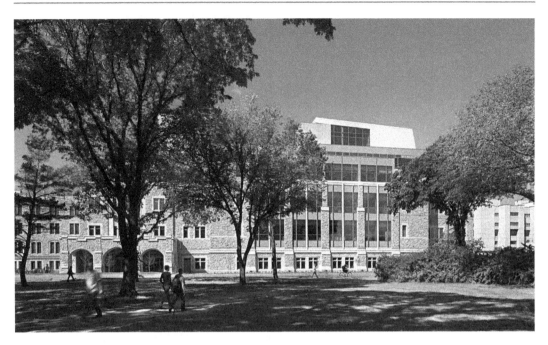

Fig. 40.7 View from east to research addition for AHS. The Tyndall Stone exterior is detailed in traditional masonry techniques which are sympathetic to the historic structures on the campus quad while defining a leading-edge research facility

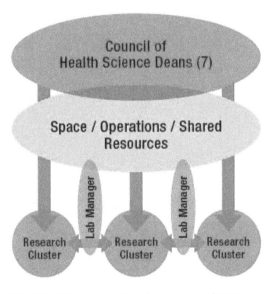

Fig. 40.8 First restructuring of governance of space

tive support to the leader and group for its growth. Department Heads/Associate Deans of Research and Deans in the Health Science Colleges need to work with research cluster leaders within the AHSC to provide appropriate research space for new hires into the research clusters.

The space management process will be overseen by the new Associate Dean of Interdisciplinary Research for the Health Sciences. As the new AHSC provides many laboratory and non-laboratory spaces for undergraduate and graduate research interaction, Team Science training programs need to be established so that students are aware of best practices of working in collaborative research settings. As noted, education and training will be needed for Departmental, Health Colleges and University promotion, tenure, and merit committees of the future to appropriately assess research endeavors of health science faculty working in team settings of the AHSC. That process will benefit from recommendations by the current University Task Force studying the Rewards and Recognition for all researchers conducting collaborative research on campus.

Fig. 40.9 New
governance model

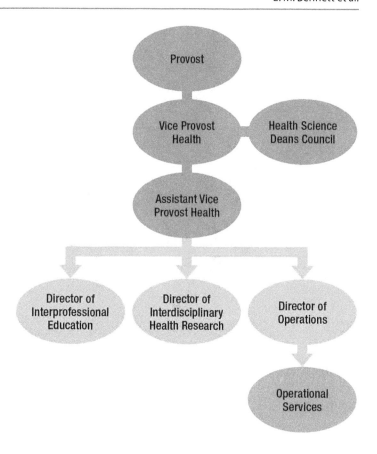

The institutional commitment to Team Science success has not wavered through these early years; from the Provost to the Health Science Deans, faculty, and students, all are realizing benefits from the AHS progress thus far. Our future holds, and will depend on, collective vigilance in ensuring that our leadership, space, and operations are working to enable our people to succeed.

The Development of a New Interdisciplinary Field: Active Living Research—A Foundation-Supported Interdisciplinary Research Funding Program

41

James F. Sallis and Myron F. Floyd

Contents

41.1 Introduction

In this chapter, we report on experiences with team science in the Active Living Research Program, illustrating how a private funding initiative can advance team science. The first section is written from the perspective of leadership of a national funding program[1] and explains how Active Living Research's intentional approach to building a new interdisciplinary field and supporting new teams of investigators was implemented across several phases of a team science life cycle. The chapter is organized around the life cycle of an interdisciplinary research program, from conceptualizing the relevant fields, to building teams of scientists, to supporting the teams and their research, to translating the findings to practitioners and policy-makers in the relevant sectors. The second section is written from the perspective of an Active Living Research grantee[2] whose Active Living Research support allowed him to lead or co-lead two interdisciplinary teams. The impact on his approach to research, lessons, and recommendations are summarized according to phases of a team science life cycle. This chapter represents "voices from the field" because the authors are practitioners and participants in team science, not scholars in the Science of Team Science (SciTS). We hope that lessons from our specific experiences will be useful for those who fund, practice, and study team science.

J. F. Sallis (✉)
Department of Family Medicine and Public Health, University of California, San Diego, CA, USA
e-mail: jsallis@ucsd.edu

M. F. Floyd
Department of Parks, Recreation and Tourism Management, North Carolina State University, Raleigh, NC, USA

---

[1] James F. Sallis
[2] Myron F. Floyd

© Springer Nature Switzerland AG 2019
K. L. Hall et al. (eds.), *Strategies for Team Science Success*,
https://doi.org/10.1007/978-3-030-20992-6_41

41.2   Building and Nurturing an Interdisciplinary Field: Active Living Research

41.2.1 Origins and Goals of Active Living Research

By the late 1990s, physical inactivity was well established as a major public health challenge, as documented in a report from the US Surgeon General (US Department of Health and Human Services 1996), and public health recommendations for physical activity had been issued (Pate et al. 1995). However, national efforts to fill gaps in research and increase the prevalence of physical activity in the US population were largely missing (Yancey and Sallis 2009). Leaders at the Robert Wood Johnson Foundation (RWJF) identified physical activity as an opportunity to provide needed leadership on a topic of clear public health significance. The Foundation developed a $90 million portfolio of programs on active living around the strategic goals of building evidence, supporting action in communities, and building demand for change (Orleans et al. 2009). Active Living Research (ALR) was initiated as a National Program by the Robert Wood Johnson Foundation in 2001 to build an evidence base to inform environmental and policy solutions to the epidemic of inactive lifestyles in the entire population (Sallis et al. 2009).

The Active Living Research National Program Office was established at San Diego State University and moved to University of California, San Diego in 2012. In 2008, Active Living Research became part of the Robert Wood Johnson Foundation commitment to reverse the epidemic of childhood obesity, and the program was supported until early 2016. The three goals of Active Living Research remained largely unchanged over 15 years (Sallis et al. 2014).

1. Establish a strong research base to identify and evaluate solutions to increase physical activity and reverse childhood obesity;
2. Build a vibrant interdisciplinary and diverse field of researchers;

3. Facilitate the use of research to guide and accelerate effective policy and practice change.

Thus, Active Living Research was an explicitly applied research program, and use of research to inform changes in policy and practice was seen as the ultimate goal.

41.2.2 Active Living Research's Interdisciplinary Approach

Active Living Research emphasized environment and policy research to fill a gap between public health recommendations that emphasized the necessity of environment and policy solutions to the problem of physical inactivity and lack of research on these topics. Behavioral research on physical activity was generally guided by theories and models that stated psychological and social factors were the primary influences on health behaviors, including physical activity. Active Living Research was based on multilevel ecological models of behavior that incorporated environmental and policy influences in addition to psychological and social factors (Sallis et al. 2006). Active Living Research's funding priorities were designed to build evidence about promising environmental and policy solutions that would complement existing literature on individual and social influences and interventions.

In the 1990s and before, most physical activity research was conducted by exercise scientists (mainly trained in physiology), behavioral scientists, and epidemiologists. None of these disciplines provided strong training in environmental or policy research. Physical activity was done in, and shaped by, specific environmental settings. The main physical activity environments were considered to be neighborhoods, parks and public spaces, transportation systems, schools, and buildings. The most relevant disciplines with expertise in these environments were city planning, parks and leisure studies, landscape architecture, transportation, education, and architecture. With the exception of a small number of transportation and city planning investigators who studied walking and bicycling for transportation, very few researchers in these fields studied physical activity. Active Living Research's second goal of building an interdisciplinary field of researchers recognized that a team approach would be needed to provide the combination of expertise in physical activity and setting-specific knowledge. Additional disciplines with highly relevant expertise included economics, geography, policy studies, criminology, and health disparities (Sallis et al. 2006).

The number of disciplines and range of expertise engaged in active living research appears to be greater than for other areas of health behavior. For example, almost all the disciplines involved in the large National Cancer Institute-funded Transdisciplinary Tobacco Use Research Centers (TTURC) and Transdisciplinary Research on Energetics and Cancer Centers (TREC) initiatives would traditionally be considered part of the health field though they represented a wide spectrum from basic biology to behavioral and population science. By contrast, most of the active living-related fields would be considered "nonhealth" fields, and few researchers in city planning, transportation, parks, and the other fields had a central interest in the health implications of their work. In the early days of Active Living Research, we heard many comments along these lines. Thus, Active Living Research faced an additional hurdle of informing researchers their expertise was relevant to health, as a preliminary step to recruiting them to interdisciplinary teams to apply for funding from a health-focused organization.

41.2.3 Organization and Leadership of Active Living Research

Virtually every element of Active Living Research was designed to welcome participation of diverse disciplines, create equal opportunities for leadership and obtaining grants, and encourage respect for the skills, perspectives, and traditions of each participating discipline. It was important for National Program Office staff to represent a diversity of disciplines, and those included health

psychology, public health, law, city and regional planning, parks and leisure studies, and sociology. The staff diversity facilitated connections and communications with the targeted disciplines and served as a model of interdisciplinary collaboration that was apparent to grantees.

A National Advisory Committee was assembled that consisted mostly of senior leaders of key disciplines. We expected participation of well-known leaders to enhance credibility of Active Living Research among others in their fields, especially in the early years. National Advisory Committee roles included assisting in recruiting grant applicants from their disciplines, advising about policies and key research questions relevant to active living, and guiding the communication of research to decision makers in their fields. Disciplines and expertise represented by the National Advisory Committee included transportation, economics, policy studies, health disparities, environmental justice, landscape architecture, environmental psychology, obesity, and urban design. Some advisors were recruited from advocacy groups and government agencies to provide perspectives of "research users." National Advisory Committee members served as grant reviewers and made recommendations about grant funding.

41.2.4 Strategies for Recruiting Diverse Disciplines to Research Teams

As a new program Active Living Research faced the challenge of informing investigators from a very wide range of disciplines about the importance of a new interdisciplinary research field, notifying them of funding opportunities, and recruiting them to participate. The idea of working with unfamiliar disciplines was new to almost all the audiences, and two main communication strategies were pursued. The first strategy was called "academic diplomacy," whereby an Active Living Research leader sought opportunities to present the new funding program to interested groups at national conferences. National Advisory Committee members helped identify appropriate organizations, made introductions to organizational leaders, advocated for Active Living Research-related events, and sometimes participated. Events ranged from invited breakfasts and advertised evening receptions to workshops and participation in symposia. Journal commentaries and newsletter articles reached wider audiences, and Calls for Proposals were distributed via mailing lists to reach all the relevant disciplines. These methods attracted large and diverse pools of grant applicants. However, these activities required substantial staff time and travel costs, so the Robert Wood Johnson Foundation-supported National Program Office was an essential component of creating a viable funding program.

A second recruitment method was the Seminar program, in collaboration with academic societies. Seminars were designed to develop leaders in active living research who would help generate interest within key disciplines. Respected members of an organization with an interest in active living were identified from Active Living Research grant applicants or referral by a National Advisory Committee member. Active Living Research staff collaborated with the discipline representative to plan a Seminar at the annual meeting targeting the needs of the audience and including at least one speaker from an "external" discipline. The discipline representative would then be recognized as a leader in the new field of active living research, and the Seminar program demonstrated interdisciplinary collaboration. Depending on the audience, the Seminar could present unfamiliar measurement or statistical methods or offer a workshop on building interdisciplinary teams. From 2003 to 2007, Active Living Research sponsored 15 workshops with academic societies (Sallis et al. 2009).

was a strong criterion in grant application reviews. The guiding assumption was that environment and policy studies were complex enough that no single investigator or discipline was expected to possess the range of needed skills. A team for a built environment study might include a city planner with GIS skills, an epidemiologist with accelerometer skills, and a psychologist with survey development skills. Active Living Research offered limited support for assembling interdisciplinary teams. Teleconferences in advance of each Call for Proposal included encouragement and guidance for finding suitable collaborators. We clarified that because the grant program was very competitive, collaborators with high-level skills should be sought, and the team should be assembled well in advance of the deadline so agreement could be reached on study aims and methods. We encouraged investigators to search outside their departments and universities to find the most appropriate collaborators, not just the most familiar or conveniently located. However, we resisted requests to host a "matchmaking" service through the Active Living Research website, because we were concerned that listing investigators seeking collaboration on the website would imply endorsement.

Active Living Research's Annual Conferences have become an important venue for finding promising collaborators, as well as exposing attendees to an unusually broad array of conceptual models, study topics, measurement methods, and analytic approaches. Attendees routinely identified more than 30 disciplines, creating a uniquely diverse mix. In post-conference evaluations, between 84% and 94% of respondents agreed the meeting provided an opportunity to make new contacts that might lead to collaborations (Sallis et al. 2009).

41.2.5 Supporting Development of Interdisciplinary Teams

The National Program Office provided an explicit incentive for forming interdisciplinary teams by emphasizing that inclusion of relevant expertise

41.2.6 Supporting Effective Functioning of Interdisciplinary Teams

Over time, Active Living Research Conferences served as a support community for improving the functioning of interdisciplinary teams. Because team science was a common experience of attendees, it was easy to share stories, concerns, and solutions. However, SciTS was young, so there was little evidence on which to base guidance. At the first Active Living Research Conference in 2004, Daniel Stokols was a keynote speaker. He presented early research findings about variations in the effectiveness of interdisciplinary TTURC teams, drew lessons for consideration by active living researchers, and published a summary (Stokols et al. 2005).

In later years, grantee meetings featured panels and interactive sessions that allowed grantees to share their perceptions of effective and ineffective collaboration strategies. Grantee meetings included breakout groups to discuss collaboration issues, facilitated by experienced investigators. At the conferences, thematic breakfast roundtables often served as a venue for sharing experiences. Active Living Research staff monitored the progress of grant teams, inquired periodically about the functioning of teams, and offered telephone consultations with senior investigators upon request. The Active Living Research approach to team functioning was supportive but informal, because staff was not aware of any educational materials that would be appropriate for the disparate teams that were common among Active Living Research grantees. Active Living Research was launched in the early days of the SciTS field, prior to journal special issues on team science and creation of the NCI Team Science Toolkit (https://www.teamsciencetoolkit.cancer.gov/Public/Home.aspx) that made research findings, best practices, and resources more accessible.

41.2.7 Engaging Research Teams in Research Translation

Communicating research to policy and practice audiences was a primary goal of Active Living Research, and several methods were implemented, including a few innovations. Substantial program resources were devoted to promoting the application of research findings. Active Living Research was defined as an applied

research program in Calls for Proposals and other materials, with a stated intention of communicating research to policy-makers and practitioners and encouraging the use of research in decision-making, also known as research translation. Conceptual models of Active Living Research identified "research user" groups in diverse sectors corresponding to the academic fields targeted for participation in research teams. Grant proposals included required sections for describing dissemination plans to both academic and "research user" audiences. Applicants were encouraged to include potential research users in investigative teams to enhance the prospects for implementation of results. One of the benefits of interdisciplinary teams was that members from each discipline provided leadership for communication and research translation activities to researchers, policy-makers, and practitioners in their sectors.

Training and support in research translation was provided to grantees during annual grantee meetings and via consultation opportunities with communications consultants. Annual conferences open to all attendees featured invited plenary sessions and workshops with policy-makers, practitioners, and advocates from multiple sectors. These sessions included instruction in communicating with non-researchers, encouragement to engage non-researchers in research teams, and examples of more policy-relevant study questions and research methods. Several sessions about research translation were published as commentaries in Active Living Research-sponsored journal special issues (e.g., Goldstein 2009; Moodie 2009). Starting in 2014, Active Living Research Conferences added an abstract track for policy and practice-oriented presentations and workshops. Research and practice-based presentations were integrated in the same sessions, so Active Living Research Conference provided more opportunities for research translation and reciprocal learning between researchers and non-researchers.

"Translating Research Into Policy" Awards were instituted to recognize excellent examples, build a norm for researchers engaging in these activities, and stimulate engagement by others.

Nominations were solicited in Annual Conference announcements, a committee selected winners, and the winning team presented at the Annual Conference and wrote a commentary for the Active Living Research special issue (e.g., Haggerty and Melnick 2013).

In the latter years of Active Living Research, the Seminar program shifted from targeting research audiences to communicating lessons of research to policy, practice, and advocacy audiences. Active Living Research staff and grantees either submitted proposals or were invited to speak at meetings or on webinars, many of which were conducted in collaboration with Dialogue4Health.org. Examples of Seminar partners were Education Commission of the States, Environmental Justice in America Conference, Urban Affairs Association, Pro/Walk Pro/Bike Conference, and National Medical Association. (Sallis et al. 2014).

The Active Living Research program office led development of about 40 research briefs to summarize lessons of research for nontechnical audiences. Briefs were generally written by researchers from the same disciplines as the target audiences of "research users," illustrating another value of the team science approach. Experts from diverse fields wrote the briefs that were edited by communication professionals, and each brief included implications or recommendations for policy and practice. Based on feedback, infographics were created to accompany many briefs, to make the content more widely accessible, especially to community-based groups. Briefs and infographics were widely used, including incorporation into national organizational and governmental communications.

Even when research produces policy-relevant findings and investigators are motivated to engage in research translation, there were common barriers such as lack of institutional support, finances, and skill. Thus, Active Living Research Translation Grants were instituted, and grantees with "actionable" findings were invited to apply for small grants. Proposals were required to describe a communication plan, with key policy-relevant messages, defined target audiences, and communication plans that included permanent products such as briefs, videos, and webinars. Applicants were encouraged to include a communication professional on the team, Active Living Research provided a communications consultant, and group teleconferences with grantees were scheduled to share lessons and build skills. Research translation activities and evaluations of some components have been published (Barker and Gutman 2014; Sallis et al. 2014, 2016). Research Translation Grants, along with communications support, could be adopted by other funding organizations to enhance the societal impact of research and to build a culture of research translation among investigators.

41.2.8 Leadership Development and Recognition

We viewed leadership development as necessary to achieve Active Living Research's goals and establish a sustained interdisciplinary research effort. Participation of effective leaders was needed to establish the legitimacy of the new field of active living research, to promote engagement of investigators from each relevant discipline, to ensure functioning of each interdisciplinary research team, to model research translation, and to act as mentors for junior investigators in this new field. Specific activities were undertaken to build leadership in each of these areas.

The interdisciplinary National Advisory Committee consisted of established leaders in their fields, and National Advisory Committee members helped build relationships with professional organizations and recruit investigators from their fields. Conference Chairs and program committee members were selected to represent key academic disciplines as well as non-researchers. Conference Chairs also guest co-edited the resulting journal special issues (http://activelivingresearch.org/resourcesearch/journalspecialissues). Emphasis was placed on ensuring racial-ethnic, age, and disciplinary diversity in leadership positions. These high-visibility positions helped individuals build their careers, establish records of leadership, and enhance their identification with the active living field.

Additional opportunities for leadership were incorporated into Active Living Research Conferences and Grantee Meetings. Leaders of breakfast and lunch theme tables either volunteered or were recruited to lead discussions on topics of interest. Diverse moderators of oral presentation sessions gained visibility. These modest leadership activities allowed many people to assemble leadership profiles.

Active Living Research staff and National Advisory Committee members identified topics of relevance to active living research that were unfamiliar to many of the involved investigators, gaps in research, methods with the potential to be improve the research, or a body of findings that were ready for translation to practitioners and policy-makers. A leader in the topic of interest was identified and invited to write a paper, prepare a report, or draft a research brief. These commissioned products were meant to establish the author(s) as a leader on this topic for the active living field. These products were used to bring concepts, methods, and findings from one discipline to the interdisciplinary field of active living research, with the goal of enriching the research and improving translation of research to policy and practice (Hack 2013; Bushnell et al. 2013). The leadership profile of the authors was often enhanced through presentations at Active Living Research conferences, and these leaders were sometimes invited to become collaborators and consultants.

It was essential for leadership roles to be distributed across the many disciplines engaged in active living research. The observable diversity of leaders reinforced messages about the interdisciplinary nature of the field. The Active Living Research approach was to provide many opportunities for large and small leadership roles and to allow many people, at all stages of their careers, to be recognized for their leadership. This strategy helped build the new interdisciplinary field by generating a commitment to the field among the many people whose leadership was recognized.

Active Living Research's efforts to build an interdisciplinary field were complemented by actions taken to ensure effective functioning of each interdisciplinary team. The next section describes and discusses experiences with specific interdisciplinary teams supported by Active Living Research.

41.3 Perspectives on Team Science from One Active Living Research Grantee

Participating in team science with talented partners from multiple disciplines offers challenge and intellectual tension that most scientists find stimulating and rewarding. Active Living Research was my (MFF) introduction to this research approach. Prior to becoming an Active Living Research grantee, I managed a visible and productive research program focused on racial and ethnic patterns in park use and recreation behavior. My specific interest centered on racial inequality in access to parks and public leisure services. At that time, my publications could be found within a handful of academic journals, most with *parks*, *leisure*, or *recreation* in their titles. Naturally, my collaborators were primarily other social scientists with expertise in recreation and leisure studies. Funding for my research came largely from state and federal recreation providers (e.g., state park agencies and USDA Forest Service) where data on user preferences and patterns of behavior were integral to recreation planning and visitor management.

Becoming an Active Living Research grantee was a major turning point in my career. In retrospect, it was a privilege to be an early recruit of the Active Living Research leadership and to be at the leading edge of a rapidly emerging new interdisciplinary field. As Robert Wood Johnson Foundation and Active Living Research sought to build health research expertise in multiple disciplines such as parks, recreation, and leisure studies as well as disparities, opportunities for new ways to apply my expertise were created and my network of collaborators expanded greatly. Although my research continues to focus on racial and ethnic inequality related to park use, my experience in Active Living Research has expanded topics in my research that I would not have considered earlier in my career (or now): these include *built environment, physical activity, overweight* and *obesity, measurement strategies,* and *research translation to policy*, among others.

Collaborators in recent years have been from disciplines of forest sciences, public health, landscape architecture, medicine, exercise science, sociology, urban planning, and psychology to name a few examples. My publications have appeared in a wider variety of health-related journals such as *American Journal of Preventive Medicine, American Journal of Health Promotion,* and *Journal of Physical Activity and Health* in addition to discipline- or field-specific journals in parks, recreation, and leisure studies. Perhaps, the most important outcome of my immersion into team science and interdisciplinary research within Active Living Research was the numerous leadership opportunities afforded from the experience.

41.3.1 Leadership Development

Leading an interdisciplinary Active Living Research team enhanced my standing as a recognized leader within the active living research community and within my own discipline. This experience is an excellent example of the Active Living Research goal to identify and develop emerging leaders and to increase identification with the active living research field. It began with an Active Living Research sponsored workshop in 2003 that brought together a small group of researchers from non-health disciplines. Through the workshop Active Living Research staff provided an orientation to active living concepts, measurement methods to assess physical activity and the built environment, and an overview of the multiple disciplines needed in childhood obesity and built environment research. Having this opportunity gave a clearer understanding of what made an Active Living Research grant proposal competitive. Two years later, I was PI on an Active Living Research-funded grant.

I was invited to be Conference Chair for the 2007 Active Living Research Annual Conference. This role came with the responsibility to help plan and shape the conference agenda. The theme selected for the conference was "Active Living in Diverse and Disadvantaged Communities" in alignment with my own research. As Conference Chair, I had the opportunity to give an opening plenary presentation and later served as guest editor for an *American Journal of Preventive Medicine* supplement containing the highest rated papers from the conference. As guest editor, I coauthored the lead article and introduction to the issue (Floyd et al. 2008) and helped select the conference chair for the following year. Being from a non-health discipline and named Conference Chair of the Active Living Research conference demonstrated the Active Living Research strategy of broadening representation of researchers from diverse backgrounds and disciplines. It was also a clear signal that parks, recreation, and leisure sciences researchers were essential partners in active living research.

Other leadership opportunities resulted from my Active Living Research involvement. These included being invited to coauthor a commissioned analysis on disparities (Whitt-Glover et al. 2009), an invitation to provide expert commentary on measurement of parks and recreation in low-income and minority communities at a National Cancer Institute workshop which led to a contributed a paper to a special issue of *American Journal of Preventive Medicine* on measurement of the built environment (Floyd et al. 2009), and contributing position papers and panel presentations that encouraged greater collaboration between the parks, recreation and leisure studies field and public health (e.g., Taylor et al. 2007).

As the health benefits of parks have become more widely reported, Active Living Research experiences gave me credibility to take on leadership roles in research within my own profession and discipline. Two key examples were being recruited to be coinvestigator on a large team to evaluate the implementation of the *HealthierUS Initiative* in the National Park System (Hoehner et al. 2010) and participation in the development of a science plan for the National Park Service to guide implementation and evaluation of its *Healthy Parks Healthy People Initiative* (Department of Interior, National Park Service). Opportunities outside of Active Living Research events show the success of the Active Living Research strategy to engage key leaders and policy officials from other sectors to promote the field of active living.

41.3.2 Experiences in and Reflections on Team Science and Interdisciplinary Research

In large part, the opportunities described resulted from participating in research teams funded by Active Living Research. What follows are a few reflections drawn from two Active Living Research grant experiences. The section is organized by the stages of collaboration (proposal, study implementation, and dissemination) including challenges and lessons learned related to each stage.

41.3.2.1 Proposal Stage and Team Composition

My first Active Living Research award came about as a response to the Round 3 Call for Proposals on understudied populations. The project examined physical activity in parks in racially diverse communities. The research team included a PI and co-PI from parks and leisure studies; coinvestigators were a landscape social scientist and two health psychologists with expertise in direct observation measurements for physical activity. How did this team come about? We implemented advice from reviewers and Active Living Research staff given on a previously submitted unsuccessful proposal. Positive comments were given to the study rationale and study aims of our failed proposal. However, a glaring limitation was the lack of state of the science measurement strategies used in physical activity research. Even though survey methods and self-report measures of behavior are standard tools in studies of park users and leisure participants, these would not be adequate. Two

immediate challenges were presented. One, where do you find the expertise to apply for future grants? Two, how do you "get up to speed" fairly quickly on a completely new literature and methodology? Fortunately, the first challenge was resolved by following up on Active Living Research staff recommendations to contact two health psychologists with expertise on observational measures health behaviors.

A key lesson from this experience was that to be successful in an interdisciplinary team, there is no getting around reading outside of your own discipline. During proposal development, it was important for the parks and leisure studies team members to dig into the literature to trace the development of physical activity observation systems, because this was necessary to understand our primary method of data collection. Furthermore, we needed to understand why direct observation and objective measures were recommended, and how to manage, analyze, and interpret the data generated. The benefit to our colleagues from health psychology was the opportunity to apply their methods in parks and recreation environments.

The second Active Living Research interdisciplinary collaboration originated closer to home. It presented a different kind of challenge. The project focused on park and neighborhood factors associated with children's and adolescents' use of parks. Unlike the first grant, the entire team was composed of faculty researchers from the same university campus, North Carolina State University. The two co-PIs were me in parks and recreation and Robin Moore, professor of landscape architecture, who had an international reputation and strong record of research on children's use of parks and public space. We were joined by other colleagues from parks, recreation, and leisure studies, geospatial sciences, sociology, and design. This team formed around mutual interests and was not influenced by Active Living Research. Because of Moore's reputation as a leading scholar and design professional combined with my background and expertise and knowledge of the Active Living Research review process, we were confident in our ability to submit a "winning" proposal.

One challenge encountered very early was differences in opinions about study methods. In the first grant, we took advice from the reviewers to add experts in systematic direct observation. On the second grant, there was less "buy in" of methods endorsed by Active Living Research staff. For example, team members from landscape architecture initially opposed the use of SOPARC (System for Observing Physical Activity and Recreation in Communities; an observational measure of physical activity in parks) and EAPRS (Environmental Assessment of Public Recreation Spaces; a park audit tool). From the previous grant experience, I knew our proposal would not be reviewed favorably if it did not use SOPARC or another method for obtaining objective measures of physical activity. My colleagues in landscape architecture were emphatic about the weaknesses of SOPARC such as the inability to collect detailed contextual information (e.g., locating children's behaviors in relation to specific park features). The lack of detail, it was argued, would not inform questions related to the design or management of park spaces. They favored behavioral mapping, the "go-to" preferred method from their discipline. Behavioral mapping does provide more detailed assessments of how people use public spaces. Decisions about methods generated intense but constructive debates on the merits of one discipline's approach over another. A breakthrough occurred with a collective realization that measures with established protocols and evidence of validity and reliability must be used to derive the best evidence on how parks help children get physical activity. Such evidence would be most persuasive to policy-makers. Looking back, key to this outcome was the trust my colleagues placed in the knowledge gained from my previous Active Living Research grant.

41.3.2.2 Study Implementation

Any project requires clear assignments of roles and responsibilities to meet study objectives and the goals of the sponsor. It is the PI who provides oversight and accountability. This can be made difficult when roles are not clearly defined. Roles and responsibilities were assigned differently in the two projects. Role assignments were made in the proposal. In the first, project roles were clearly defined according to expertise. The health psychologists and measurement experts were responsible for adapting their protocols for parks, training data collectors, and developing analysis plans. Team members in parks and recreation made contacts with local parks departments to gain permission for the study, directed park audits, developed the GIS data, and supervised field staff. Nonoverlapping roles reduced chances for conflicts and redundant work. Clear separation of responsibilities contributed to the project's success. This collaboration was also successful because the disciplines involved were so different. On the one hand, having very distinct disciplines on a team seems like it would create more conflict compared to a team composed of researchers in similar fields. But our experience was the clear separation of responsibilities removed that potential for conflict.

In the second project, even though roles were assigned during the proposal stage, there was more diffusion of responsibilities during study implementation because our fields were not all that distinct. While they are recognized fields, parks and recreation and landscape architecture have an overlapping history and draw on similar literature. This was an obvious benefit. There were few barriers to communication when discussing research concepts. But it also meant that we were not as quick to defer to each other when decisions needed to be made—we were all experts in the field. For example, although the proposal identified the roles for each team member, we tended to challenge each other on how data collection training should be conducted, or how the parks should be audited, and on what type of supplemental data should be collected (e.g., should we supplement systematic observations with behavioral mapping?). In essence, changes to the study design were being proposed. Making such changes during the course of a study can lead to project delays. Fortunately, there were no serious setbacks. To keep the team focused required reminding team members of the project objectives and of the importance of setting aside disciplinary preferences to meet the needs of our sponsor.

41.3.2.3 Dissemination Phase

The main challenge at this stage was adjusting to journal standards within different fields. Most leisure studies journals limit manuscripts to 9000 words or 25 double-spaced pages. Like most social science journals, the introduction devotes significant space to the literature review and theoretical model used in the study. My public health colleagues were less accustomed to preparing manuscripts to suit these requirements, particularly elaboration on theoretical background. Many health journals limit authors to 3000–4000 words, and little space is given to theoretical background. Typically, there is a quick reference to the ecological model followed by a concise literature review. During the first submissions of our Active Living Research manuscripts to leisure studies journals, editors and reviewers were not receptive to physical activity studies and papers that did not include social psychological outcomes (e.g., perceived benefits of park use). Although the field of parks, recreation and leisure studies had a long history of studying health and well-being (Henderson and Bialeschki 2005), the field had not yet made an explicit connection to research on active living and preventing obesity. Active Living Research leadership was instrumental in helping to lower barriers that may have existed to publishing active living research in leisure studies journals (and journals in other disciplines). For example, Robert Wood Johnson Foundation and Active Living Research co-sponsored a special issue of *Leisure Sciences* (2005, Vol. 27, Issue 5) that highlighted the connection between active living research and the parks, recreation and leisure studies field. Active Living Research also sponsored a panel on interdisciplinary research at the 2006 National Recreation and Park Association Annual Meeting.

41.3.3 Benefits of Team Science and Interdisciplinary Research

In addition to the leadership opportunities, participation in team science with interdisciplinary partners advances the development of individual scientists as well as disciplines. My Active Living Research experiences (and the experiences of other researchers in my field of parks, recreation, and leisure studies (PRLS)) brought new theory and methods into more common use in our field. These experiences raised the visibility of parks, recreation, and leisure studies and integrated it into active living research and the larger field of public health. As the active living research field has grown, more opportunities have been created for other PRLS researchers to participate in Active Living Research teams. PRLS has also benefitted from emphasis given to dissemination and translation research in Active Living Research. Researchers typically include a section on management or policy implications at the end of journal articles, yet practitioners rarely have access to scientific papers and few read them. The strategy of commissioning researchers to translate their work into nontechnical research briefs brought attention to the need to be more deliberate about informing policy-makers with data to support their decisions.

41.3.4 Lessons from These Experiences in Team Science

In summary, four points highlight key lessons learned from these experiences. First, the PI must articulate the expectations of the sponsor and hold team members accountable to meeting the aims of the project. Differences in opinions about disciplinary approaches should be recognized, but when they begin to undermine success, they must take a back seat to fulfilling the aims of the project. Team members must show flexibility and be adaptive. At the same time, it is important to be a strong representative of your discipline. As my Dean often reminds us, "Strong disciplines make strong interdisciplinary partners." Second, and related, trust is vital within large teams. It is essential when working with new collaborators who bring unfamiliar methods or when working with new sponsors as was the case in the examples I described. There will be members who are more familiar with an approach or with a funder. Trusting the expertise of the PI who has earned credibility through performance, or trusting an unfamiliar method to do what it has been documented to be capable of, makes it possible to work through the more difficult differences of opinion. Third, researchers on interdisciplinary teams should read journals from other fields to become familiar with disciplinary norms and expectations of their collaborators. Fourth, faculty researchers should involve their students in all stages of interdisciplinary research, from proposal writing to dissemination. Research is moving toward team science, so doctoral programs should prepare students for interdisciplinary collaborations. Topics and concerns in many disciplines demand interdisciplinary teams and commitments to work in this way. Many funders also require interdisciplinary teams. Graduate students will be better prepared for successful research careers if they get this exposure during their programs.

Involvement in team science and the Active Living Research program changed the trajectory of my research program. The most notable influence of Active Living Research was the exposure to the interdisciplinary team approach. This experience provided new areas to apply my scientific expertise and connected me to an expanded network of interdisciplinary partners. Becoming comfortable working in interdisciplinary teams and increasingly confident about the expertise parks and recreation researchers bring to active living research are direct results of my experience as an Active Living Research grantee. This had led to several subsequent publications and grants with interdisciplinary collaborators. Another important and related aspect taken from the Active Living Research experience is publishing in "high impact" health-related journals outside of my field. Publication in high quality journals helps to ensure that the best evidence on parks and physical activity is more widely visible so it can be used to inform intervention strategies. In addition, by publishing in journals in other disciplines, awareness of the role parks and recreation research play in active living can be increased.

41.4 Conclusion

Because of the major impacts of physical activity on health and disease, as well as the high prevalence of physical inactivity (Sallis and Carlson 2015), it is important that physical activity research continues to draw upon the diverse talents and contributions of investigators from diverse fields. The necessity of interdisciplinary research is based on the documented influences of practices and policies in several "non-health" sectors (Sallis et al. 2012) as well as the social, environmental, and economic benefits of designing environments that support active living (Sallis et al. 2015). Interdisciplinary research teams are likely to advance research and support translation of research findings to policy and practice better than teams from a single discipline.

The active living field is notable because of the unusually broad range of "non-health" disciplines involved in the research and its translation. We are not aware of another health topic that is directly related to such a wide range of major academic disciplines and societal sectors, such as city planning, education, transportation, parks and recreation, sports, recreation industry, health care, public health, geography, policy studies, and economics. The Active Living Research program was created by the Robert Wood Johnson Foundation to fill important gaps in not only the broad topic of environments and policies related to active living, but also the highly diverse interdisciplinary teams needed to conduct the research. The consensus of Robert Wood Johnson Foundation leaders in the early 2000s was that the National Institutes of Health was unlikely to invest sufficiently in this nascent field of research that differed in so many ways from the dominant biomedical model. Thus, a private foundation was willing to take a risk by "seed funding" a new interdisciplinary field, which has become mainstream and now attracts substantial NIH support. This role of "pioneering" a new research area is a valuable and appropriate one for foundations.

Recruiting investigators from such diverse fields and forming effective interdisciplinary teams was a special challenge. Many investigators did not perceive their prior research as being related to health. Fortunately, Active Living Research had the resources to reach out to many disciplines, invite them to participate in health-related research, support a culture of respectful interdisciplinary collaboration, and build skills in collaborative research. One indicator that Active Living Research had an impact on building a new field was a remarkable increase in publications on physical activity policy and environment research in the literature in general (Sallis et al. 2014) and in papers presented at the interdisciplinary Society of Behavioral Medicine (Sallis et al. 2013). Another indicator was documentation that principal investigators of Active Living Research grants came from 31 disciplines (Barker and Gutman 2014). About 57% of grantees reported that Active Living Research stimulated new interdisciplinary collaboration within their institution, and 71% reported new collaborations with other disciplines outside their institution (Barker and Gutman 2014). We consider this good evidence that an interdisciplinary field has been established.

Active Living Research was a laboratory for team science, because approximately 200 interdisciplinary teams were supported by grants. The case studies of interdisciplinary teams in this chapter provide rich examples of the experiences of two teams. The cases illustrate that each team had different dynamics, strengths, and challenges, even when some of the members overlapped. Lessons from these cases are not expected to generalize in all aspects to other teams. However, the richness of case studies can complement quantitative research on team science by illustrating findings from the evaluations and generating hypotheses to be tested in future SciTS studies.

A culture and expectation of interdisciplinary research was established in Active Living Research that is likely to persist, even as Active Living Research no longer funds teams to conduct studies, especially among those investigators who experienced the benefits of interdisciplinary collaboration. But the extent of persistence and advancement of interdisciplinary research will depend on support from funders, academic institutions, and professional organizations, all of which tend to be discipline-centric. We perceive little evidence that governmental or private research funders have adopted goals of prioritizing interdisciplinary health research, especially when the disciplines are as disparate as those in active living research. Most journals are dedicated to serving their disciplinary subscribers. Barriers to interdisciplinary collaboration remain in universities. Given the ongoing challenges, resources to encourage and support interdisciplinary research also need to be ongoing. We encourage public and private funders, journal editors, and university administrators to adopt goals and implement methods to support interdisciplinary research, and we believe there are lessons from the Active Living Research experience that could be fruitfully applied to other topic areas.

> **Box: Lessons and Recommendations from Active Living Research**
>
> When problems are complex and solutions need to be multidimensional, then team science may be required to make progress.
>
> The institutional barriers to team science among public and private funders, universities, professional organizations, and journals are so ingrained that study of these problems using a SciTS model is needed. It would be most appropriate if multiple scientific, governmental, nongovernmental, and academic organizations worked together on such a study and produced a high-profile report, then committed themselves to implementing the recommendations.
>
> Active Living Research demonstrated that a multifaceted approach to team science can be successful in recruiting diverse disciplines, nurturing interdisciplinary teams, generating new measures, producing

influential scientific papers, and building a culture of interdisciplinary respect and collaboration. It is likely Active Living Research could have been more effective if the lessons of the SciTS had been available at the beginning of Active Living Research.

Applied research should be judged not only by the quantity, quality, and impact of its scientific products, but by the impact of the science on practice, policy, and society. In interdisciplinary research areas, the challenges of translating the lessons of research to multiple sectors are magnified. Though Active Living Research's efforts to enhance research translation—including briefs, Research Translation Grants, and commissioned reports—appeared to be useful, they were not formally evaluated. This is another topic for which SciTS approaches could be usefully applied.

An important shortcoming of Active Living Research was the program was not subject to evaluation using SciTS approaches. Because Active Living Research had more diversity of disciplines than NIH-supported team science initiatives, an evaluation of Active Living Research might have produced complementary findings.

Many of the methods used by Active Living Research are likely to be adaptable to other team science programs. Fortunately, the methods have been described (Sallis et al. 2009, 2014, 2016) and evaluated (Barker and Gutman 2014; Gutman et al. 2009; Ottoson et al. 2009) in multiple journal articles so they will be available for future funders to consider.

References

Barker DC, Gutman MA. Evaluation of active living research: ten years of progress in building a new field. Am J Prev Med. 2014;46:208–15.

Bushnell MA, Poole BW, Zegeer CV, Rodriguez DA. Costs for pedestrian and bicyclist infrastruc-ture improvements: a resource for researchers, engineers, planners, and the general public. Report commissioned by active living research. 2013. http://activelivingresearch.org/costs-pedestrian-and-bicy-clist-infrastructure-improvements-resource-research-ers-engineers-planners.

Floyd MF, Crespo CJ, Sallis JF. Active living research in diverse and disadvantaged communities: stimulating dialogue and policy solutions. Am J Prev Med. 2008;34:271–4.

Floyd MF, Taylor WC, Whitt-Glover M. Measurement of park and recreation environments that support physical activity in low-income communities of color: highlights of challenges and recommendations. Am J Prev Med. 2009;36(4, Suppl):S156–60.

Goldstein H. Commentary: translating research into public policy. J Public Health Policy. 2009;30:S16–20.

Gutman MA, Barker DC, Samples-Smart F, Morley C. Evaluation of active living research: progress and lessons in building a new field. Am J Prev Med. 2009;36(2Suppl. 2):S22–33.

Hack G. Business performance in walkable shopping areas. Report commissioned by active living research. 2013. http://activelivingresearch.org/business-performance-walkable-shopping-areas.

Haggerty B, Melnick A. Translating research to policy through health impact assessment in Clark County, Washington: a commentary to accompany the active living research supplement to annals of behavioral medicine. Ann Behav Med. 2013;45:6–8.

Henderson KA, Bialeschki MD. Leisure and active lifestyles: research reflections. Leis Sci. 2005;27:355–65.

Hoehner CM, Brownson RC, Allen D, Gramann J, Behrens TK, Floyd MF, et al. Parks promoting physical activity: synthesis of findings from interventions in seven national parks. J Phys Act Health. 2010;7(Suppl):S67–81.

Moodie R. Commentary: where different worlds collide: expanding the influence of research and researchers on policy. J Public Health Policy. 2009;30:S33–S7.

Orleans CT, Leviton LC, Thomas KA, et al. History of the Robert Wood Johnson foundation's active living research program: origins and strategy. Am J Prev Med. 2009;36(2Suppl):S1–9.

Ottoson JM, Green LW, Beery WL, Senter SK, Cahill CL, et al. Policy-contribution assessment and field-building analysis of the Robert Wood Johnson foundation's active living research program. Am J Prev Med. 2009;36(2 Suppl):S34–43.

Pate RR, Pratt M, Blair SN, Haskell WL, Macera CA, et al. Physical activity and public health: a recommendation from the centers for disease control and prevention and the american college of sports medicine. J Am Med Assoc. 1995;273:402–7.

Sallis JF, Bull F, Burdett R, Frank LD, Griffiths P, Giles-Corti B, Stevenson M. Using science to guide city planning, policy and practice: achieving health and sustainable future cities. Lancet. 2016;388:31–41.

Sallis JF, Carlson JA. Physical activity: numerous benefits and effective interventions. In: Kaplan RM, Spittel

ML, David DH, editors. Population health: behavioral and social science insights. Rockville, MD: US Government Printing Office: Agency for Healthcare Research and Quality; 2015. p. 169–84.. http://www.ahrq.gov/professionals/education/curriculum-tools/population-health/index.html.

Sallis JF, Carlson JA, Mignano AM, Lemes A, Wagner N. Trends in presentations of environmental and policy studies related to physical activity, nutrition, and obesity at society of behavioral medicine, 1995-2010: a commentary to accompany the active living research supplement to annals of behavioral medicine. Ann Behav Med. 2013;45(1, Suppl 1):14–7.

Sallis JF, Cervero RB, Ascher W, Henderson KA, Kraft MK, Kerr J. An ecological approach to creating more physically active communities. Annu Rev Public Health. 2006;27:297–322.

Sallis JF, Cutter CL, Lou D, Spoon C, Wilson AL, et al. Active living research: creating and using evidence to support childhood obesity prevention. Am J Prev Med. 2014;46:195–207.

Sallis JF, Floyd MF, Rodriguez DA, Saelens BE. The role of built environments in physical activity, obesity, and CVD. Circulation. 2012;125:729–37.

Sallis JF, Linton LS, Kraft MK, Cutter CL, Kerr J, et al. The active living research program: six years of grant-making. Am J Prev Med. 2009;36(2 Suppl.2):S10–21.

Sallis JF, Spoon C, Cavill N, Engelberg J, Gebel K, et al. Co-benefits of designing communities for active living: an exploration of literature. Int J Behav Nutr Phys Act. 2015;12:30.. http://www.ijbnpa.org/content/pdf/s12966-015-0188-2.pdf

Stokols D, Harvey R, Gress J, Fuqua J, Phillips K. In vivo studies of transdisciplinary scientific collaboration: lessons learned and implications for active living research. Am J Prev Med. 2005;28(suppl 2):202–13.

Taylor WC, Floyd MF, Whitt-Glover MC, Brooks J. Environmental justice: a framework for collaboration between the public health and parks and recreation fields to study disparities in physical activity. J Phys Act Health. 2007;4(Supp 1):S50–63.

U.S. Department of Health and Human Services. Physical activity and health: a report of the Surgeon General. Atlanta, GA: U.S. Department of Health and Human Services, Centers for Disease Control and Prevention, National Center for Chronic Disease Prevention and Health Promotion; 1996.

Whitt-Glover MC, Taylor WC, Floyd MF, Yore MM, Yancey AK, Matthews CE. Disparities in physical activity and sedentary behaviors among US children and adolescents: prevalence, correlates, and intervention implications. J Public Health Policy. 2009;30(1):S309–34.

Yancey AK, Sallis JF. Physical activity: Cinderella or Rodney Dangerfield? Prev Med. 2009;49:277–9.

Part XI

Technological Supports for Team Science

The Power of Research Networking Systems to Find Experts and Facilitate Collaboration

42

Griffin M. Weber and Leslie A. Yuan

Contents

42.1 Introduction

The scientific workforce requires teams to solve the most critical intellectual and social problems that confront us today. Though, in order to form teams, investigators must first be able to find each other. With scientific teams in recent years becoming increasingly interdisciplinary and multi-institutional (Wuchty et al. 2007, Jones et al. 2008), searching for collaborators is more challenging than ever before. To address this problem, there has been a rapid emergence of "research networking systems" (RNSs) that help users identify investigators with particular areas of expertise, affiliations, interests, resources, or other characteristics that would make them potential collaborators (Kahlon et al. 2014).

42.1.1 Distinguishing Research Networking Systems from Other Collaboration Tools

RNSs are distinct from Internet search engines and general-interest social networking platforms, in that they are typically implemented by organizations, such as universities or research centers, to create online profiles of their own investigators. Organizations can use local administrative databases to populate their RNSs with authoritative up-to-date information about investigators, such as their positions and job titles, academic ranks, training, and contact information. Many RNSs can automatically use this to discover additional details about investigators' scholarly activities, such as their publications, patents, courses, or funded projects. The prestige of an organization adds credibility to its RNS, leading visitors of the website to trust the content and motivating investigators themselves to ensure the accuracy of their data.

G. M. Weber (✉)
Beth Israel Deaconess Medical Center and
Harvard Medical School, Boston, MA, USA
e-mail: griffin_weber@hms.harvard.edu

L. A. Yuan
University of California San Francisco,
San Francisco, CA, USA

© Springer Nature Switzerland AG 2019
K. L. Hall et al. (eds.), *Strategies for Team Science Success*,
https://doi.org/10.1007/978-3-030-20992-6_42

The result is that RNSs provide visitors with a targeted search of investigators within a pre-defined community, using data that has been aggregated from multiple sources, supplemented with additional content not available on other websites, and curated and backed by an established research organization (Friedman et al. 2000, Schleyer et al. 2008). While an Internet search for "social and behavioral health" returns a mixture of educational programs, departments, job postings, news articles, and journals, an RNS takes users directly to the list of people who have expertise in that area. Furthermore, RNSs can filter and sort the list of investigators based on criteria that are important to users, such as institution or academic rank; or, they can help users expand their searches to individuals who have expertise in related research topics. These features of RNSs are grounded on principles of Team Science and distinguish those websites from other types of social networking platforms.

ResearchGate and Mendeley are examples of large-scale commercial collaboration tools, with accounts created by millions of scientists worldwide (Gewin 2010; ResearchGate 2016; Mendeley 2016). RNSs provide similar functionality, but are centered on an organization and its investigators. Investigators generally do not have to sign up for a research networking site. The software can automatically create a profile based on information contained with the organization's administrative databases. As a result, RNSs have a complete list of the institution's investigators, with accurate data presented and updated in a consistent way.

Large intellectual capital-driven companies, such as IBM (DiMicco et al. 2008) and Deloitte Consulting (Riemer and Scifleet 2012), have implemented "expertise location" and "social networking" systems to facilitate knowledge sharing and team building (Dorit et al. 2009). The motivations are similar to RNSs, but the industry versions of these tools are closed systems, available only to company employees. In contrast, RNSs are meant to be public, to expose information about an organization's investigators to a wide audience, and to encourage collaboration across institutional boundaries (Kahlon et al. 2014).

RNSs are complementary to "groupware" tools, such as Google Docs, SharePoint, and Slack, but serve a distinct purpose (Google Docs 2016; SharePoint 2016; Slack 2016). RNSs aid in locating experts and forming new collaborations, while groupware helps teams that have already formed work together more effectively.

42.1.2 Chapter Overview

The goal of this chapter is to provide organizations with an overview of the capabilities of RNSs (Sect. 42.2), the wide range of use cases (Sect. 42.3), and techniques for successfully implementing RNSs and encouraging their adoption (Sect. 42.4). It draws from our own personal experiences of building an open-source system at Harvard University called Profiles Research Networking Software (Profiles RNS) and installing and enhancing it at other institutions, such as the University of California, San Francisco (UCSF). We touch upon the many obstacles we have faced along the way, ranging from specific issues related to privacy and data quality, to larger questions about the overall impact and return on investment from RNSs. We conclude with an overview of the current state of RNSs and where they will be heading in the future (Sect. 42.5).

There are various stakeholders within an organization who can benefit from the different types of knowledge we present in this chapter. For example, leaders of science teams will learn how to use RNSs to assemble teams and how to advocate to their organizations' administrations for the development and implementation of RNSs; administrators who read this chapter will gain an understanding of how these tools can be used and the value-add of RNSs; and implementers will have a better sense of what needs to be considered to launch and maintain one. Although investigators are the ones being featured in RNSs, their profiles are typically created for them automatically, and they do not necessarily have to participate in the implementation process in order to benefit from RNSs. However, investigators who read this chapter will be shown why their organizations are adopting RNSs and how the websites can help them disseminate their research, build new collaborations within academia, and form partnerships with commercial entities such as pharmaceutical companies.

Although our original intent in developing an RNS was to facilitate team science, many other uses cases for RNSs have emerged in recent years. For example, efficiencies can be gained within organizations by repurposing the data collected about investigators in RNSs for departmental websites, library archives, conflict of interest systems, mentoring tools, promotion and tenure committees, public access compliancy checks, and many other administrative applications. Public relations offices are discovering that news stories linking directly to investigators' RNS pages are driving up Internet traffic to their organization's websites and increasing their rankings in search engines like Google. Pharmaceutical companies are leveraging the RNSs at academic research centers to learn about possible new drug targets that are being studied and to find sites to conduct clinical trials. Last, but not least, patients are using RNSs to find clinicians and read about their areas of expertise. These and other examples described throughout this chapter speak to the larger audience of individuals who might not yet realize the benefits that RNSs can provide to them.

42.2 Profiles Research Networking Software (Profiles RNS)

This section presents a brief history of why we developed an RNS and an overview of its features.

42.2.1 Origins of a Research Networking System

Harvard Medical School (HMS) has more than 20,000 faculty, though most are spread across 15 affiliated hospitals and academic health centers, with offices scattered throughout New England. As a result, people are separated both organiza-

tionally and physically, leading to numerous silos within the research community and creating barriers to collaboration and Team Science. In 2008 we sought to fix this problem when Harvard received a 5-year $120 million grant from the National Institutes of Health (NIH) to establish a Clinical and Translational Science Center (CTSC) (Harvard Catalyst 2019). It was one of 60 CTSCs across the United States funded by the NIH through its Clinical and Translational Science Award (CTSA) program, with the goal of accelerating the process of turning basic science discoveries into interventions that improve human health (Zerhouni 2005, Woolf 2008, Reis et al. 2010).

A key component of Harvard's CTSC was developing infrastructure to facilitate and encourage collaboration, so that laboratory scientists and clinical investigators could come together and more easily conduct research that leveraged the resources and patient populations across our different affiliated institutions. This involved tasks such as streamlining regulatory workflows, creating shared research core facilities, and providing funding for pilot studies to newly formed interdisciplinary teams. However, we quickly recognized that in order for these programs to reach their full potential, investigators must first be able to find each other.

Our solution was to develop a website called Profiles Research Networking Software (Profiles RNS), which creates searchable online "profiles" of all HMS investigators (Fig. 42.1) (Profiles RNS 2016). In designing the software, an objective was to automate as much of the website as possible, since it would be nearly impossible to collect information manually from 20,000 faculty and keep the data up-to-date. We began by obtaining names, positions, contact information, and ID photos from Harvard's human resources databases. Mentored projects, research resources, and other content are also imported from internal Harvard systems. This is supplemented with external sources of data, such as publications from the U.S. National Library of Medicine's (NLM) MEDLINE database (MEDLINE 2016) and

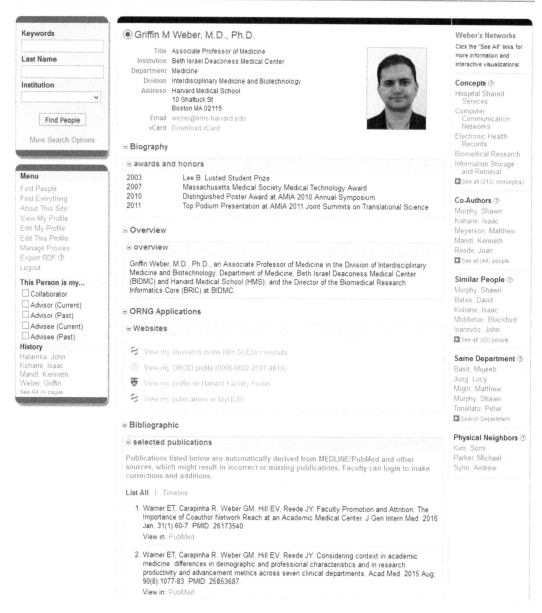

Fig. 42.1 Profiles Research Networking Software (RNS). Investigator profile page, with "active" networks on the left sidebar and "passive" networks on the right sidebar. The main section in the center contains content aggregated from multiple sources, including contact information from internal administrative systems, a custom photo provided by the investigator, an OpenSocial gadget with links to external websites, and publications automatically imported from MEDLINE

grants from NIH ExPORTER (ExPORTER 2016). Investigators can login to Profiles RNS to edit any of their profile content, manage privacy settings, or enter additional information, such as awards and honors, videos, presentations, a descriptive narrative, or links to other personal websites. Profiles RNS also has a proxy feature, which enables authorized users, such as a department administrator, to edit investigators' profiles on their behalf.

42.2.2 Passive and Active Networks

Visitors to the Profiles RNS website can search for investigators by keywords or name, and filter and sort the search results by institution, department, and academic rank. Once on an investigator's profile page, in addition to the main profile content, users are presented with links to interactive network visualizations that show how that person is connected to others within the HMS community. These connections are determined in two different ways. "Passive" network visualizations are based on existing relationships among investigators, such as common research interests, past collaborations, or physically nearby offices (Fig. 42.1, right sidebar). The networks are passive because Profiles RNS automatically discovers them using data mining techniques and machine learning algorithms. In contrast, "active" networks are generated by investigators themselves as they search the website, view different profile pages, or explicitly flag a person as a collaborator, mentor, or advisee (Fig. 42.1, left sidebar).

There were three motivations behind the idea of adding passive and active network visualizations to Profiles RNS. First, users might not always know what to search for, especially if they are seeking a collaborator from another discipline. The network visualizations help them branch out from an investigator or topic that they are familiar with and browse profiles of related people whose expertise might be more relevant to their particular problems. Second, the investigators with the most expertise (e.g., the most publications or grants) might be too busy, too far away, have conflicts of interest, or be unwilling to collaborate. The network visualizations help users look for alternatives and incorporate personal preferences into their search. Finally, it makes the website interesting and fun to use. Simply posting 20,000 resumes online would not engage investigators in the way we wanted. The network visualizations, though, enable users to explore the *relationships* among investigators; and, this is much more exciting since the visualizations often reveal facts about users' colleagues (or about themselves) that were unexpected. The automated passive networks provided a rich set of information to users the day we launched Profiles RNS, and the active networks collect data that helps us improve the website over time.

42.2.3 Discovering and Visualizing Networks

This section describes several types of data-derived passive network visualizations (Fig. 42.2). Each network has multiple visualizations to highlight different dimensions of the data; and, many visualizations are applied to different types of networks.

"Concept" networks reflect investigators' areas of expertise. For biomedical researchers, Profiles RNS uses the Medical Subject Headings (MeSH) "descriptors" linked to investigators' publications as their concept network. MeSH is a controlled vocabulary initially developed in 1960 by the NLM as a way of indexing biomedical publications (MeSH 2016). Today, there are more than 25,000 descriptors, and NLM assigns several descriptors to most articles in MEDLINE. In Profiles RNS, users can click any concept listed on an investigator's profile page and view other investigators with publications linked to that same MeSH descriptor.

In a concept "cloud" visualization (Fig. 42.2a), concepts are ranked based on their relative importance in the network, with highly ranked concepts displayed in large bold font, and low ranked concepts in a small font. The ranking is based on many factors, including the number of articles the investigator has published about the concept, how many years ago the articles were written, and whether the investigator was the first or senior author of the article. A uniqueness score is also included in the ranking, based on the number of other investigators with that concept. This emphasizes investigators' particular areas of expertise that are less common among their colleagues. In other words, highly ranked concepts indicate knowledge that an investigator can uniquely bring to a new collaboration.

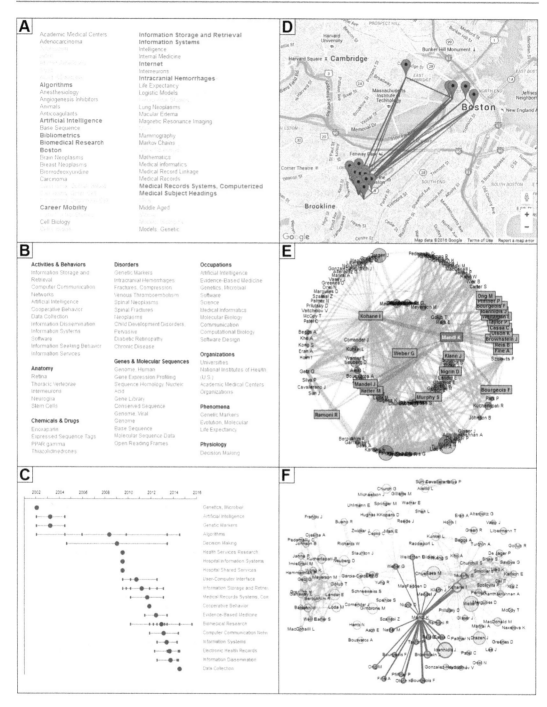

Fig. 42.2 Interactive network visualizations in profiles RNS. (**a**) Concept Cloud, (**b**) Concept Categories, (**c**) Concept Timeline, (**d**) CoAuthor Map, (**e**) CoAuthor Radial Graph, (**f**) CoAuthor Cluster Graph

In a concept "categories" visualization (Fig. 42.2b), concepts are grouped into semantic clusters, with diseases, for example, in one category, and chemicals in another. The "timeline" visualization creates a timeline for each concept, showing when each article linked to that concept was published (Fig. 42.2c). A circle on each timeline marks the mean publication date of those articles. The timelines are sorted by the average publication date, so that concepts investigators wrote about early in their careers are at the top, and concepts associated with more recent articles are at the bottom.

"Coauthor" networks connect investigators who have previously collaborated on a publication. The timeline visualization can be used with coauthor networks; however, in this case, each timeline corresponds to a different coauthor, rather than a concept. The visualization shows how investigators' collaborators change over time. In a "map" visualization (Fig. 42.2d), the coauthors' office addresses are converted to latitude and longitude coordinates and plotted on a Google map to show where investigators' collaborators are located geographically. An interactive "radial" graph (Fig. 42.2e) plots an investigator in the center of the visualization with her coauthors in a surrounding inner ring, and the coauthors of those coauthors in an outer ring. These are individuals the investigator can easily reach out to, either because they have worked together in the past, or because they share a collaborator who can make an introduction. This same group of people can be viewed in a force-directed "cluster" graph (Fig. 42.2f), in which investigators who have coauthored more articles together are placed closer to each other in the visualization. The cluster graph groups investigators into the teams in which they typically collaborate; yet, it also shows the connections between the teams.

"Similar People" networks connect investigators, who are not necessarily coauthors, but who are conducting similar research, as defined by having multiple concepts in common. There are many use cases for similar people networks beyond searching for a research collaborator. For example, they can be used to find a group of people doing related research to teach a course, present at a symposium, or serve on a review committee. "Same Department" networks

show organizational relationships among people, which is particularly useful in large institutions like Harvard, where a single department can have over a thousand investigators. "Physical Neighbor" networks indicate the people whose offices are physically nearest to an investigator, which is important because proximity can affect the performance of a team (Lee et al. 2010).

Each of these networks also has a "Details" view, which lists each item in the network, along with summary information and a "Why?" link, which leads to a "Connection" page. The Connection page lists the sources of information that Profiles RNS used to discover that the item is part of the network. For example, the connection page of a coauthor network lists the publications that the two people coauthored; and, the connection page of a similar person network lists the concepts that the two people have in common. Connection pages also display a "connection score," which is proportional to the number and types of items listed on that page. For example, the more publications two people wrote together, the higher their coauthor connection score.

42.3   Use Cases for Research Networking

In this section, we look at several examples of successful implementations of RNSs, with an emphasis on who initiated the efforts, what were the intended use cases, and how these influenced the design, software architecture, policies, and governance of the websites. What is remarkable is how varied the resulting websites can be, even when they are based on the same underlying data or software. Our objective is not to provide a comprehensive list of all use cases for RNSs, but rather to encourage organizations to think creatively about how they might benefit from RNSs and which stakeholders to engage.

42.3.1 University Relations Office: Publicize Faculty and Their Research

In 2010, Harvard Medical School made the underlying source code of Profiles RNS freely available to other institutions through an open-source software license. In the years since then, dozens of organizations have adopted Profiles RNS and customized it for different use cases. These customizations include simple user interface changes and branding, additional sources of data, new functionality, and even completely different software architectures.

The Clinical and Translational Science Institute (CTSI) at University of California, San Francisco (UCSF) was the first institution outside Harvard to use Profiles RNS (UCSF Profiles 2016). Although their initial goal, like Harvard, was to help their internal investigators build new collaborations, they saw visits from external users rapidly grow until their "UCSF Profiles" website had almost one-fifth the site traffic of their established UCSF campus website (Kahlon et al. 2014). They attributed this, in part, to a strategic partnership with their University Relations office to use UCSF Profiles to publicize university faculty and their research. This involved adding links in press releases and news stories about faculty to their UCSF Profiles pages, linking the university directory to UCSF Profiles, integrating data from UCSF Profiles into department websites, and applying various search engine optimizations approaches to the UCSF Profiles website. The result was that 75% of visitors to UCSF Profiles came directly from external search engines (91% from Google, 4% from search on the UCSF campus website, and 5% from Bing, Yahoo, and other websites), and 17% of visitors were referrals from other websites linking to individual faculty profile pages.

A significant enhancement UCSF CTSI made to the Profiles RNS software was adding support for OpenSocial, an Internet standard for developing cross-platform modular plugins, or "gadgets," for social networking applications (ORNG 2016). OpenSocial was originally developed by Google and MySpace and later expanded to enterprise social networking systems from IBM, Cisco, and other companies (OpenSocial Wikipedia 2016). OpenSocial gadgets for UCSF Profiles enable investigators to post mentoring opportunities, link to news stories, list their education and degrees, and embed content from external websites, such as their Twitter streams (Twitter 2016), presentations from SlideShare (SlideShare 2016), and videos from YouTube (YouTube 2016). Gadgets can be shared across different websites and applications supporting the OpenSocial framework. This includes not only other organizations using Profiles RNS, but also sites using other RNSs such as VIVO that support the standard. The addition of OpenSocial to UCSF Profiles provided faculty with an opportunity to post rich multimedia content about their research to their profile pages. This draws additional traffic to the website and has made UCSF Profiles the link of choice for external media outlets. For example, New York Times (Hafner 2012) and other news media have linked to UCSF Profiles when referencing UCSF faculty (Kahlon et al. 2014).

In addition to the University Relations Office, the faculty themselves also view Profiles RNS as a way to inform the public of their discoveries and publicize their accomplishments. Having an attractive profile on an official university website becomes a valuable resource for faculty in helping them "be found." This can be especially true for junior faculty and investigators new to a field.

42.3.2 University Library: Provide Access to the Scholarly Works of Faculty

In 2007, the Marston Science Library at the University of Florida (UF) began using a program called VIVO (VIVOWeb 2016), which was initially developed by the Cornell University Library, to record information about research faculty from UF's Institute of Food and Agricultural Sciences, including their publications, awarded grants, and areas of expertise (de Farber 2016). Like other research networking tools, VIVO can generate searchable online faculty profile pages. However, a key innovation of VIVO was its use of Semantic Web standards, which promote common data formats and exchange protocols (Berners-Lee et al. 2001).

Semantic Web applications use the Resource Description Framework (RDF), which is a method of expressing information in the form of subject–predicate–object "triples," such as "a researcher publishes an article," "an agency funds a grant," or "an instructor teaches a course" (RDF Wikipedia 2016). By linking thousands or millions of triples, the complexity of an entire research organization can be represented using an extremely simple data model. Information within Semantic Web applications can be published online as Linked Open Data and connected to many other linked open datasets that exist around the world, such as DBpedia (based on data extracted from Wikipedia), GeoNames (a database with more than 7.5 million geographical features), and data.gov (more than 1000 datasets from the United States government) (LOD Wikipedia 2016).

Semantic Web applications are based on an ontology, which defines different kinds of objects, attributes, and relationships in the model. VIVO combined and extended several existing Semantic Web ontologies to create a new VIVO ontology, which could better represent the activities and accomplishments of academic research communities (VIVOWeb 2016). Institutions whose RNSs published linked open data using the VIVO ontology can exchange structured information about their investigators in a common way and build new applications that leverage these data using a semantic query language called "SPARQL" (SPARQL Wikipedia 2016).

In 2009, UF, in collaboration with the Cornell University Library and five other academic libraries at Washington University, Scripps Research Institute, Indiana University, Ponce School of Medicine, and Weill Medical College of Cornell University, was awarded a $12 million grant through an NIH initiative to expand the use of RNSs (VIVOWeb 2016). Central to the project was the pivotal roles of libraries, which could not only implement the website and curate the data, but also had extensive experience supporting faculty, dissemination of knowledge, and perform-

ing community outreach (de Farber 2016). The result was a rapid growth in both the awareness and use of RNSs, as well as the adoption of the VIVO ontology in other research networking platforms. For example, Profiles RNS was rewritten in 2012 as a Semantic Web application based on the VIVO ontology (Profiles RNS 2016), and Elsevier's commercial research networking products can publish VIVO-compatible linked open datasets (Elsevier Pure 2016).

42.3.3 University Provost Office: Facilitate Cross-Discipline Initiatives

Harvard University has 11 schools in addition to its medical school, including a law school, business school, school of education, and undergraduate college. The Office of the Provost oversees university-wide activities, including fostering interfaculty collaboration, supporting a diverse pipeline of scholars at all stages of the academic career ladder, and advancing innovations in teaching and learning (Harvard Provost 2016). Within the Office of the Provost, the Faculty Development & Diversity (FD&D) office guides institutional policies and practices in all areas of faculty affairs, including providing leadership and coordination for faculty appointments, retention, and promotion (Harvard FD&D 2016).

In 2012, FD&D began a project to determine whether there was interest in consolidating faculty information across the university. While the medical school used Profiles RNS, the other schools used a combination of homegrown and commercial products to generate online profiles of their faculty. An early idea proposed implementing a new RNS, possibly based on Profiles RNS or another system, which would include faculty from all Harvard schools. There were numerous objections to this, with schools concerned that having multiple profiles for faculty (e.g., a university profile and a school profile) would both be confusing to users and pull Internet traffic away from the school-based websites.

Further discussions between FD&D and key stakeholders at the schools led to the conclusion that a university-wide faculty search tool was needed, but without the generation of faculty profile pages. Profiles RNS was selected as the software platform because of its ability to integrate disparate data sources, but nearly all the functionality except the search page was removed, and the website was named Harvard Faculty Finder (HFF) to emphasize its primary function as a search tool (HFF 2019). At first glance, HFF appears like an ordinary RNS. Users can search for faculty across all Harvard schools by keyword or name, view a list of all matching people, and filter and sort the search results in different ways. However, instead of clicking a person and being shown a profile of that faculty member within the HFF website, users are taken to that faculty member's profile page on her school's local website. This approach not only addressed the Provost Office's need to highlight the expertise that exists across the entire university, but it could also draw Internet traffic to the school websites rather than away from them.

Once there was general agreement on the structure of HFF as a search tool, the next challenge was concerns from schools that their faculty members' expertise would not be fairly represented in search results. For example, senior biomedical researchers at the medical school have hundreds of publication abstracts easily accessible and freely available through MEDLINE/PubMed, while the focus of other faculty might be teaching, performance, community service, or other scholarly activities where

data about them are more difficult to obtain. Therefore, the search engine might rank faculty from some disciplines as having more expertise, on average, than other faculty, simply because the software can find more things about them. Simply indexing the existing school-based faculty websites was not sufficient because they varied greatly, even by department within a school, in the types, quantity, and format of the data they contained. Also, asking thousands of busy faculty to provide resumes or manually enter data was infeasible.

Eventually, three steps were taken to avoid discipline bias in the website. First, publication data were purchased from a commercial vendor. MEDLINE mostly contains biomedical journal articles. In contrast, commercial databases such as Clarivate Analytics' Web of Science and Elsevier's Scopus include publications across all disciplines. Futhermore, in addition to journal articles, commercial databases index conference proceedings, books, and other publication formats. Nearly all Harvard faculty have at least a few publications of some form; and, therefore, commercial publication data could be a starting point for HFF.

In general, faculty with few publications have other types of scholarly works. Thus, the second step was identifying what these were (Table 42.1). This required domain expertise, and representatives from each of the Harvard schools were consulted. Based on the results of those interviews, numerous data sources were linked to HFF, each

Table 42.1 Harvard Faculty Finder—fraction of faculty with different content types

School	Articles	Books	Patents	Projects	Courses	Websites
Arts & Sciences	0.742	0.145	0.022	0.065	0.730	0.628
Business	0.869	0.131	0.012	**0.508**	0.385	0.912
Dental	0.602	0.006	0.025	0.003	0.012	**1.000**
Design	0.529	0.076	0.017	0.067	0.034	0.731
Divinity	0.597	0.153	0.000	0.028	0.486	0.431
Education	0.699	0.096	0.000	0.059	**0.772**	0.912
Engineering	0.870	0.083	**0.204**	0.028	0.759	0.713
Government	0.731	0.170	0.005	0.154	0.143	0.769
Law	0.661	**0.188**	0.010	0.057	0.693	0.891
Medicine	0.810	0.021	0.026	0.003	0.037	0.999
Public Health	**0.902**	0.074	0.029	0.133	0.133	**1.000**

The values indicate the fraction of faculty from each Harvard school with journal articles, books, patents, international projects, courses taught, and local school or departmental websites. The highest values for each content type are in bold benefitting different groups of faculty to varying degrees. For example, 10 years of data from the Harvard Course Catalog revealed the extensive teaching history of many of the faculty, especially at the college and the school of education; although a search of the United States Patent and Trademark Office (USPTO) database (USPTO 2016) found patents for only 1–2% of Harvard faculty overall, the rate increased to 20% for faculty at the engineering school; and more than half the faculty at the business school were listed in the Harvard Worldwide database of international projects.

Quantity does not equal quality. One faculty member might be able to write several journal articles in the same amount of time another faculty member spends developing and teaching a new course. The third step was to compensate for this discrepancy. The Profiles RNS search engine can be configured to weight each type of item that it indexes differently. In HFF, the weights were initially set inversely proportional to the number of items of a particular type. For example, because there were approximately ten times as many journal articles as courses in the database, courses were given ten times as much weight. These numbers were then adjusted based on feedback from a committee of Faculty Affairs deans from each school, who tested the HFF website using a combination of broad and specific search terms, such as "energy," "China," and "Shakespeare," to see which faculty matched and how they were ranked by the website.

With the launch of HFF, the Office of the Provost and FD&D provided students, investigators, and others, for the first time, a searchable interface to all Harvard faculty based on research and teaching expertise. HFF linked multiple websites and databases across the university, and through HFF's web service interfaces, the connected Linked Open Data could be extracted and used in a wide range of cross-school and cross-discipline applications.

42.3.4 Using Research Networking to Help Patients

The RNSs of a physician network, government agency, and pharmaceutical company illustrate three ways in which these systems can directly or indirectly help patients.

The Undiagnosed Disease Network (UDN) is an NIH-funded collaboration between seven U.S. clinical sites to help patients with rare or hard-to-diagnose diseases (UDN 2016). These patients often suffer for years without a diagnosis and are unable to find a physician who can treat them. The UDN performs a complete clinical evaluation of its patients, including genomic analyses, metabolic studies, and evaluation of environmental exposures. They then seek to match the patients with the best possible physicians within their network. "UDN Profiles" is a single website containing physicians from multiple UDN hospitals across the country, which enables users to search for individuals with expertise in rare or complex conditions.

The United States Food & Drug Administration (FDA) regularly assembles committees of scientists within the FDA's Office of Science and Engineering Laboratories (OSEL) to review new medical devices. Specialized knowledge about particular materials or technologies is often needed for this. The best source of information about who has this expertise is an internal FDA database describing past device reviews and the members of those committees. These records were loaded into an "FDA Profiles" website to help FDA administrators identify OSEL scientists for future device reviews (FDA Profiles 2013). Because of the narrow use case and the sensitive nature of the FDA's device review database, the FDA Profiles site is protected behind a firewall and access is restricted to a small number of users within the FDA.

Pharmaceutical companies have a dual need for research networking tools. The first is to understand what expertise exists within their company. Many have thousands of employees, spread across multiple countries, and divided into independent groups working on different diseases or biochemical pathways. As a result, these groups might have little knowledge about what other groups are doing. The second major use case is looking outwards to investigators in academic health centers who are conducting research relevant to the company. In the early stages of drug development, they are interested in basic scientists exploring new potential drug targets, and in later stages they seek collaborators to assist with clinical trial recruitment or post-market surveillance. Creating an RNS for this second use case is difficult because the population of investigators to include in the website is not well defined, and the pharmaceutical company might have little data about those people. One approach is simply to query publicly available RNSs that already exist at many universities.

42.3.5 Using Research Networking for Reporting and Analysis

RNSs contain vast amounts of data about an organization, which can be used for portfolio analysis and strategic planning. For example, Elsevier offers a commercial RNS called Pure, which is part of a suite of "research intelligence" products, which includes Scopus and SciVal (Elsevier Pure). Scopus, which is one of the largest abstract and citation databases of peer-reviewed literature, is used to obtain publication data for investigator profiles in Pure. SciVal also uses data from Scopus and other sources to generate metrics about the research performance of 7500 institutions and 220 nations worldwide. Combined, these tools provide research administrators with a wide range of functionality, such as benchmarking their investigators' research against peer institutions, identifying the most productive investigators and rising stars, and matching targeted funding opportunities to investigators.

Profiles RNS contains a specialized module that calculates several metrics based on social network analysis (SNA) of the coauthor network that it derives from publication data. SNA is a method of quantitatively characterizing the structure of a social network for a variety of purposes, such as identifying key individuals who connect different parts of an organization and testing hypotheses of how new collaborations form. An example of an SNA metric available in Profiles RNS is coauthor "reach," which is the number of coauthors an investigator has plus the number of coauthors the investigator's coauthors have. The

radial and cluster graphs in Profiles RNS are visual representations of coauthor reach. At Harvard Medical School, the Office for Diversity Inclusion & Community Partnership used the coauthor reach metric in Profiles RNS to show how collaboration patterns among faculty differ across fields (Warner et al. 2015) and between men and women faculty (Warner et al. 2016).

42.3.6 Cross-Institution Research Networking Applications

In 2010, the Research Networking Working Group of the national NIH CTSA Consortium launched an initiative called Direct2Experts to develop a cross-institution search tool, which could locate investigators across multiple universities' RNSs. Despite the fact that these websites were public, at first nearly all participating universities expressed concerns about privacy issues and competitive intelligence that could result from sharing data. As a result, the focus for the initial Direct2Experts pilot was on simply gaining institutional buy-in to the general idea of a national network, even if that meant greatly limiting the functionality of the system (Weber et al. 2011).

The agreed upon software architecture for the pilot had two general principles. First, there would be no central data repository of investigator data. Users enter keywords into a search form on the Direct2Experts website, and those keywords are broadcast to each institution's RNS and processed locally. Second, only the aggregate count of the number of investigators matching the search keywords would be returned to the Direct2Experts website (Fig. 42.3). Institutions would not have to share data on any individual people. Users can click an aggregate count on the Direct2Experts website and be taken to the corresponding institution's local RNS to view the list of people who matched the query.

By creating a low barrier to joining the Direct2Experts network, interest rapidly grew; and, within 6 months, seven major research networking products supported the Direct2Experts technical requirements, and 28 universities connected their websites to the network. Despite

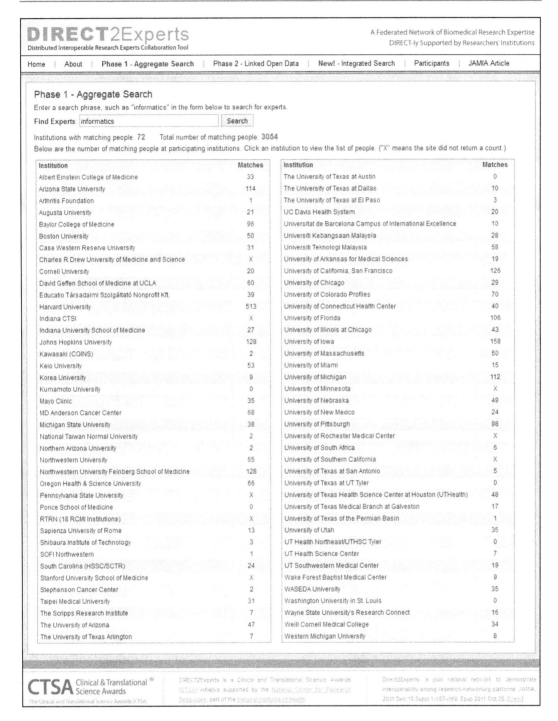

Fig. 42.3 Direct2Experts. Federated search across 80 institutions using 8 different RNS platforms. Shown are the number of people who match the search term "infor-matics" at each participating institution. Clicking an institution name reveals the list of matching people

the minimal capabilities of Direct2Experts, it established a path forward for future efforts to build cross-institution research networking applications. VIVO further helped to change institutions' attitudes toward sharing data; and, within a couple years, many universities supported a new website called CTSAsearch, which copied the institutions' faculty information into a central database and included advanced research networking functionality such as coauthor network graphs (CTSAsearch 2016). As of mid-2016, there were 80 institutions worldwide in the Direct2Experts network (Direct2Experts 2016), and nearly the same number, 74, in CTSAsearch.

42.4   Guide to Success

Here we list frequently asked questions about research networking, which organizations can use as a guide before, during, and after they implement a system. It is well worth the effort to take the time to think about each of these. Often the focus is on selecting the right product. However, today the major research networking platforms, such as Profiles RNS, VIVO, and Elsevier Pure, are mature enough that they have far more similarities than differences; and, all of them have been highly successful at some institutions and failures at others. The way institutions approach establishing governance, determining policies, setting expectations, promoting use, and providing ongoing support of their RNSs is what really determines the outcomes.

42.4.1 Questions to Consider Before Implementing a Research Networking System

42.4.1.1   What Problem Is My Organization Trying to Solve?

Implementing an RNS requires a significant institutional investment, in both cost and human time, even for freely available open-source products. There are usually many other projects competing for the same resources that have higher priority within a research organization, such as regulatory and compliance applications, financial systems, and data storage solutions. You will not gain institutional support for an RNS if the arguments are limited to "other institutions have them," "the visualizations are interesting," or "they will create new collaborations." You need to show how the website will solve a specific problem that is already viewed within the organization as high priority. As was the case with HFF, this might not be obvious at first, and could require some exploration.

42.4.1.2   What Other Faculty Information Websites Already Exist at My Organization?

It is rare today to find a large research organization that does not already have some website with information about its investigators, even if it is as simple as an online phone directory. It is essential to identify these systems, determine who their owners are, and figure out if a new research networking website will replace or be complementary to those existing systems. We often see organizations with multiple RNSs set up independently by different groups. The result is that investigators don't know which of their several profiles to update, and the future of all the websites remain in doubt.

42.4.1.3   Who Should Be the Business Owner?

The business owner of the research networking website is not necessarily the group that implements it. The business owner should be at a high level within the organization, have well-established relationships with investigators, be able to commit a large amount of effort to the project, and be the person or group ordinarily responsible for the problem the research networking website is intended to address. As was illustrated in the previous examples, the appropriate business owner varies depending on the use case. Possibilities include an organization's Public Relations office, Provost Office, Faculty Affairs office, or library. Information Technology and Human Resources departments often implement the websites or provide the data for them, but might not be the best business owner. There might be specialized groups within an organization, like Clinical and Translational Science Institutes, whose mission includes facilitating collaboration and Team Science. They are often the ideal home for RNSs, but they benefit from strategic partnerships with other parts of the organization. An example is UCSF CTSI's alliance with the University Relations office.

42.4.1.4 How Should We Think About Governance?

Avoid too much of it. Assembling a large committee with representatives from both the faculty and administration to review and approve each step of the implementation process will slow things down to the point where the website will never be launched. An alternative strategy is to identify key stakeholders, and work with them individually to gain their support. These people include data owners, such as the Chief Information Officer and Head of Human Resources, and individuals responsible for faculty career advancement and research, such as the Faculty Affairs Dean and Vice President for Research. As you get closer to launching the website, you can begin looking for a small number of friendly senior investigators who can provide constructive feedback, serve as advocates for the website, and encourage their colleagues to use the website.

42.4.1.5 What Factors Are Important in Selecting a Research Networking Product?

Most of the major products share a core set of functionality, such as combining local administrative data with publications and other external data sources, various search options, and methods of extracting the data. They differ in small ways, largely depending on the initial use case that led to the creation of the system. For example, Profiles RNS has multiple network analysis and visualization modules because of its original goal of using the existing connections between investigators as a way of guiding users towards new potential collaborators. VIVO, which promoted the use of Semantic Web standards in RNSs, includes sophisticated tools for managing and extending the ontology. Elsevier's Pure benefits from synergies with Elsevier's commercial databases. The best product for an organization often depends on which system aligns best with their use case. A Wikipedia page provides a detailed comparison of several RNS platforms and related collaboration tools (RNS Wikipedia 2016).

42.4.1.6 Who Should Lead the Implementation?

If managed internally, it is typically the Information Technology (IT) department, an Informatics group, or the library which leads the technical part of the implementation of the research networking website. Other institutions work with an external vendor, in which case the business owner might be the local point of contact for the implementation. A common mistake is placing the one analyst in the business owner's department, the person who "knows some HTML," or the summer student in charge of the implementation. RNSs should be treated in the same way as other enterprise mission critical software applications in an organization.

42.4.1.7 Should We Implement the Research Networking Website Ourselves or Hire a Vendor?

Both Profiles RNS and VIVO have partnered with a commercial company, Symplectic, which can assist institutions in installing, customizing, and managing their RNSs (Symplectic 2016). Institutions using Elsevier's Pure automatically get support from Elsevier. Although working with a vendor costs money, the vendor's experience with the software enables them to implement the software more efficiently than an organization's own staff, potentially reducing the overall cost to the organization. As organizations gain familiarity with the websites over time, they may choose not to renew annual support contracts.

42.4.1.8   How Much Do RNSs Cost?

The more you put into an RNS, the more you will get out of it. For example, Profiles RNS is free, and it can be installed in 1 day. However, that alone will not get anyone to visit the website. The benefits of an RNS increase greatly if resources are put into curating the data, acquiring additional data sources, building custom extensions to the software, and developing a comprehensive marketing strategy. Typically, the costs can be divided into a technical component (e.g., computer servers to host the website and IT staff to manage the software) and a business analyst component (e.g., the staff within the business owner's office who will meet regularly with stakeholders and investigators). A small organization might only require fractional effort of two people. A large organization doing significant software development to customize or extend the functionality of their research networking website might have several dedicated staff. The overall costs can range from tens of thousands to hundreds of thousands of dollars per year. In some cases, working with a commercial vendor can be less expensive than implementing the system entirely in-house.

42.4.1.9   How Do We Estimate a Return on Investment?

This is an extremely difficult question to answer. It makes sense that an RNS could help create a new collaboration that results in being awarded a grant, convince a high net-worth philanthropist to make a large donation to the organization, or attract new patients seeking care. However, the website alone does not make these things happen. Many factors lead to these outcomes, and the website likely only played a very small role. Though, note that a large number of people often visit these websites. Profiles RNS at Harvard and UCSF, for example, each get more than a million visitors per year. Thus, the websites probably benefit many people in small incremental ways. Adding this up in a quantitative way is challenging. It is also important to consider secondary uses for RNSs. For example, we built Profiles RNS at Harvard to facilitate new collaborations. However, it also has streamlined many administrative workflows, such as assembling committees, matching students with faculty mentors, and

identifying speakers for conferences and other events. These unintended uses might have greater overall benefit to the university than the new collaborations.

42.4.1.10   Do RNSs Reduce Administrative Burden on Investigators?

Globally, not yet. This is a commonly described use case for RNSs. The idea is that once investigators curate their profile page, they will never again have to enter their publication lists into another system, generate a biosketch for a grant proposal, or email a headshot to an event. All the information should be available as Linked Open Data. However, two things must happen before this becomes a reality. First, systems like ORCID (Open Research and Contributor Identifier) (ORCiD 2016), which attempt to solve the name disambiguation problem by creating unique author identifiers, must become more widely used in order to improve the accuracy of the data in RNSs. Second, funding agencies and others who frequently request faculty information must have simple tools to extract the data from RNSs. But, the good news is that locally, within an institution, headway has been made. Harvard, UCSF, and Duke, to name just a few, offer a variety of technical approaches that allow their RNS data to be syndicated across their respective institutions with heavy uptake from department websites and various administrative systems.

42.4.2   Questions to Consider While Implementing a Research Networking System

42.4.2.1   Which People Should Have Profiles in the Website?

This appears to be a simple question, with the obvious answer being the organization's investigators. However, it often becomes much more complicated when attempting to design the specific query to run against the human resources database to obtain that list of people. Do you want to include only faculty or also the staff and trainees working in the research laboratories? Are postdoctoral fellows, emeritus faculty, visiting professors, and part-time employees considered faculty? Should you include faculty who primarily teach or treat patients instead of doing research? Should both a person's academic and administrative titles be displayed on the website, or just the academic titles? How should investigators at closely affiliated centers or institutes that are not officially part of the organization be handled?

42.4.2.2 Should There Be an Opt-out or Opt-in Policy?

In an opt-out policy, a profile is automatically created for all investigators unless an individual investigator requests that it be removed. In an opt-in policy, profiles are only created for investigators who ask for one. In almost all cases, organizations should strive for opt-out (or even mandatory), despite the increased privacy risks. This is because many of the use cases for research networking depend on a large fraction of investigators within an organization having profiles. This is difficult to achieve with an opt-in policy. The policy at Harvard is that faculty cannot opt out of the Profiles RNS website; however, they can hide everything on their profile except their name, affiliation, title, and mailing address. The rationale is that the person's job as a Harvard faculty member "belongs" to Harvard and must be shown, but all the scholarly works (e.g., publications, awards, etc.) belong to the person. Students are not included in the website because their data are protected by Federal FERPA (Family Educational Rights and Privacy Act) laws (FERPA 2016). Organizations in the United States must use an opt-in policy for students.

42.4.2.3 How Will Human Resources Data About Investigators Be Obtained on a Regular Basis?

Human resources data contain sensitive information, such as social security numbers and salaries. As a result, the owners of the data are usually cautious about giving the data to others, even within the same organization. Furthermore, there might be technical challenges of extracting the

information, and the data might be coded in a way that needs to be transformed for a public website (e.g., converting "Sr Fac Dept Med" to "Department of Medicine"). It is important to begin working with the Human Resources department early in the implementation process to resolve these issues.

42.4.2.4 What Other Types of Data Need to Be Included in the Website Before Launching It?

HFF illustrates an extreme case, where the research networking website contained a diverse population with many different forms of scholarly work and key stakeholders expected a high degree of data completeness. Numerous data sources had to be integrated into the website before it could be launched. This added a great deal of complexity to the system and makes ongoing support of the website difficult. In general, it is better to start simple. Publications alone might be sufficient for an initial version of a website, and users can be given a timeline of when other types of data will be added.

42.4.2.5 Do We Have Permission to Use the Data?

Make sure you confirm that you have permission to display your different data sources on a public research networking website. For example, an organization might object to using email address on a public website because of the potential for increased email spam. Also, licenses for commercial data might prohibit redistribution of the data, which could prevent its use in an RNS.

42.4.2.6 How Often Do the Data Need to Be Updated?

Different types of data in an RNS should be updated according to how rapidly the data change and an acceptable time lag for updates. For example, at Harvard, we aim to update human resources information and privacy settings on a nightly basis; publications and grants weekly; and course catalog data once a semester.

42.4.2.7 How Do We Deal with Incorrect or Missing Data?

Set appropriate expectations. The best automated algorithms in the world for matching publications to people are only about 85% accurate. At Harvard Medical School, with 20,000 faculty, this means that thousands of them will look at their profile pages for the first time and see either missing or incorrect publications. Investigators with common names, such as "John Smith," will be more likely to have data errors than those with unusual names. Be sure to have disclaimers on the website explaining how the data were generated and provide contact information for someone who can help the investigator correct her data. Also, determine what types of errors are most tolerable for your use cases. For example, is it worse for investigators to be missing publications or to have someone else's publications on their profile pages? In Profiles RNS, organizations can set their preference, with the default keeping incorrect publications at a low rate with the trade-off being a higher rate of missing publications.

42.4.2.8 Should the Website Be Public or Private?

If at all possible public! Requiring a login eliminates many of the privacy concerns and enables more detailed tracking of how investigators use the site. However, it removes much of the benefit of the website. The login creates a barrier that discourages investigators within an institution from using the website, and it completely blocks all the potential external collaborators. If there is a particular data type in the system, such as awarded grants, which is raising privacy concerns, then consider the harm of removing those data compared to blocking the entire website from the public. It should also be noted that many RNSs provide investigators with privacy settings that give them granular control over which data on their profiles can be accessed publicly.

42.4.2.9 What Should the URL of the Website Be?

Keep it short and easy to remember. For individual investigator profile pages, include the name of the person in the URL if possible, since it increases the rank of the page in search engines such as Google, and it makes it more likely that other websites will link to that page. In addition, academic institutions should use the organization's .edu domain in the URL.

42.4.3 Questions to Consider When Launching a Research Networking System and Beyond

42.4.3.1 What Is a Good Rollout Strategy?

This must be carefully planned and customized for each organization. One approach is to launch the website in a single department, and make changes based on user feedback before expanding to the entire organization. Another is to make the website private for a brief period of time to give investigators a chance to review their profile content before it becomes available to the public. The launch of the website can be accompanied with a simultaneous marketing campaign; or, it can be done as a "silent release." The slower more gradual rollout options are safer, but they might hurt in the long run by potentially decreasing enthusiasm for the website as it lingers in state where traffic to the website is intentionally reduced.

42.4.3.2 How Do We Encourage Use and Adoption of the Website?

UCSF Profiles provides examples of effective approaches to encouraging use and adoption. First, as described above, a partnership with the University Relations Office led to other UCSF websites linking to investigator profiles. This increased use of UCSF Profiles from within the organization. Second, search engine optimization strategies, such as simple descriptive URLs and page titles, resulted in an increase in external visitors to the website. Third, several techniques were used to encourage investigators themselves to visit the website and add content to their profile pages: (a) Investigators were told that they would be eligible to win a free iPod if they added a research narrative to their profile. They were not required to do anything else, but since they had already logged into the site and navigated to the editing interface to write the research narrative, many took the opportunity to complete other portions of their profiles. (b) Newly hired investigators are sent welcome emails to introduce them to UCSF Profiles and to let them know that they have a profile page. (c) Once a year, investigators are emailed a summary of the number and types of people who visited their profile page. They can login to their profile to view a full report based on website usage data collected by Google Analytics.

42.4.3.3   How Do We Evaluate Success?

This question, like return on investment, is complicated to answer. Because RNSs are typically public and do not require a login, it is usually not possible to know exactly who visited the website by analyzing web logs. The total number of visitors to the website and the fraction of investigators who update their profiles pages provide quantitative measures of adoption, but adoption alone usually is not the main goal of the website. Anecdotal stories from investigators or formal surveys might be the only way of understanding how the website is really being used. Another approach is to do before-and-after comparisons or compare your organization to a similar one that does not have an RNS. For example, at Harvard, we could look at whether the coauthor network of faculty has more connections now than before we built Profiles RNS. However, there are so many other variables, such as changes in NIH funding rates, faculty turnover, and organizational changes (e.g., the creation of a new department), that it

becomes impossible to determine what to attribute to the research networking website. Although calculating the impact of RNSs on team science is complicated, other benefits of RNSs can be simpler to identify, such as when data from RNSs are used by other systems within an organization (e.g., department websites, research compliance tools, etc.).

42.4.3.4   When Should We Upgrade to the Latest Version of the Software?

Research networking products often have one or two major software updates per year. Organizations would like to have the latest new features, but upgrading can be difficult. Especially with open-source applications, institutions might implement numerous customizations and software extensions over time. Upgrading to a new version of the software may require reapplying all those changes. Ontology changes that modify the data can be even more of a challenge since they can affect all other systems that utilize investigator information from the website. As a result, organizations are often several versions behind because the new features are not worth the effort needed to upgrade.

42.4.3.5   How Do We Connect to Cross-Institution Networks?

Two cross-institution networks are Direct2Experts and CTSAsearch. Their respective websites provide information on how to join the networks. Elsevier has an additional network just for its Pure websites.

42.4.3.6   What Opportunities Are There to Learn More About Research Networking?

Profiles RNS, Elsevier Pure, and VIVO each have active user communities, with mailing lists and regular webinars. VIVO hosts an annual conference to bring together both implementers and users of RNSs (VIVOConference 2016).

42.5   The Current State of Research Networking and Future Directions

A survey of 61 CTSA sites was conducted in 2012 to assess the state of adoption of RNSs (Obeid et al. 2014). Among these large academic health centers, nearly all respondents (47 of 48) were in different stages of selecting or implementing an RNS. Half (24) had a live production website, with three institutions having implemented two separate websites, and one institution having implemented three different research networking products. Elsevier Experts (its predecessor to Pure), Profiles RNS, and VIVO were each used in approximately a quarter of the institutions, with several other products distributed among the remaining institutions. The majority of institutions (54%) were already publishing faculty information as Linked Open Data or had plans to do so within 2 years.

The survey showed types of people and data included in the RNSs varied greatly between institutions. Tenured faculty were included in 92% of the websites, while only 35% had postdoctoral fellows, 26% had research staff, and 11% had graduate students. Publications were included in 85% of the websites, while 60% had funded grants, 23% had courses taught, and 17% had patents. Investigators outside of the biomedical sciences were included in 36% of websites; though, another 36% were planning or considering to add them later. In the majority of websites (53%), investigators were required to have a profile page, while 33% had an opt-out policy, 10% were opt-in, and 4% had no response.

The landscape of RNSs has transformed remarkably over the past decade. In 2007, the software tools were in their infancy, and institutions were hesitant to expose information about their investigators online, despite the fact that data about their scholarly works (e.g., publications, funded grants, etc.) were already in the public domain. In the 5 years that followed, new products emerged, and attitudes towards data privacy and the importance of data sharing shifted rapidly as a result of multi-institutional initiatives such as VIVO, Direct2Experts, and CTSAsearch. By 2016, the products have matured, and organi-

zations have discovered a wide range of applications for RNSs, beyond just helping investigators find new collaborators.

The next 5 years will likely see an increase in the use of analytical tools and reporting modules integrated within RNSs. While in the past the emphasis was on simply identifying the scholarly works of investigators, greater access to citation data and altmetrics (AltMetric 2016) will enable users to understand the impact and significance of investigators' research. With several years of website usage data, institutions will have a better idea about who is visiting their RNSs and will be able to analyze the impact of past efforts to increase adoption. Additional knowledge about how RNSs are used will lead to the development of personalized search tools and "recommendation systems" (Fazel-Zarandi et al. 2011) which will intelligently adjust search result rankings based on investigators' discipline, career stage, and preferences. Finally, RNSs will increasingly become the primary source of data about investigators, replacing the traditional biosketch, reducing administrative burden on investigators, and presenting metrics that accurately reflect investigators' contributions to collaborations and Team Science activities.

We hope that our experience with RNSs and the examples we presented in this chapter have provided stakeholders with a better understanding of the features of RNSs, ideas on how they might use RNSs within their organizations, and an appreciation for what factors contribute to their success.

Acknowledgments This work was conducted with support from Harvard Catalyst | The Harvard Clinical and Translational Science Center and the UCSF Clinical and Translational Science Institute (National Center for Research Resources and the National Center for Advancing Translational Sciences, National Institutes of Health Awards UL1 TR001102 and UL1 TR001872) and financial contributions from Harvard University and its affiliated academic healthcare centers. Additional funding was provided by National Institutes of Health awards UL1TR000004, DP4GM096852, R01GM111563, and U01GM112623 and National Science Foundation awards #1238469 and #1360042. The content is solely the responsibility of the authors and does not necessarily represent the official views of Harvard Catalyst, Harvard University and its affiliated academic healthcare centers, UCSF, the National Institutes of Health, or the National Science Foundation.

References

Altmetrics Wikipedia. 2016. https://en.wikipedia.org/wiki/Altmetrics. Accessed 1 Jul 2016.

Berners-Lee T, Hendler J, Lassila O. The semantic web: a new form of web content that is meaningful to computers will unleash a revolution of new possibilities. Basingstoke: Scientific American; 2001.

CTSAsearch. 2016. http://research.icts.uiowa.edu/polyglot. Accessed 1 Jul 2016.

de Farber BG. Collaborative grant-seeking: a practical guide for librarians. Volume 24 of practical guides for librarians. Lanham, MA: Rowman & Littlefield; 2016.

DiMicco J, Millen DR, Geyer W, Dugan C, Brownholtz B, Muller M. Motivations for social networking at work. In: Proceedings of the ACM Conference on Computer Supported Cooperative Work, San Diego, CA, USA. 2008. pp. 711–720.

Direct2Experts. 2016. http://Direct2Experts.org. Accessed 1 Jul 2016.

Dorit N, Benbasat I, Wand Y. Who knows what? Wall Street Journal/Sloan Management Review. 2009. http://online.wsj.com/news/articles/SB100014240529 70203946904574302032097910314. Accessed 1 Jul 2016.

Elsevier Pure. 2016. https://www.elsevier.com/solutions/pure. Accessed 1 Jul 2016.

ExPORTER. 2016. https://exporter.nih.gov. Accessed 1 Jul 2016.

Fazel-Zarandi M, Huang Y, Contractor N. Expert recommendation based on social drivers, social network analysis, and semantic data representation. In: Proceedings of the 2nd International Workshop on Information Heterogeneity and Fusion in Recommender Systems. 2011: pp. 41–48.

FDA Profiles. 2013. http://lj.libraryjournal.com/2013/03/people/movers-shakers-2013/jessica-hernandez-movers-shakers-2013-community-builders. Accessed 1 Jul 2016.

FERPA. 2016. http://www2.ed.gov/policy/gen/guid/fpco/ferpa/index.html. Accessed 1 Jul 2016.

Friedman PW, Winnick BL, Friedman CP, Mickelson PC. Development of a MeSH-based index of faculty research interests. Proc AMIA Symp. 2000:265–269.

Gewin V. Collaboration: social networking seeks critical mass. Nature. 2010;468(7326):993–4. https://doi.org/10.1038/nj7326-993a.

Google Docs. 2016. https://www.google.com/docs. Accessed 1 Jul 2016.

Hafner K. For second opinion, consult a computer? New York, NY: New York Times; 2012. http://www.nytimes.com/2012/12/04/health/quest-to-eliminate-diagnostic-lapses.html?pagewanted=all. Accessed 1 Jul 2016.

Harvard Catalyst. 2019. https://catalyst.harvard.edu. Accessed 8 Jul 2019.

Harvard FD&D. 2016. http://faculty.harvard.edu. Accessed 1 Jul 2016.

Harvard Provost. 2016. http://provost.harvard.edu. Accessed 1 Jul 2016.

HFF. 2019. http://facultyfinder.harvard.edu. Accessed 8 Jul 2019.

Jones BF, Wuchty S, Uzzi B. Multi-university research teams: shifting impact, geography, and stratification in science. Science. 2008;322(5905):1259–62. https://doi.org/10.1126/science.1158357.. http://www.sciencemag.org/cgi/pmidlookup?view=long&pmid=18845711

Kahlon M, Yuan L, Daigre J, Meeks E, Nelson K, Piontkowski C, Reuter K, Sak R, Turner B, Weber GM, Chatterjee A. The use and significance of a research networking system. J Med Internet Res. 2014;16(2):e46. https://doi.org/10.2196/jmir.3137.

LOD Wikipedia. 2016. https://en.wikipedia.org/wiki/Linked_data. Accessed 1 Jul 2016.

Lee K, Brownstein JS, Mills RG, Kohane IS. Does collocation inform the impact of collaboration? PLoS One. 2010;5(12):e14279.

MEDLINE. 2016. http://www.medline.com. Accessed 1 Jul 2016.

MeSH. 2016. https://www.nlm.nih.gov/mesh. Accessed 1 Jul 2016.

Mendeley. 2016. https://www.mendeley.com. Accessed 1 Jul 2016.

Obeid JS, Johnson LM, Stallings S, Eichmann D. Research networking systems: the state of adoption at institutions aiming to augment translational research infrastructure. J Transl Med Epidemiol. 2014;2(2):1026.

ORCiD. 2016. http://orcid.org. Accessed 20 Dec 2016.

ORNG. 2016. http://www.orng.info. Accessed 1 Jul 2016.

OpenSocial Wikipedia. 2016. https://en.wikipedia.org/wiki/OpenSocial. Accessed 1 Jul 2016.

Profiles RNS. 2016. http://profiles.catalyst.harvard.edu. Accessed 1 Jul 2016.

RDF Wikipedia. 2016. https://en.wikipedia.org/wiki/Resource_Description_Framework. Accessed 1 Jul 2016.

Reis SE, Berglund L, Bernard GR, Califf RM, Fitzgerald GA, Johnson PC, et al. Reengineering the national clinical and translational research enterprise: the strategic plan of the national clinical and translational science awards consortium. Acad Med. 2010;85:463–9.

ResearchGate. 2016. https://www.researchgate.net. Accessed 1 Jul 2016.

Riemer K, Scifleet P. Enterprise social networking in knowledge-intensive work practices: a case study in a professional service firm. ACIS; Australasian Conference on Information Systems; December 3–5, 2012; Geelong, Australia. 2012, pp. 1–12.

RNS Wikipedia. 2016. https://en.wikipedia.org/wiki/Comparison_of_research_networking_tools_and_research_profiling_systems. Accessed 1 Jul 2016.

SPARQL Wikipedia. 2016. https://en.wikipedia.org/wiki/SPARQL. Accessed 1 Jul 2016.

Schleyer T, Spallek H, Butler BS, Subramanian S, Weiss D, Poythress ML, Rattanathikun P, Mueller G. Facebook for scientists: requirements and services for optimizing how scientific collaborations are established. J Med Internet Res. 2008;10(3):e24. https://doi.org/10.2196/jmir.1047.. http://www.jmir.org/2008/3/e24/

SharePoint. 2016. https://products.office.com/en-us/sharepoint/collaboration. Accessed 1 Jul 2016.

Slack. 2016. https://slack.com. Accessed 1 Jul 2016.

SlideShare. 2016. http://www.slideshare.net. Accessed 1 Jul 2016.

Symplectic. 2016. http://symplectic.co.uk/services/open-profile-services. Accessed 1 Jul 2016.

Twitter. 2016. https://twitter.com. Accessed 1 Jul 2016.

UCSF Profiles. 2016. http://profiles.ucsf.edu. Accessed 1 Jul 2016.

UDN. 2016. https://undiagnosed.hms.harvard.edu. Accessed 1 Jul 2016.

USPTO. 2016. http://www.uspto.gov. Accessed 1 Jul 2016.

VIVOConference. 2016. http://vivoconference.org. Accessed 20 Dec 2016.

VIVOWeb. 2016. http://vivoweb.org. Accessed 1 Jul 2016.

Warner ET, Carapinha R, Weber GM, Hill EV, Reede JY. Considering context in academic medicine: differences in demographic and professional characteristics and in research productivity and advancement metrics across seven clinical departments. Acad Med. 2015;90(8):1077–83. https://doi.org/10.1097/ACM.0000000000000717.

Warner ET, Carapinha R, Weber GM, Hill EV, Reede JY. Faculty promotion and attrition: the importance of coauthor network reach at an academic medical center. J Gen Intern Med. 2016;31(1):60–7. https://doi.org/10.1007/s11606-015-3463-7.

Weber GM, Barnett W, Conlon M, Eichmann D, Kibbe W, Falk-Krzesinski H, Halaas M, Johnson L, Meeks E, Mitchell D, Schleyer T, Stallings S, Warden M, Kahlon M. Direct2Experts collaboration Direct2Experts: a pilot national network to demonstrate interoperability among research-networking platforms. J Am Med Inform Assoc. 2011;18(Suppl 1):i157–60. https://doi.org/10.1136/amiajnl-2011-000200.. http://jamia.bmj.com/cgi/pmidlookup?view=long&pmid=22037890

Woolf SH. The meaning of translational research and why it matters. JAMA. 2008;299:211–3.

Wuchty S, Jones BF, Uzzi B. The increasing dominance of teams in production of knowledge. Science. 2007;316(5827):1036–9.

YouTube. 2016. https://www.youtube.com. Accessed 1 Jul 2016.

Zerhouni EA. Translational and clinical science-time for a new vision. N Engl J Med. 2005;353:1621–3.

Strategies for Success in Virtual Collaboration: Structures and Norms for Meetings, Workflow, and Technological Platforms

43

Nicholas Berente and James Howison

Contents

43.1 Introduction

Science is moving increasingly to team collaboration at distance (Olson et al. 2008; Olson and Olson 2013), or "virtual collaboration" (Jarvenpaa et al. 1998). Organization science has studied virtual collaboration and can provide a variety of useful insights.[1] In this chapter, we draw on findings from this research to help scientists increase the likelihood of leading successful, effective virtual collaboration. In particular, we emphasize how discussion (in the form of conference calls and emails) is, on the one hand, a critical, valuable, and unavoidable mechanism for coordinating virtual collaborations. However, discussion is often the primary mode of coordination, and this can be problematic. Virtual collaborations absolutely need to mitigate these negative consequences of discussion-based coordination in order to thrive.

Organization science has a long tradition of studying the mechanisms through which work can be coordinated. These mechanisms include markets, hierarchical supervision and authority, occupational roles, project management, work structuring, plans, routines, norms, conventions, culture, technology platforms, visioning, and direct communication or "discussion" (Mintzberg 1979; Srikanth and Puranam 2011). Unfortunately, those new to virtual collaborations often emphasize the "discussion" mechanism for coordination almost exclusively. This discussion takes the form of virtual meetings, particularly long conference calls; and emails that can involve long unstructured and meandering conversational streams.

---

[1] For scholarly reviews of this abundant literature, see Gilson et al. 2015; see also Powell et al. 2004; Hertel et al. 2005; D'Urso et al. 2015; Scott and Wildman 2015.

N. Berente (✉)
Mendoza College of Business, University of Notre Dame, Notre Dame, IN, USA
e-mail: nberente@nd.edu

J. Howison
School of Information, University of Texas at Austin, Austin, TX, USA

© Springer Nature Switzerland AG 2019
K. L. Hall et al. (eds.), *Strategies for Team Science Success*,
https://doi.org/10.1007/978-3-030-20992-6_43

Table 43.1 Potential problems with overreliance on discussion (conference calls and emails) as a coordination mechanism for virtual collaboration

Inefficiency	Spending unnecessary time and resources on meetings and emails
Ineffectiveness	Difficult to schedule or convey appropriate communications
Poor resource utilization	Requiring participation in communications not relevant
Delays	Time waiting for others to communicate
Lack of attention	Not paying attention to relevant communications

Table 43.2 Tactics for mitigating the problems with overreliance on discussion (conference calls and emails) as a coordination mechanism for virtual collaboration

Structuring work	• Structure the work based on discrete deliverables • Schedule deliverable-focused meetings including only those responsible for the deliverable • In kickoff meeting, include everyone in goal-setting
Technology platform	• Choose a platform for its simplicity, accessibility, and inclusiveness—don't choose one that gets in the way • Include transactive memory system (knowledge directory), particularly for larger collaborations • In kickoff meeting, spend time developing norms and using the platform
Meetings	• Deliverable-focused • Emphasize inclusion, bonding among participants, and identification with the team • Targeted communications only, respect time of participants

Discussion is a critically important coordination mechanism—one that is absolutely essential for virtual organizations. However, there are a variety of problems with an overreliance on discussion as a primary source of coordination (see Table 43.1). First is efficiency, particularly for well-defined work. Discussions are often significantly less efficient for coordinating well-defined work than other forms of coordination. Further, when synchronous communication is desirable, particularly in a distributed team often across time zones, it is difficult to schedule those communications (O'Leary and Cummings 2007; Srikanth and Puranam 2011). Another problem involves human resource utilization, including wasting time in irrelevant communications such as documentation that nobody reads (Berente et al. 2009), and reading that documentation or long emails trails that are not relevant to a person's tasks (Whittaker and Sidner 1996; Dabbish and Kraut 2006). Also there is the problem of waiting for communication and decision-making bottlenecks. When discussion is taking place, there are also issues with attention; for example, people may not always pay attention to a conference call at the right times, or they may not pay attention to emails, even when the content directly applies to their work (Wasson 2004).

Science teams do not want to eliminate meetings and emails, certainly. But there are a number of lessons that we can take from organization science to help coordinate work and reserve time and energy for improved discussions when they are necessary. In the following pages, we address three general categories for coordinating work

and reducing some of the downside of open-ended discussion: (1) structuring the work, (2) technological platforms and associated norms; and (3) meetings and associated norms (see Table 43.2).

The suggestions in this essay are not silver-bullets for effective collaboration. Instead, we propose these guidelines as practices that leaders should think about and apply when structuring their collaborations. In particular, we focus on minimizing the negative consequences of too much reliance on discussion in virtual collaboration among science teams. In our research into science, we have found a significant reliance on discussion as the primary coordination mechanism—in particular conference calls and emails. Certainly these are important for coordinating work, but they are often overused or misused, leading to a variety of dysfunctions. These practices can help mitigate the dysfunctions of overreliance on discussion throughout a virtual collaboration.

We encourage teams to attend very explicitly to each of these categories up-front, in a face-to-face kickoff meeting to reduce coordination costs throughout the collaboration while still maximizing outcomes. Particularly in science work, however, not everything can be planned, so discussion remains a valuable way of dealing with unexpected interdependencies among people and tasks (i.e., when someone needs the input of someone else, or another task to be accomplished, before that person can complete a task). Discussion can also help with disseminating learning outcomes from different tasks in a distributed project. The overall goal of this chapter is to provide actionable advice, grounded in organization science, for reducing reliance on discussion as a coordination mechanism, and at the same time improving those discussion-based communications that do need to take place and improve project outcomes.

43.2 Structuring Work

The formal structuring of work has been found to be particularly useful in coordinating virtual collaboration (Hoch and Kozlowski 2014; Steinhardt and Jackson 2014). Virtual collaboration means working at a distance, across organizations or labs, and relying on information technologies to make work possible. A key challenge of any collective activity is the challenge of coordination, by which we mean managing dependencies between people and between tasks (Malone and Crowston 1994). Dependencies are what gives working in teams its power, especially in the larger, diverse teams made possible in virtual collaborations, but dependencies are also what makes teamwork problematic. A number of problems result from coordination failure, including problems like slowing work due to waiting, unnecessary work due to poor communication, time and money spent re-working contributions to match those of others, and time wasted by participants attempting to rectify problems and continually re-adjust.

The first step in formal structuring to better coordinate work involves "goal setting"—which is the process through which team members identify and agree to overall goals and subgoals for the project. Goal setting is perhaps the most well-

established factor for better performance among innovative teams in the existing body of research (Hoegl and Parboteeah 2003). Once goals and subgoals are established, the team needs to figure out how to accomplish these goals—how to structure work to meet these goals. This involves breaking tasks down into discrete, manageable chunks. This notion of task decomposition is at the root of everything from the division of labor to the work breakdown structure process in project management (March and Simon 1958; PMBOK 2001). Once tasks are identified and aligned with subgoals, it is important to coordinate across these tasks to accomplish higher level goals. The principles of modularity, which involve breaking up of work into well-defined chunks with specific interfaces, are particularly critical for accomplishing this coordination and managing complex science tasks in virtual collaborations.

Research into the many forms of virtual collaboration emphasize the power of modularity. For example, modularity is critical to successful distributed technological innovation, outsourcing relationships, and distributed software development (Baldwin and Clark 2000), including open-source software projects (MacCormack et al. 2006). The key to modularity are the two components: (1) break up work into discrete tasks, and (2) create well-defined interfaces between these tasks.

The first step involves hierarchical task decomposition—to take the complex task and divide it up into smaller tasks. In project management, this step is often referred to as creating the work breakdown structure. Take large tasks and break them up into smaller tasks, and break these up to even smaller tasks until you find the appropriate unit of work. Hierarchically enumerate these tasks. In project management practice, one then typically takes this work breakdown structure and organizes it according to a schedule in a Gantt chart (PMBOK 2001).

Of course, this process sounds simpler than it actually is in scientific projects. In scientific research, goals and outputs are not well defined in advance and often change throughout the course of the product (Turner and Cochrane

1993). Simply, it is typically not apparent how to break down a team's work in advance. A best practice for dealing with this is to identify key deliverables and the information requirements for those deliverables (Turner 2000). In an exploratory situation, one can never perfectly predict things like the information content nor the duration of tasks, but one can predict the sorts of information that will be needed for subsequent steps. Deliverables of data collection involve the data. Deliverables of analysis may involve lab reports or statistical analyses. These deliverables can be further broken down.

An important note about deliverables is that they do not just mark the end and completion of a task, but that deliverables are used for many and multiple subsequent tasks. If one thinks about deliverables as the interface between tasks (i.e., all subsequent tasks), then the conversation moves to structuring the sorts of information—or the information requirements—of all subsequent tasks. It is critical to align leadership responsibilities, communication, and incentives (such as reward systems) with deliverables to drive better performance (Hoch and Kozlowski 2014). See Fig. 43.1 for a conceptual depiction of task decomposition in a work breakdown structure liked to goals and information requirements.

Even if work breakdowns can only be projected out for a short period of time, beyond which tasks are unknowable, work breakdown can be worthwhile for its side effects. This is because working to accomplish simple tasks in a way that is visible to others in the initial stages of a collaboration can provide trust and knowledge of each other's skills that can enable the group to adjust their work over time (Iacono and Weisband 1997; Mitchell and Zigurs 2009). Thus establishing a set of simple tasks whose accomplishment and deliverables are visible to each other is worthwhile almost regardless of the specific content of the tasks; certainly visible, structured, work is a promising alternative to long meetings early in a project. Further, science teams will have difficulty developing an accurate project schedule from a work breakdown structure, but the exercise of creating and targeting dates and date ranges for deliverables assists in coordination of a project. As indicated above, goal setting is invaluable for innovative team performance (Hoegl and Parboteeah 2003), and the act of breaking down work, defining deliverables, and determining initial schedules are the fundamental activities in goal setting.

So how does this all translate into structuring a virtual collaboration? First, it is well established that face-to-face kickoff meetings are particularly important for virtual team success (Hertel et al. 2005; Ferrazzi 2014). Kickoff meetings help build interpersonal relationships and

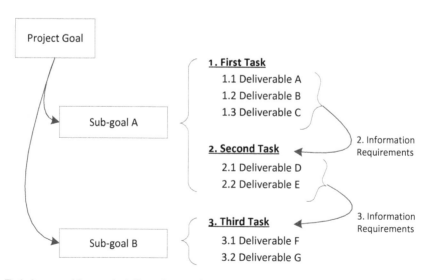

Fig. 43.1 Task decomposition, goals, information requirements

trust that will be invaluable throughout the collaboration. But, as we discuss further below, the kickoff meeting should not be unstructured. During that kickoff meeting, it is important to structure the work and to involve project participants in goals setting. The main tasks in the kickoff meeting involve (1) agreeing to goals and subgoals, (2) identifying key deliverables, (3) breaking down these deliverables into their lower level tasks, (4) identifying information requirements of tasks and codifying them as standards for deliverables, and (5) assigning team members to the different tasks.

Focus the subsequent virtual meetings and documentation on deliverables with participants from the appropriate teams responsible for these deliverables. Team members do not need to participate in meetings, conference calls, or email chains, unless they are specifically associated with a given task for a deliverable. To the extent possible, schedule meetings around deliverables and include only those assigned to particular deliverables for those meetings and included in those tasks.

It is important to note that complex tasks like science projects can rarely be considered to be perfectly modular. They inevitably involve unforeseen interdependencies with other tasks in unanticipated ways. Nobel prize winning economist Herb Simon referred to this as the "near decomposability" of complex systems (Simon 1962). So it is important to realize that a perfectly modular work breakdown is likely unattainable and no team will get it right the first time. So teams should occasionally coordinate across modules. This cross-module coordination involves periodic cross-team meetings, but these cross-team meetings should focus on deliverables and information requirements to reduce unnecessary discussion. Broader meetings across groups (i.e., meetings across groups responsible for different deliverables) should be scheduled before, during, and after deliverable handoffs, and when interdependencies become evident.

An important note is that the coordination requirements of virtual collaboration scales with the size of the virtual team (Boh et al. 2007; O'Leary and Cummings 2007); bigger teams,

teams with more diverse expertise, and teams from different organizations and in different time zones all require more structure to avoid the inefficiency of too much ad-hoc, discussion-focused coordination that may be fine for smaller, homogenous teams (Cummings et al. 2013; Nguyen-Duc et al. 2015).

43.3 Technological Platforms and Associated Norms

Technological platforms make virtual collaboration possible. It is imperative that virtual teams take the technological platform seriously, because platforms do not just enable virtual collaboration, but they can also get in the way of virtual collaboration (Gilson et al. 2015). By platforms, we mean a wide variety of technologies, including email, video conferencing tools, shared document storage, shared document editors, content management systems, project hosting services, and commercial software suites marketed as "groupware" systems.

Despite marketing hype, platforms by themselves don't do anything: what matters is the ways in which they are used (DeSanctis and Poole 1994). For example, in case of open-source software development, platforms offer a number of different tools to help with collaboration and development, but not all projects that use the platform use all of the tools and different open-source projects, and tools are used in much different ways in different projects. Successful projects establish and maintain norms around platforms. Norms are simply the established or standard ways of working on a platform. For example, a collaboration may develop a naming convention for versions of documents (such as including a date and last author's initials), or develop a norm about using comments in an online editor.

Collaboration platforms are effective when they are a central meeting place for participants and when participants learn shared norms and conventions for their use (Maruping and Magni 2015). New platforms are constantly being created, and they make it easy to get started. Often it only takes a single member of the collaboration to sign up and send out a link to others. This can quickly lead to a fracturing of a collaboration's records and documents, with multiple semi-abandoned platforms associated with a single ongoing collaboration. Chopping and changing platforms leads to fractured attention. Even worse, it undermines the time and shared experience needed to evolve and learn shared ways of using platforms. There is value in establishing and maintaining a specific platform long enough for norms for its use to emerge and to become shared. As frustrating as older platforms can seem in comparison to shiny new platforms, having a single, well-practiced, platform is likely of more value in the long run than any enticing features of a new platform. Some of the most successful open-source teams, for example, only use email lists, even for practices such as voting (Crowston et al. 2012). New features are seen to solve immediate problems, but adopting a platform is a key decision with important consequences for the whole collaboration and should be undertaken rarely and with the involvement of all participants.

Holding a collaboration focused on learning and using a particular platform is an important leadership role. As with most pieces of technology, there is a well-understood tendency for the most powerful members of an organization to use their status to resist using unfamiliar technologies (Grudin 1988; Lapointe and Rivard 2005). It is difficult for less powerful members of a collaboration to influence the more powerful to work in particular ways. Conversely, visible and enthusiastic use of a platform by the leaders of a virtual collaboration sends a powerful message and shapes use of the platform throughout the team. Scholars refer to these effects as a form of "social proof" (Cialdini and Goldstein 2004) and the ability of leaders to drive uptake as "information cascades" (Bikhchandani et al. 1992).

Finally, virtual collaborations have fluid and partial memberships, and it is important to keep this in mind when thinking about the role of technical platforms. This means that all participants are unlikely to be working on virtual collaboration full-time and that their involvement will be sporadic, with a lot of activity during certain times, but inactivity for long periods (Ahuja et al. 2003; Steinhardt and Jackson 2014). Moreover, the power of a virtual collaboration comes from being able to access diverse skills and experience, which means being able to bring new members on board quickly and easily, often from new organizations, and to identify skills and experience of these new and existing team members. A directory of such capabilities—sometimes referred to as a "transactive memory system"—helps virtual organizations to perform better (Choi et al. 2010). It is imperative that virtual teams keep a current directory of "who knows what" and "who is responsible for what" over the course of a project, particularly for larger, more complex virtual teams, and those that are entirely virtual (Kanawattanachai and Yoo 2007).

Fluid and partial memberships also influence the impact of pricing schemes for virtual collaboration platforms. Some commercial platforms are expensive, requiring fees that give access to a particular number of users (often called per-seat pricing). These do not match fluid and bursty participation well because the collaboration has to pay for seats even during the times of low participation. Similarly, per-seat licensing often has steep pricing threshold built in, such as free for up to 10 users and $1000 per user once you go over 10 users. Pricing schemes like that can make growing virtual collaborations, or replacing members, very painful. Similarly, platforms (e.g., Microsoft Sharepoint) are sometimes available free to members of particular universities through site-licensing. Yet building a virtual collaboration means extending across organizations, but if a platform is limited to one set of users adding users from other organizations means adding on new platforms, undermining the centrality of any platform and disrupting the norming process that leads to effective platform use.

Further, because virtual team membership tends to be fluid and partial, it is critical that the team develop norms and expectations associated with the use of platforms and other collaborative activity. Since this partial and fluid membership and attention is so prevalent in virtual teams, the role of central people in the project is even more important (Ahuja et al. 2003). Central people, such as leaders and administrative support who schedule and lead the activities, must be fully engaged and consistent with coordinating all activity and setting a good example, reinforcing the norms of collaboration. A key critical finding of virtual teams literature highlights the importance of leadership to both setting the stage for effective collaboration with strong norms and conventions, and constantly monitoring and reinforcing those norms (Bell and Kozlowski 2002).

There are platforms for synchronous work, involving simultaneous interaction, and asynchronous work, which does not occur at the same time. For synchronous work such as meetings, conference calls, and web conferences, it is imperative that the medium both scale to the appropriate number of users and provide reliability at that scale. Many free web conferencing platforms that are fine for small groups do not scale well to bigger groups and can have issues with reliability. Similarly, for small groups, well-defined version control practices can help with asynchronous work, but the larger the group scales, the more likely that a technological system for version control and associated approvals are in order. It is important that the team standardize the platforms and use the same platform across the collaboration as a part of admission.

Thus there are a number of important platform-related activities that must take place during the startup meeting. First, it is important to choose platform and begin using it at the face-to-face meeting. It is particularly tempting, since we are used to meeting face to face, to treat the startup meeting for a virtual collaboration like any other meeting. Yet it is important to remember that the working circumstances of the startup meeting will not continue: rather than being nearby, after the meeting participants will be at distance. Rather than all being present for long periods of time, participants will be returning to their busy work lives. Participants at ApacheCon, a meeting of a very successful open-source community, had a norm for scheduling meetings when all members of a collaboration were available. Yet when they met, they continued to (and practiced) using the platforms they used when at distance

(Crowston et al. 2007). The startup meeting, therefore, should focus on learning to use the platform that will enable ongoing work after the meeting. Simply, projects should seek to start as they will continue. Being together but using platforms designed for remote work will seem strange at first, but will build norms to make working at distance more effective.

43.4 Meetings and Associated Norms

Discussion can be frustrating, but it is a catch-all fallback coordination mechanism. Here we review how successful virtual collaborations use meetings and how to improve them.

Meetings, particularly synchronous meetings at distance, such as conference calls, should be regularly scheduled to lead up to deliverables for the teams generating those deliverables. In general, virtual teams need to create a schedule of regular, synchronous virtual meetings, accompanied by task-focused asynchronous communications in between (Maznevski and Chudoba 2000). Successful collaborations schedule the meetings around deliverables and teams responsible for the deliverables. Outside of this schedule, meetings should be thought of as a fallback coordination mechanism and should be infrequent.

There are a number of simple practices that can make any online meeting more effective. The website "Distributed Science"[2] draws together lessons from practice: establish common ground prior to the meeting (e-introductions or profiles that can be consulted), establish a shared agenda (perhaps through a shared document), stick to the agenda in the meeting, have a designated note taker focused on recording commitments of different team members, and circulate these commitments following the meeting. If you must schedule another meeting, try to do this early in the call, rather than at the very end, when relevant people may have already left.

A strong team culture is critical for virtual team outcomes (Scott and Wildman 2015), par-

---

[2] http://distributedscience.ischool.utexas.edu/

ticularly for innovative projects like those of science teams (Hoegl and Gemuenden 2001). It is imperative for team meetings to avoid establishing any sort of "us" and "them" subgrouping because such subgroupings undermine attention to the meeting and commitment to the team (Cramton and Hinds 2004; O'Leary and Mortensen 2010). A key finding from research is that it is easy to undermine common ground in synchronous teleconferences by highlighting differences in geography, including countries and timezones (Olson and Olson 2013). People are social beings and intensely affected by symbols and cues. It is imperative for virtual teams to intentionally be aware of symbolic communication to drive identification and bonding with the virtual team to guide team outcomes (Fiol and O'Connor 2005; O'Leary et al. 2014). A strong bond among virtual team members can avoid multiple coordination problems and reduce the negative consequences of conflict (Hinds and Mortensen 2005). Thus, virtual team leadership cannot underemphasize the symbolic and social identification elements of team meetings.

There are a variety of simple practices that can take place in meetings to encourage inclusiveness. Some small practices such as beginning meetings with standard greetings such as "good morning" can make participants for whom it is not morning feel excluded (make them feel "peripheral" rather than "central"). Participant's circadian rhythms are also relevant to scheduling meetings: if a meeting is always at the end of the workday for one group, they may be less likely to generate new ideas or if it always falls immediately before lunch, one group may be particularly impatient (Danziger et al. 2011). One strategy is to find two or three times for meetings and rotate them rather than sticking with a single time more convenient to one, usually powerful, subgroup.

Even within conference calls or face-to-face meetings, the usefulness of routines and technological platforms should not be discounted. For example, establishing a well-defined and practiced structure for calls helps participants under-

stand what to do. Similarly, using a central, shared document before and during a call allows the group to establish an agenda, take shared notes, and to quietly share resources (such as links, papers, data) while others are talking. It is important to establish strict norms to avoid social loafing in team meetings. One tactic for this is for team members to make a deal to avoid social loafing (i.e., foregoing active engagement in a meeting and thereby increasing the workload of those who participate) and split attention (i.e., only partial engagement in the meeting, and partial engagement with something else—such as reading email during a conference call) in return for minimizing the amount of time in meetings. Members might cheat from time to time, but establishing a norm guides behavior and provides a resource for recovering from breakdowns.

As with the structure of the collaboration and the appropriate use of standard technological platforms, it is imperative to use the kickoff meeting to discuss the norms for conducting meetings, expectations in those meetings, and conventions for interacting with technology and changing routines. Research in organizational scholarship refers to practices that change existing norms, conventions, and routines as "meta-routines" (Pentland et al. 2012). Meta-routines are necessary over the course of a collaboration to assess how things are going with the formal and informal norms that the team has been using, and to change them as needed. Some time in periodic meetings should be spent assessing the norms for discussions—both synchronous and asynchronous—to reinforce and assess the effectiveness of the way that the project does things. One way to accomplish this is to actually walk through the problems with effective discussion (Table 43.1) and ask if team members are experiencing these and if they see ways to improve the norms. One cautionary note is not to attempt too many improvements at once. Stability is essential to the propagation of team identification and predictability.

Further, as improvements or ideas for new tasks will undoubtedly emerge over the course of the collaboration, teams should resist the temptation of allocating the task to the person who contributed the idea; a principle established in the "brainstorming" literature. This can kill the flow of ideas and people might actually refrain from contributing. Instead, team coordinators should keep a running list of ideas, and have people revisit them from time to time and see if they are now motivated and able to do them (Howison and Crowston 2014).

The most important thing to remember is that meetings should be task-focused. The bulk of virtual meetings should focus on specific deliverables, and these meetings should actively respect the time of the meeting participants. One strategy is to have leaders check in with everyone 5–10 min short of the scheduled end of the meeting, offering to wrap up and checking whether short continuation is possible (but never assuming that a rushed continuation is better than continuing offline or rescheduling). Meetings should be no longer than necessary, should only include the team members involved with the task at hand and related tasks, and should actively look to minimize social loafing and split attention.

Box 43.1 Key terms and definitions

Key term	Definition
Coordination	Managing dependencies between activities
Coordination failure	Failure in managing dependencies, leading to delays, low quality work, or having to repeat work
Dependencies	Shared resources, Producer/Consumer relations (e.g., prerequisite activities, standardization), Simultaneity constraints, Task/subtask. See Malone and Crowston (1994)
Discussion	Unstructured verbal communication between people involved in tasks
Goal-setting	The process through which team members identify and agree to overall goals and subgoals for the project. Goal setting is perhaps the most well-established factor for better performance among innovative teams

Key term	Definition
Information requirements	Data required from other tasks in order to accomplish a task
Meta-routines	Routines for changing organizational routines
Modularity	Degree to which task components are encapsulated into independent units
Organizational routines	Common processes, practices, and procedures repeatedly followed by organizations to accomplish tasks
Task decomposition	Dividing larger into relatively independent subtasks
Technology platform	The combination of networks, hardware, software, people, and associated norms and practices that support a work team
Transactive memory system	Directory of "who knows what" in an organization
Virtual collaboration	Working together at distance, typically using an online platform
Work breakdown structure	Organization of tasks and subtasks in a hierarchical and sequential order

43.5 Conclusion

In this chapter, we provide some ideas for increasing the likelihood of successful virtual coordination. Of course, there have now been roughly two decades of intensive research on virtual collaboration, given the emergence of the Internet. This has resulted in thousands of scientific publications on the topic, including review articles (see Powell et al. 2004; Olson et al. 2008; Hertel et al. 2005; Olson and Olson 2013; Gilson et al. 2015; D'Urso et al. 2015; Scott and Wildman 2015). We have mentioned a number of key findings from this body of research, including the importance of structuring work, the criticality of the face-to-face kick-off meeting (particularly for goal-setting and establishing trust), establishing and reinforcing team norms, nurturing strong team identification, and other important elements. But in such a short essay we cannot do justice to the entirety of the research from organization science in all of its nuance. (See resources listed in Box 43.2 for further readings.)

Box 43.2 Further Reading

Evidence-based guidance summaries on virtual collaborations:
Getting VirtualTeams Right.
Ferrazzi, Keith. (2014)
Harvard Business Review
Leading virtual teams.
Malhotra A, Majchrzak A, Rosen B. (2007).
Academy of Management Perspectives
Principles for effective virtual teamwork.
Nunamaker Jr., Jay F., Bruce A. Reinig, and Robert O. Briggs. (2009).
Communications of the ACM
Working together apart: Collaboration over the Internet.

Olson, J. S., & Olson, G. M. (2013)
Synthesis Lectures on Human-Centered Informatics.
The management of virtual teams and virtual meetings
White M. (2014)
Business Information Review
Additional resources:
Team Science Toolkit, browse by "Collaborate Virtually."
http://www.teamsciencetoolkit.cancer.gov/
Distributed Science.
http://distributedscience.ischool.utexas.edu/
Collaboration Readiness.
http://hanalab.ics.uci.edu/wizard/

It is important to appreciate that virtual collaborations represent a complex social system, deeply situational, and it is a moving target—technologies and ways of collaborating are always changing, and so are social systems, institutions, and other contextual factors. So much about effective virtual collaboration hinges on the very specific nature of the work, and on strong leadership and fit among the styles and preferences of the team members and their leaders (Hoegl and Gemuenden 2001; Potter and Balthazard 2002). One approach, led by Judy and Gary Olson, has been to provide a pre-collaboration survey to assess "collaboration readiness" (The "Collaboration Success Wizard") and thus identify areas to improve.[3]

One of the things we highlight is the importance of team norms for coordinating work. Violating community norms can lead a loss of support from the community including loss of focus as splinter projects emerge (Garud et al. 2002). There is a delicate equilibrium between maintaining community values and the overarching desire for value creation. Clear communication of vision and adopting a consensus-driven approach to accomplishing, or even changing, high-level goals are important for success. One

cannot underestimate the impact of strong, well-established norms for coordinating work.

With this emphasis on norms—particularly in both the use of technological platforms and in running meetings—it is important to understand that virtual collaborations evolve over a life-cycle (see Sarker and Sahay 2003; D'Urso et al. 2015). Early in the collaboration, during the kickoff meeting and in the initial team meetings, it is critical to set expectations for contribution and a laser-like focus on deliverables—thus establishing and reinforcing the norms that were established early on, and also setting expectations, building trust, and forming a cohesive identity. In subsequent phases, teams can selectively re-evaluate elements of the project, including the structure, norms, and conventions. Research is now also addressing the wind-down phase, highlighting the manner in which these can be highly emotional and affect future collaborations (Steinhardt 2016).

A frequent source of frustration with virtual collaboration is an excess of discussion, especially long tele-conferences or meandering email threads. In this essay we draw on the organization science literature to highlight and analyze alternatives to discussion and tactics to improve discussion when it is necessary.

---

[3]http://hanalab.ics.uci.edu/wizard/

References

Ahuja MK, Galletta DF, Carley KM. Individual centrality and performance in virtual R&D groups: an empirical study. Manag Sci. 2003;49(1):21–38.

Baldwin CY, Clark KB. Design rules: the power of modularity, vol. Vol. 1. Cambridge, MA: MIT Press; 2000.

Bell BS, Kozlowski SW. A typology of virtual teams implications for effective leadership. Group Org Manag. 2002;27(1):14–49.

Berente N, Vandenbosch B, Aubert B. Information flows and business process integration. Bus Process Manag J. 2009;15(1):119–41.

Bikhchandani S, Hirshleifer D, Welch I. A theory of fads, fashion, custom, and cultural change as informational cascades. J Polit Econ. 1992;100:992–1026.

Boh WF, Ren Y, Kiesler S, Bussjaeger R. Expertise and collaboration in the geographically dispersed organization. Organ Sci. 2007;18(4):595–612.

Choi SY, Lee H, Yoo Y. The impact of information technology and transactive memory systems on knowledge sharing, application, and team performance: a field study. MIS Q. 2010;34:855–70.

Cialdini RB, Goldstein NJ. Social influence: compliance and conformity. Annu Rev Psychol. 2004;55:591–621.

Cramton CD, Hinds PJ. Subgroup dynamics in internationally distributed teams: ethnocentrism or cross-national learning? Res Organ Behav. 2004;26:231–63.

Crowston K, Wei K, Howison J, Wiggins A. Free (Libre) open source software development: what we know and what we do not know. ACM Comput Surv. 2012;44(2):7.

Crowston K, Howison J, Eseryel UY, Masango C. The role of face-to-face meetings in technology-supported self-organizing distributed teams. IEEE Trans Prof Commun. 2007;50(3):185–203.

Cummings JN, Kiesler S, Zadeh RB, Balakrishnan AD. Group heterogeneity increases the risks of large group size a longitudinal study of productivity in research groups. Psychol Sci. 2013;24(6):880–90.

Dabbish LA, Kraut RE. Email overload at work: an analysis of factors associated with email strain. In: Proceedings of the 2006 20th Anniversary Conference on Computer Supported Cooperative Work. New York, NY: ACM; 2006. p. 431–40.

Danziger S, Levav J, Avnaim-Pesso L. Extraneous factors in judicial decisions. Proc Natl Acad Sci. 2011;108(17):6889–92. https://doi.org/10.1073/pnas.1018033108.

DeSanctis G, Poole MS. Capturing the complexity in advanced technology use: adaptive structuration theory. Organ Sci. 1994;5(2):121–47.

D'Urso PA, Graham D, Krell R, Maul JP, Pernsteiner C, Shelton DK, Piercy GW. An Exploration of Organizational Structure and Strategy in Virtual Organizations: A Literature Review. J Perspectives in Organizational Behavior, Management, & Leadership, 2015;1(1):25–40.

Ferrazzi K. Getting virtual teams right. Harvard business review. 2014.

Fiol CM, O'Connor EJ. Identification in face-to-face, hybrid, and pure virtual teams: untangling the contradictions. Organ Sci. 2005;16(1):19–32.

Garud R, Jain S, Kumaraswamy A. Institutional entrepreneurship in the sponsorship of common technological standards: the case of sun microsystems and java. Acad Manag J. 2002;45(1):196–214.

Gilson LL, Maynard MT, Young NCJ, Vartiainen M, Hakonen M. Virtual teams research 10 years, 10 themes, and 10 opportunities. J Manag. 2015;41(5):1313–37.

Grudin J. Why CSCW applications fail: problems in the design and evaluation of organizational interfaces. In: Proceedings of the 1988 ACM Conference on Computer-Supported Cooperative Work. New York, NY: ACM; 1988. p. 85–93.

Hertel G, Geister S, Konradt U. Managing virtual teams: a review of current empirical research. Hum Resour Manag Rev. 2005;15(1):69–95.

Hinds PJ, Mortensen M. Understanding conflict in geographically distributed teams: the moderating effects of shared identity, shared context, and spontaneous communication. Organ Sci. 2005;16(3):290–307.

Hoch JE, Kozlowski SW. Leading virtual teams: hierarchical leadership, structural supports, and shared team leadership. J Appl Psychol. 2014;99(3):390.

Hoegl M, Gemuenden HG. Teamwork quality and the success of innovative projects: a theoretical concept and empirical evidence. Organ Sci. 2001;12(4):435–49.

Hoegl M, Parboteeah KP. Goal setting and team performance in innovative projects: on the moderating role of teamwork quality. Small Group Res. 2003;34(1):3–19.

Howison J, Crowston K. Collaboration through open superposition: a theory of the open source way. MIS Q. 2014;38(1):29–50.

Iacono CS, Weisband S. Developing trust in virtual teams. In: System Sciences, 1997, Proceedings of the Thirtieth Hawaii International Conference on (Vol. 2). Piscataway, NJ: IEEE; 1997. p. 412–20.

Jarvenpaa SL, Knoll K, Leidner DE. Is anybody out there? Antecedents of trust in global virtual teams. J Manag Inf Syst. 1998;14(4):29–64.

Kanawattanachai P, Yoo Y. The impact of knowledge coordination on virtual team performance over time. MIS Q. 2007;31:783–808.

Lapointe L, Rivard S. A multilevel model of resistance to information technology implementation. MIS Q. 2005;29:461–91.

MacCormack A, Rusnak J, Baldwin CY. Exploring the structure of complex software designs: an empirical study of open source and proprietary code. Manag Sci. 2006;52(7):1015–30.

Maznevski ML, Chudoba KM. Bridging space over time: global virtual team dynamics and effectiveness. Organ Sci. 2000;11(5):473–92.

Malone TW, Crowston K. The interdisciplinary study of coordination. ACM Computing Surveys (CSUR). 1994;26(1):87–119.

March JG, Simon HA. Organizations. University of Illinois at Urbana-Champaign's Academy for Entrepreneurial Leadership Historical Research Reference in Entrepreneurship. 1958.

Maruping LM, Magni M. Motivating employees to explore collaboration technology in team contexts. MIS Q. 2015;39(1):1–16.

Mintzberg H. Structuring of organizations: a synthesis of the research. In: Mintzberg H, editor. Theory of management policy series. Upper Saddle River, NJ: Prentice-Hall; 1979.

Mitchell A, Zigurs I. Trust in virtual teams: solved or still a mystery? ACM SIGMIS Database. 2009;40(3):61–83.

Nguyen-Duc A, Cruzes DS, Conradi R. The impact of global dispersion on coordination, team performance and software quality–a systematic literature review. Inf Softw Technol. 2015;57:277–94.

O'Leary MB, Cummings JN. The spatial, temporal, and configurational characteristics of geographic dispersion in teams. MIS Q. 2007;31(3):433–52.

O'Leary MB, Mortensen M. Go (con) figure: subgroups, imbalance, and isolates in geographically dispersed teams. Organ Sci. 2010;21(1):115–31.

O'Leary MB, Wilson JM, Metiu A. Beyond being there: the symbolic role of communication and identification in perceptions of proximity to geographically dispersed colleagues. MIS Q. 2014;38(4):1219–43.

Olson GM, Zimmerman A, Bos N. Scientific collaboration on the internet. Cambridge, MA: MIT Press; 2008.

Olson JS, Olson GM. Working together apart: collaboration over the internet. Synt Lect Human Centered Inform. 2013;6(5):1–151.

Pentland BT, Feldman MS, Becker MC, Liu P. Dynamics of organizational routines: a generative model. J Manag Stud. 2012;49(8):1484–508.

PMBOK. Project management body of knowledge (PMBOK® GUIDE). In Project Management Institute. 2001.

Potter RE, Balthazard PA. Virtual team interaction styles: assessment and effects. Int J Hum Comput Stud. 2002;56(4):423–43.

Powell A, Piccoli G, Ives B. Virtual teams: a review of current literature and directions for future research. ACM Sigmis Database. 2004;35(1):6–36.

Sarker S, Sahay S. Understanding virtual team development: an interpretive study. J Assoc Inf Syst. 2003;4(1):1.

Scott CP, Wildman JL. Culture, communication, and conflict: a review of the global virtual team literature. In: Leading global teams. New York, NY: Springer; 2015. p. 13–32.

Simon HA. The architecture of complexity. Proc Am Philos Soc. 1962;106(6):467–82.

Srikanth K, Puranam P. Integrating distributed work: comparing task design, communication, and tacit coordination mechanisms. Strateg Manag J. 2011; 32(8):849–75.

Steinhardt SB. Breaking down while building up: design and decline in emerging infrastructures. In: Proceedings of the 2016 CHI Conference on Human Factors in Computing Systems. New York, NY: ACM; 2016. p. 2198–208. https://doi.org/10.1145/2858036.2858420.

Steinhardt SB, Jackson SJ. Reconciling rhythms: plans and temporal alignment in collaborative scientific work. In: Proceedings of the 17th ACM Conference on Computer Supported Cooperative Work & Social Computing. New York, NY: ACM; 2014. p. 134–45. https://doi.org/10.1145/2531602.2531736.

Turner JR, Cochrane RA. Goals-and-methods matrix: coping with projects with ill defined goals and/ or methods of achieving them. Int J Proj Manag. 1993;11(2):93–102.

Turner JR. Do you manage work, deliverables or resources? Int J Proj Manag. 2000;18(2):83–4.

Wasson C. Multitasking during virtual meetings. People Strategy. 2004;27(4):47.

Whittaker S, Sidner C. Email overload: exploring personal information management of email. In: Proceedings of the SIGCHI Conference on Human Factors in Computing Systems. New York, NY: ACM; 1996. p. 276–83.

Open Sharing of Behavioral Research Datasets: Breaking Down the Boundaries of the Research Team

Rick O. Gilmore and Karen E. Adolph

Contents

44.1 Introduction

Behavior is the lynchpin underlying many of the most vexing problems in public health. Behavior can contribute to the progression or prevention of disease, define a disorder or mark recovery, and provide mechanisms for therapeutic intervention. Clinicians and health researchers have many robust and reliable tools at hand—from blood assays to

---

The original version of this chapter was revised. The correction to this chapter is available at https://doi.org/10.1007/978-3-030-20992-6_46

R. O. Gilmore (✉)
Department of Psychology, The Pennsylvania State University, PA, USA
e-mail: rick.o.gilmore@gmail.com

K. E. Adolph
Department of Psychology, Applied Psychology, and Neural Science, New York University, New York, NY, USA

brain or whole body images—for measuring people's physical health. But the tools for measuring healthy and at-risk behaviors in the contexts where they naturally occur are markedly limited.

Nevertheless, a readily available, inexpensive, and profoundly powerful tool already exists to capture the complexity and richness of many health-related human behaviors— video recording. Video captures subtle, real-time dimensions of behavior that standardized observational or self-report instruments ignore or grossly simplify. Video captures the nuances and vital details of experimental procedures more completely and accurately than do written protocols or the "methods sections" of published articles (Adolph et al. 2017; Gilmore et al. 2018). Although video contains identifiable information such as faces and voices, video data can be securely but openly shared with other researchers by adapting existing policy frameworks and building on proven technology. In this chapter, we introduce Databrary (databrary.org), a digital data library that is specialized for storing and sharing video recordings of behavior and experimental procedures. In doing so, we describe the benefits of open video sharing, barriers to its widespread adoption, and solutions that Databrary has devised to overcome these barriers. We argue that by making commonplace secure video sharing about health-related behaviors and empirical procedures, we can break down barriers between diverse and geographically dispersed research teams, increase scientific transparency, improve the reproducibility of research results, and hasten the pace of disease prevention and health promotion.

44.2   Behavior and Public Health

Researchers have long recognized the central role of behavior in public health (Committee on Health and Behavior: Research, Practice, and Policy 1982). Unintentional injury—the result of risky behavior—is the leading cause of death through middle age (Centers for Disease Control n.d.). In older adults, heart, lung, cerebrovascular, and liver disease are leading causes of mortality—all diseases strongly associated with behaviors involving diet, exercise, and substance use. One in five Americans suffers from mental illness each year, and 1 in 25 suffers from a serious form of mental illness (Serious Mental Illness (SMI) Among U.S. Adults n.d.)—illnesses in part defined by, caused by, and treated by behavior. Developmental disabilities affect about one in six children (Developmental Disabilities Prevalence Trends | Key Findings | NCBDDD | CDC n.d.), and characteristic patterns of behavior distinguish the leading types of health problems including learning disabilities, attention deficit hyperactivity disorder, developmental delay, and autism spectrum disorder. Across health problems, medication is a primary source of treatment, but fewer than 50% of patients comply with recommended patterns of prescription drug therapies (WHO | Adherence to long-term therapies n.d.).

Despite the central role of behavior in health risk, assessment, and treatment, current tools used to capture health-relevant patterns of behavior have substantial weaknesses. Most tools do not rely on direct behavioral observation. Instead, the tools involve self-report questionnaires or reports by others (family members, teachers, co-workers), making such questionnaires susceptible to the vagaries of human memory and veracity (e.g., Boase and Ling 2013; Schoeller et al. 2013). Most tools are standardized instruments (patients or participants are assigned a normed summary score or set of scores) that can mask important dimensions of individual and cultural variation (Deevybee 2011). And even those tools that do involve direct behavioral assessments out-

side the clinical context may suffer from questionable reproducibility (Open Science Collaboration 2015; Gilbert et al. 2016). Video has largely untapped potential to overcome many of these weaknesses and thereby enhance and advance the study of behavior.

44.2.1   Making Video a Pillar of Social and Behavioral Research

Researchers who study human or animal behavior (Egnor and Branson 2016) have recognized the power of visual media to capture the richness and complexity of behavior as it unfolds in real time (Adolph 2016; Gesell 1946, 1991). Video closely mimics the visual and auditory experiences of live human observers, so recordings collected by one researcher for a particular purpose may be readily understood and reused by a different researcher for a different purpose. Behavioral video has research life and potential long after the original study is completed. This makes video an especially valuable raw material for discovery and treatment, especially *if it can be shared*.

Currently, video is the backbone of research for thousands of behavioral scientists who study learning and development, each of whom collects hundreds to thousands of hours of video each year. The scale and breadth of video data collection in the developmental and learning sciences is vast. For example, the Databrary Project has collected 45,000+ hours of video from 900+ research studies of infants, children, and adults in its first 5 years of operation. The Measures of Effective Teaching Project, funded by the Gates Foundation, generated more than 1000 videos from 3000 K-12 classrooms over a 3-year period. The data, constituting tens of terabytes of storage, are streamed to registered viewers across the country. The NSF-funded HomeBank project and TalkBank/CHILDES archive are collecting and sharing thousands of hours of audio recordings of language by and to children, some of which are accompanied by video. The Autism and Beyond Project at Duke University has deployed an iPhone application that will collect video images of thousands of children's facial expressions to evaluate the feasibility of using computer vision techniques to screen children in their homes for developmental disorders and risk of mental illness. Clearly, the widespread availability of low-cost, high-resolution cameras has made video a large and rapidly growing source of information about behaviors relevant to child development, classroom learning, language learning, and the prevalence of health risk. Video has also proven its utility in medicine as a diagnostic aid in telemedicine (mHealthIntelligence 2015), as a mnemonic aid for patients (Meeusen and Porter n.d.), and as a tool for medical training (JBJS Video Supplements n.d.).

44.2.2 Video Facilitates Transparency

Video has unique virtues for addressing researchers' growing concerns about reproducibility, transparency, and openness (Adolph et al. 2017 and Gilmore et al. 2018; Open Science Collaboration 2015; Gilbert et al. 2016; Gilmore and Adolph 2017; Nosek and Bar-Anan 2012; Nosek et al. 2012). Video documents the interactions between people and their physical and social environment unlike any other form of measurement. It captures when, where, and how people look, gesture, move, communicate, and interact (Adolph 2016; Curtis 2011; Derry 2007; Gesell 1946, 1991; Goldman et al. 2014). As such, video can capture essential details about empirical procedures that are overlooked or omitted in the most detailed and carefully written methods sections of scientific papers. Video can record how people gave consent to participate in research, what tasks participants performed, and in what order. Video can capture behavior in laboratory and classroom settings, at home, and in more public settings. It can capture the dynamics of computer-based tasks and displays used in laboratory research.

Videos of empirical procedures can and should be viewed as the gold standard of documentation across the behavioral sciences. Indeed, were the use of video for this purpose more widespread, many disagreements about whether empirical replications truly reproduced the original experimental conditions would be moot (Open Science Collaboration 2015; Gilbert et al. 2016). The power of video to document procedures should also be an attractive solution for scientists in

fields that do not commonly collect or analyze video (Gelman 2012). The *Journal of Visualized Experiments (JOVE)* arose precisely to meet this need for making research methods more widely available, but more affordable and accessible tools for sharing videos of research methods are needed.

44.2.3 Video Poses Challenges to Sharing, but These Barriers Can Be Overcome

Personally identifiable information on video poses problems for the protection of participants' privacy. Most videos of people contain identifiable information—faces, voices, spoken names, and interiors of homes and classrooms. Removing identifiable information from video severely diminishes its value for reuse and puts additional burdens and costs on researchers. For years, policies have existed for sharing de-identified text-based data (U.S. HHS 2012), but video cannot be readily de-identified in the same ways as text data. Therefore, video sharing requires new policies that protect the privacy of research participants while preserving the integrity of raw video for reuse by others.

Large file sizes and diverse formats present technical challenges. Video files are large (1 h of HD video can consume 10 GB of storage) and come in various formats and sources (from cell phones to high-speed video). Many studies use multiple camera views to capture desired behaviors from different angles. Thus, sharing videos requires substantial storage capacity, significant computational resources, and specialized technical expertise to store and transcode videos into common formats that can be preserved over the long term.

Video sharing poses practical challenges of data management. Researchers lack time and resources to find, label, clean, organize, link, and convert files into formats that can be used and understood by others (Ascoli 2006). Most researchers lack training and expertise in standard practices of data curation (Gordon et al. 2015). Video coding tools represent the correspondence between video and coding files in tool-specific ways, or not at all. Few researchers reliably or reproducibly document workflows or data provenance. When researchers do share, standard practice involves organizing data after a project is finished, perhaps when a paper goes to press. This "preparing for sharing" after the fact presents a difficult and unrewarding chore for investigators, one that often exceeds the cost and time frame contemplated under federal data-sharing policies (discussed below). It also makes curating datasets a challenge for repositories.

Extracting behavioral patterns from video presents technical and practical barriers. Although machine-assisted image and video-tagging has made significant advances in recent years, it cannot yet replace the ability of human observers to recognize complex sets of behaviors (e.g., whether a mother is "responsive" to her infant's "bid" for assistance), distinguish similar behaviors (a reach versus a point), detect particular behaviors (parent and child speech amidst the noisy sea of television, music, and traffic in the everyday home), and assign new meanings to behaviors (an exploratory versus performatory action). Currently, researchers represent patterns extracted from video in a variety of ways, including paper and pencil, and so most codes cannot be easily exported to other tools. In principle, researchers could build on the videos and tags generated by others. But in practice, most researchers do not share coding files with researchers outside their labs. Moreover, coding files often contain proprietary and incompatible data formats making them difficult to push along the analysis pipeline and to share with other researchers. As a result, the hard-won, expensive-to-acquire human insights about behaviors extracted from research video remain difficult to analyze and largely hidden from the greater scientific community.

44.2.4 Federal and Journal Data-Sharing Policies Largely Ignore Video

Both NSF and NIH have had data-sharing policies in place for some time. NSF expects investigators to share with other researchers "primary data, samples, physical collections, and other supporting materials" associated with NSF-funded work "at no more than incremental cost and within a reasonable timeframe" (National Science Foundation n.d.). Since 2003, NIH has required grantees seeking more than $500,000 in direct costs in any single year to include in their application a plan for data sharing or a statement about why sharing is not possible (NIH 2003). NIMH has made data sharing an especially high priority, providing support for a specific repository infrastructure—the NIMH Data Archive (NDA)—that NIMH grantees are now required to use for depositing de-identified research data (NIMH 2015). In light of increased concern about transparency and reproducibility of published results, many journals have begun to enforce data-sharing requirements. Nonetheless, current data-sharing policies from research funders and publishers largely ignore video because recordings often contain potentially identifiable faces and voices. Until recently, requiring videos to be shared has seemed at best impractical. We describe in the next section how Databrary has overcome barriers to widespread video data sharing among researchers, making it easy and practical surprisingly straightforward (Gilmore et al. 2018).

44.3 Databrary Facilitates Sharing and Reuse of Research Video

Databrary is a digital data library that is specialized for the storage, management, and sharing of research video. It arose to meet the needs of researchers who collect video in laboratory, home, classroom, or museum contexts. The project is supported by awards from the National Science Foundation (BCS-1238599), the National Institute of Child Health and Human Development (NICHD U01-HD-076595 and R01-HD-094830), the Society for Research in Child Development, the LEGO Foundation, the James S. McDonnell Foundation, and the Alfred P. Sloan Foundation. The project team and digital library are housed at New York University. In launching and growing Databrary over the past several years, the PIs overcame critical barriers to sharing video, including solutions for respecting participants' privacy; for storing, streaming, and sharing video; and for managing video datasets and associated metadata (Gordon et al. 2015). Databrary's technology and policy framework established the foundation for securely sharing research videos. As of late 2019, more than 1,400 researchers from some 500+ institutions around the world have authorization to access more than 42,000 hours of video stored in Databrary. The files depict more than 11,400 research participants from 3 weeks to 60 years of age representing diverse racial, ethnic, and cultural backgrounds engaging in a wide range of behaviors. Databrary has also developed a free, open-source, video-coding tool called Datavyu (http://datavyu.org) to enable researchers to add annotations that are time-locked to individual frames or video segments. Databrary has targeted the developmental and learning sciences community because it is the PIs' intellectual home and a substantial source of research video, but we have specifically designed Databrary to be adapted for and used by other researchers in the behavioral sciences.

Databrary permits users to upload, store, organize, and share data with collaborators, the restricted community of authorized Databrary users, or the public, depending on the level of sharing permission granted by participants. Users may also search for, browse, view, and download videos stored on the site. They may view specific metadata such as participants' ages or recording context (e.g., home, lab, or school) for recoding and reanalysis. Databrary also empowers users to create, view, or download highlights—video excerpts that can be shown for educational or research purposes. Thus, Databrary supports sharing, reanalysis, and pre- or non-research uses of video while simultaneously solving some of the thorniest problems associated with sharing data that contain personally identifiable information.

44.3.1 Databrary's Policies Enable Sharing of Identifiable Data

Databrary's policy framework recognizes that the content of recordings must not be altered if we wish to maximize the potential for reuse. Thus, Databrary does not attempt to de-identify videos. However, to enable sharing of unaltered research video containing identifiable information, Databrary developed new policies to protect participants' privacy. First, Databrary restricts access to researchers who register and secure formal authorization from their institutions. These "authorized investigators," primarily faculty members, are eligible to conduct independent research at the institution, have research ethics training, and their institution accepts responsibility for the researcher's actions related to the use of Databrary. Second, Databrary shares identifiable data only with the explicit permission of the participants, and only at the level the participants specify. Databrary has created template language for seeking participants' permission to share data, which researchers may adapt for their own use. An online user guide fully describes these policies.

Unique among data repositories, Databrary authorizes both data use and contribution. However, users agree to store on Databrary only materials for which they have IRB/ethics board approval. Data may be stored on Databrary for the contributing researcher's use regardless of whether the records are shared with others. When a researcher chooses to share, Databrary makes the data available to the community of authorized researchers. We note that a 1000 researchers and their institutions have agreed to Databrary's framework.

44.3.2 Databrary Overcomes Technical Barriers to Video Data Sharing

To address the problem of diverse video formats, Databrary uses New York University's high-performance computing services to automatically transcode each recording into a common format suitable for web-based streaming (currently H.264 + AAC in MP4 for video). The system maintains a copy in the original format for long-term preservation. To address local file storage limitations, Databrary does not currently place limits on the number or size of files that can be uploaded. As a web-based application fully compatible with modern web-browsers, Databrary does not require special software for access. Databrary's assets total more than 65 TB and are stored on New York University's central IT storage, which provides one off-site mirror and regular long-term tape backups.

44.3.3 Databrary's Design Overcomes Practical Barriers to Sharing

All data types are enhanced when accompanied by rich and informative metadata, and Databrary supports the storage and sharing of multiple data types beyond video. But unlike other forms of data, video requires relatively little metadata to be useful to others. The only metadata that are strictly required are participants' preferences about sharing. Because many researchers find post hoc data curation to be aversive (Ascoli 2006), Databrary developed a novel "active-curation" framework that reduces the burden (Gordon et al. 2015). The system empowers researchers to upload and organize data as it is collected. Immediate uploading reduces the workload on investigators, minimizes the risk of data loss and corruption, and accelerates the speed with which materials become available.

To encourage immediate uploading, Databrary provides a complete set of controls so that researchers can restrict access to their own labs or to other users of their choosing prior to sharing. Datasets can be shared with the broader research community at a later point when data collection and ancillary materials are complete, whenever the contributor is comfortable sharing, or when journals or funders require it. Furthermore, any de-identified data associated with a dataset, including demographic and study metadata, stimuli or displays, coding manuals, and coding data, may be shared publicly, substantially broadening the availability of these materials.

To encourage active curation, Databrary employs familiar, easy-to-use spreadsheet and timeline-based interfaces that allow users to upload videos, add metadata about tasks, set-

tings, and participants, link related coding files and manuals, and assign appropriate permission levels for sharing. Users can view videos, create highlights from them, and tag them in the web browser. Shared materials must be made available in findable, accessible, interoperable, and reusable formats to be maximally useful to others (Wilkinson et al. 2016). To that end, Databrary allows researchers to search for videos that meet their particular specifications. Each data set or study on Databrary has its own unique web page that when shared receives its own persistent identifier (DOI) that may be used to cite the resource.

Active curation poses few new burdens on researcher's time beyond current practices while offering significant benefits. In effect, Databrary acts as a researcher's personal lab file server and cloud storage, enabling web-based sharing among research teams and ensuring secure off-site backup. Moreover, by entering participant- and study-level metadata into Databrary, researchers make it possible for others to search for participants or studies that meet specific criteria. Thus, researchers who wish to reuse materials from Databrary for new studies can find exactly the videos and related metadata they need to address their question.

44.3.4 Video Coding Tools Enable Discovery

Most researchers who collect video deploy trained human observers to view the recordings and annotate them with specific tags that label the onset and offset of particular behaviors or events, the category or type of behavior, transcriptions of speech, and qualitative judgments about mood or other psychological characteristics. In the developmental sciences, spreadsheet software and paper-and-pencil are the most commonly used tools for annotating video, but an increasing number of researchers use specialized tools for video and audio annotation. The tools allow coders to play video forward and backward at varied speeds time-locked to the codes. This enables researchers to unpack the multi-layered complex patterns of human behavior as it unfolds in time. Following one or more coding passes, each of which focuses on a subset of behavioral dimensions, the tags or annotations are then exported for visualization and analysis using other tools.

One of us (Adolph) has pioneered the use of video coding tools for mining the data contained in video, and so the development of and support for video coding tools has been integral to the Databrary project from the beginning. To that end, Databrary has published a web-based best practices guide for coding video that is agnostic about the tool or tools a researcher chooses to use (Databrary n.d.). We have also continued to develop Datavyu, making it suitable for a variety of video coding use cases. Datavyu's Ruby scripting API makes it possible for users to customize the program and automate many routine tasks that would otherwise require significant time investment and often error-prone human intervention. Datavyu files, called spreadsheets, may be uploaded to Databrary and shared along with the videos they are linked to. This allows research teams in geographically separate locations—across campus or across the globe—to share video coding files and to validate or build upon each other's codes.

The rich set of time-locked annotations contained in the Datavyu files can be visualized on the Databrary timeline, but not easily searched. But empowering Databrary to import, display, make searchable, and export annotation from Datavyu and related video coding tools remains an important project goal. In the near future, a researcher will be able to search across Databrary for specific time segments in which a particular type of behavior occurred. For example, a researcher could search for all instances of crying, or all instances of vocalizations by English-speaking children between 12 and 24 months of age. To our knowledge, Databrary is the only data library in the social and behavioral sciences that stores individual- and session-level metadata in this way. We believe that indexing video and associated data elements by individual participant characteristics has the potential to break down boundaries between research teams and also to make it possible to ask and answer new important research questions that seem completely impractical today.

For example, imagine convening a team of experts representing a wide range of topical domains—e.g., language, emotion, cognition, physical activity, the environment—and asking them to develop a set of foundational codes that can be applied to video recordings collected from some form of natural human behavior. The joint time series of these moment-by-moment codes across domains, if openly and widely shared, would constitute a valuable resource for new discovery about patterns of behavior—within and across domains—especially if it were coupled with other traditional self-report and observational measures and individual-specific metadata. By committing to making video recordings of all procedures and using video exemplars to demonstrate code definitions, the team could substantially advance the transparency of its research innovations and ensure highly reproducible procedures are implemented even across geographically dispersed data collection sites.

As it happens, the authors and their colleagues have embarked on such an endeavor. The Play & Learning Across a Year (PLAY) project aims to collect, code, and share hour-long videos of 900 12-, 18-, and 24-month-old infants and their mothers engaged in natural home activities. A team of more than 65 experts representing diverse content domains has contributed to planning the protocol and designing the coding passes. All aspects of project planning, coding, and grant writing have relied upon and been documented with video stored on Databrary. Datavyu has been updated with features that make certain types of coding—especially speech transcription—easier. A web (wiki)-based protocol has been created that couples text- and static image descriptions of procedures and codes with video exemplars. So, our vision of how shared research video can transform team-based behavioral research is based on our own personal experiences. We are optimistic that other research teams will find value in making video a cornerstone of their behavioral research programs.

44.4 Conclusions

Biomedical research faces many challenges in the era of "Big Data" (Gilmore 2016), including the very real problem of meeting the public's high expectations about what ought to be achieved versus what actually can be achieved. Multidisciplinary, geographically dispersed research teams in the biomedical and health sciences face many barriers to collaborative discovery. Yet, we argue that researchers across the health sciences might take this moment to renew an interest in the complexities and marvels of behavior in all of its manifest forms, especially those that relate directly to the central questions about how to promote human health. Focusing on the limits of current measures in capturing essential properties of human behavior will help us ask better, more informed questions about what combination of factors leads to which health outcomes.

A curated, sharable, and reusable repository of video-recorded behavior could shed light on some of the most vexing issues in biomedical research. Researchers are already using video to record natural sleep behaviors in the homes of new parents (Batra et al. 2016), discovering that most parents put infants to sleep in environments with established risk factors even when they know they are being recorded. Video recordings of people with anorexia show differences in meal-time eating behaviors relative to healthy controls that could be important targets for therapeutic intervention (Gianini, et al. 2015). Video recordings of movement are being used in the diagnosis and treatment of Parkinson's disease (Reich et al. 2014). And video has even become part of an effort to make biomedical wet lab research protocols more reproducible through the Aquarium Project (http://klavinslab.org/aquarium-about.html).

To our knowledge, no one has yet proposed to measure the human "behavior-ome," but someone should. The PLAY project is our attempt to jumpstart a behavior-ome by focusing on a population we know about best and care about most. Our experiences thus far suggest that video recordings and tools for storing, managing, coding, and sharing videos like Databrary and Datavyu will be essential for comparable efforts with other target populations that intend to share data and procedures widely and openly. Policies for the sharing of identifiable data with the permission of research participants among a restricted group of authorized researchers who promise to uphold the highest ethical standards

will also be needed. We believe that the infrastructure Databrary and Datavyu have established in the developmental and learning sciences—and which other data repositories are establishing in other fields—will help to break down barriers that confine the membership of research teams and limit the questions they can pursue. With a rich array of videos of actual human behavior accessible openly and readily alongside other types of measures, research team members can be located anywhere, and ask questions that are limited only by their own imaginations.

References

Adherence to long-term therapies: evidence for action. n.d.. http://www.who.int/chp/knowledge/publications/adherence_report/en/. Accessed 19 Aug 2016.

Adolph KE. Video as data—association for psychological science. 2016. http://www.psychologicalscience.org/index.php/publications/observer/2016/march-16/video-as-data.html.

Adolph KE, Gilmore RO, Freeman C, Sanderson P, Millman D. Toward open behavioral science. Psychol Inq. 2012;23(3):244–7. https://doi.org/10.1080/1047840X.2012.705133.

Adolph KE, Gilmore RO, Kennedy JL. Video as data and documentation will improve psychological science. 2017. https://www.apa.org/science/about/psa/2017/10/video-data.

Ascoli GA. The ups and downs of neuroscience shares. Neuroinformatics. 2006;4(3):213–5. https://doi.org/10.1385/NI:4:3:213.

Batra EK, Teti DM, Schaefer EW, Neumann BA, Meek EA, Paul IM. Nocturnal video assessment of infant sleep environments. Pediatrics. 2016;138:e20161533. https://doi.org/10.1542/peds.2016-1533.

Boase J, Ling R. Measuring mobile phone use: self-report versus log data. J Comput-Mediat Commun. 2013;18(4):508–19. https://doi.org/10.1111/jcc4.12021.

Centers for Disease Control. Health United States. n.d.. http://www.cdc.gov/nchs/data/hus/hus15.pdf#019.

Committee on Health and Behavior: Research, Practice, and Policy. Health and behavior: the interplay of biological, behavioral, and societal influences: Institute of Medicine; 1982.

Curtis S. "Tangible as tissue": Arnold Gesell, infant behavior, and film analysis. Sci Context. 2011;24(3):417–42.

Databrary (n.d.) Best Practices for Coding Behavioral Data From Video, http://datavyu.org/user-guide/best-practices.html.

Deevybee. BishopBlog: are our "gold standard" autism diagnostic instruments fit for purpose? 2011. http://deevybee.blogspot.com/2011/05/are-our-gold-standard-autism-diagnostic.html.

Derry SJ. Guidelines for video research in education: recommendations from an expert panel. Chicago, IL: Data Research and Development Center; University of Chicago; 2007.. http://drdc.uchicago.edu/what/video-research-guidelines.pdf

Developmental Disabilities Prevalence Trends | Key Findings | NCBDDD | CDC. (n.d.). https://www.cdc.gov/ncbddd/developmentaldisabilities/features/birth-defects-dd-keyfindings.html. Accessed 19 Aug 2016.

Egnor SER, Branson K. Computational analysis of behavior. Annu Rev Neurosci. 2016;39:217–36. https://doi.org/10.1146/annurev-neuro-070815-013845.

Gelman S. Technology could help. 2012. http://www.psychologicalscience.org/index.php/publications/observer/scientific-rigor.html#gelman.

Gesell A. Cinematography and the study of child development. Am Nat. 1946;80(793):470–5.

Gesell A. Cinemanalysis: A method of behavior study. *Journal of Genetic Psychology. 1935*;47:3-16. https://doi.org/10.1080/00221325.1991.9914712.

Gianini L, Liu Y, Wang Y, Attia E, Walsh BT, Steinglass J. Abnormal eating behavior in video-recorded meals in anorexia nervosa. Eat Behav. 2015;19:28–32. https://doi.org/10.1016/j.eatbeh.2015.06.005.

Gilbert DT, King G, Pettigrew S, Wilson TD. Comment on "estimating the reproducibility of psychological science". Science. 2016;351(6277):1037–7. https://doi.org/10.1126/science.aad7243.

Gilmore RO. From big data to deep insight in developmental science. Wiley Interdiscip Rev Cogn Sci. 2016;7(2):112–26. https://doi.org/10.1002/wcs.1379.

Gilmore RO, Adolph KE. Video can make behavioural science more reproducible. Nat Hum Behav. 2017;1:128. https://doi.org/10.1038/s41562-017-0128.

Gilmore, RO, Kennedy, JL, Adolph, KE. Practical solutions for sharing data and materials from psychological research. *Advances in Methods and Practices in Psychological Science*, 2018:1(1):121–130 https://doi.org/10.1177/2515245917746500.

Goldman R, Pea R, Barron B, Derry SJ. Video research in the learning sciences. Abingdon: Routledge; 2014.

Gordon AS, Millman DS, Steiger L, Adolph KE, Gilmore RO. Researcher-library collaborations: data repositories as a service for researchers. J Libr Sch Commun. 2015;3(2):eP1238. https://doi.org/10.7710/2162-3309.1238.

JBJS Video Supplements. n.d.. http://www.vjortho.com/about/jbjs-video-supplements/. Accessed 1 Sept 2016.

Meeusen AJ, Porter R. Patient-reported use of personalized video recordings to improve neurosurgical patient-provider communication. Cureus. n.d.;7(6):e273. https://doi.org/10.7759/cureus.273.

mHealthIntelligence. How telemedicine, video recording promotes patient care. 2015. http://mhealthintelligence.com/news/how-telemedicine-video-recording-promotes-patient-care. Accessed 1 Sept 2016.

National Institute of Health. Final NIH statement on sharing research data. 2003. https://grants.nih.gov/grants/guide/notice-files/NOT-OD-03-032.html. Accessed 16 Mar 2017.

National Institute of Mental Health. Data sharing expectations for clinical research funded by NIMH. 2015. https://grants.nih.gov/grants/guide/notice-files/NOT-MH-15-012.html. Accessed 16 Mar 2017.

National Science Foundation. Dissemination and sharing of research results. n.d.. https://www.nsf.gov/bfa/dias/policy/dmp.jsp. Accessed 16 Mar 2017.

Nosek BA, Bar-Anan Y. Scientific utopia: I. Opening scientific communication. Psychol Inq. 2012;23(3):217–43. https://doi.org/10.1080/1047840X.2012.692215.

Nosek BA, Spies JR, Motyl M. Scientific utopia: II. Restructuring incentives and practices to promote truth over publishability. Perspect Psychol Sci. 2012;7(6):615–31. https://doi.org/10.1177/1745691612459058.

Open Science Collaboration. Estimating the reproducibility of psychological science. Science. 2015;349(6251):aac4716. https://doi.org/10.1126/science.aac4716.

Reich MM, Sawalhe AD, Steigerwald F, Johannes S, Matthies C, Volkmann J. The pirouette test to evaluate asymmetry in parkinsonian gait freezing. Movement Disorders Clinical Practice. 2014;1(2):136–8. https://doi.org/10.1002/mdc3.12018.

Schoeller DA, Thomas D, Archer E, Heymsfield SB, Blair SN, Goran MI, et al. Self-report–based estimates of energy intake offer an inadequate basis for scientific conclusions. Am J Clin Nutr. 2013;97(6):1413–5. https://doi.org/10.3945/ajcn.113.062125.

Serious Mental Illness (SMI) Among U.S. Adults. n.d.. http://www.nimh.nih.gov/health/statistics/prevalence/serious-mental-illness-smi-among-us-adults.shtml. Accessed 19 Aug 2016.

U.S. Department of Health and Human Services. Methods for de-identification of PHI [Text]. 2012. http://www.hhs.gov/hipaa/for-professionals/privacy/special-topics/de-identification/index.html. Accessed 1 Sept 2016.

Wilkinson MD, Dumontier M, Aalbersberg IJJ, Appleton G, Axton M, Baak A, Blomberg N, et al. The FAIR guiding principles for scientific data management and stewardship. Scientific Data. 2016;3:160018. https://doi.org/10.1038/sdata.2016.18.

Comprehensive Collaboration Plans: Practical Considerations Spanning Across Individual Collaborators to Institutional Supports

45

Kara L. Hall, Amanda L. Vogel, and Kevin Crowston

Contents

The original version of this chapter was revised.
The correction to this chapter is available at
https://doi.org/10.1007/978-3-030-20992-6_46

K. L. Hall (✉)
Division of Cancer Control and Population Sciences,
National Cancer Institute, Bethesda, MD, USA
e-mail: hallka@mail.nih.gov

A. L. Vogel
Clinical Monitoring Research Program Directorate,
Frederick National Laboratory for Cancer Research
sponsored by the National Cancer Institute,
Frederick, MD, USA

K. Crowston
School of Information Studies, Syracuse University,
Syracuse, NY, USA

45.1 Introduction

Team science has a unique role to play in addressing challenging scientific and societal problems, most notably by bringing to bear a range of expertise to generate novel solutions. Team science can be especially effective in the context of scientific initiatives that aim to integrate disciplines, cross levels of analysis, enhance comprehensiveness, or stimulate innovation, as it can harness and integrate the knowledge and creativity of team members with wide ranging disciplinary, professional, and "real-world" expertise.

When the conditions in which science is conducted, align with team science approaches, teams thrive, and research outcomes are enhanced (Hall et al. 2018). These include the right mix of team members, effective leadership, strong team functioning supported by appropriate communication and coordination mechanisms, and supportive organizational environments that help to facilitate team science. Yet all too often collaborators find they face barriers to team effectiveness across all levels, from individuals to organizations. Furthermore, project collaborators as well as administrators and leaders may be unaware that some of the conditions under which they operate are misaligned with the team science approach.

Collaboration Planning is a deliberative approach to assessing the state of a team's environment(s) for a range of factors that may influence the likelihood and degree of its scientific and collaborative success. Collaboration Planning can help collaborators plan for how to make the most of facilitators and address anticipated challenges. Doing so can help lay the groundwork for success by supporting effective team functioning, identifying needed changes, and preventing or mitigating what are often predictable challenges.

Longstanding strategies to plan for scientific collaboration include informal discussions or agreements among future collaborators, memoranda of agreement (MOAs), and documentation that fulfills grant application requirements such as letters of support from participating institutions. MOAs and grant supporting documents typically reflect a commitment to collaborate or address a specific issue such as access to specialized laboratory equipment or access to particular patient populations. Collaborative research agreements also may be focused on specific topics such as intellectual property.[1] Yet these documents frequently include little or no content addressing how such collaborations will be carried out. Further, such agreements typically address one or two aspects of a collaboration, failing to address many other factors that influence the success of science teams.

In recent years, a number of new approaches have emerged that focus on enhancing team dynamics. For example, a "Welcome to My Lab" letter to new lab members lays out expectations of team membership (Bennett et al. 2014). This type of onboarding document may address a wide range of topics such as the goals of the research group, roles and responsibilities of team members and leadership, team interactions, authorship and credit, career development, mentoring, and institutional and local resources. Pre-collaboration agreement templates include sets of questions for potential future collaborators to discuss (NIH Office of the Ombudsman 2017) related to topics such as the overall goals and vision for the collaboration, collaborator roles and responsibilities, authorship and credit, contingencies and communication, and potential

conflicts of interest. In addition, the National Institutes of Health requires that multiple principal investigator (PI) grant applications include a leadership plan identifying the roles and responsibilities of each co-PI (NIH Office of Extramural Research 2017).

We believe there is a need for a comprehensive resource that guides potential or future collaborators in systematically considering the complete range of influences on the success of a science team, including individual team members' attitudes and competencies, team interactions, and institutional factors, as documented in the literature on science teams, and reflected in this volume (c.f., Hall et al. 2018). In response, we created an approach called Collaboration Planning, described in the remainder of this chapter. The Collaboration Planning Approach is designed to support the development of a document called a Collaboration Plan that lays out a holistic plan for addressing the range of influences on team science. It serves as a guide to navigating the collaborative process and maximizing the likelihood of success.

45.1.1 The Collaboration Planning Approach

The Collaboration Planning Approach refers to the process of considering the specific conditions associated with a set of key influences for a given research team, center, or initiative. A primary step in the Collaboration Planning Approach involves documenting the key influences and agreed upon actions to address each influencing factor. This process results in a written Collaboration Plan that is tailored to a given team science effort.

Ten key influences on team science were identified to guide the Collaboration Planning process. These ten influences range from the initial scientific rationale for a team approach to the collaboration readiness of participating individuals and institutions to team communication and coordination mechanisms to approaches to quality improvement for team functioning (Fig. 45.1). The Collaboration Planning framework serves

---

[1] http://www.iphandbook.org/handbook/ch07/p04/

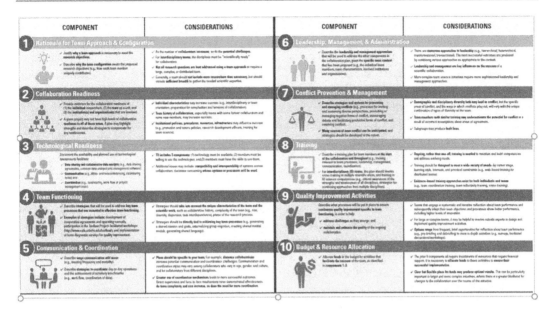

Fig. 45.1 Ten components of the Collaboration Plan (Hall et al. 2015; https://www.teamsciencetoolkit.cancer.gov/public/TSResourceBiblio.aspx?tid=3&rid=3261)

to guide collaborators through dialogue and planning around each influence and draws their attention to key issues for consideration related to each influence. Decisions are captured in the written Collaboration Plan.

In the Collaboration Plan, each component documents the collaborators' plans to maximize success related to this component, for example, by dedicating resources, leveraging facilitating factors, or addressing known challenges. All told, the Collaboration Plan summarizes the various ways the group will build the foundation for, and support, effective collaboration across the lifespan of the team science initiative, in light of these ten key influences. Given the comprehensive range of influences that are addressed, and the various factors included within each component, the Collaboration Planning approach may incorporate any of the aforementioned strategies (MOAs, grant supporting documents, Welcome to My Lab letters, and pre-collaboration agreement templates), among others, to help plan for success.

45.1.2 Origins of the Collaboration Planning Approach

The origins of the Collaboration Planning framework began in the context of the Subcommittee on Team Science of the Networking and Information Technology Research and Development (NITRD) Program of the President's Office of Science and Technology Policy (OSTP). The NITRD Program provides a forum in which many federal agencies come together to coordinate their networking and information technology (IT) research and development (R&D) efforts (NITRD, n.d.). Given the virtually mediated nature of almost all collaboration in science, NITRD established a subcommittee on Team Science, with members from government, industry, and academia. Two of the authors of this chapter (KLH and KC) were co-chairs of the subcommittee, and one author (ALV) was a member of the subcommittee.

The authors initially proposed the concept of the Collaboration Plan, and its general structure and content, while participating in the subcommittee Input into the key elements of Collaboration Planning from members across numerous federal agencies enhances its potential applicability and relevance across a broad array of sciences. Subcommittee members agreed that Collaboration Planning represented a common need across agencies and that such an approach would be valuable for investigators conducting research. Furthermore, the subcommittee considered the approach promising for enhancing the grant application process, such that investigators could use the approach to write a Collaboration Plan to include in an application for funds and reviewers and agency officials could use the framework to help assess applicants' readiness to participate in team science grant initiatives. Guest speakers from a range of federal agencies and from the external scientific community were brought in to speak to the subcommittee to inform the development of the framework. Thereby informed by their expertise in the Science of Team Science (SciTS) field, the evidence in the team science literature (c.f., Stokols et al. 2008; NRC 2015), as well as the NITRD subcommittee guest speakers and group discussions as part of a year-long set of activities, the co-authors developed the Collaboration Planning framework (Hall et al. 2014, 2015).

45.1.3 Collaboration Plans Are Critical for Complex Teams

While Collaboration Plans can benefit teams of any size, the larger and more complex the team, the greater the number of potential challenges that may arise, in turn increasing the potential benefits of advance planning. As the size and complexity of the team grows, so does the likelihood of encountering challenges related to team formation, leadership and management, and team functioning (Hall et al. 2018; Cummings et al. 2013; Cummings and Kiesler, 2007). Evidence from complex teams highlights the fact that poorly managed collaboration can negatively impact the quality of the science that is produced, whereas well-managed science teams have the potential to accelerate science (Hall et al. 2012a, 2018; Cummings et al. 2013).

The National Academy of Sciences report *Enhancing the Effectiveness of Team Science* (National Research Council 2015) identifies seven "complexity dimensions" of science teams: diversity of membership, degree of needed knowledge integration (from unidisciplinarity to transdisciplinarity integration), team size, degree of goal alignment, permeability of team boundaries, geographic dispersion of team members, and degree of task interdependence. Complexity on any of these dimensions may be critical to enhance the science (e.g., by bringing diverse perspectives to bear on a problem), but also can increase the challenges for team functioning. For example, the geographic distribution of team members introduces challenges for communication and coordination. The disciplinary diversity of a team introduces challenges in terms of developing shared goals for the collaboration, shared terminology, and mutually agreed-upon and understood approaches to conducting the science.

There are many additional factors that can add complexity in science teams. These include the aims of the science; the resources needed to achieve these aims (e.g., nonscientist collaborators, specialized technical infrastructure); intrapersonal factors such as members' attitudes toward collaboration; interpersonal factors such as members' history of collaboration with one another; organizational factors such as policies related to cross-departmental or cross-institutional collaboration; technological factors such as the degree to which collaborators have access to compatible technology for data sharing, communication, and coordination of work tasks, and their comfort with using these technologies; the diverse physical and cultural environments of the institutions where the participating individuals are employed; and societal and political influences such as funding opportunities that support team science approaches.

To be effective, a Collaboration Plan must take into account the unique combination of complexity dimensions and other influencing factors that shape the planned scientific collaboration. As a result, each Collaboration Plan will be unique. In addition, a Collaboration Plan likely will require more details and elements as the size and complexity of the initiative increases. For example, three co-PIs from the same department who have worked together successfully in the past might need a modest Collaboration Plan that outlines practices that have worked for them during previous projects, while emphasizing additional plans around elements that are needed to address unique aspects of the new project. In contrast, a newly established multidisciplinary multi-institutional collaboration would likely require a lengthier Collaboration Plan that includes more extensive details associated with all ten components. Such a collaboration would likely benefit from a Collaboration Plan that gives special consideration to how the team will navigate disciplinary differences in terminology and scientific methods, and how the participating institutions will work together, including how they will address relevant policies and procedures as well as technological issues. Similarly, an international collaboration involving investments by multiple academic institutions and governments (e.g., the Human Genome Project, the Large Hadron Collider) would benefit from an even more sophisticated Collaboration Plan establishing the roles and responsibilities of each participating organization as well as procedures for communication and decision making, approaches for sharing resources, and many other aspects of the functioning of the scientific collaboration.

45.2 Ten Key Components to Address in a Collaboration Plan

This portion of the chapters lays out the ten influences that are addressed in the Collaboration Plan and highlights factors for consideration related to each influence.

45.2.1 Rationale for Team Approach and Team Composition

Scientific considerations should be primary when determining, first, whether an individual or team-based approach is best, and second, the composition of the team. The Collaboration Plan will need to justify how the team approach, as well as the team size and composition, is required for scientific success, in light of such complexity dimensions as geographic dispersion and disciplinary diversity, which can introduce challenges to team functioning (NRC 2015; O'Rourke et al. 2019; Gibbs et al. 2019).

45.2.1.1 Team Approach

The Collaboration Plan should begin by justifying why the particular scientific questions and goals require a team approach. For example, it may be that experts from diverse disciplines may be needed on the research team to answer a question beyond the scope of an individual discipline. Alternatively, a research question may require that a team rely on equipment or infrastructure located at multiple institutions, within multiple centers or labs. Or a team may require the involvement of nonscientists, for example, if the goals of the project involve applications within specific cultures or communities or for translations into interventions, practices, or policies (O'Rourke et al. 2019; Pohl and Wuelser 2019; Kiviniemi 2019).

It is also critical to consider and address whether the disciplines and fields to be included on the team will be able to work together successfully to achieve the scientific objectives. Hays notes that if the participating disciplines or "fields of science have not sufficiently evolved toward one another or their underlying support structures are incongruous, it may be difficult or impossible to initiate and maintain cross-disciplinary research even though the participants are eager and other readiness challenges have been successfully met" (Hays 2008). This is known as "scientific readiness" for cross-disciplinary or cross-field integration (c.f., James and Redline 2019; Falcone et al. 2019).

45.2.1.2 Team Size and Composition

Given that coordination costs can increase with team size and diversity of expertise (Cummings et al. 2013, Hall et al. 2012a, b), the Collaboration Plan should justify how both the proposed mix of expertise and the team size are necessary to provide the expertise and time investment required to achieve the scientific goals (Cummings and Haas 2012). Recent literature has found that different team compositions may be effective for different team goals. For example, the ideal composition and size may differ for a team that is focused on incremental change within a field versus a team focused on translational science versus a team focused on radical innovation (Hall et al. 2018). Recent findings suggest that ideal team size also varies based on the disciplines involved, the scientific questions being explored, and contextual factors (Hall et al. 2018). In addition, research has documented certain advantages of diversity in a science team, including disciplinary and demographic diversity, as well as the mix of academic ranks and professional roles on the team, with different compositions producing different benefits (Hall et al. 2018; Gibbs et al. 2019). Researchers may draw on guiding principles by O'Rourke et al. (2019) when considering which experts to choose.

Finally, particularly for large and/or complex collaborations, consideration should be given to whether there is a need for team members whose roles are specific to project management, scientific governance, cross-disciplinary integration, translational science, or cross-initiative integration to help support effective team functioning. New roles in team science are now being developed and recognized as specialized professional roles and are increasingly understood to be critical to the success of large and/or complex science teams (e.g., Hendren and Ku 2019).

45.2.2   Collaboration Readiness

The Collaboration Plan should provide evidence for the collaboration readiness of the individual participating investigators, the team as a unit, and the institutions that are involved. It can be expected that not all individuals, teams, and institutions will be entirely prepared for the range of potential demands involved in complex collaborations. This is especially the case for organizational or individual members whose primary mission is not research. Therefore, the Collaboration Planning process also should iden-

tify potential challenges to collaboration readiness, and whenever possible, the Collaboration Plan should identify steps that will be taken to address these challenges and enhance collaboration readiness. Researchers can consider established guiding questions to help assess a team's readiness for integration and draw on a range of readiness tools to bolster collaborative capacity (O'Rourke et al. 2019).

45.2.2.1   Individual Collaboration Readiness

Individual characteristics related to team science, such as interest in and motivation to engage in collaboration, perceived threats of collaboration, and past experiences with collaboration, influence collaboration readiness (Mallinson et al. 2016; Stokols et al. 2008; Hall et al. 2008b, Stipelman, et al. 2010). It is important to consider strategies to support collaboration readiness given the wide range of personalities, work styles, experiences, and attitudes that team members bring to the collaboration (e.g., See Bennett et al. 2018; Stipelman et al. 9). In the Team Science Field Guide,[2] Bennett and colleagues offer case studies and guiding questions for considering one's readiness to participate in or lead a research team and help to bolster researchers' readiness to collaborate.

45.2.2.2   Team Collaboration Readiness

Team-level influencing factors such as the mix of collaboration histories of proposed team members, and team leaders' past experience with leading teams. For example, teams with a mix of prior and new collaborators may be most successful because they can benefit from the good working relationships of prior collaborators as well as the new perspectives injected by new team members (Uzzi and Spiro 2005). Teams may enhance their collaborative readiness by using tools like the Team Diagnostic Survey[3] and the associated feedback report, which together

---

[2] https://www.cancer.gov/about-nci/organization/crs/research-initiatives/team-science-field-guide

[3] https://www.teamdiagnosticsurvey.com/the-tds/

have been found to improve team effectiveness (Eisele 2013, Wageman et al. 2005).

45.2.2.3 Institutional Collaboration Readiness

This refers to the resources, infrastructure, and policies that each of the participating institutions has in place to support the collaboration. Institutions may provide support relevant to many of the key influences on team science that are described in this document. Examples include promotion and tenure policies that recognize participation in science teams; research development professionals[4] and Intereach professionals[5] whose work supports team formation and nurtures ongoing collaborations; and consultants who can enhance leadership and management skills and facilitate quality improvement activities. This section of the Collaboration Plan should address each of the institutions involved in the proposed collaboration. It should identify indicators of readiness, highlight potential challenges in the institutional environments, and describe plans to address these challenges. For instance, collaborating organizations that are primarily service oriented often require explicit reassurances concerning the minimization of burdens and disruptions created by research collaboration. Protocols to initiate discussions among organizations and document strategies to address specific collaborative concerns between organizations are a means to demonstrate an institutional collaborative readiness. A university might consider an assessment to identify existing strengths and opportunities for enhancing its collaboration readiness, such as the National Organization of Research Development Professionals' (NORDP) Program for External Evaluation of Research Development,[6] to identify and utilize tools, best practices, and guidance for enhancing institutional facilitators of team science.

45.2.3 Technological Readiness

The Collaboration Plan should document the availability and planned use of technological resources to support the scientific collaboration (Stokols et al. 2008). These may include mechanisms to support both scientific and collaborative processes.

45.2.3.1 Scientific Processes

Mechanisms to support the scientific process may include approaches for data sharing and collaborative analysis (e.g., data sharing agreements, shared databases, web-based collaborative data analysis platforms) as well as issues of confidentiality and intellectual property associated with technologies used or produced by the collaborative research. In diverse teams, some issues that may be "obvious" to one researcher may be new to another. For instance, while some collaborators may regularly develop new technologies or apply for patents, others may have never dealt with technology transfer issues. Outlining key elements related to relevant aspects of research such as intellectual property[7] or data management[8] can help ensure all collaborators are aware of, and may plan for, potential issues involved in the planned research, thus reducing the likelihood of related conflicts (see Conflict Prevention and Management, below).

45.2.3.2 Collaborative Processes

Mechanisms to support collaborative processes include research networking and profiling tools (see comprehensive online resource for comparison of tools[9]), communication technologies (e.g., videoconferencing, teleconferencing, instant messaging), and coordination technologies (e.g., calendaring and workflow or project management tools). To support collaboration, researchers may use collaborative platforms, which may include multiple features specifically designed to support scientific collaboration (e.g., HubZero, Trellis), or leverage collaboration software designed for any work environment (e.g., Jive, Microsoft SharePoint). Many collaborations will use multiple types of tools to meet a range of needs.

---

[4] c.f., http://www.nordp.org/

[5] c.f., https://www.intereach.org/

[6] http://www.nordp.org/peerd-consulting-program

[7] http://www.iphandbook.org/handbook/ch07/p04/

[8] https://www.nsf.gov/news/news_summ.jsp?cntn_id= 118038

[9] https://en.wikipedia.org/wiki/Comparison_of_research_ networking_tools_and_research_profiling_systems

Researchers may adopt collaborative editing tools (e.g., Google Docs/Sheets, Zoho, Nuclino) as stand-alone tools or on an ad hoc basis during particular phases of the research process or they may adopt a strategy designed to integrate multiple applications (e.g., Slack). These technologies may be provided by the team lab, department, or host institution(s). A growing number of resources exist that provide guidance for choosing collaborative technologies (e.g., Berente and Howison 2019; Distributed Science website[10]).

An important consideration is whether members of the team are ready to use the available technologies, including having both the willingness and skills. Training on the use of collaborative technologies may warrant specific training time or budgetary allocations (see Training and Budget sections below). Another important consideration is the interoperability of systems, as members of the group may have trouble working together if they are using different systems (e.g., different videoconferencing systems, different databases, different data analysis packages). Institutional policies and procedures should also be considered (e.g., a firewall blocking system access by nonlocal team members). In addition, cultural factors can enhance or complicate collaboration, especially when norms of collaboration processes are not explicitly considered and respected. Collaboration Planning should address each of these issues.

45.2.4 Team Functioning

The Collaboration Plan should describe plans for carrying out key processes that underlie effective team functioning. These include generating a shared vision, mission, and goals; creating shared mental models of the team structure and the collaborative scientific project; and externalizing group cognition throughout the collaboration (e.g., by generating visual schematics that capture the group's understanding of the scientific problem space, the research question(s), and the

collaborative workflow). The Collaboration Plan also should describe approaches that will be used to support key team processes that help to develop team-level understanding of each team member's areas of expertise, roles on the team, and contributions to the science, i.e., developing shared understanding of who knows what (compilational transactive memory), who does what (compositional transactive memory), and how things get done (task work transactive memory) on the team (Hall et al. 2012, b; Kozlowski and Bell 2019; Berente and Howison 2019).

Strategies may include a kickoff meeting to develop a shared vision that involves developing a vision statement, sharing team members' reflections on how their work contributes to the vision, and discussing responsibility and accountability for helping achieve the team's overall goals (e.g., Bennett et al. 2018)

To facilitate the behavioral and cognitive team processes described above, motivational and affective processes are critical. These help to create a supportive context for team functioning. Consideration of processes including developing team cohesion, providing a psychologically safe environment, and engendering confidence in the team's ability to attain shared goals is useful (team efficacy; Hall et al. 2012a, b; Kozlowski and Bell 2019). The literature on science teams has pointed to the importance of trust among team members to support knowledge sharing, coordination, and conflict resolution (Hall et al. 2012a, b, 2018). The Collaboration Plan may describe strategies for supporting an environment of psychological safety in the team context, which includes supporting team members to take ownership for mistakes, display scientific humility, cultivate appreciation of others' contribution, and help one another address scientific or collaborative challenges. In addition, multiple studies have shown the importance of face-to-face meetings to the success of science teams (Hall et al. 2018). These may be located at a partnering institution, conference, or other setting. For geographically dispersed collaborations, the Collaboration Plan might describe how face-to-face interactions might be supported, virtually or in person.

---

[10]http://distributedscience.ischool.utexas.edu/node/104.html

Regular engagement in iterative reflection can help to maintain highly functioning teams and enhance performance. In the context of such reflection, teams systematically consider team performance and participate in related adaptation of team goals and processes (West et al. 2011; West and Lyubovnikova 2012). The Collaboration Plan should describe approaches for team-level reflection. Strategies may involve macro-level opportunities, for instance, to reflect on how team processes are supporting or hindering progress toward overall project or institute goals (e.g., at annual strategic planning meetings) and ways in which improvements can be made. Teams may also plan for strategies at a more micro-level (e.g., day-to-day activities), such as intermittently leaving time at the end of regular meetings to reflect on team efficiency and effectiveness (e.g., Is the group meeting too frequently? Are there ways the group could better prepare for meetings?).

Collaboration Plans for cross-disciplinary teams also should include plans for fostering team processes needed specifically for cross-disciplinary work, such as critical awareness of the strengths and weaknesses of contributing disciplines, a shared team vocabulary that bridges disciplinary differences, and integration of diverse perspectives, as needed (Hall et al. 2012a, b; Marino et al. 2019). For example, the creation of glossaries of key terms or summaries of key concepts/theories for speakers to distribute during cross-disciplinary seminars can help facilitate shared understanding of language and terminology (Hall et al 2012b; Falcone et al 2019). A cross-disciplinary orientation among team members, which includes an understanding of the potential contributions and limitations of each participating discipline, has been found to support more creative and cross-disciplinary products with greater anticipated translational impact (Hall et al. 2018).

Suggestions for integrating disciplinary perspectives include the use of metaphors, perspective taking, and mapping conceptual ideas (Salazar et al. 2019; Gehlert 2019; Fiore et al. 2019). Furthermore, there are numerous approaches that can be used to facilitate the integration of the perspectives of a wide range of stakeholders, such as patients, citizens, and community leaders (e.g., Johnson and Smalley 2019; Couch et al. 2019; Wallerstein et al. 2019), including more than a dozen methods described in td-net's toolbox for co-production of knowledge.[11]

In addition, teams can facilitate iterative reflection by periodically revisiting their Collaboration Plans and reflecting on what is working and what can be improved (e.g., team structure, coordination, communication, leadership, available resources), which can help to support quality improvement in team functioning and identify needed resources. Strategies should be selected based on the characteristics of the collaboration, such as phase of the research process (Hall et al. 2012a, b), interpersonal relationships and collaborative history of team members (Stokols et al. 2008), and complexity factors (e.g., multi-team system such as a center initiative; Carter et al. 2019a). Professional consultation or facilitation may be helpful to support some of these strategies, especially when there are significant cultural differences among team members. Furthermore, advisory boards can provide valuable perspectives for helping teams identify gaps and opportunities for new connections, partnerships, and integration of ideas as well as recommendations for team process and institutional supports (Gehlert et al. 2019).

45.2.5 Communication and Coordination

Team science requires that effort be invested in supporting effective communication and coordination of tasks. As team size increases, so does the needed level of investment in team communication and coordination. Given the infrastructure and resources associated with communication and coordination, these two team processes are addressed separately, here.

---

[11] https://naturalsciences.ch/topics/co-producing_knowledge/about

45.2.5.1   Communication

The Collaboration Plan should describe plans for effective communication within the team, including meeting frequency and modality (e.g., teleconference, in-person) and asynchronous communications (e.g., email use or document sharing). Teams that are particularly diverse in terms of team members' geographic locations, languages, cultures, or disciplinary training (e.g., authorship traditions, work styles, terminology, preferred methods) typically face increased communication challenges. A key problem is bridging different assumptions and understandings in multidisciplinary teams. Explicitly identifying potential differences and identifying approaches to bridge them can be helpful. The Toolbox Dialogue Initiative[12] provides a set of prompts for guided discussions among collaborators, with the goals of rooting out unrecognized differences, and enhancing communication about their shared work (O'Rourke and Crowley 2013).

45.2.5.2   Coordination

Greater use of coordination mechanisms has been found to be related to more successful outcomes in large teams (Cummings and Kiesler 2005). The Collaboration Plan should describe strategies to coordinate day-to-day operations and approaches, such as how tasks get allocated, how resources get shared, and how work gets integrated into the collaborative effort. Strategies may include workflow coordination software, data sharing agreements, and procedures for data integration. As always, the strategies adopted must be tailored to the particular collaboration, addressing such factors as the number and distribution of team members and needed equipment and technologies, as well as the design of team tasks (e.g., Berente and Howison 2019). For large and/or complex collaborations, it may be particularly helpful to formalize coordination strategies. This sort of attention to coordination in the Collaboration Plan is particularly helpful for collaborations that include multiple institutions with different policies, procedures, and resources to be

navigated and leveraged. Coordination centers or shared administrative supports can play key roles in supporting team science (Rolland 2019).

45.2.6   Leadership, Management, and Administration

Providing vision, direction, and representation for an initiative is critical to success, particularly in team science. The more complex the team science initiative, the greater the demands on leadership and management, and the greater the potential impact of effective or ineffective leadership. The Coordination Plan should describe the leadership and management approaches that will be used to facilitate the other components of the plan, given the specific scientific, team, and institutional contexts involved.

45.2.6.1   Leadership

There are numerous approaches to leadership (e.g., hierarchical, heterarchical, transformational, transactional; Gray 2008; Hall et al. 2018). A leader's approach will depend on the particular characteristics of the scientific initiative, including scientific goals, team composition and size, resources, and institutional factors, among others, as well as the personalities of the leader and other team members (c.f., Berger 2019). A Collaboration Plan can help in conceptualizing what strategies will be effective given these characteristics, as a primary goal of the leader in a scientific collaboration is to help inspire and empower team members to engage in and support team processes integral to team function. When considering leadership specifically for cross-disciplinary teams, Salazar et al. (2019) describe five key integrative leadership capabilities: (a) visioning, (b) reflexivity, (c) perspective-seeking, (d) conflict management, and (e) coordination. Approaches for each capacity are described; for instance, to support reflexivity it is recommended that leaders discuss errors, create an environment for exploration and experimentation, and promote respect among team members (Salazar et al. 2019). When more than one leader is identi-

---

[12]http://toolbox-project.org/

fied for a collaboration, shared leadership governance strategies are needed (c.f., sample NIH multiple PI leadership plans[13]; Fiore et al. 2019).

45.2.6.2 Management

Ensuring that the vision for the scientific work is carried out requires roles to be established, tasks to be identified and assigned, and research plans to be executed, as well as changed as needed. The Collaboration Plan should outline strategies for managing personnel, processes, and procedures within the team and across institutions (e.g., for collaborative activities or for subcontracts). For example, the Collaboration Plan should identify how key decisions will be made about changes in the direction of the science and in team personnel. This section of the Collaboration Plan might also include a projected schedule for the project, including both managerial and scientific benchmarks. It might also include an analysis of risks and limitations facing the project and discuss how these will be addressed or managed should they arise. Finally, the Collaboration Plan should address where responsibility lies for financial management and resources available for this task. Coordination centers can play an important role in management, for example, in negotiating questions of roles and responsibilities, prioritizing projects in view of limited resources, coordinating protocol development, and managing IRB applications (Rolland 2019).

45.2.6.3 Administration

As team size increases, administrative tasks become increasingly important to team coordination. Collaboration Plans should consider the need for administrative support for the team. Administrative activities of critical importance to large teams include recruitment, hiring, annual reporting, support for organizing meetings and conference calls, and other activities. This section of the Coordination Plan should also consider administrative support for coordination and communication mechanisms.

Leadership, management, and administration need to be addressed regardless of the size and scope of a project, team, center, or initiative. Small teams may require only a leader to handle the full range of tasks. As projects grow in size and complexity, leaders may distribute these tasks across collaborators or resources may be available to bring on team members to take on management and administrative roles. Additionally, individuals with experience in emerging career paths such as the Interdisciplinary Executive Scientist may be brought on to combine disciplinary expertise with competencies for facilitating boundary-spanning collaborations such as translational skills and skills for effective knowledge synthesis among disciplines. These individuals balance intellectual leadership with key administrative responsibilities (Hendren and Ku 2019).

45.2.7 Conflict Prevention and Management

Some degree of conflict within a collaboration is inevitable. While some types of conflict are highly disruptive, conflict need not be seen as all negative. Indeed, scientific conflict may be helpful for the team to achieve its goals, for example, by leading to new avenues of thought for everyone involved. But relational conflict may undermine team functioning and ultimately negatively impact the science, so efforts to avoid and ameliorate such conflict are critical.

The Collaboration Plan should identify strategies that will be used to identify factors that might lead to conflict (e.g., ownership of data, intellectual property rights, authorship order, potential faultlines on the team, scientific challenges) and prevent, manage, and resolve conflicts that emerge. Many sources of team conflict can be anticipated (e.g., scientific differences of opinion due to disciplinary differences, authorship order in large teams). But conflicts may arise even when not expected. For example, investigators with similar training may underestimate the potential for conflict due to incorrect assumptions about areas of agreement.

---

[13] http://grants.nih.gov/grants/multi_pi/sample_leadership_plans.pdf

The potential for conflict, and how conflict plays out, will depend on the characteristics of the team, including team composition, scientific goals, and the environments in which team members work (Eigenbrode et al. 2007). Two common sources of conflict on science teams are demographic diversity (e.g., age, gender, culture) and disciplinary diversity. The existence of team subgroups, along either of these lines, may produce faultlines along which conflicts emerge (Bezrukova 2013).

45.2.7.1 Conflict Prevention

Strategies to prevent conflict can be implemented at the individual, team, and initiative levels. For instance, at the individual level an onboarding letter (e.g., "Welcome to my Team" Letter; Bennett et al. 2014) provides a scaffold for building trust by outlining for new team members from the outset what they can expect of the team, what the team expects of new members, and what to do if members disagree. An example of a team-level conflict prevention strategy is the use of a pre-collaboration agreement template, also sometimes called a "prenuptial agreement for scientists" (Gadlin and Jessar 2002). The template agreement can guide discussion among potential or current collaborators around issues that are typical sources of conflict, such as scientific and other goals, expected contributions of each collaborator, authorship/credit, ownership of data and patent rights, as well as conflict management and resolution approaches. These discussions may take place informally or serve as the basis for a written document that documents agreed-upon elements and can be referenced and modified as the collaboration progresses.

At the initiative level, pre-collaboration agreements can be elaborated to incorporate elements that address multiple projects and organizations. Leaders can facilitate discussions among members and develop a formal agreement document to be used by all members of an initiative. Large initiatives may warrant an initiative-level agreement as well as a team-level agreement that specifically addresses the unique needs of a given team. Furthermore, for large-scale collaborations, operating manuals (c.f., TREC Manual of Operations[14]) may include a pre-collaboration agreement, while also outlining a full range of policies and procedures (e.g., policies and approaches for sharing data, findings, and credit across multiple teams in an initiative). Operating manuals should be developed and approved early in the life of a collaboration, though they should be considered living documents to be modified as needed. Overall, documenting collaborative decisions helps to ensure members have a shared understanding of agreements and can serve as an effective strategy to prevent and manage conflict over key issues over the life cycle of the collaboration.

45.2.7.2 Conflict Management

Despite efforts to prevent conflict, conflicts often still arise. To be successful, an initiative must have approaches in place for managing conflicts. These include processes for encouraging scientific debate and facilitating productive scientific conflict while preventing and/or managing negative interpersonal conflict as well as processes and procedures for resolving detrimental conflicts. These may call upon preexisting institutional resources for conflict management and resolution, utilize outside resources (e.g., mediation), and/or introduce team-level responses. The approaches taken should be commensurate with the characteristics of the proposed collaboration (e.g., size, geographic dispersion of members, cross-cultural makeup) and available resources.

All members of a team play a critical role in preventing and managing conflict, while leaders play an important role in helping to create norms and serve as role models to support conflict prevention and management (Salazar et al. 2019; Bennett and Gadlin 2019).

45.2.8 Training

The Collaboration Plan should outline training strategies to enhance the scientific collaboration among participating investigators. This may

---

[14] http://www.teamsciencetoolkit.cancer.gov/public/TSResourceTool.aspx?tid=1&rid=371

include training for investigators for whom collaboration is new as well as more advanced training for investigators with prior experience with team science. Training may be provided at the start of the initiative and/or at any time during the collaboration. As with other aspects of the Collaboration Plan, the training plan should consider how training approaches, including both content and format, will be tailored to the particular characteristics of the team, including the type of science (e.g., level of integration, diversity of disciplines), team traits (e.g., new vs. long-standing collaborators, proximal vs. distributed), and institutional characteristics (e.g., availability of training resources). Training needs may span from bolstering team science competencies to learning how to use new collaborative technologies.

45.2.8.1 Training Content

Training for scientific collaboration can help to build skills across the key areas identified in this document (e.g., team processes, leadership, management, communication, coordination, technologies, and quality improvement activities). For cross-disciplinary collaborations, training might also include a focus particular to cross-disciplinary work, such as building critical awareness of the strengths and weaknesses of participating disciplines, and strategies for combining approaches (e.g., theories, concepts, methods) from two or more disciplines. Training may also focus on enhancing knowledge and

skills specific to the science in the proposed collaboration, for example, knowledge of a particular scientific area of interest, and/or skills related to using platforms or software that will be used in the particular collaboration (e.g., shared databases and data management/analysis software).

45.2.8.2 Training Approaches

Team science training may be packaged together in a retreat, workshop, or course explicitly devoted to team science and can be incorporated into coursework, on-the-job training, and mentoring using team-oriented approaches. Relevant pedagogical approaches may include problem-based, team-based, studio learning and include small-group work, meta-cognitive techniques, or interactions among learners and instructors (Fiore et al. 2019). Taking time to consider which key complexity dimensions may be at play and what strategies can be implemented to address them can help increase the efficiency and effectiveness of training (Table 45.1). For instance, in order to facilitate goal alignment, team members must develop a shared vision and goals; thereby, visioning and goal setting and team reflexivity training can enhance the likelihood of a team achieving its desired outcomes.

45.2.8.3 Training Format

A range of formats can be used to deliver team science training. The format of a training program can be designed to meet a wide variety of investigator circumstances and needs, including

Table 45.1 Mapping of types of training that can be used to enhance skill and processes across key team science dimensions

Dimension	Skills/Processes	Type of training
Diversity	Communication and interpersonal interactions	ID educational seminars, interpersonal skills training
Integration	Coordination and communication, shared mental models	Cross-training, knowledge-sharing training, coordination training
Size	Compositional, taskwork, and teamwork transactive memory	Positional clarification, communication, coordination training
Proximity	Compilational, compositional transactive memory, team cohesion/self-efficacy	Team reflexivity training, positional clarification training
Boundaries	Team-specific knowledge/goals	Cross-training, knowledge development
Task interdependance	Taskwork transactive memory	Team reflexivity training

different career stages, learning styles, training interests and needs, and practical constraints. For example, online tutorials or interactive web-based training may be most appropriate for geographically distributed teams. Training can be carried out at the individual level and for team units. Training might be formal (e.g., online courses, such as teamscience.net,[15] which provides a completion certificate) or informal (e.g., seminar series featuring the work of all participating team members, to build cross-disciplinary awareness and greater mutual understanding).

Consideration should be given to identify which training format can best support the collaborative needs and team goals. For instance, cross-learning through cross-disciplinary seminar series or journal clubs can be bolstered by using techniques such as providing glossaries of terms or implementing a yellow card strategy (i.e., yellow card raised when a term is used that is unknown to audience members to ensure effective knowledge transfer). Learning to integrate knowledge across disciplines can be supported through collaborative writing retreats that structure opportunities for simultaneous and sequential writing time. The use of research pilot funds to support opportunities for development of scientific leadership skills can be structured to require junior faculty to lead projects with collaborators from other disciplines, domains, and/or universities. This offers the added benefit of providing experience across multiple collaborative dimensions (e.g., degree of integration, cross-institutional, geographic distribution, etc.; Hall et al. 2018; Vogel et al. 2012; Fiore et al. 2019).

Training content, approaches, and format will vary depending on the features of the collaboration and experience of the collaborators. Although there are common sets of competencies (Fiore et al. 2019) that are relevant across team science, training content and strategies will vary for graduate students (e.g., Klein 2019), postdoctoral fellows (e.g., Bachrach et al. 2019), and senior scientists (e.g., Spring et al. 2019).

The Collaboration Plan should address how the training content, approach, and format will be decided upon given the circumstances of the specific collaboration. Plans should explicitly map training goals, skills, approaches, and formats and outline expectations for participation in training (e.g., the frequency and type of training members should participate in) or agreements by those involved in providing training or mentorship (e.g., how often a mentor may meet with trainees or co-mentors).

45.2.9 Quality Improvement Activities

Teams that engage in systematic and iterative reflection about team performance and subsequently adapt their team objectives and processes show better performance, including higher levels of innovation (West et al. 2011; West and Lyubovnikova 2012). The Collaboration Plan should describe plans for activities that will be implemented over the course of the research initiative to facilitate reflection about team performance (e.g., pre-briefing and debriefing). It should also describe how the resulting information will be used for quality improvement, to help address challenges and improve the quality of the collaboration, including the science and team interactions, as necessary. For a large and complex initiative, it may be helpful to involve outside experts to design and implement these reflection and quality improvement-oriented activities (e.g., facilitators, evaluators). Commercial products also may support reflection and quality improvement (e.g., the Team Diagnostic Survey[16] and the Collaboration Success Wizard[17]) (Bietz et al. 2012; Wageman et al. 2005).

45.2.10 Budget/Resource Allocation

Successful collaborations require investments of both time and funds to support technological infrastructure (e.g., for coordination, communication, and scientific data sharing and analysis),

[15] www.teamscience.net

[16] https://www.teamdiagnosticsurvey.com/the-tds/
[17] http://hana.ics.uci.edu/wizard/

training of team members, management and administration of the team, and quality improvement-oriented activities. The Collaboration Plan should identify the specific budget lines or items needed to support the activities included in the plan. Clear but flexible plans for funds can allow optimal preparation for and facilitation of collaboration. This can be particularly important in large and complex initiatives where directions can change during the course of the initiative (e.g., scientific objectives, team members, involved institutions).

45.3 How to Use a Collaboration Plan

The work of writing a Collaboration Plan can be used as a start to the collaborative process, as it begins to establish shared goals and mutual understanding, and lays the groundwork for systems of communication and coordination. It can also be an opportunity to lay the groundwork for how technologies will be used, how conflict will be managed, and how the collaborators will engage in quality improvement-related activities. Table 45.2 highlights the ten Collaboration Plan components and provides examples of subcomponents and key considerations. Additionally, the table provides examples of chapters throughout this book that address elements of each of the 10 Collaboration Plan components, which offer additional guidance for relevant policies and practices.

Once developed, Collaboration Plans serve as roadmaps to facilitate effective team formation and functioning. Yet these documents should not be treated as static or prescriptive, but as "living documents" that may be revised periodically to reflect the evolving characteristics, functioning, needs, and goals of the team, as well as changes in influencing conditions that may positively or negatively affect the success of the collaboration. Collaboration Plans also can be used to establish benchmarks to support quality improvement.

Collaboration Plans also can be used to communicate a team's likelihood of collaborative success, goals and expectations, and needs to a wide variety of stakeholders with varied goals. For example, Collaboration Plans can be shared with (a) funders to demonstrate readiness for team collaboration; (b) current and future team members and other stakeholders (e.g., academic administrators, funders) to share information about team roles, functioning, and resources; and (c) organizational leaders to make the case for needed resources or changes in policy or procedures to support effective team functioning and, ultimately, scientific success.

A Collaboration Plan can be developed at any stage in the life cycle of a collaboration to serve needs particular to that stage. For example, a Collaboration Plan may be developed by potential collaborators before the start of an initiative to help guide their future collaboration. This can be provided as part of a grant application for team-based research, where application rules allow, to demonstrate readiness for collaboration. Alternatively, a Collaboration Plan may be developed at the launch of a new collaboration, after funding has been awarded, and simultaneous with team formation, to help plan for success. A Collaboration Plan also may be developed at any time during an ongoing collaboration, when involved parties recognize that additional attention to key influences may help to enhance the team's functioning and performance. For example, team members may find that certain aspects of team interactions, leadership and management, resources, or infrastructure are in need of further development, standardization, or specific improvements.

Collaboration Plans can also be used to assess and improve upon the evolving development and functioning of the team. They may help to pose and answer questions such as: Does the ultimate makeup of the team reflect the goals for team composition? And is there a need to add other expertise to the team? Do the individual members of the team demonstrate readiness to collaborate with one another, across the various areas of diversity on the team—including disciplines, fields, demographics, etc.? And is there a need to enhance readiness, and, if so, what strategies might be successful? Has the team procured the necessary technical resources for data sharing, collaborative data analysis, virtual

Table 45.2 Key considerations for the 10 Collaboration Planning components and related book chapters

Ten components	Key considerations	Related book chapters (selected)
1. Rationale for team approach and team composition		
Team approach	***Justify*** why a team approach is necessary to meet the research objectives	Pohl and Wuesler (Chap. 8) Kiviniemi (Chap. 11)
Team size and composition	***Describe*** how the team configuration meets the proposed research objectives (e.g., how each team member contributes uniquely)	O'Rourke et al. (Chap. 2) Gibbs et al. (Chap. 15) Hendren and Ku (Chap. 27) Sallis and Floyd (Chap. 40)
Team assembly	***Discuss*** considerations for assembling the team (e.g., what expertise is needed, history of collaboration)	Twyman and Contractor (Chap. 17) Berger (Chap. 25) Salis and Floyd (Chap. 41) Weber and Yaun (Chap. 42)
	Specify key stakeholders and relevant contributions of team members across the research phases	O'Rourke et al. (Chap. 2) Pohl and Wuesler (Chap. 8) Arriaga and Abowd (Chap. 5) Kiviniemi (Chap. 11) Couch et al. (Chap. 12)
2. Collaboration readiness		
	Provide evidence for collaborative readiness associated with…	
Individual collaboration readiness	Intrapersonal skills and characteristics of research members	Nurius and Kemp (Chap. 13) Stipelman et al. (Chap. 14)
Team collaboration readiness	Interpersonal skills and capacity of the team as a unit	Ranwala et al. (Chap. 20) O'Rourke et al. (Chap. 2)
Institutional collaborative readiness	Institutions and organizations involved	Winter (Chap. 35) Carter, Carlson et al. (Chap. 28) Crow and Dabars (Chap. 37) Brown et al. (Chap. 38)
	Alignment of rewards and recognition for team-based research	Berger (Chap. 26) Carter, Carlson et al. (Chap. 28) Gehlert et al. (Chap. 31) Vogel et al. (Chap. 39)
	Availability and planned use of shared resources	Hurn and Traystman (Chap. 6) Rolland (Chap. 32)
	Strategic planning	Gehlert (Chap. 30) Brown et al. (Chap. 38)
3. Technological Readiness		
	Document the availability and planned use of technological resources to facilitate:	
Scientific and collaborative processes	Data sharing and collaborative data analysis	Berente and Howison (Chap. 43) Rolland (Chap. 32) Gilmore and Adolph (Chap. 44)
	Communication	Berente and Howison (Chap. 43) Rolland (Chap. 32) Fiore et al. (Chap. 33) Winter (Chap. 37)
	Coordination	Berente and Howison (Chap. 43) Rolland (Chap. 32) Fiore et al. (Chap. 33)
	Provide evidence for institutional support related to…	

(continued)

Table 45.2 (continued)

Ten components	Key considerations	Related book chapters (selected)
Institutional resources	Interoperability of proposed technology systems	Winter (Chap. 25) Rolland (Chap. 32)
	Policies	Winter (Chap. 25) Crow and Dabars (Chap. 37) Vogel et al. (Chap. 39)
	Physical space designed for collaboration	Bennett et al. (Chap. 40)
4. Team functioning		
	Document strategies for supporting team functioning, including strategies to…	
General	Identify gaps in team functioning processes and competencies	Kozlowski and Bell (Chap. 21) Fiore et al. (Chap. 33) Nurius and Kemp (Chap. 13)
Cognitive/behavioral processes	Develop shared vision, mission and goals	Falcone et al. (Chap. 4) Jain and Klein (Chap. 23) Carter, Carlson et al. (Chap. 28)
	Create shared mental models of the team structure and collaborative scientific project	Gehlert (Chap. 30) Bennett and Gadlin (Chap. 22)
	Externalize group cognition throughout the collaboration	Pohl and Wuelser (Chap. 8) Fiore et al. (Chap. 33) Falcone et al. (Chap. 4)
	Foster team-level understanding of each team member's areas of expertise, roles on the team, and contributions to the science	Kozlowski and Bell (Chap. 21) Twyman and Contractor (Chap. 17)
	Encourage perspective taking	Salazar et al. (Chap. 24) O'Rourke et al. (Chap. 2)
	Engage in on-going iterative reflection	Gehlert (Chap. 30) Salazar et al. (Chap. 25) Fiore et al. (Chap. 33)
	Clarify roles and expectations	Bennett and Gadlin (Chap. 22); Rolland (Chap. 32) Sallis and Floyd (Chap. 41)
Affective/motivational processes	Foster team cohesion	Bennett and Gadlin (Chap. 22) Kozlowski and Bell (Chap. 21) Salazar et al. (Chap. 24)
	Provide a psychologically safe environment	Kozlowski and Bell (Chap. 21) Bennett and Gadlin (Chap. 22) Gehlert (Chap. 30)
	Engender confidence in team's ability to attain shared goals	Kozlowski and Bell (Chap. 21) Bennett and Galdin (Chap. 22)
	Bolster trust among team members	Kozlowski and Bell (Chap. 21) Bennett and Gadlin (Chap. 22) Jain and Klein (Chap. 23)

(continued)

Table 45.2 (continued)

Ten components	Key considerations	Related book chapters (selected)
Cross-disciplinarity/convergence	Foster interactions among diverse contributors to create new collaborations and/or advance existing teams	Gehlert et al. (Chap. 31) Bennett and Gadlin (Chap. 22) Christen and Levine (Chap. 19) Ranwala et al. (Chap. 20)
	Develop critical awareness of the strengths and weaknesses of contributing disciplines	O'Rouke et al. (Chap. 2) Kiviniemi (Chap. 11) Nurius and Kemp (Chap. 13)
	Create shared understanding of key disciplinary-specific terms and develop shared team vocabulary	Marino et al. (Chap. 18) Carter, Carlson et al. (Chap. 28) O'Rourke et al. (Chap. 2) Falcone et al. (Chap. 4)
	Foster cross-disciplinary orientation	Fiore et al. (Chap. 33)
	Share knowledge	Falcone et al. (Chap. 4) Berger (Chap. 26)
	Integrate and co-produce knowledge	Pohl and Wuelser (Chap. 8) O'Rourke et al. (Chap. 2)
	Integrate knowledge across stakeholders (e.g., non-academic and academic)	Wallerstein et al. (Chap. 9) Johnson and Smalley (Chap. 10) Kiviniemi (Chap. 11) Couch at al. (Chap. 12) Blot et al. (Chap. 16)
	Embrace opportunities for serendipity	Hurn and Traystman (Chap. 6) Madden et al. (Chap. 7) Bennett et al. (Chap. 40)

5. Communication and coordination

	Provide plans and strategies for…	
Communication	Communication across the team and among team members	O'Rourke et al. (Chap. 2) Carter, Asencio et al. (Chap. 29)
Coordination	Coordination of day-to-day operations and the on-going achievement of scholarly benchmarks	Wallerstein et al. (Chap. 9) Rolland (Chap. 32)

6. Leadership, management, and administration

	Provide descriptions of…	
Leadership	Leadership approaches to address the components in the Collaboration Plan; include the ways all team members will serve to lead (e.g., within roles/expertise) and how the team will work/lead together to achieve mission/vision/goals	Salazar et al. (Chap. 24) Berger (Chap. 26) Carter, Asencio et al. (Chap. 29) Gehlert (Chap. 30) Winter (Chap. 25) Klein (Chap. 36)
Management	Management approaches to address the components in the Collaboration Plan; include ways all team members will contribute to and support overall management	Twyman and Contractor (Chap. 17) Carter, Carlson et al. (Chap. 28) Carter, Asencio et al. (Chap. 29) Rolland (Chap. 32) Fiore et al. (Chap. 33) Winter (Chap. 25)
Administration	Strategies for recruitment, hiring, and daily administration of the team	Winter (Chap. 25) Hendren and Ku (Chap. 27) Rolland (Chap. 32)

7. Conflict prevention and management

	Describe strategies for…	
Conflict prevention	Preventing conflicts	Bennett and Gadlin (Chap. 22) Stipelman et al. (Chap. 14) Sallis and Floyd (Chap. 41)
Conflict management	Managing conflicts	Bennett and Gadlin (Chap. 22)

(continued)

Table 45.2 (continued)

Ten components	Key considerations	Related book chapters (selected)
8. *Training*		
	Provide description of, and implementation strategies for, …	
Training content	Training plans for the team and team members at the start of the collaboration and throughout, including strategies to identify gaps competencies and skills relevant to the team	Nurius and Kemp (Chap. 13) Fiore et al. (Chap. 33) Klein (Chap. 36)
Training approaches	Training approaches to enhance the relevant competencies and skill of the team	Bachrach et al. (Chap. 35) Madden et al. (Chap. 7) Brown et al. (Chap. 38)
Training format	Type of training format and how it incorporates the needed training content and proposed approaches	Kozlowski and Bell (Chap. 21) Spring et al. (Chap. 34) Klein (Chap. 36) Brown et al. (Chap. 38)
9. *Quality improvement activities*		
Processes and metrics	*Describe* the processes and metrics that will be put in place to ensure continuous quality improvement	Nurius and Kemp (Chap. 13) Stipelman et al. (Chap. 14) Gibbs et al. (Chap. 15) Blot et al. (Chap. 16) Carter, Carlson et al. (Chap. 28) Carter, Asencio et al. (Chap. 29) Winter (Chap. 25) Weber and Yuan (Chap. 42)
10. *Budget/resource allocation*		
Allocation of funds	*Allocate* funds in the budget for activities that facilitate the success of the team, as identified in components 1–9	Carter, Carlson et al. (Chap. 28) Winter (Chap. 25)

communication, and coordination of tasks? What additional technologies might facilitate the team's scientific goals and processes, based on the team's experiences to date? To what extent has the team implemented the strategies proposed in the Collaboration Plan, for each component? Why or why not? Have these been sufficient? What can be done to build upon successes and address gaps? Have training plans been put into action, and how have these impacted team functioning? What else might be needed in the way of training or professional development? Are current financial and other resources adequate to support the activities proposed in the Collaboration Plan, and, if not, what gaps exist? Can the Collaboration Plan facilitate communications with the participating institutions around requests for additional needed resources?

45.3.1　The Role of Academic Institutions

As investigators gain experience in developing Collaboration Plans, approaches to the document may become standardized for a research group or institution. This may lead to the development of model language that reflects particular institutional approaches, resources, and policies. Having such language to draw upon, in addition to examples of prior Collaboration Plans, and information about what strategies were successful and unsuccessful for past science teams at the institution, can greatly facilitate the development of future Collaboration Plans. Ultimately, however, each plan should be tailored to the unique circumstances of the proposed collaborative initiative.

One university resource to support the development of Collaboration Planning is Research Development Professionals (RDPs). RDPs are a growing group of academic administrators with specialized skills in supporting the efforts of faculty to initiate and nurture scientific collaborations and to secure extramural research funding for team collaborations. Their ultimate goals are to enable competitive team-based research and facilitate research excellence. Key activities of RDPs in team science include helping scientists to form collaborations, build cross-disciplinary and cross-institutional bridges, create cross-disciplinary and cross-field research concepts, and craft collaborative funding applications (Carter et al. 2019b). RDPs are therefore in the position to help investigators identify and address potential challenges to their collaborations, develop strategies to maximize success and mitigate challenges, and develop Collaboration Plans that capture this knowledge.

University administrators (e.g., VPs of Research, Department Chairs, Deans, Chancellors) are key to facilitating changes that align resources and policies to support team science (Hurn and Traystman 2019. Faculty, staff, and administrators can work together to help identify, support, and advocate for common needs to strengthen a university's capacity for collaboration (e.g., changes to promotion and tenure policies). For instance, the RDP, while helping teams across the university, may recognize the need for specialized team science training, policies to support distribution of indirect funds to collaborating schools or departments, or promotion and tenure policies that align with team-based research. They may effect changes in these areas via efforts that reach beyond the university to support the development of these resources. For instance, RDPs may work together nationally through NORDP to share resources that support collaboration activities, including model Collaboration Plans (NORDP, n.d.). Faculty may take action through their positions as journal editors to implement authorship contribution statements to increase the transparency of contributions among collaborators (or on boards of professional organizations) (c.f., McNutt et al. 2018).

45.3.2 Role of Collaboration Plans in the Peer Review of Grant Applications and Development of Funding Initiatives

Funding agencies currently emphasize evaluation of the technical and scientific merit of funding applications, but only rarely do they bring reviewers' attention to the collaborative merit of the application (e.g., demonstration of readiness to collaborate, and plans for maximizing the success of the future collaboration). But literature has shown (Guthrie et al. 2017) that scientific merit alone may not be predictive of the future success of the proposed research. These findings speak to the multiple hidden factors influencing the success of a research project that are not captured in the documentation submitted under current grant application requirements. We propose that the ten key components recommended for inclusion in Collaboration Plans can help provide additional important information about the potential success of a proposed team science initiative. Especially for large, complex team science applications, the merit of the Collaboration Plan may be as important as the merit of the scientific plan, when aiming to assess the prospective success of the scientific endeavor.

When included in funding applications, Collaboration Plans provide applicants with the opportunity to demonstrate their preparedness for the team science that is being proposed. They offer a structured opportunity to articulate the often-unstated assumptions about the visible and invisible work that needs to be done to lead, manage, and engage in a successful team science initiative, as well as the resources needed (infrastructure, technology, staffing, and funding) to support the team functioning essential for the science to proceed effectively.

The 10 components of the Collaboration Plan described in this chapter offer funding agencies and investigators guidance for considering specific requirements or templates for Collaboration Plans. This can help structure proposal content around planning for team science and can serve to guide reviewers in evaluating the collaborative aspects of a team science proposal. To enhance the success of funded team science, we anticipate that funding agencies will begin to more regularly ask investigators to submit Collaboration Plans, in addition to the required research plans, as part of their funding applications. Currently, funding agencies require some documentation of pre-planning for team science in funding applications, though typically the required documentation is narrow in scope. For instance, NSF requires collaboration plans for some large proposals, but give little guidance about what those should include or how to review them.[18] And although NIH requires a Leadership Plan for any Multiple-Principal Investigator (MPI) submission, the NIH leadership plan simply requires the MPIs to document how they will address issues specific to the leadership team, such as the division of leadership responsibilities and communication among the multiple designated PIs. As agencies fund more team science and have become more familiar with Collaboration Plans, requests for more robust plans have increased; for instance, one recent funding announcement states, "In addition to the required multiple PD/PI leadership plan, applications are expected to develop a comprehensive team management plan."[19]

Consideration of the support needed for collaboration has implications for how funding for team science is structured. An example of how this is implemented in practice is the center grant initiatives supported by the National Cancer Institute (NCI; e.g., CPHHD, CECCR, TREC, TTURC). These initiatives provide funds specifically for "cores" and/or coordination centers that offer resources and support across funded research centers (e.g., training in cross-disciplinary collaboration, biostatistics support). They also provide funding to support communication and coordination in cross-research center working group teams, and funding for each center director to coordinate the work of three to five large

research projects housed within the center, each of which is equivalent in scope and size to an R01 grant. One of the most successful enterprises of the NCI is the Cancer Center Support Grant (P30). Over the history of this program, which now supports seventy centers, requirements concerning transdisciplinary team science and collaboration have been steadily strengthened. Heightened attention to Collaboration Planning in the grant application and review process reflects the increasing attention to collaboration infrastructure in large initiatives such as these.

45.4 Conclusion

This chapter provides a structured process for systematically considering the key influencing factors for enhancing team science addressed throughout this book (Table 45.2). It provides a rationale for investigators, universities, and funding agencies to attend to the process of developing and documenting a Collaboration Planning. It illuminates the value of Collaboration Plans at the beginning and throughout a collaboration as well as the value of incorporating Collaboration Plans as part of the grant application and review process. Further, the chapter highlights the importance for all parts of the scientific enterprise (e.g., funding agencies, professional organizations, universities) to align practices and policies to support team science and the need for resources to be developed and shared. Resources and training that address the components discussed in the Collaboration Plan, such as effective communication and coordination; leadership, management, and administration; conflict prevention and management; training for team science; and quality improvement activities, continue to be sorely needed. As the scientific enterprise works together to support the alignment of team science, Collaboration Plans will help to highlight ongoing needs and serve to guide researchers to maximize collaborative success in order to realize the scientific breakthroughs we need to enhance the health and well-being of our society.

---

[18] https://www.nsf.gov/news/news_summ.jsp? cntn_id=118038

[19] https://grants.nih.gov/grants/guide/pa-files/PAR-17-340.html

Acknowledgments This project has been funded in whole or in part with federal funds from the National Cancer Institute, National Institutes of Health, under Contract No. HHSN261200800001E. The content of this publication does not necessarily reflect the views or policies of the Department of Health and Human Services, nor does mention of trade names, commercial products, or organizations imply endorsement by the US Government.

References

Arriaga RI, Abowd GD. The intersection of technology and medicine: ubiquitous computing and human computer interaction driving behavioral intervention research to address chronic care management. In: Hall KL, Vogel AL, Croyle RT, editors. Strategies for team science success: handbook of evidence-based principles for cross-disciplinary science and practical lessons learned from health researchers. New York, NY: Springer; 2019.

Bachrach C, Robert SA, Thomas Y. Training for interdisciplinary research in population health science. In: Hall KL, Vogel AL, Croyle RT, editors. Strategies for team science success: handbook of evidence-based principles for cross-disciplinary science and practical lessons learned from health researchers. New York, NY: Springer; 2019.

Bennett LM, Gadlin H. Conflict prevention and management in science teams. In: Hall KL, Vogel AL, Croyle RT, editors. Strategies for team science success: handbook of evidence-based principles for cross-disciplinary science and practical lessons learned from health researchers. New York, NY: Springer; 2019.

Bennett LM, Gadlin H, Marchand C. Collaboration and team science: a field guide (DHHS Publication No. 18–7660). Bethesda, MD: U.S. Government Printing Office; 2018.

Bennett LM, Maraia R, Gadlin H. The 'Welcome Letter': a useful tool for laboratories and teams. J Transl Med Epidemiol. 2014;2(2):1035.

Bennett LM, Nelan R, Steeves B, Thornhill J. The interrelationship of people, space, operations, institutional leadership, and training in fostering a team approach in health sciences research at the University of Saskatchewan. In: Hall KL, Vogel AL, Croyle RT, editors. Strategies for team science success: handbook of evidence-based principles for cross-disciplinary science and practical lessons learned from health researchers. New York, NY: Springer; 2019.

Berente N, Howison J. Strategies for success in virtual collaboration: structures and norms for meetings, workflow, and technological platforms. In: Hall KL, Vogel AL, Croyle RT, editors. Strategies for team science success: handbook of evidence-based principles for cross-disciplinary science and practical lessons learned from health researchers. New York, NY: Springer; 2019.

Berger NA. How leadership can support attainment of cross-disciplinary scientific goals. In: Hall KL, Vogel AL, Croyle RT, editors. Strategies for team science success: handbook of evidence-based principles for cross-disciplinary science and practical lessons learned from health researchers. New York, NY: Springer; 2019.

Bezrukova K. Understanding and addressing faultlines. Santa Clara, CA: Santa Clara University; 2013.. http://sites.nationalacademies.org/cs/groups/dbassesite/documents/webpage/dbasse_083763.pdf

Bietz MJ, Abrams S, Cooper DM, Stevens K, Puga F, Patel DI, Olson GM, Olson JS. Improving the odds through the collaboration success wizard. Transl Behav Med. 2012;2(4):480–6. https://doi.org/10.1007/s13142-012-0174-z.

Blot WJ, Hargreaves M, Zheng W. The added value of team member diversity to research in underserved populations. In: Hall KL, Vogel AL, Croyle RT, editors. Strategies for team science success: handbook of evidence-based principles for cross-disciplinary science and practical lessons learned from health researchers. New York, NY: Springer; 2019.

Brown SA, Leinen MS, Strathdee SA. Building a cross-disciplinary culture in academia through joint hires, degree programs, and scholarships. In: Hall KL, Vogel AL, Croyle RT, editors. Strategies for team science success: handbook of evidence-based principles for cross-disciplinary science and practical lessons learned from health researchers. New York, NY: Springer; 2019.

Carter D, Asencio R, Trainer H, DeChurch L, Zaccaro S, Kanfer R. Best practices for researchers working in multi-team systems. In: Hall KL, Vogel AL, Croyle RT, editors. Strategies for team science success: handbook of evidence-based principles for cross-disciplinary science and practical lessons learned from health researchers. New York, NY: Springer; 2019a.

Carter S, Carlson S, Crockett J, Falk-Krzensinski HJ, Lewis K, Walker BE. The role of research development professionals in supporting team science. In: Hall KL, Vogel AL, Croyle RT, editors. Strategies for team science success: handbook of evidence-based principles for cross-disciplinary science and practical lessons learned from health researchers. New York, NY: Springer; 2019–b.

Christen SP, Levine AJ. Facilitating cross-disciplinary interactions to stimulate innovation: Stand Up To Cancer's matchmaking convergence ideas lab. In: Hall KL, Vogel AL, Croyle RT, editors. Strategies for team science success: handbook of evidence-based principles for cross-disciplinary science and practical lessons learned from health researchers. New York, NY: Springer; 2019.

Couch J, Theisz K, Gillanders E. Engaging the public: citizen science. In: Hall KL, Vogel AL, Croyle RT, editors. Strategies for team science success: handbook of evidence-based principles for cross-disciplinary science and practical lessons learned from health researchers. New York, NY: Springer; 2019.

Crow MM, Dabars WB. Restructuring research universities to advance interdisciplinary collaboration. In: Hall KL, Vogel AL, Croyle RT, editors. Strategies for team science success: handbook of evidence-based principles for cross-disciplinary science and practical lessons learned from health researchers. New York, NY: Springer; 2019.

Cummings JN, Haas MR. So many teams, so little time: time allocation matters in geographically dispersed teams. J Organ Behav. 2012;33:316–41. https://doi.org/10.1002/job.777.

Cummings J, Kiesler S. Collaborative research across disciplinary and organizational boundaries. Soc Stud Sci. 2005;35(5):703–22.

Cummings JN, Kiesler S. Coordination costs and project outcomes in multi-university collaborations. Res Policy. 2007;36:1620–34. https://doi.org/10.1016/j.respol.2007.09.001.

Cummings JN, Kiesler S, Zadeh R, Balakrishnan A. Group heterogeneity increases the risks of large group size: a longitudinal study of productivity in research groups. Psychol Sci. 2013;24(6):880–90. https://doi.org/10.1177/0956797612463082.

Eigenbrode SD, O'Rourke M, Wulfhorst JD, Althoff DM, Goldberg CS, Merrill K, Bosque-Perez NA. Employing philosophical dialogue in collaborative science. Bioscience. 2007;57(1):55–64. https://doi.org/10.1641/B570109.

Eisele P. Validation of the team diagnostic survey and a field experiment to examine the effects of an intervention to increase team effectiveness. Group Facilitation. 2013;12:53–70.

Falcone M, Loughead J, Lerman C. The integration of research from diverse fields: transdisciplinary approaches bridging behavioral research, cognitive neuroscience, pharmacology and genetics to reduce cancer risk behavior. In: Hall KL, Vogel AL, Croyle RT, editors. Strategies for team science success: handbook of evidence-based principles for cross-disciplinary science and practical lessons learned from health researchers. New York, NY: Springer; 2019.

Fiore SM, Gabelica C, Wiltshire T, Stokols D. Training to be a (team) scientist. In:In: Hall KL, Vogel AL, Croyle RT, editors. Strategies for team science success: handbook of evidence-based principles for cross-disciplinary science and practical lessons learned from health researchers. New York, NY: Springer; 2019.

Gadlin H, Jessar K. Preempting discord: prenuptial agreements for scientists. NIH Catal. 2002;10(3). http://nihsearch.cit.nih.gov/catalyst/2002/02.05.01/page6.html

Gehlert S. Developing a shared mental model in the context of center initiative. In: Hall KL, Vogel AL, Croyle RT, editors. Strategies for team science success: handbook of evidence-based principles for cross-disciplinary science and practical lessons learned from health researchers. New York, NY: Springer; 2019.

Gehlert SJ, Bowen D, Martinez ME, Hiatt R, Marx C, Colditz G. The value of advisory boards to increase collaboration and advance science. In: Hall KL, Vogel AL, Croyle RT, editors. Strategies for team science success: handbook of evidence-based principles for cross-disciplinary science and practical lessons learned from health researchers. New York, NY: Springer; 2019.

Gibbs K, Han A, Lun J. Demographic diversity in teams: the challenges, benefits, and management strategies. In: Hall KL, Vogel AL, Croyle RT, editors. Strategies for team science success: handbook of evidence-based principles for cross-disciplinary science and practical lessons learned from health researchers. New York, NY: Springer; 2019.

Gilmore RO, Adolph K. Open sharing of behavioral research datasets—breaking down the boundaries of the research team. In: Hall KL, Vogel AL, Croyle RT, editors. Strategies for team science success: handbook of evidence-based principles for cross-disciplinary science and practical lessons learned from health researchers. New York, NY: Springer; 2019.

Gray B. Enhancing transdisciplinary research through collaborative leadership. Am J Prev Med. 2008;35 (Suppl. 2):S124–32. https://doi.org/10.1016/j.amepre.2008.03.037.

Guthrie S, Ghiga I, Wooding S. What do we know about grant peer review in the health sciences? F1000 Res. 2017;6:1335. https://doi.org/10.12688/f1000research.11917.2.

Hall K, Crowston K, Vogel A. How to write a collaboration plan. Team Science Toolkit. 2014. https://www.team-sciencetoolkit.cancer.gov/public/TSResourceBiblio.aspx?tid=3&rid=3119.

Hall KL, Stokols D, Moser RP, Taylor BK, Thornquist MD, Nebeling LC, Jeffery RW. The collaboration readiness of transdisciplinary research teams and centers: findings from the National Cancer Institute's TREC year-one evaluation study. Am J Prev Med. 2008b;35(Suppl. 2):S161–72. https://doi.org/10.1002/job.777.

Hall KL, Stokols D, Stipelman BA, Vogel AL, Feng A, Masimore B, Berrigan D. Assessing the value of team science: a study comparing center- and investigator-initiated grants. Am J Prev Med. 2012a;42:157–63. https://doi.org/10.1016/j.amepre.2011.10.011.

Hall KL, Vogel AL, Huang GC, Serrano KJ, Rice EL, Tsakraklides SP, Fiore SM. The Science of Team Science: a review of the empirical evidence and research gaps on collaboration in science. Am Psychol. 2018;73(4):532–48.

Hall KL, Vogel AL, Stipelman B, Stokols D, Morgan G, Gehlert S. A four-phase model of transdisciplinary team-based research: goals, team processes, and strategies. Transl Behav Med. 2012b;2:415–30.

Hall KL, Vogel A, Crowston K. Collaboration plans: planning for success in team science. Poster Presentation at Science of Team Science (SciTS) 2015 Conference, Bethesda, Maryland. 2015. https://www.teamsciencetoolkit.cancer.gov/public/TSResourceBiblio. aspx?tid=3&rid=3261.

Hays T. The Science of Team Science: commentary on measurements of scientific readiness. Am J Prev Med. 2008;35(2S):S193–5.

Hendren CO, Ku S. The Interdisciplinary Executive Scientist: connecting scientific ideas, resources, and people. In: Hall KL, Vogel AL, Croyle RT, editors. Strategies for team science success: handbook of evidence-based principles for cross-disciplinary science and practical lessons learned from health researchers. New York, NY: Springer; 2019.

Hurn PD, Traystman RJ. Research spanning animal and human models: the role of serendipity, competition, and strategic actions in advancing stroke research. In: Hall KL, Vogel AL, Croyle RT, editors. Strategies for team science success: handbook of evidence-based principles for cross-disciplinary science and practical lessons learned from health researchers. New York, NY: Springer; 2019.

Jain P, Klein D. Precollaboration framework: academic/industry partnerships: mobile and wearable technologies for behavioral science. In: Hall KL, Vogel AL, Croyle RT, editors. Strategies for team science success: handbook of evidence-based principles for cross-disciplinary science and practical lessons learned from health researchers. New York, NY: Springer; 2019.

James P, Redline S. The introduction of a new domain into an existing area of research: novel discoveries through integration of sleep into cancer and obesity research. In: Hall KL, Vogel AL, Croyle RT, editors. Strategies for team science success: handbook of evidence-based principles for cross-disciplinary science and practical lessons learned from health researchers. New York, NY: Springer; 2019.

Johnson LB, Smalley JB. Engaging the patient: patient-centered research. In: Hall KL, Vogel AL, Croyle RT, editors. Strategies for team science success: handbook of evidence-based principles for cross-disciplinary science and practical lessons learned from health researchers. New York, NY: Springer; 2019.

Kiviniemi M. Engaging the practitioner: "but wait, that's not all!"—collaborations with practitioners and extending the reasons you started doing research in the first place. In: Hall KL, Vogel AL, Croyle RT, editors. Strategies for team science success: handbook of evidence-based principles for cross-disciplinary science and practical lessons learned from health researchers. New York, NY: Springer; 2019.

Klein W. Cross-disciplinary team science with trainees: from undergraduate to post-doc. In: Hall KL, Vogel AL, Croyle RT, editors. Strategies for team science success: handbook of evidence-based principles for cross-disciplinary science and practical lessons learned from health researchers. New York, NY: Springer; 2019.

Kozlowski SWJ, Bell BS. Evidence-based principles and strategies for optimizing team functioning and performance in science teams. In: Hall KL, Vogel

AL, Croyle RT, editors. Strategies for team science success: handbook of evidence-based principles for cross-disciplinary science and practical lessons learned from health researchers. New York, NY: Springer; 2019.

Madden GJ, McClure S, Bickel WK. Collaborating to move laboratory findings into public health domains: maxims for translational research. In: Hall KL, Vogel AL, Croyle RT, editors. Strategies for team science success: handbook of evidence-based principles for cross-disciplinary science and practical lessons learned from health researchers. New York, NY: Springer; 2019.

Mallinson T, Lotrecchiano GR, Schwartz LS, Furniss J, Leblanc-Beaudoin T, Lazar D, Falk-Krzesinski HJ. Pilot analysis of the motivation assessment for team readiness, integration, and collaboration (MATRICx) using Rasch analysis. J Investig Med. 2016;64:1186–93.

Marino AH, Suda-Blake K, Fulton KR. Innovative collaboration formation—The National Academies Keck Futures Initiative. In: Hall KL, Vogel AL, Croyle RT, editors. Strategies for team science success: handbook of evidence-based principles for cross-disciplinary science and practical lessons learned from health researchers. New York, NY: Springer; 2019.

McNutt K, Bradford M, Drazen JM, Hanson B, Howard B, Jamieson KH, Kiermer V, Marcus E, Pope BK, Schekman R, Swaminathan S, Stang PJ, Verma IM. Transparency in authors' contributions and responsibilities to promote integrity in scientific publication. Proc Natl Acad Sci. 2018;115(11):2557–60. https://doi.org/10.1073/pnas.1715374115.

National Research Council. Enhancing the effectiveness of team science. Washington, DC: The National Academies Press; 2015. https://doi.org/10.17226/19007.

NIH Office of Extramural Research. Examples of project leadership plans for multiple PI grant applications. 2017. https://grants.nih.gov/grants/multi_pi/sample_leadership_plans.pdf.

NIH Office of the Ombudsman. Questions for scientific collaborators. 2017. https://ccrod.cancer.gov/confluence/display/NIHOMBUD/Collaborative+Agreement+Template.

NITRD. The networking and information technology research and development program. n.d. https://www.nitrd.gov/about/about_nitrd.aspx.

NORDP. The National Organization of Research Development Professionals. n.d. http://www.nordp.org/.

Nurius PS, Kemp SP. Individual level competencies for team collaboration with cross-disciplinary researchers and stakeholders. In: Hall KL, Vogel AL, Croyle RT, editors. Strategies for team science success: handbook of evidence-based principles for cross-disciplinary science and practical lessons learned from health researchers. New York, NY: Springer; 2019.

O'Rourke M, Crowley S. Philosophical intervention and cross-disciplinary science: the story of the toolbox project. Synthese. 2013;190(11):1937–54. https://doi.org/10.1007/s11229-012-0175-y.

O'Rourke M, Crowley S, Laursen B, Robinson B, Vasko SE. Disciplinary diversity in teams: integrative approaches from unidisciplinarity to transdisciplinarity. In: Hall KL, Vogel AL, Croyle RT, editors. Strategies for team science success: handbook of evidence-based principles for cross-disciplinary science and practical lessons learned from health researchers. New York, NY: Springer; 2019.

Pohl C, Wuelser G. Methods for co-production of knowledge among diverse disciplines and stakeholders. In: Hall KL, Vogel AL, Croyle RT, editors. Strategies for team science success: handbook of evidence-based principles for cross-disciplinary science and practical lessons learned from health researchers. New York, NY: Springer; 2019.

Ranwala D, Alberg AJ, Brady KT, Obeid JS, Davis R, Halushka PV. Retreats to stimulate cross-disciplinary translational research collaborations: Medical University of South Carolina CTSA Pilot Project Program Initiative. In: Hall KL, Vogel AL, Croyle RT, editors. Strategies for team science success: handbook of evidence-based principles for cross-disciplinary science and practical lessons learned from health researchers. New York, NY: Springer; 2019.

Rolland B. Designing and developing coordinating centers as infrastructure to support team science. In: Hall KL, Vogel AL, Croyle RT, editors. Strategies for team science success: handbook of evidence-based principles for cross-disciplinary science and practical lessons learned from health researchers. New York, NY: Springer; 2019.

Salazar M, Widmer K, Doiron K, Lant T. Leader integrative capabilities: a catalyst for effective interdisciplinary teams. In: Hall KL, Vogel AL, Croyle RT, editors. Strategies for team science success: handbook of evidence-based principles for cross-disciplinary science and practical lessons learned from health researchers. New York, NY: Springer; 2019.

Sallis JF, Floyd MF. The development of a new interdisciplinary field: active living research—a foundation-supported interdisciplinary research funding program. In: Hall KL, Vogel AL, Croyle RT, editors. Strategies for team science success: handbook of evidence-based principles for cross-disciplinary science and practical lessons learned from health researchers. New York, NY: Springer; 2019.

Spring B, Pfammatter A, Conroy DE. Continuing professional development for team science. In: Hall KL, Vogel AL, Croyle RT, editors. Strategies for team science success: handbook of evidence-based principles for cross-disciplinary science and practical lessons learned from health researchers. New York, NY: Springer; 2019.

Stipelman B, Feng A, Hall KA, Stokols D, Moser RP, Berger NA, Goran MI, Jeffrey R, McTiernan A, Thornquist M, Nebeling L, Vogel AL. The relationship between collaborative readiness and scientific productivity in the transdisciplinary research on energetics and cancer (TREC) centers. Poster Presentation at the 31st Annual Meeting of the Society of Behavioral Medicine. 2010.

Stipelman B, Rice E, Vogel AL, Hall KL. The role of team personality on team effectiveness and performance. In: Hall KL, Vogel AL, Croyle RT, editors. Strategies for team science success: handbook of evidence-based principles for cross-disciplinary science and practical lessons learned from health researchers. New York, NY: Springer; 2019.

Stokols D, Misra S, Moser R, Hall K, Taylor B. The ecology of team science: understanding contextual influences on transdisciplinary collaboration. Am J Prev Med. 2008;35(Suppl. 2):96–115.

Twyman M, Contractor N. Team assembly. In: Hall KL, Vogel AL, Croyle RT, editors. Strategies for team science success: handbook of evidence-based principles for cross-disciplinary science and practical lessons learned from health researchers. New York, NY: Springer; 2019.

Uzzi B, Spiro J. Collaboration and creativity: the small world problem. Am J Sociol. 2005;111(2):447–504.

Vogel AL, Feng A, Oh A, Hall KL, Stipelman BA, Stokols D, Nebeling L. Influence of a National Cancer Institute transdisciplinary research and training initiative on trainees' transdisciplinary research competencies and scholarly productivity. Transl Behav Med. 2012;2(4):459–68.

Vogel AL, Hall KL, Klein JT, Falk-Krzensinski HJ. Broadening our understanding of scientific work for the era of team science: implications for recognition and rewards. In: Hall KL, Vogel AL, Croyle RT, editors. Strategies for team science success: handbook of evidence-based principles for cross-disciplinary science and practical lessons learned from health researchers. New York, NY: Springer; 2019.

Wageman R, Hackman JR, Lehman EV. Team Diagnostic Survey: development of an instrument. J Appl Behav Sci. 2005;41(4):373–98.

Wallerstein N, Calhoun K, Eder M, Kaplow J, Wilkins CH. Engaging the community: community-based participatory research and team science. In: Hall KL, Vogel AL, Croyle RT, editors. Strategies for team science success: handbook of evidence-based principles for cross-disciplinary science and practical lessons learned from health researchers. New York, NY: Springer; 2019.

Weber G, Yuan L. The power of research networking systems to find experts and facilitate collaboration. In: Hall KL, Vogel AL, Croyle RT, editors. Strategies for team science success: handbook of evidence-based principles for cross-disciplinary science and practical lessons learned from health researchers. New York, NY: Springer; 2019.

West M, Dawson J, Admasachew L, Topakas A. NHS staff management and health service quality: results from the NHS staff survey and related data. 2011. https://www.gov.uk/government/publications/nhs-staff-management-and-health-service-quality. Accessed 27 Jul 2016.

West MA, Lyubovnikova J. Real teams or pseudo teams? The changing landscape needs a better map. Ind Organ Psychol. 2012;5:25–8.

Winter S. Organizational perspectives on leadership strategies for the success of cross-disciplinary science teams. In: Hall KL, Vogel AL, Croyle RT, editors. Strategies for team science success: handbook of evidence-based principles for cross-disciplinary science and practical lessons learned from health researchers. New York, NY: Springer; 2019.

Correction to: Strategies for Team Science Success

Kara L. Hall, Amanda L. Vogel, and Robert T. Croyle

Correction to:
K. L. Hall et al. (eds.), Strategies for Team Science Success,
https://doi.org/10.1007/978-3-030-20992-6

- The published version of the book has missed to include the corresponding authors' e-mail address for chapters 14, 35 and 44.
- Affiliation correction provided for the author Dr. Milton Eder in chapter 9 has been missed to update in the list of contributors.
- The affiliation detail for the author Dr. Stephen M were published incorrectly in chapter 33. Also, the text in the Abstract section which reads "(cite other chapters in team science book)," was not removed during the copy editing stage.

These errors have been corrected, and the text has been updated in the book.

Chapter 45:

This chapter was previously published non-open access. It has now been changed to open access under a CC BY 4.0 license and the copyright holder has been updated to "The Author(s)". The book has also been updated with these changes.

The updated online version of this book can be found at
https://doi.org/10.1007/978-3-030-20992-6
https://doi.org/10.1007/978-3-030-20992-6_9
https://doi.org/10.1007/978-3-030-20992-6_14
https://doi.org/10.1007/978-3-030-20992-6_15
https://doi.org/10.1007/978-3-030-20992-6_33
https://doi.org/10.1007/978-3-030-20992-6_35
https://doi.org/10.1007/978-3-030-20992-6_44
https://doi.org/10.1007/978-3-030-20992-6_45

© Springer Nature Switzerland AG 2020
K. L. Hall et al. (eds.), *Strategies for Team Science Success*,
https://doi.org/10.1007/978-3-030-20992-6_46

Index

A
Academic-community research collaborations, 130
Academic diplomacy, 525
Academic Health Centers, 100
Academic Health Science Complex (AHSC), 509, 520, 521
Academic/industry partnerships
  behavioral and social sciences, 303
  behavioral science forward, 303
  companies and universities, 303
  evidence-based principles, 303
  external partners, 303
  framework, 304
  industrial R&D, 303
  innovative hypertension intervention, 307
  intellectual property, 308, 309
  joint mission statement, 307, 308
  matching expectations, 308
  mHealth interventions, 304
  mindful of risks, 308
  mobile and wearable technologies, 304
  motivation, 308
  partnering pillars, 305–307
  process of sharing, 307
  technology development, 303
  time-sensitive product development projects, 303
  translational science partnership framework, 304, 305
Academic researchers, 124
Academic Senate leadership, 490
Accelerometer, 56, 58, 60
Across disciplinary content, 426
Actigraphs, 60
Actionable research, 54
Active living research
  academic diplomacy, 525
  advisors, 525
  annual conferences, 527
  behavioral mapping, 532
  collaborators, 530
  communications, 528
  conceptual models, 526, 527
  disciplines, 524, 525
  environment and policy, 524

  goal, 524, 527
  health behaviors, 531
  health-related journals, 534
  infographics, 528
  interdisciplinary, 530
  interdisciplinary collaboration, 531
  interdisciplinary field, 529
  interdisciplinary research field, 525
  interdisciplinary teams, 525, 526, 529, 534
  leadership, 525, 528, 533
  leadership opportunities, 530, 533
  literature review, 533
  match-making, 526
  National Program Office staff, 525
  nontechnical audiences, 528
  physical activity, 524, 531
  physical inactivity, 524
  policy and practice, 527
  presentations and workshops, 527
  PRLS, 533
  racial inequality, 529
  recreation planning and visitor management, 529
  responsibilities, 532
  San Diego State University, 524
  SciTS, 527
  Seminar program, 526
  SOPARC, 532
  staff, 527
  team members, 533
  team science, 529, 534
  training and support, 527
  TTURC teams, 527
  US population, 524
Active Living Research Program, 523
Active Living Research review process, 531
Actor constellation, 118, 119
Advisory board
  collaborations, 411
  EAB and IAB meeting, 411
  expectations and requirements, 411
  shared conceptual/mental model, 411
  TREC conceptual model, 411
  viewed and evaluated, 411
  WU TREC conceptual model, 411

© Springer Nature Switzerland AG 2019
K. L. Hall et al. (eds.), *Strategies for Team Science Success*,
https://doi.org/10.1007/978-3-030-20992-6

CPSIA information can be obtained
at www.ICGtesting.com
Printed in the USA
LVHW020823280122
709473LV00006B/396